Manual of
High Risk
Pregnancy
&Delivery

FOURTH EDITION

Elizabeth Stepp Gilbert, RNC, MS, FNPC
Certified Family Nurse Practitioner in Private Practice
Associate Professor
Associate Dean of the Graduate Program
Grand Canyon University
Phoenix, Arizona

MOSBY
ELSEVIER

11830 Westline Industrial Drive
St. Louis, Missouri 63146

MANUAL OF HIGH RISK PREGNANCY & DELIVERY

ISBN-13: 978-0-323-04016-7
ISBN-10: 0-323-04016-0

Copyright © 2007 by Mosby, Inc., an affiliate of Elsevier Inc.

Notice

Knowledge and best practice in this field are constantly changing. As new research and experience broaden our knowledge, changes in practice, treatment and drug therapy may become necessary or appropriate. Readers are advised to check the most current information provided (i) on procedures featured or (ii) by the manufacturer of each product to be administered, to verify the recommended dose or formula, the method and duration of administration, and contraindications. It is the responsibility of the practitioner, relying on their own experience and knowledge of the patient, to make diagnoses, to determine dosages and the best treatment for each individual patient, and to take all appropriate safety precautions. To the fullest extent of the law, neither the Publisher nor the Authors assumes any liability for any injury and/or damage to persons or property arising out or related to any use of the material contained in this book.

The Publisher

Previous editions copyrighted 2003, 1998, 1993

ISBN-13: 978-0-323-04016-7
ISBN-10: 0-323-04016-0

Acquisitions Editor: Catherine Jackson
Developmental Editor: Laurie K. Gower
Publishing Services Manager: John Rogers
Senior Project Manager: Helen Hudlin
Design Direction: Amy Buxton
Cover Designer: Melissa Walter
Text Designer: Amy Buxton

Working together to grow libraries in developing countries

www.elsevier.com | www.bookaid.org | www.sabre.org

ELSEVIER   BOOK AID International   Sabre Foundation

Printed in the United State of America

Last digit is the print number: 9 8 7 6 5 4 3 2 1

To my husband, Robert, and my son, Michael
who support me in all my professional and personal endeavors

Contributors & Reviewer

CONTRIBUTORS

Marsha L. Ramstad, RN, LCCE
Assistant Professor
Grand Canyon University
Phoenix, Arizona

Barbara Oxley, NMD, RN, BSN, IBCLC
Director
Bethany Ranch Health Clinic
Phoenix, Arizona

REVIEWER

Rhonda R. Martin, RN, MS
Clinical Assistant Professor of Nursing
University of Tulsa
Tulsa, Oklahoma

Preface

Today's technologic advances make it possible to offer the woman and her family, who are experiencing a high risk pregnancy and delivery, a good chance for a positive outcome. The nursing and medical literature abound with evidence-based practice recommendations from sources such as *Best Practice in Labor Ward Management* (Kean, Baker, & Edelstone, 2000), the easily accessible version of *The Cochrane Database* (2006), and evidence-based clinical guidelines such as Agency for Healthcare Research and Quality (AHRQ), National Guideline Clearinghouse (NGC), Institute for Clinical Systems Improvement (ICSI), and Society of Obstetricians and Gynaecologiest of Canada (SOGC) as well as references from professional organizations such as AWHONN and ACOG. As nurses, nurse practitioners, and nurse midwives, we each have a responsibility to keep our practices up-to-date and evidence-based. Nurses play a key role in ensuring that women and their fetuses receive the best possible care. Perinatal nurses in all obstetric facilities must know about screening for risk factors; they must provide preventive management using effective alternative and complementary therapies and appropriately intervene when complications develop. Unfortunately, many women do not receive adequate prenatal care and enter the health care system only after complications occur. Because these women seek assistance from various types of facilities, nurses who practice in clinics, emergency rooms, and primary care settings must also be alert to perinatal complications and be prepared to provide immediate stabilizing care in ambulatory or other inpatient care settings.

Manual of High Risk Pregnancy & Delivery is designed to provide comprehensive information in a concise, portable, and accessible format. Clearly written text and numerous tables and boxes enhance comprehension and facilitate easy retrieval of information. The nursing process serves as the organizational framework for discussions of both preventive and emergent care for a wide range of topics. Nursing interventions are grounded in evidence-based practice recommendations.

The coverage of the various problems includes incidence, etiology, physiology, pathophysiology, as well as the usual, expected, and intensive care management protocols for advanced nurse practitioners. Management and intervention protocols are addressed for high risk and critical care obstetric care. Psychosocial implications and family considerations are incorporated throughout. A unique, contributed chapter discusses and emphasizes how advance practice nurses can access relevant alternative and complementary therapies, which are evidence-based for high risk pregnancy and delivery care.

Manual of High Risk Pregnancy & Delivery is organized into seven units to facilitate easy retrieval of critical content. Unit I presents physiologic considerations and identification of high risk pregnancy, fetal assessment and monitoring, technologic advances in perinatal nursing, and an emphasis on alternative and complementary therapies. Unit II addresses the psychologic implications and adaptation to a high risk pregnancy. A chapter within this unit covers pregnancy loss and grief. Unit III discusses ethical dilemmas and legal considerations in perinatal nursing. Separate chapters in Unit IV focus on the effects of diabetes, as well as cardiac, renal, connective tissue, and pulmonary diseases and their effects on pregnancy, with emphases on preventing complications, delivering care in the inpatient environment, and setting the stage for critical care. Unit V deals with spontaneous abortion, ectopic pregnancy, gestational trophoblastic disease, placental abnormalities, disseminated intravascular coagulopathy, hemolytic incompatibility, hypertensive disorders of pregnancy, and preterm labor. Chapters in this unit present the latest information on multiple gestation, premature rupture of membranes, and trauma during pregnancy, with emphases on ambulatory care prevention and inpatient care with critical care protocols, as appropriate. Unit VI discusses the effects of sexually transmitted diseases and substance abuse on both mother and fetus. Unit VII focuses on alterations in the mechanics of labor and delivery, with a strong emphasis on the prevention of complications and the use of alternative and complementary therapies in the prevention and treatment of labor dystocia.

It is my conviction that with thorough, knowledgeable, and evidence-based care of the mother and fetus, neonatal morbidity and mortality can be considerably decreased, and complications for the mother can be lessened. It is my intent and hope that this text will enable health care professionals to provide optimal care for mother, fetus, and family from ambulatory, preventive, inpatient, and critical care arenas through the early postpartum period.

Elizabeth Stepp Gilbert

Contents

UNIT VI   TERATOGENS AND SOCIAL ISSUES COMPLICATING PREGNANCY

UNIT VII   ALTERATIONS IN THE MECHANISM OF LABOR

I

Physiologic Considerations, Assessments, and Integrative Therapies

S ignificant physiologic changes occur in a woman's body during pregnancy. Within a very few weeks, alterations are measurable in many body systems. The mother acquires and circulates more nutrients for herself and the fetus. Her body forms and maintains a new organ, the placenta. Through the placenta, her body disposes of fetal waste products and provides fetal nutrition and respiration. Throughout pregnancy, homeostatic mechanisms adapt to protect the fetus and to guard against its rejection as a foreign substance.

When caring for the high risk pregnant woman, the nurse considers numerous physiologic aspects, such as adaptations in maternal body functions and development of the maternal-fetal unit. By analyzing these physiologic aspects, specific antenatal assessments of maternal and fetal health are made and high risk pregnancies are identified. Special methods of assessing fetal health, including fetal monitoring, fetal surveillance testing, diagnostic studies, and evolving evidence-based therapies such as fetal surgery and complementary therapies are discussed in the five chapters in this unit.

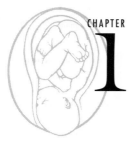

1

Physiologic and Nutritional Adaptations to Pregnancy

The foundation of high risk pregnancy management is based on careful, thorough physiologic and nutritional assessments. The nurse caring for the high risk expectant mother must have a thorough understanding of the anatomic and physiologic changes that occur in a pregnant woman's body to be able to recognize normal as well as abnormal responses.

ADAPTATIONS

Cardiovascular

The most dramatic changes during pregnancy involve the cardiovascular system. These changes are anatomic and hemodynamic. The following normal hemodynamic changes occur during pregnancy:

- *Hypervolemia*. Blood volume increases 48%, leading to such auscultatory changes as S_1 splitting, auditory S_3 by 20 weeks of gestation, systolic murmur, and, occasionally, a transient diastolic murmur.
- *Hemodilution*. Plasma volume increases approximately 50%, whereas red blood cell volume increases only 20%, causing hemodilution. This leads to a lower colloid osmotic pressure (COP), which is the force that holds fluid in the capillaries. The opposing force, capillary hydrostatic pressure measured as pulmonary capillary wedge pressure (PCWP), which moves fluid out of the capillaries into the interstitial space, remains the same. COP is dependent on the plasma concentration of colloids, plasma proteins such as albumin, and to a lesser extent, globulin and fibrinogen. Because the hemodilution of the plasma colloids causes the COP to decrease while there is no change in the PCWP, there is a tendency to develop dependent edema. During a pregnancy coupled with a high risk condition that further decreases the COP or increases the PCWP, the risk for pulmonary edema is greater.
- *Hyperdynamic state*. Cardiac output increases 40% by 36 to 38 weeks of gestation (cardiac output = heart rate × stroke volume). Both stroke volume and heart rate increase 20% by this point in gestation.

- *Low resistance.* Normally, systemic vascular resistance decreases 20%, and pulmonary vascular resistance decreases 35% related to progesterone, local prostaglandins such as prostacyclin, and nitric oxide. This lowered systemic vascular resistance usually causes the baseline blood pressure to decrease at the end of the first trimester and throughout the second trimester and to return to the nonpregnancy baseline during the third trimester.

Anatomically, the heart is displaced upward and to the left throughout pregnancy, changing the location of the point of maximum impulse (PMI) from the fifth intercostal space (ICS) to approximately the fourth ICS and moving it more lateral to the midclavicular line. This results in electrocardiogram changes such as a left axis deviation of the QRS complex, a nonspecific S-T segment, and an abnormal T wave.

Respiratory

The normal respiratory changes follow:

- *Thoracic breathing.* During pregnancy, the mother changes from being an abdominal breather to being a thoracic breather. This is because the diaphragm raises 4 to 7 cm and the ribs flare, increasing the anterior to posterior diameter.
- *Improved oxygen delivery.* Oxygen consumption increases by 20% to meet fetal growth and development needs and increased maternal growth and basal metabolism. Oxygen consumption further increases during labor, and it is higher during pregnancy with multiples.
- *Hyperventilation.* Maternal tidal volume (volume of air that is exchanged with each breath) increases 40% related to progesterone. Maternal functional residual capacity (volume of air that remains in the lung on expiration) decreases 25%. The result is increased depth of respirations because there is increased oxygenated air mixed with a smaller amount of carbon deoxygenated air. For high risk management, note that hyperventilation lowers oxygen reserve and that hypoxia can develop more rapidly in a high risk condition. This can enhance induction of and recovery from general anesthesia.
- *Compensatory respiratory alkalosis.* Because of the hyperventilation effect of pregnancy, the arterial oxygen tension is increased (normal Po_2, 100 to 108 mm Hg) and the arterial carbon dioxide tension is reduced (normal Pco_2, 27 to 32 mm Hg) because the excess CO_2 is exhaled, decreasing carbonic acid. Maternal serum bicarbonate decreases (normal, 18 to 22 mEq/L) to maintain the maternal acid-base balance. Therefore the normal arterial blood gases of pregnancy reflect the state of chronic compensatory respiratory alkalosis. Women with high risk pregnancies can develop respiratory and metabolic acidosis rapidly.

Hematologic

The normal hematologic changes during pregnancy follow:

- *Hypercoagulation.* During pregnancy, the equilibrium for coagulation-fibrinolysis is skewed toward coagulation. Plasma fibrinogen rises throughout pregnancy. The fibrinogen clotting factors are increased, and the fibrinolytic activity is suppressed because there is a decrease in circulatory plasminogen activators. Platelet count either remains normal or is reduced insignificantly.

- *Leukocytosis, especially neutrophils.* White blood cells, or leukocytes, are primarily responsible for fighting infections. Leukocytes are either granulocytes or nongranulocytes. When infection occurs, granulocytes increase and nongranulocytes migrate to inflammatory areas by way of the circulatory system. During pregnancy, the number of neutrophils that are granulocytes increases. This increase is stimulated by estrogen and plasma cortisol.

Renal

- *Hypervolemia.* Increased blood volume circulates through the kidneys. Renal blood flow constitutes about one fifth of the cardiac output; therefore it is increased 50% to 80%. The entire plasma volume is filtered about 60 times per day.
- *Hyperdynamics.* Substances to be retained by the body are first filtered and then reabsorbed in the tubules. Substances to be excreted are added to the fluid and flow to the distal portion of the tubules. During pregnancy, larger quantities are filtered in the glomerulus because of the greater capillary pressures associated with the increased blood flow; the glomerular filtration rate increases about 50%. Glucose, nitrogenous waste products of metabolism, and bicarbonate are therefore excreted in the urine in greater quantities. In turn, blood levels of nitrogenous waste products decrease. During pregnancy, normal laboratory values indicating renal function must be adjusted. A blood urea nitrogen level higher than 12 mg/dl is abnormal even though it is within the nonpregnant normal range. Serum creatinine levels higher than 0.8 mg/dl are considered abnormal for pregnancy. Creatinine clearance levels are normally elevated (110 to 160 ml/min) during pregnancy.
- *Physiologic hydroureter and hydronephrosis.* As the gravid uterus displaces other organs in the abdomen, it causes a physiologic hydroureter and hydronephrosis. It is usually more pronounced on the right side than on the left. The dilation of the ureters is further facilitated by estrogen. During pregnancy, the bladder has decreased tone because of hormonal influences. This factor and the distended ureters cause the pregnant woman to be more vulnerable to urinary tract infections. The increased glucose excretion into the urine also promotes bacterial growth.

Gastrointestinal

The predominant gastrointestinal change is hypotonic. A hypotonic gastrointestinal tract leads to decreased gastric motility and a prolonged stomach-emptying time, resulting primarily from the anatomic shifting of abdominal contents. Constipation is frequently a problem during pregnancy.

The gallbladder is influenced by estrogen and becomes hypotonic. This causes an increased concentration of bile. An increased incidence of gallstones can result. Acute cholecystitis can lead to the second most common nonobstetric surgical condition of pregnancy, following appendicitis. Intrahepatic cholestasis of pregnancy, the most common liver disorder unique to pregnancy, is the result of retained bile in the liver. Pruritus is the predominant presenting factor.

For high risk management, it is important to note that giving an order for nothing by mouth before surgery does not necessary mean an empty stomach. Gastric pH is normally more acid during pregnancy because of the hypertonic states of the gastrointestinal system. Therefore there is an increased risk for aspiration of high acidic gastric content in the event of general anesthesia.

Metabolic

The predominant metabolic change during pregnancy is hyperinsulinemia, causing a diabetogenic state. This is related to the increased insulin resistance caused by the placental hormone and lactogen and by prolactin, cortisol, and glucagon.

DEVELOPMENT OF THE MATERNAL-FETAL UNIT

Knowledge of the growth and development of the maternal-fetal unit provides a basis for care of the mother or fetus at risk for disease or for treatment of pregnancy complications. This knowledge provides a basis for early detection of maternal or fetal problems, enabling more serious complications to be prevented.

Embryo

During the luteal phase of the menstrual cycle, cervical mucus becomes receptive to spermatozoa. Ejaculation of sperm into the vagina is aided by mucoid receptivity, which allows rapid migration of spermatozoa through the cervix, into the uterine cavity, and into the fallopian tube.

Active spermatozoa can reach the outer portion of the fallopian tube within 75 minutes. The sperm and ovum meet in the distal portion of the fallopian tube. Fertilization occurs when the sperm penetrates the vitelline membrane of the ovum. Cell division begins, forming a small cell mass called the *morula.*

The morula passes through the fallopian tube by way of tubal peristalsis and ciliary propulsion. The outer cell layer of the morula secretes a fluid that pools in a segmentation cavity. Now the cell mass is called a *blastocyst.*

The blastocyst takes approximately 6 to 7 days to form. Implantation takes place at the blastocyst stage, usually occurring high in the uterine fundus. At this time, the outer cells on the blastocyst are called *trophoblasts.*

The trophoblasts then invade the endometrium. It is thought that the reason the trophoblast cells are not treated as foreign and rejected by the mother is because there is an exchange of fetal and maternal cytoplasmic and nuclear material from the trophoblastic cells. This exchange allows the maternal immunologic system to tolerate the fetus as a part of the body rather than as foreign to it.

Progesterone from the corpus luteum provides stored nutritive substances in the endometrium, called the *decidua*. The trophoblasts secrete proteolytic and cytolytic enzymes, permitting them to destroy vessels, glands, and stroma in the endometrium.

Placenta

The trophoblasts proliferate rapidly after implantation, and three layers of cells appear. These send out fingerlike projections called *villi*. The outer layer of cells (syncytiotrophoblast), the inner layer (orcytotrophoblast), and the dividing layer of thin connective tissue (mesotrophoblast), are formed within these fingerlike projections. The mesotrophoblast forms the support for the villi and fetal vascular tissue. The syncytial cells then synthesize proteins, glucose, and hormones for use by the embryo.

After 2 or 3 weeks, the chorion begins to develop within the villi. While the chorion is developing, the amnion and its cavity are forming. Two cavities form in the embryonic pole. The ventral cavity is the yolk sac. The dorsal cavity becomes the amniotic cavity. As the chorion enlarges, it forces the formation of the body stalk, the allantois, the blood vessels, and the beginning of the umbilical cord.

The decidua basialis, the layer beneath the embryoblast tissue, comes into contact with the villi, which then multiply rapidly. During villi multiplication, the decidua basialis is called the *chorion frondosum*.

By 14 weeks, the chorion frondosum organizes into the discrete organ called the *placenta*. The placenta has segments, called *cotyledons*, which are connected by vascular channels to the umbilical cord. The placental surface is exposed to the maternal blood in the intervillous space and thins to a single layer of cells called the *placental membrane*. The exposure of fetal blood to maternal blood across this membrane provides for fetal oxygenation, nutrition, and excretion of fetal wastes. The two umbilical arteries carry CO_2 and other waste from the fetus to the mother. The vein carries nutrition and oxygen to the fetus.

Transfer of O_2, CO_2, nutrition, and waste depends on molecular size. Smaller molecules, such as O_2, CO_2, electrolytes, and water, transfer by simple diffusion, moving passively from the side of greater to the side of lesser molecular concentration. Their transfer largely depends on the adequacy of uterine blood flow into the intervillous space.

A more complex process called *facilitated diffusion* selectively transfers larger molecules, such as glucose. This process occurs against a large concentration gradient and requires a carrier system. Energy expenditure can also provide for selective transfer. Facilitated diffusion and selective transfer depend primarily on placental surface area and thickness for their diffusion.

In addition to simple and complex diffusion, the placenta also adopts an endocrine function. Early in pregnancy, it assumes responsibility for maintenance of the pregnancy. The principal hormones produced by the placenta are estrogen, progesterone, human chorionic gonadotropin, and human placental lactogen.

Amniotic Fluid

Origin

Initially, the amnion fetal membrane primarily produces the amniotic fluid by actively transporting solute and passively transporting water from maternal serum to the amniotic fluid space. As the fetus develops, the amnion fetal membrane makes a significant contribution by excreting urine into the amniotic fluid.

Functions

Amniotic fluid is normally swallowed by the fetus and absorbed in the gastrointestinal tract. If there are abnormalities of the fetal gastrointestinal tract or renal system, neurotube defects, or ruptured membranes, amniotic fluid may be excessive, deficient, or absent. Sufficient amounts of amniotic fluid provide a buoyant medium, which does the following:

- Permits symmetric growth and development
- Prevents adherence of the amnion to embryo or fetal parts
- Cushions the fetus against jolts by distributing impacts the mother may receive
- Helps control the fetal body temperature by maintaining a relatively constant temperature
- Enables the fetus to flex, extend, and move freely, thus aiding musculoskeletal development
- Provides fetal nutritional development
- Allows the umbilical cord to be relatively free of compression

Fetus

The first trimester is a period of tremendous growth and organogenesis from an embryo into a fetus. By the end of the second week, the three embryologic germ layers develop to form body organs and systems. The formation of these layers is called *gastrulation.*

The ectoderm gives rise to the skin, hair, and nails; the epithelium of the internal and external ear, nasal cavity, mouth, and anus; the nervous system tissues; and the glands. The mesoderm forms the connective tissue, blood vessels, lymphatic tissue, kidneys, pleura, peritoneum, pericardium, muscles, and skeleton. The endoderm forms the respiratory tract, bladder, liver, pancreas, and digestive tract.

By 6 weeks, a single-chamber heart is functioning and lung buds appear, as do a rudimentary kidney and gut. By the end of the first trimester, the heart has compartmentalized into four chambers; the lungs have bronchi; the gut, liver, pancreas, and spleen have developed; and the gender can be distinguished.

During the second trimester, facial features become defined. Fine body hair, called *lanugo,* appears, and vernix is produced to protect fetal skin. Meconium begins to appear in the gut. Maturation of organs allows some immature functioning.

In the third trimester, the fetus rapidly gains weight and the final maturation of the organs for extrauterine life occurs. Subcutaneous fat deposits appear, and the body has a rounded appearance.

Assessing fetal well-being has become sophisticated. In addition to estimating fetal well-being by examining maternal well-being, it can be estimated biochemically by using laboratory studies and physically by observing fetal heart activity on the fetal monitor and by visualizing the fetus using ultrasound techniques.

EXERCISE AND BEDREST

For healthy women with a normal pregnancy, exercise is safe and promotes the health and well-being of the mother and fetus (Talmadge, Kravitz, and Robergs, 2000; ACOG, 2002). Exercise has been shown to improve a woman's fitness and comfort during pregnancy, to decrease the risk for gestational diabetes and hypertension, and to enhance her postpartum recovery because muscle loss and excessive fat gain are minimized.

In general, the following exercise guidelines are recommended by the American College of Obstetricians and Gynecologists (ACOG, 2002) for healthy pregnant women:

- Moderate exercise for 30 minutes or more is recommended throughout pregnancy. The exercise heart rate is the same as for a nonpregnant woman. That rate is 60% to 80% of the maximum heart rate (200 minus age). Although the fetal heart rate increases similarly, no negative effects have been shown (ACOG, 2002).
- Exercise is modified based on maternal symptoms such as shortness of breath, lightheadedness, and nausea.
- Exercise is stopped when the woman is fatigued, and she must never exercise to exhaustion.
- No exercise is performed in a supine position after the third month. Exercise positions must be modified by inserting support under the head, neck, and shoulders and by tilting the abdomen to the left.
- Breathing must be regular at all times during exercise. The Valsalva maneuver is to be avoided.
- Caloric intake should be adequate to meet the demands of both the pregnancy and the exercise. The pregnant woman who exercises regularly needs about 300 additional calories.
- Prevent dehydration by frequently drinking fluids.
- Movements are to be smooth at all times. Jerky, bouncy motions must be avoided to prevent injury.
- Avoid long periods of motionless standing since this position decreases cardiac output.
- Avoid contact sports, scuba diving, and exertion at high altitudes.

Women with a preexisting medical condition involving the heart, kidney, lungs, or thyroid should be referred to a specialist for appropriate, individualized exercise plans. Contraindications to exercise are listed below (ACOG, 2002):

- Incompetent cervix or cerclage
- Intrauterine growth-restricted fetus
- Preeclampsia
- Preterm premature rupture of membranes
- History of preterm labor or current preterm labor symptoms, indicating high risk for preterm labor
- Persistent second or third trimester bleeding

In the event the pregnancy becomes high risk, restricting activity to varying degrees or prescribing bedrest is frequently part of the management plan. It is estimated that nearly 20% of all women who deliver each year in the United States were prescribed bedrest by their physicians for some period during their pregnancy after 20 weeks of gestation (Maloni and Kutil, 2000; Sprague, 2004). The benefits of this liberal use of bedrest during pregnancy are under review. There is conclusive evidence of adverse physical and psychosocial effects in both women and their families when compliance with bedrest was reported.

Negative physical effects of bedrest include the following (Maloni and others, 1993; Maloni and Kutil, 2000; Maloni, 2002; Sprague, 2004):

- Skeletal muscle atrophy within 6 hours, with greatest progression of atrophy in 3 to 7 days
- Muscle volume loss of more than 25% to 30% in 5 weeks
- Weight loss despite reduced activities and controlled calorie intake
- Plasma and blood volume decrease by approximately 7% of body weight
- Increased blood coagulation
- Heartburn and reflux
- Decreased cardiac output and stroke volume
- Glucose intolerance and insulin resistance
- Prolonged postpartum physical recovery, including symptoms of muscular and cardiovascular deconditioning

Negative psychosocial effects of bedrest on pregnant women and their families include the following (Maloni and others, 1993; Maloni and Kutil, 2000; Maloni and others, 2001):

- Increased stress, family and marital
- Specific increased concerns about family status, emotional changes, health and body image
- Loss of financial support
- Disruption of routine

Except in the high risk conditions that are serious enough to be life-threatening to the mother or fetus, the benefits of bedrest is not evidence-based. High risk conditions that do require bedrest include serious kidney, hypertension, and heart disease and placental abnormalities such as abruptio placenta or placenta previa (Schroeder, 1998). Because studies of newborns do not show improved outcomes and some studies suggest deleterious physical and psychosocial effects with antenatal home or hospital bedrest, we must reevaluate the frequent recommendations for these expensive measures. This is especially true for otherwise healthy women who experience preterm labor or who are pregnant with multiples (Crowther and Dodd, 2005).

The nurse's focus should be one of preventive counseling, thereby decreasing the development or severity of the high risk condition that predisposes that woman to bedrest. Furthermore, nurses can be advocates of evidence-based practice to promote changes in the prescription of bedrest (Sprague, 2004). If bedrest becomes necessary—that is, it is related to a life-threatening risk— then the nurse should implement care to decrease the physical effects of bedrest with isometric exercises. The isometric exercises listed in Box 1-1 can help prevent some of these problems for women who must have long-term bedrest or severely curtailed exercise. These exercises are not aerobic, but they do maintain conditioning and provide a sense of physical well-being. A support group or a referral to the national bedrest support group Sidelines can reduce the psychosocial stress of bedrest. See the Sidelines website *(http://sidelines.org)*.

ANTEPARTUM NUTRITION

Nutrition plays a significant role in fetal well-being and in the prevention and treatment of a high risk pregnancy. To give adequate counseling, the nurse caring for high risk patients must know about nutrition needs, modifications, and risks for potential deficiencies. Utilize the new U.S. Department of Agriculture (USDA, 2005) food guide pyramid *(http://www.mypyramid.gov)* and the Department of Health and Human Services (HHS) and U.S. Department of Agriculture (USDA) Dietary Guidelines for Americans, 2005 *(http://www. healthierus.gov/dietaryguidelines)*.

Nutrient Needs

Adequate nutrients are critical for cell growth to take place during pregnancy. A 25% deficit in needed calories and protein can interfere with the synthesis of DNA. The cells that are undergoing rapid division at the time of insult are the ones most damaged (Reifsnider and Gill, 2000).

During the first 2 months of pregnancy, a deficit in adequate nutrients can have teratogenic effects or cause a spontaneous abortion. After the second month, a nutritional deficit can impede fetal growth, causing a small-for-gestational-age infant or a small-brain-growth infant (Kretchmer and Zimmermann, 1997). These infants may, as a consequence, have limited stature, intellect, and future health (Kretchmer and Zimmermann, 1997; International Food Information Council Foundation and March of Dimes [2003]).

After 24 weeks of gestation, a nutritional deficit is associated with significantly increased preterm delivery and decreased fetal stores of nutrients, especially calcium, magnesium, and iron (Kretchmer and Zimmermann, 1997).

Cell division occurs by two processes: (1) hyperplasia, or an increase in cell number, and (2) hypertrophy, or an increase in the size of the cell. If the insult occurs during hyperplastic cell division, the number of cells will be permanently reduced. This can cause mental retardation, even in developed countries, where nutritional concerns are frequently overlooked. Malnutrition during pregnancy can also increase the risk for preeclampsia, premature rupture of membranes, and preterm labor. Excessive weight gain can have deleterious effects as well. Gestational diabetes, preeclampsia, deep venous thrombosis, and labor dystocia are

Box 1-1   Isometric Exercises for Pregnant Women on Therapeutic Bedrest

Kegel Exercise
Lying on your back at a left tilt or sitting up, tighten your pelvic floor muscles (as if stopping and starting your urine). Hold for three counts and then relax.

Abdominal Breathing
Lying on your back at a left tilt with knees bent, breathe in deeply, letting your abdominal wall rise. Exhale slowly through your mouth as you tighten your stomach muscles.

Bridging
Lying on your back at a left tilt with knees bent, raise your hips off the bed while keeping your shoulders down (see figure below).

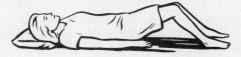

Curl-Ups
Lying on your back at a left tilt with knees bent, put your hands on your stomach. Lift your head and shoulders up (tuck your chin). Keep small of your back against the bed (see figure below).

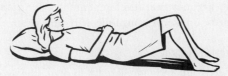

Leg Sliding
Lying on your back at a left tilt with knees bent, slide your legs out slowly, straightening your knees. Keep small of your back flat against the bed. Slowly pull both knees back up (see figure below).

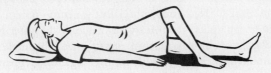

Modified Leg Raises
Lying on your back at a left tilt with one knee bent, bend opposite knee up toward your chest. Then straighten leg by kicking it up toward the ceiling and lower it to bed. Repeat with first bent knee.

Abduction
Lying on your back at a left tilt with knees bent, let your knees come apart and then squeeze them back together.

Continued

Box 1-1	Isometric Exercises for Pregnant Women on Therapeutic Bedrest—cont'd

Ankle Circles

Pump ankles up and down. Circle the foot first in one direction, then in the other while resting your right ankle on left knee. Repeat with left ankle on right knee.

Arm Lifts

Exhale deeply through your nose as you lift one arm up to the side over your head. The sides of your chest should expand. Exhale as you bring your arm down. Repeat with opposite arm.

deleterious effects related to high birth weight. These infants tend to be at greater risk for obesity, type 2 diabetes, hypertension, and hyperlipidemia in later life (Reifsnider and Gill, 2000; Barker and others, 2002; Chauhan and Henrichs, 2003).

Protein: Body's Basic Building Blocks

Protein, 70 g daily or about 1 g/kg per day (Institute of Medicine, 2002), is very important to support the increased embryonic-fetal cellular growth, promote the increased maternal blood volume, and possibly facilitate the prevention of preeclampsia. To prevent the development of anemia, pregnant women also require an adequate intake of iron, folic acid, and vitamins B_6 and B_{12}.

Carbohydrates: Provides Energy

Carbohydrate needs are individualized based on the woman's recommended weight gain and her level of exercise. However, the Institute of Medicine (2002) recommends an average intake of 175 g per day.

Fat: Promotes Proper Central Nervous System Development

Essential fatty acids such as linoleic (omega 6) and alpha-linolenic (omega 3) acids are important for tissue formation, especially the neuron system and the eyes. Food sources include egg yolks, green-leafy vegetables, cold water fatty fish, and oils such as canola, flaxseed, soybean, corn, or safflower. The intake of these essential fatty acids should be increased slightly for the singleton pregnancy and even more for the multifetal pregnancy (Monti, 2003).

Iron

Iron deficiency anemia is a serious condition during pregnancy and has been associated with preterm labor, decreased fetal iron stores resulting in anemia during the first year of life, and increased risk for hypertension in adulthood (Hindmarsh and Others, 2000; Reifsnider and Gill, 2000; Strong, 2005). To prevent iron deficiency during pregnancy, women need 27 mg of iron per day but should not to exceed 45 mg daily (Institute of Medicine, 2001; ODS and NIH, 2005). Foods high in iron include meats and plant foods such as legumes, dried fruits, whole grains, and green leafy vegetables. Iron from plants (non-heme iron) is less well absorbed by the body, but absorption can be improved by eating these foods along with a food high in vitamin C. Caffeinated beverages should be avoided or consumed between meals because they interfere with iron absorption.

All pregnant women on their first prenatal visit should be screened for iron deficiency anemia. It is estimated that in the United States 12% of pregnant women are iron deficient (Cogswell and others, 2003). The initial screen usually is best made by the hemoglobin, hematocrit, and serum ferritin values. The serum ferritin value reflects iron reserves. A ferritin value lower than 12 mcg/dl in the presence of a low hemoglobin value (11.0 g/dl in the first trimester, 10.5 g/dl in the second, and 11 g/dl in the third) indicates iron deficiency anemia. Then 60 to 120 mg of iron per day is usually prescribed in divided doses to increase absorption (CDC, 1998; Kaiser and Allen, 2002). Excessive iron levels can lower zinc absorption and increase the risk for free radicals and oxidative damage resulting possibly in cardiac disease (Strong, 2005).

Prophylactic iron supplementation can be given selectively or routinely. Very little information is available on pregnancy outcome with its use according to the Cochrane Reviews (Mahomed, 1998; Mahomed, 2000). Currently, the CDC, IOM, and ACOG recommend iron supplementation use during pregnancy starting after the first prenatal visit (Lee, 2004). When prophylactic iron supplementation is used, 30 mg of ferrous iron in the form of ferrous gluconate, 300 mg daily, or ferrous sulfate, 150 mg daily, is given. For best absorption, instruct the woman to take the supplemental iron between meals. Ascorbic acid does not increase absorption of iron supplements in ferrous form.

Folate

Folic acid, one of the most important vitamins during pregnancy, is intimately involved in all DNA synthesis and functions as a coenzyme in amino acid metabolism. Therefore this vitamin is essential to all cell division such as the fetus, placenta, and maternal red blood and protein synthesis (Mahomed, 1997). Folic acid deficiency has been associated with an increased occurrence of neural tube defects (AAP, 1999; ACOG, 2003). The ACOG (2003) recommended that all women of childbearing age capable of becoming pregnant consume 400 mcg of folic acid daily. Folic acid is commonly found in dark green leafy vegetables, citrus fruits, eggs, legumes, and whole grains. In January 1998, the U.S. Food and Drug Administration (FDA) established rules under which specified grain products are fortified with approximately 140 mcg of folic acid.

During pregnancy the RDA for folic acid increases to 600 mcg/day (IOM, 1998). Therefore if the woman is eating at least five servings of fruits and vegetables and includes whole or fortified grains in her diet, supplementation is not necessary. If the diet is inadequate or if the patient is at risk for folic acid deficiency because of cigarette smoking or drug or alcohol abuse, a folic acid supplement is recommended (Reifsnider and Gill, 2000). If the mother has a personal obstetric history of a major central nervous system anomaly, such as a neural tube defect, a 4 mg/day dosage of folate is recommended. The woman should start taking the folate before conception and continue through the first three gestational months (International Food Information Council Foundation and March of Dimes, 2003; ICSI, 2004).

Zinc

Zinc is an essential mineral for normal growth and development, DNA synthesis, and immune function. During pregnancy, the diet should contain between 11 and 40 mg of zinc each day (IOM, 2001). Zinc is commonly found in nuts, meats, whole grains, legumes, and dairy products. A deficiency of zinc during pregnancy increases the risk for intrauterine growth restriction, mental retardation, hearing and speech disorders, birth defects, premature rupture of membranes, and preterm labor (Long, 1995; Steegers-Theunissen, 1995). Other risks that increase with zinc deficiency in the mother include postdate pregnancy, bleeding disorders, protracted labor related to uncoordinated uterine activity, and increased cervical and vaginal lacerations.

Sodium

Restricted sodium intake, as well as excessive intake, can cause problems during pregnancy. Restricted sodium intake can interfere with adequate maternal blood volume increase. Excessive sodium intake can increase the sensitivity of the blood vessel wall to angiotensin, causing vasoconstriction. Thus an average sodium intake of 1.5 to 2.3 g/day is considered therapeutic during pregnancy (IOM, 2004; Duley, Henderson-Smart, and Meher, 2005).

Calcium

According to the new dietary reference values, the pregnant woman needs 1000 mg of calcium and the pregnant adolescent needs 1300 mg/day (IOM, 1997). Intakes greater than 2500 mg/day are associated with increased incidence of kidney stones.

Fluids

Hofmeyr and Gulmezoglu (2002) indicated that oral hydration is important for amniotic fluid volume. In the presence of oligohydramnios, oral fluids appear to increase the amniotic fluid volume by increasing maternal plasma volume, thereby improving uteroplacental blood flow. Decreased fluids also increase the risk for uterine irritability and urinary tract infections. The amount of fluid is unique to each individual, but the dietary reference intake (DRI) for water during pregnancy is 3 liters/day (IOM, 2004).

Assessment

To determine whether the pregnant woman is obtaining adequate nutrition and to prevent nutrition-related complications, the nurse must conduct an ongoing assessment. To assess the nutritional needs and status of the pregnant woman, her pattern of weight gain, prepregnancy weight, daily activities, and dietary intake should be evaluated throughout the pregnancy. The formation of fatty and lean body tissues is important. These act as a reserve for energy that the fetus can draw on during the last part of pregnancy and provide a source of energy during labor and delivery and lactation.

Weight Gain for Singleton Pregnancy

An average weight gain during a normal singleton pregnancy (Table 1-1) is between 25 and 35 pounds, according to the U.S. Department of Health and Human Services, Healthy People 2010 document (USDHHS, 2000) and the Food and Nutrition Board of the National Academy of Science (Institute of Medicine, 1998). During the first 2 months, a 2- to 4-pound weight gain is considered average, with a gain of about 1 pound per week during the remainder of the pregnancy. Differences in fat deposition and water retention, as well as in body frame, influence the amount and rate of gain. Tall, thin women tend to gain more fat. Overweight women tend to gain fluid.

According to the Food and Nutrition Board of the National Academy of Science (Institute of Medicine, 1998; USDHHS, 2000), a woman whose prepregnancy weight is 90% of the standard weight for her height and age (BMI below 19.8) should gain more than the average (28 to 40 pounds) to offset the increased risk for fetal mortality and maternal complications of pregnancy. During the first 2 months, the woman should gain the pounds she is underweight, with a gain of 1 pound or more per week during the remainder of the pregnancy.

A woman whose prepregnancy weight is 120% to 135% of standard weight for her height and age (BMI 26–29) needs to gain less than average (15 to 25 pounds). She needs to gain only a couple of pounds during the first trimester and then approximately 2/3 pound per week for the remainder of the pregnancy.

If she is more than 135% of standard weight (BMI above 29), a gain of approximately 15 pounds is recommended in the U.S. Department of Health and Human Services, *Healthy People 2010* document (USDHHS, 2000), and by the Food and Nutrition Board of the National Academy of Science (Institute of Medicine, 1998). However, because of the increased risk for macrosomia related to a prepregnancy maternal overweight state (above 135% of standard weight for height), some health care providers recommend for these women a nutritious diet that maintains their prepregnancy weight instead of a weight gain.

Table 1-1   Weight Gain During Pregnancy

Weight Before Pregnancy	Recommended Weight Gain During Pregnancy (Pounds)
Underweight	28–40
Normal weight	25–35
Moderate overweight (120%–135% of standard)	15–25
Severe overweight (more than 135% of standard)	15

Table 1-2   Dietary Requirements for Pregnancy*

*Because we are interested in helping you, through good nutrition, to produce a
healthy baby and experience an optimally healthy pregnancy, some of these
guidelines may need to be adjusted for your usual weight, pregnancy
complications, and food preferences or religious or other dietary habits. This is
intended as a guideline. The recommendations will be discussed with you, your
questions will be answered, and any specific modifications you require will be
made with you.*

Nutrients	Nonpregnant	Singleton	Twins	Triplets	Quadruplets
Proteins, fats, calories, and carbohydrates per day	2200	2500	3500	4000	4500
Recommended weight gain before 24 weeks		½ lb/wk	1 lb/wk	1½ lb/wk	2 lb/wk
Recommended weight gain after 24 weeks		1 lb/wk	2 lb/wk	2½ lb/wk	3 lb/wk
Optimal total weight gain		25–30 lb	40–50 lb	50–60 lb	65–80 lb
Average length of gestation		40 wk	36 wk	32 wk	30 wk

*Gaining the recommended amount of weight from recommended nutrients can help prevent some preterm and premature labor and extremely premature deliveries.

Weight Gain in Multifetal Pregnancy

In multifetal pregnancies, early weight gain is important, with a recommended
gain of 1.5 pounds per week in the second and third trimesters (Brown and
Carlson, 2000). In a twin pregnancy, a weight gain of 35 to 45 pounds has been
associated with improved outcomes (Brown and Carlson, 2000; Suitor, 1997). In
triple gestation, a weight gain of 50 pounds improves outcome (IFICF and
MOD, 2003). Just as in a singleton gestation, underweight women should gain
at the high end, 1.75 to 2.0 pounds per week, and overweight women should gain
somewhat less (Table 1-2).

Food Groups

To ensure that the body receives the needed additional nutrients, a pregnant
woman is encouraged to select nutrient-rich foods using the guide to daily food
choices. She should select servings from each of the food groups: protein,
grains, milk and milk products, fruits, and vegetables (Table 1-3). Fried foods
and calorie-laden foods that are void of nutrients should be avoided. These
foods increase the number of calories but do not supply the body with any
nutrients. Thus they promote an abnormal weight gain. In addition, social

Table 1-3   Guide to Daily Food Choices

Food Groups	Adolescents (Under 17 yr)	Adults (Over 18 yr)
Protein	6 oz	6 oz
Grains	6–11 servings	6–11 servings
Fruits and vegetables	5–9 servings	5–9 servings
1 yellow fruit or vegetable		
1 vitamin C fruit or vegetable		
1 green leafy vegetable		
Dairy	5 servings	4 servings
Fats and sweets	Cautious use	Cautious use

habits such as drinking alcohol, smoking cigarettes, and abusing drugs, if continued during pregnancy, interfere with adequate absorption and intake of various nutrients (see Chapter 26).

According to the Institute of Medicine (1990), women with multifetal pregnancy should eat a healthy diet (Table 1-4). In addition, they should receive a supplement that contains the following (Brown and Carlson, 2000):

- Iron 30 mg
- Zinc 15 mg
- Copper 2 mg
- Calcium 250 mg

- Vitamin B_6 2 mg
- Folate 300 mg
- Vitamin C 50 mg
- Vitamin D 5 mcg or 200 international units

Referrals

When obvious deficiencies cannot be met using a balanced meal plan, arrange a consultation with a registered dietitian. Cultural or religious practices can also influence and complicate nutritional intake. Careful planning in these situations may allow for alternative food selections that provide adequate nutrition while still meeting cultural and religious practices. Financial aid agencies, such as the Special Supplementary Food Program for Women, Infants, and Children (WIC), can be used if income is inadequate to purchase healthful foods.

Hyperphenylalaninemia

Women with phenylketonuria (PKU) are put on a dietary phenylalanine restriction before conception and throughout pregnancy (AAP, 2001). According to the National Institutes of Health (2000), levels of the amino acid phenylalanine (Phe) are recommended to be below 6 mg/dl for at least 3 months before conception. This decreases the risk for PKU-related teratogenic effects of high level of phenylalanine. The dietary modification normally excludes all high-protein foods such as meat, milk, eggs, and nuts as well as wheat products. Throughout pregnancy, the Phe levels are monitored at least once but preferably twice a week. The recommended level is 2 to 6 mg/dl during pregnancy (National Institutes of Health, 2000).

Table 1-4   Menu Guidelines

Food Group	Serving Size	Singleton	Twins	Triplets	Quads
Dairy	8 oz milk 8 oz cottage cheese 8 oz ice cream 1 oz hard cheese 1 cup yogurt*	6 servings per day	8 servings per day	10 servings per day	12 servings per day
Meats, fish, poultry	1 oz	6 servings per day	10 servings per day	10 servings per day	12 servings per day
Eggs	1	1 per day	2 per day	2 per day	2 per day
Vegetables	1/2 cup cooked or 1 cup fresh	4 per day	4 per day	5 per day	6 per day
Fruits	1/2 cup or 1 fresh	4 per day	7 per day	8 per day	8 per day
Grains and breads	1 oz; 1/2 cup cooked or 1 slice	8 per day	10 per day	12 per day	12 per day
Fats, oils, and nuts	1 T oil 1 pat butter 1 oz nuts	5 per day	6 per day	7 per day	8 per day

Fats and oils are heroes, not villains, for expectant Moms.
Stock cupboards, refrigerator, and freezer with the basics.
Do not disparage fast foods.
Practice on-the-job snacking savvy.
Eat right, on the job and at home.

Adapted from Luke B, Johnson T, Petrie R: *Clinical maternal-fetal nutrition*, Boston, 1993, Little, Brown.
*Contains 2 times the calcium, ounce-per-ounce, compared with other dairy servings listed.

Hyperemesis Gravidarum

Hyperemesis is a condition characterized by severe nausea and vomiting with weight loss and dehydration. It may be seen more frequently in patients with hydatidiform mole, advanced diabetes, anorexia nervosa or bulimia, or gastrointestinal diseases such as peptic ulcers. Many explanations have been postulated in the literature, including the following:

- High levels of human chorionic gonadotropin
- High levels of estrogen
- Increased glucose drain on maternal metabolism
- Family history (genetics)
- Psychogenic factors

To date, these explanations have not proved to be causes because these same factors are present in women without hyperemesis and in women who have mild early pregnancy nausea with or without vomiting.

One major nutritional concern with severe nausea and vomiting is the vitamin B complex and protein deficiency. Various therapies have been tried. Therapies that correlate with supportive therapy seem to be the most effective (Box 1-2). The few women who experience intractable vomiting need close nutritional supervision. Therapy involves lifestyle changes and the following approach:

- Prevention—Multivitamin at time of conception (ACOG, 2004).
- Increased dietary sources of potassium and magnesium (Boxes 1-3 and 1-4).
- Ginger 1 g (Smith and others, 2004).
- Acupressure to stimulate the P6 acupuncture site (3 fingerwidths above the wrist on the anterior side) with a wristband-type, miniaturized, battery-operated transcutaneous electrical nerve stimulator called *Reliefbanc* (Davis, 2004).
- Acupuncture at the P6 acupuncture point (Smith and others, 2002).
- Phridoxine (Vitamin B_6) 25 mg every 8 hours with or without doxylamine; one half of a scored 25-mg tablet orally (ACOG, 2004). According to the Cochrane Review, pyridoxine may be the most effective in reducing the severity (Jewell and Young, 2003).
- Antiemetic pharmacologic management, including prochlorperazine (Compazine), trimethobenzamide (Tigan), or ondansetron (Zofran).
- Antihistamines such as diphenhydramine (Benadryl), meclizine (Antivert), or dimenhydrinate (Dramamine).
- Motility drugs that increase GI motility through the stomach, such as metoclopramide (Reglan).
- Intravenous formula for nutrients and supplementation as follows: add one multivitamin injection, 10 mg pyridoxine, and 2 g magnesium sulfate (192 elemental magnesium) to 1 L of lactated Ringer's solution; administered for 2 hours (Table 1-5).
- Enteral feeding.

With any of these therapies or interventions, the goal is for the woman to obtain food, nutrients, vitamins, and protein from oral intake.

Box 1-2   Managing Morning Sickness

- Rest and eat a small amount of carbohydrates such as biscuits.
- Follow the salty and sweet approach—even so-called junk foods are okay.
- Eat frequently, at least every 2–3 hours. Separate liquids from solids and alternate every 2–3 hours.
- Eat protein after sweets.
- Be aware that foods normally liked may have no appeal at this time.
- Some find that dairy products stay down most easily.
- If you vomit even when your stomach is empty, try sucking on a popsicle.
- Try ginger tea. Peel and finely dice a knuckle-sized piece of ginger and place it in a mug of boiling water. Steep for 5–8 minutes and add brown sugar to taste.
- Try warm ginger ale (with sugar, not artificial sweetener) or ginger tea.
- Try acupressure or antinausea wristbands advertised for motion sickness. When they are worn, they apply acupressure to point P6.
- In general, eat what sounds good, rather than trying to balance your meals. Nongreasy, dry, sweet, and salty may sound good to you.

Turbo-boosters *(assist in adding calories fast)*

Sweet Success	Ensure
Instant Breakfast	ReSource
Boost	Sustacal-Plus
Sustacal	Ensure-Plus

Adapted from Jewell D, Young G: Interventions for nausea and vomiting in early pregnancy, *Cochrane Database Syst Rev*, Issue 4, 2003; and Luke B, Eberlein T: *When you're expecting twins, triplets, and quads*, New York, 1999, Harper & Row.

Box 1-3   Foods Rich in Potassium

Fruits	Fruit Juices	Vegetables
Avocados	Apricot nectar	Broccoli
Bananas	Grapefruit juice	Cooked dry beans
Cantaloupes	Orange juice	Peanuts
Dates	Pineapple juice	Potatoes
Dried figs	Prune juice	Spinach
Prunes	Tomato juice	Dark yellow or orange
Raisins		squashes
Watermelons		Yams
Dried apricots		

Box 1-4   Food Sources of Magnesium

Foods Rich in Magnesium	Foods Moderately Rich in Magnesium
Vegetables	*Fruits*
Spinach	Avocados
Swiss chard	*Vegetables*
Nuts and Seeds	Beans, including garbanzo, kidney,
Nuts	navy, pinto, or soy
Pumpkin seeds	Beet greens
Sunflower seeds	Broccoli
	Lima beans
	Tofu
	Cereals and Grains
	Cereal: bran or whole wheat
	Wheat germ
	Whole wheat bread or muffin
	Nuts and Seeds
	Peanuts
	Peanut butter

Table 1-5   Nutrient Composition of One Suggested Formula for Intravenous Supplementation

Nutrients	Pregnancy RDA	Actual Intake Using D_5 Lactated Ringer's Solution
Vitamin A (international units)	4000	3300
Vitamin B_{12} (mcg)	2.2	5
Vitamin C (mg)	70	100
Vitamin D (international units)	400	200
Vitamin E (international units)	15	10
Calcium (mg)	1200	80
Niacinamide (mg)	17	40
Potassium (mg)	2000	156
Magnesium (mg)	320	192
Thiamine (mg)	1.5	3.0
Riboflavin (mg)	1.6	3.6
Folic acid (mcg)	400	400
Sodium (mg)	500	3381
Biotin (mcg)	30–100	60
Pantothenic acid (mg)	447	15
Pyridoxine (mg)	2.2	14
Dextrose (kcal)		170
Chloride (mg)	750	5538

Data from Newman V, Fullerton J, Anderson P: Clinical advances in the management of severe nausea and vomiting during pregnancy, *J Obstet Gynecol Neonatal Nurs* 22(6):483–490, 1993.
RDA, Recommended daily allowance.

CONCLUSION

Knowledge of maternal physiology and the normal adaptations to pregnancy is essential in the management of high risk and complicated pregnancy. Nutrition and fitness play a significant role in fetal well-being and in prevention and treatment of a high risk pregnancy. The content in this chapter provides the foundation for optimal high risk pregnancy and delivery care.

BIBLIOGRAPHY
General

Cunningham F and others: *Williams obstetrics*, ed 22, Norwalk, Conn, 2005, Appleton & Lange.

Exercise and Bedrest

American College of Obstetricians and Gynecologists (ACOG) Committee on Obstetric Practice: ACOG Committee Opinion: Exercise during pregnancy and the postpartum period, Number 267, *Int J Gynaecol Obstet* 77(1):79–81, 2002.

Chauhan S, Henrichs C: Obesity in pregnancy: risks and interventions by gestational stage, *OBG Management Online*, 2003. Retrieved from *http://www.obgmanagement.com/content*

Crowther C, Dodd J: Multiple pregnancy. In James D and others, editors: *High risk pregnancy: management options*, ed 3, Philadelphia, 2005, Saunders.

Heffernan A: Exercise and pregnancy in primary care, *Nurse Pract* 25(3):42, 2000.

Institute for Clinical Systems Improvement (ICSI): *Health care guidelines: routine prenatal care*, Bloomington, Minn, 2004, ICSI. Retrieved from *http://www.icsi.org*

Maloni J: Astronauts and pregnancy bed rest, *AWHONN Lifelines* 6(4):319, 2002.

Maloni J: Bed rest during pregnancy: implications for nursing, *J Obstet Gynecol Neonatal Nurs* 22(5):422–426, 1993.

Maloni J: Averting the bed rest controversy: preventive counseling can help avoid the issue, *AWHONN Lifelines* 2(4):64, 61, 1998.

Maloni J: Bed rest and high-risk pregnancy: differentiating the effects of diagnosis, setting, and treatment, *Nurs Clin North Am* 31(2):313–325, 1996.

Maloni J: Home care of the high risk pregnant woman requiring bed rest, *J Obstet Gynecol Neonatal Nurs* 23(8):696–706, 1994.

Maloni J, Kutil RL: Antepartum support group for women hospitalized on bed rest, *MCN Am J Matern Child Nurs* 25(4):204–210, 2000.

Maloni J and others: Physical and psychosocial side effects of antepartum hospital bed rest, *Nurs Res* 42(4):197–203, 1993.

Maloni J, Brezinski-Tomasi J, and Johnson L: Antepartum bed rest: effect upon the family, *J Obstet Gynecol Neonatal Nurs* 30(2):165–173, 2001.

Schroeder C: Bed rest in complicated pregnancy: a critical analysis, *MCN Am J Matern Child Nurs* 23(1):45–49, 1998.

Sprague A: The evolution of bed rest as a clinical intervention, *J Obstet Gynecol Neonatal Nurs* 33(5):542–549, 2004.

Talmadge A, Kravitz L, and Robergs R: Exercise during pregnancy: research and application, *IDEA Health and Fitness Source* 18:28–35, 2000.

Nutrition

American Academy of Pediatrics (AAP) Committee on Genetics: maternal phenylketonuria, *Pediatrics* 107(2):427–428, 2001.

American Academy of Pediatrics (AAP) Committee on Genetics: folic acid for the prevention of neural tube defects, *Pediatrics* 104(2 Pt 1):325–327, 1999.

American College of Obstetrics and Gynecology (ACOG): Nausea and vomiting of pregnancy, *Practice Bulletin*, No. 52, Washington, April, 2004, ACOG.

American College of Obstetrics and Gynecology (ACOG): Neural tube defects, *Practice Bulletin,* No. 44, Washington, July, 2003, ACOG.

Barker D and others: Fetal origins of adult disease: strength of effects and biological basis, *Int J Epidemiol* 31(6):1235–1239, 2002.

Barrett J and others: Absorption of non-haem iron from food during normal pregnancy, *BMJ* 309(6947):79–82, 1994.

Brown J, Carlson M: Nutrition and multifetal pregnancy, *J Am Diet Assoc* 100(3):343–348, 2000.

Calhoun S: Focus on fluids: examining maternal hydration and amniotic fluid volume, *AWHONN Lifelines* 3(6):20–24, 2000.

Centers for Disease Control (CDC) and others: Recommendations to prevent and control iron deficiency in the United States, *MMWR Morb Mortal Wkly Rep* 47:1–36, 1998.

Cogswell M and others: Iron supplementation during pregnancy, anemia, and birth weight: a randomized controlled trial, *Am J Clin Nutr* 78(4):773–781, 2003.

Davis M: Nausea and vomiting of pregnancy: an evidence-based review, *J Perinat Neonatal Nurs* 18(4):312–328, 2004.

Duley I, Henderson-Smart D, and Meher S: Altered dietary salt for preventing pre-eclampsia, and its complications in women with normal blood pressure, *Cochrane Database Syst Rev,* Issue 4, 2005.

Hindmarsh P and others: Effect of early maternal iron stores on placental weight and structure, *Lancet* 356(9231):719–723, 2000.

Hofmeyr G, Gulmezoglu A: Maternal hydration for increasing amniotic fluid volume in oligohydramnios and normal amniotic fluid volume, *Cochrane Database Syst Rev,* Issue 1, 2002.

Institute of Medicine, Subcommittee on Nutritional Status and Weight Gain During Pregnancy: *Nutrition during pregnancy,* Washington, DC, 1990, National Academy Press. Retrieved from *http://www.nal.usda.gov/fnic/etext/000105.html*

Institute of Medicine: *Dietary reference intakes for calcium, phosphorus, magnesium, vitamin D and fluoride,* Washington, DC, 1997, National Academy Press. Retrieved from *http://www.nal.usda. gov/fnic/etext/000105.html*

Institute of Medicine: *Dietary reference intake for energy, carbohydrate, fiber, fat, fatty acids, cholesterol, protein, and amino acids,* Washington, DC, 2002, National Academy of Science. Retrieved from *http://www.nal.usda.gov/fnic/etext/000105.html*

Institute of Medicine: *Dietary reference intakes for thiamin, riboflavin, niacin, vitamin B_6, folate, vitamin B_{12}, pantothenic acid, biotin, and choline,* Washington, DC, 1998, National Academy Press. Retrieved from *http://www.nal.usda.gov/fnic/etext/000105.html*

Institute of Medicine: *Dietary reference intake for vitamin A, vitamin K, arsenic, boron, chromium, copper, iodine, iron, manganese, molybdenum, nickel, silicon, vanadium, and zinc,* Washington, DC, 2001, National Academy Press. Retrieved from *http://www.nal.usda.gov/fnic/etext/000105.html*

Institute of Medicine: *Dietary reference intake for water, potassium, sodium, chloride, and sulfate,* Washington, DC, 2004, National Academy Press. Retrieved from *http://www.nal.usda.gov/fnic/ etext/000105.html*

Institute of Medicine, Subcommittee for a Clinical Application Guide, Committee on Nutritional Status During Pregnancy and Lactation, Food and Nutrition Board: *Nutrition during pregnancy and lactation: an implementation guide,* Washington, DC, 1998, National Academy Press.

International Food Information Council Foundation (IFICF) and March of Dimes (MOD): *Healthy eating during pregnancy,* Washington, DC, 2003, IFIC Foundation. Retrieved from *http://www.ific.org/publications/brochures/pregnancybroch.cfm*

Jewell D, Young G: Interventions for nausea and vomiting in early pregnancy, *Cochrane Database Syst Rev,* Issue 4, 2003.

Kaiser L, Allen L: Position of the American Dietetic Association: nutrition and lifestyle for a healthy pregnancy outcome, *J Am Diet Assoc* 102(10):1479–1497, 2002.

Kretchmer N, Zimmermann M: *Developmental nutrition,* Boston, 1997, Allyn & Bacon.

Lee R: Iron deficiency anemia, IOM Food and Nutrition Board, Washington, DC, 2004. Retrieved from *http://www.mch.dhs.ca.gov/documents/pdf*

Long P: Rethinking iron supplementation during pregnancy, *J Nurse Midwifery* 40(1):36–40, 1995.

Luke B, Eberlein T: *When you're expecting twins, triplets, quads,* New York, 1999, Harper & Row.

Mahomed K: Folate supplementation in pregnancy, *Cochrane Database Syst Rev,* Issue 3, 1997.

Mahomed K: Iron supplementation in pregnancy, *Cochrane Database Syst Rev,* Issue 1, 2000.

Mahomed K: Iron and folate supplementation in pregnancy, *Cochrane Database Syst Rev,* Issue 3, 1998.

Monti D: What's so "essential" about essential fatty acids in pregnancy? *IJCE* 18:3, 2003.

National Institutes of Health: *Phenylketonuria: screening and management, Consensus development conference statement,* October 16–18, 2000. Retrieved from *http://www.consensus.nih.gov*

Newman V, Fullerton J, and Anderson P: Clinical advances in the management of severe nausea and vomiting during pregnancy, *J Obstet Gynecol Neonatal Nurs* 22(6):483–490, 1993.

Office of Dietary Supplements (ODS) and National Institutes of Health (NIH): *Dietary supplement fact sheet,* Bethesda, Maryland, 2005. Retrieved from *http://ods.od.nih.gov/factsheets/iron.asp*

Reifsnider E, Gill S: Nutrition for the childbearing years, *J Obstet Gynecol Neonatal Nurs* 29(1):43–55, 2000.

Smith C and others: Acupuncture to treat nausea and vomiting in early pregnancy: a randomized controlled trial, *Birth* 29(1):1–9, 2002.

Smith C and others: A randomized controlled trial of ginger to treat nausea and vomiting in pregnancy, *Obstet Gynecol* 103(4):639–645, 2004.

Steegers-Theunissen B: Maternal nutrition and obstetric outcome, *Baillieres Clin Obstet Gynaecol* 9(3):431–443, 1995.

Strong J: Anemia white blood cell disorders. In James D and others, editors: *High risk pregnancy: management options,* ed 3, Philadelphia, 2005, Saunders.

Suitor C: Nutritional assessment of the pregnant woman, *Clin Obstet Gynecol* 37(3):501–514, 1994.

Suitor C: *Maternal weight gain: a report of an expert work group,* Arlington, Va, 1997, National Center for Education in Maternal and Child Health. Retrieved from *http://www.ncemch.org*

US Department of Agriculture: Dietary guidelines for Americans, 2005. Retrieved from *http://www.healthierus.gov/dietaryguidelines*

US Department of Agriculture: MyPyramid Food Guide, 2005. Retrieved from *http://www.mypyramid.gov*

US Department of Health and Human Services: *Healthy People 2010: understanding and improving health,* Washington, DC, 2000, USDHHS. Retrieved from *http://health.gov/healthypeople/Document/tableofcontents.htm*

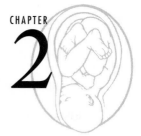

General Nursing Assessment of the High Risk Expectant Family

A pregnancy becomes high risk when the mother or fetus has a significantly increased risk for disability (morbidity) or death (mortality). To achieve an optimal perinatal outcome, high risk factors must be recognized early so that appropriate and timely treatment can be implemented.

Nursing care for the family experiencing a high risk pregnancy focuses on the nurse's independent and collaborative roles. The independent role of the perinatal nurse is to diagnose and treat the expectant family's reactions or concerns about the potential risks inherent to this condition. This role is based on the American Nurses Association's (2003) definition of the unique role of the professional nurse:

> Nursing is the protection, promotion, and optimization of health and abilities, prevention of illness and injury, alleviation of suffering through the diagnosis and treatment of human response, and advocacy in the care of individuals, families, communities, and populations.

The second and equally important role of the perinatal nurse is collaborative management of a high risk condition with other health team members in a way that facilitates health and healing. According to Carpenito (2005), the nurse's collaborative role is to monitor the high risk condition and implement physician- and nurse-prescribed interventions to minimize fetal and maternal complications. These interventions should be evidence-based whenever evidence is available.

ANTEPARTUM NURSING ASSESSMENT

We have used the problem-solving process as the framework for patient care. To make appropriate nursing diagnoses, a comprehensive nursing database must be compiled. We chose Gordon's functional health patterns (1994) because they are relevant to all conceptual nursing models and they provide a systematic way to collect data to determine an individual's or a family's functioning response to a potential or actual threat to the optimal physical and emotional pregnancy outcome.

A prenatal assessment guide using the functional health patterns has been developed (Box 2-1). This tool can help health care providers assess the expectant mother and family in the acute care setting or in home care in several ways:

- It provides a way to assess prenatal physical and emotional risks to make screening easier for a high risk complication.
- It assesses the patient's and family's reactions to hypothetical high risk conditions so that if one develops, it is easier to formulate a nursing strategy.
- It assesses the members of the support system, the resources, and the belief system of the family. This facilitates individualized care planning.
- It assesses the patient's and family's cultural beliefs and practices to enable creation of a patient care strategy that takes these important aspects into consideration. This facilitates optimal health outcomes.

ANTEPARTUM DIAGNOSTIC ASSESSMENT
Laboratory Studies

Initial laboratory studies provide baseline data about previous maternal disease, existing maternal disease, or predisposition to disease or complications during pregnancy. A typical prenatal profile includes several laboratory studies.

Complete Blood Cell Count

A complete blood cell count at the first prenatal visit provides information about leukocyte and erythrocyte levels and the plasma-to-volume ratio. It also supplies information about platelets and erythrocyte formation. If leukocyte levels are high, infection may be present and it can be treated early. Shifts in the granular and nongranular leukocyte counts can help determine whether viral or bacterial infections are present. If the erythrocyte count is low or hemoglobin and hematocrit levels are low, anemia may be a problem; it should be treated vigorously with nutritive and iron supplements. If the woman is of African or Mediterranean descent, further screening for sickle cell disease (thalassemia) may be needed.

All women should have repeat hemoglobin and hematocrit levels taken at 28 to 32 weeks. Although serum volume increases slightly more than the proportion of erythrocytes, anemia should not occur if red blood cells are normal before pregnancy and iron and folic acid intake are increased throughout pregnancy. True anemia of pregnancy is defined as a hemoglobin level lower than 11 g/dl in the first and third trimesters and lower than 10.5 g/dl in the second trimester.

Urine Culture

Urine culture and sensitivity for asymptomatic bacteriuria (ASB) is recommended on the first prenatal visit. If renal function is thought to be compromised, further evaluation may be needed to evaluate creatinine, protein, and uric acid in the urine and serum. If infection is present, treatment can be started

Text continued on p. 33

Box 2-1   Functional Health Pattern Assessment for High Risk Pregnancy

Health Perception and Health Management Pattern (i.e., the Perceived or Actual Prenatal Risks)
Individual Assessment (Ask questions in all of the following areas)
- Demographic risks: geographic location, socioeconomic status, educational attainment, marital status, age, racial or ethnic group, occupational hazards, and blood type
- Behavioral characteristics
- Time prenatal care first sought
- Usage patterns and perception of effects on health of self and fetus of alcohol, tobacco, prescription and nonprescription drugs, illegal drugs, passive smoke, and sexual contact with an illegal drug user
- Health screening patterns, such as physical, dental, and eye examinations; Pap smears; and immunizations (especially rubella)
- Seat belt use
- Breast self-examination pattern
- Current medication use—over-the-counter and prescription
- Complementary and alternative therapy use, including herbal medications, acupuncture, massage therapy, and therapeutic touch
- Current general health (any of the following health problems?)
  - Known allergies
  - Anemia (severe)
  - Cardiac disease
  - Chronic hypertension
  - Chronic lung disease
  - Diabetes
  - Emotional problems
  - Metabolic disease, such as phenylketonuria
  - Phlebitis
  - Renal disease
  - Seizure disorder
  - Thyroid disease
  - Ulcers
- Medical history, including childhood diseases
  - Sexually transmitted diseases
  - Surgeries
  - Hereditary disorders
  - Multiple births
  - Diethylstilbestrol use
  - Premature birth
- Environmental or chemical exposure
  - Heavy metals
  - Organic solvents
  - Pollutants
- Radiation or x-ray exposure
- Viral infections such as cytomegalovirus, rubella, or toxoplasmosis
- Prenatal health care resources used or planned, such as childbirth education classes, support groups, social services, and community agencies

Continued

Box 2-1   Functional Health Pattern Assessment for High Risk Pregnancy—cont'd

- Expectations of the health care providers
- Birth plan
- Need for control

Family Assessment
- What is your family medical history? (Are there any health problems in your family? If yes, what?)
- Who in the family determines such things as what the family eats, when and how they exercise, or when to visit the doctor?
- What does your family do to stay healthy?
- What are your bathing and dental hygiene practices?

Community Assessment
- What, if anything, does the community do to help or hinder your attempts to be healthy?
- What, if anything, does the community do to help or hinder you in raising children?

Cultural Practice Assessment
- Do you plan to immunize your child?
- How often do you or your family get routine checkups?
- What is your belief about health care during pregnancy?

Nutritional-Metabolic Pattern

Individual Assessment
- What is a typical daily food and fluid intake? Eating times? Food likes and dislikes? Dieting patterns? Ways you like your meat cooked (rare)?
- What is your understanding as to the needed dietary changes, especially in folic acid and calcium intake, in (use the appropriate situation) normal pregnancy/high risk pregnancy/adolescent pregnancy/multiple gestation/ lactation/postdelivery recovery?
- How is your appetite?
- What supplements do you use: iron, vitamins, minerals?
- What food restrictions or cravings are you experiencing? Are you experiencing pica?
- What eating-related discomforts, such as nausea or vomiting, leg cramps, heartburn, or bleeding gums are you experiencing?
- What is your nutritional status: height and weight, amount of weight gained or lost, condition of skin, teeth, hair, and nails?

Family Assessment
- Which family member makes the nutrition-related decisions?
- Is the cost of nutritional foods within your family's budget?

Community Assessment
- Are stores reasonably accessible to your family?
- Are any community resources such as WIC or Food Stamps needed?
- Is the water supply safe?

Cultural Practices Assessment
- Are there any cultural practices regarding foods or fluids that you and/or your family value?

Box 2-1   Functional Health Pattern Assessment for High Risk Pregnancy—cont'd

Elimination Pattern
Individual Assessment
- Urinary elimination pattern: Have you experienced changes or problems in urinating such as frequency, odor, or burning pain?
- Bowel elimination pattern: Have you experienced changes or problems such as flatulence, constipation, odor, or hemorrhoids?
- What remedies have you used?

Family Assessment
- What is the family's use of laxatives?
- Do you have an indoor cat? If so, who changes the litter box?

Pest Control and Garbage Disposal
Community Assessment
- What are the sanitation and disposal practices of the community?
- Are there any hazardous waste disposal plants near the community?
- How is the air quality?

Cultural Practices Assessment
- Are there any cultural practices in the area of elimination that you or your family value?
- When do you think a child should be toilet-trained?

Activity and Exercise Pattern
Individual Assessment
- What is your usual pattern of exercise, activity, use of leisure time, and recreation?
- Do you plan to change this pattern during pregnancy/high risk condition/postdelivery recovery in any way? Be specific.
- Are you experiencing any problems that interfere with the desired or expected pattern of activity?
- Since becoming pregnant, what has been your level of energy?
- Have you been experiencing any discomforts such as backache, round ligament pain, or varicosities?
- (If a high risk condition develops and limited physical activity or bedrest becomes necessary) Do you understand the reason for the treatment?

Family Assessment
- What are the family's activity, leisure, and recreational patterns?
- Does the family have adequate transportation available?

Community Assessment
- What activities are available in the community for an expectant and new family?

Cultural Practices Assessment
- What activities or movements are prescribed during pregnancy or puerperium?
- What activities or movements are forbidden during pregnancy or puerperium, such as bathing or type of water used?

Continued

Box 2-1   Functional Health Pattern Assessment for High Risk Pregnancy—cont'd

Sleep-Rest Pattern
Individual Assessment
- What is your pattern of sleep, rest, and relaxation? Any problems? If so, what remedies are you using?
- Which position(s) do you sleep in?

Family Assessment
- What are the family's sleeping arrangements and plans for where the new baby will sleep?
- When do you believe a child should start sleeping through the night?

Community Assessment
- Do any community activities interfere with the family's sleep?

Cultural Practices Assessment
- How much sleep should the pregnant woman get?
- In what position should one sleep?

Cognitive-Perceptual Pattern
Individual Assessment
- Do you find it easy or difficult to communicate with family members or health care providers?
- Is there any information you would like to know about the following?
  - Reproduction
  - High risk condition you are at risk for
  - Screening methods to be ordered
  - Labor and delivery
  - Postdelivery recovery
- What are your perceptions of the needs of the fetus and infant? How do you propose to meet these needs?
- Do you know how to care for an infant? Do you have prior experience? Do you have a planned method of infant feeding?
- How do you learn best? (teaching method, strategies, preferred method, level of education, language spoken, readiness, and motivation)
- What are the nature and location of your pains and discomforts?
- Are your sensory modes or the prosthesis that you use adequate?

Family Assessment (Family's decision-making process and pattern of communication)
- Which family member decides whether to attend a childbirth education class?

Community Assessment
- If community resources are needed, such as a support group, are they available if a high risk condition develops?

Cultural Practices Assessment
- What educational goals do you have for yourself? For this child?
- How should a person respond to pain?

Self-Perception/Self-Concept Pattern
Individual Assessment
- How do you feel about yourself, your general mood, body image, sense of worth, sense of control over your life?

Box 2-1   Functional Health Pattern Assessment for High Risk Pregnancy—cont'd

- How do you feel about your life situation (use appropriate situation): health status, being pregnant, physical and emotional changes that you are experiencing, parenthood, pregnancy loss?
- How would you describe your childhood?

Family Assessment

- What is your significant other's response to the present life situation (choose the appropriate situation): the pregnancy, high risk condition, your physical and emotional changes, parenthood, pregnancy loss?
- How would the father-to-be describe his childhood?
- What are the family's feelings, in general?
- What is the response of the other family members, such as your other children, to the pregnancy?

Community Assessment

- What are the housing conditions where you live?
- What would you say is the overall feeling in your neighborhood?

Cultural Practices Assessment

- Are there any cultural practices where you live that will influence parenting?

Role-Relationship Pattern

Individual Assessment

- Do you feel loved and secure in your family relationship?
- What are your home responsibilities, child care, housework?
- What is your present or former occupation?
- How would you describe your work environment, commuting distance, hours at work, stress level, involvement in work activities such as lifting or standing, exposure to chemicals or infections?
- What are your hobbies?
- What is your perception of how pregnancy or a high risk condition will affect your responsibilities?
- Anticipatory guidance: What would you do if you had to be hospitalized for a few days? Who will take care of your home or other children while you are in the hospital to have your baby?
- What is your greatest concern?

Family Assessment

- Who is in your family? What are the living arrangements?
- What are the responsibilities of each family member in the home? At work? In the community?
- What are your significant other's and your perceptions of how parenthood will affect the future activities and plans of the family?

Community Assessment

- What referral services are needed, such as homemaker, child care, and financial assistance?

Cultural Practices Assessment

- What are the family's beliefs about the role of the father during pregnancy, during labor, and in child care?

Continued

Box 2-1   Functional Health Pattern Assessment for High Risk Pregnancy—cont'd

Sexuality and Reproductive Pattern
Individual Assessment
- Are your sexual relationships satisfying during this pregnancy?
- Are you experiencing any sexuality problems?
- How are you dealing with the modified or restricted sexual activity (if indicated because of a high risk condition)?
- Menstrual history: What was the length of your menstrual cycle and period? What was the date of your last normal menstrual period? What is the estimated date of delivery?
- Contraceptive history: What method of contraception did you use? Did you experience any problems? What do you know about alternative methods? What do you plan to use for future contraception?
- What is your obstetric history?
  - Gravid/para (FPAL); dates of previous pregnancies
  - Spontaneous abortions; induced abortions; ectopic pregnancy; abruptio placentae; placenta previa
  - History of low-birth-weight or large-for-gestational-age infants
  - History of multiple birth
  - History of birth defects or intrauterine fetal death
  - History of preterm birth
  - History of labor dystocia/operative delivery/breech delivery
  - Rh or ABO incompatibility
  - High risk pregnancy complicated with gestational diabetes or preeclampsia
  - Postpartum depression
  - What is your current obstetric status?
  - Prenatal care
  - Multiple gestation
  - Fetal presentation
  - Bleeding
  - Complications
- Fundal height; quickening; gestational age when first heard FHR (correlate with gestational age)
- Diagnostic tests such as hemoglobin, urinalysis, blood sugar (within normal limits)

Family Assessment
- What is your desired family size?
- What is your significant other's sexuality response to pregnancy? (sexual restrictions, if necessary)

Community Assessment
- What are your community's patterns of reproduction? (birth rates, teenage pregnancy rate, maternal and fetal mortality)
- Are you aware of the various prenatal care alternatives, family planning, abortion services, and adoption services available? (community resources)

Cultural Practices Assessment
- Are there any beliefs about sexual practices during pregnancy that you follow?
- Where should delivery take place?
- What does the due date mean to you?

Box 2-1	Functional Health Pattern Assessment for High Risk Pregnancy—cont'd

Coping and Stress-Tolerance Pattern
Individual Assessment
Perceived life stressors
- Is there anything in particular that is worrying you about yourself? Your significant other? Your baby?
- What do you think about childbirth, high risk condition, hospitalization?
- Have you had or are you anticipating any other major life changes during this pregnancy?
- How do you feel you are doing, adjusting to the role of parent? Have you had lifestyle changes?
- Have you ever been physically, emotionally, or sexually abused by someone?
- Have you ever been forced to participate in sexual activities?

Losses Experienced
- Have you ever had an infant or a child who died?
- Have you had a recent death in your immediate family?
- Are you still grieving about the death?

Coping mechanisms used
- What do you do when you are upset?

Perception of Support System
- Who comforts you when you have a problem?
- Who do you talk with about your pregnancy?
- Fill in the blanks. The baby's father is _____ . Your mother is _____ .
- What can the nurses do to provide you with more comfort and security?

Family Assessment
- Is there anything in particular that is worrying your significant other? Your family?

Community Assessment
- Does the community where you live cause you added stress?
- Do you need any referral services? (social worker, community health nurse, mental health nurse, mental health referral, support group)

Cultural Practices Assessment
- Are there any religious practices that are important to you?
- Do you feel your faith in God is helpful to you? If so, how?
- Is prayer important to you?

before renal function is impaired and before the pregnancy is threatened by premature labor.

ABO and Rho (D) Blood Typing

ABO and D (formally Rh) blood typing are important to know to prevent and treat erythroblastosis in the fetus. Repeat Rho (D) antibody testing at 28 weeks. If the mother is Rho (D) negative and unsensitized, Rho (D) immunoglobulin should be given at 28 weeks as well as within 72 hours postpartum.

Antibody Screen

Antibody screening should be done regardless of the D type because other hemolytic incompatibilities may be present. Clinically significant disease may develop because of various blood group antigens shown in the ABO, RhD, Duffy, and Kell systems. A mnemonic device to help remember the significance of various antibodies is "Duffy dies, Kell kills, and Lewis lives."

Rubella/Rubeola/Varicella Screen

A rubella, rubeola, and varicella screen provides information about immunity against these diseases. If titers indicate lack of immunity, the patient cannot be vaccinated with the MMR or varicella vaccine during pregnancy because these vaccines contain a live virus and could cause fetal anomalies. She should be instructed to avoid contact with people who could potentially infect her. Vaccination is recommended with the use of contraception at a minimum of 3 months' postpartum.

Venereal Disease Research Laboratory (RPR or VDRL)

All mothers should receive a serologic test to screen for syphilis because presence of this disease affects the treatment of the mother and of the fetus for potential congenital syphilis caused by maternal infection. The prenatal health examination may be the first time the woman learns that she is infected. Treatment with antibiotics and follow-up serology must be undertaken.

Sexual Transmitted Infections

All patients should also be screened for venereal gonococcus and chlamydia at the first prenatal visit.

Hepatitis B Virus Screen

The Centers for Disease Control and Prevention and the American College of Obstetricians and Gynecologists (ACOG) recommend that all pregnant women be screened for hepatitis B surface antigen (HBsAg) at the initial prenatal visit (see Chapter 25).

Human Immune Deficiency Screening

HIV testing is routinely recommended. Pregnant women should be encouraged to undergo testing, and confidentiality of test results should be explained. If test results are positive, the woman can be treated with antiviral medications and combination drug therapies to prevent transmitting HIV to the fetus and to lessen the likelihood of developing overt disease or worsening disease (see Chapter 25).

Glucose Test for Gestational Diabetes

All pregnant women, except those who are at low risk, should be screened between 24 and 28 weeks of gestation for gestational diabetes. All those who are at high risk for developing gestational diabetes should be screened at the first prenatal visit and again between 24 and 28 weeks of gestation (see Chapter 10).

Papanicolaou Smear

A Pap smear should be done on all pregnant women at the time of their first prenatal visit if one was not done in the previous year. If third trimester bleeding develops, a Pap smear can be repeated to rule out bleeding caused by carcinoma. Pregnancy may increase cervical cancerous growth because of hormonal influences. In the presence of cervical cancer, pregnancy might need to be terminated so that the mother may be treated.

Other diseases, such as *Monilia* and bacterial vaginitis infections, may be detected on the Pap smear. These should be treated even if the woman is asymptomatic. Organism proliferation found on the Pap smear may become significant enough to cause miscarriage or premature rupture of membranes if left untreated.

Purified Protein Derivative Test for Tuberculosis

A purified protein derivative (PPD) screen (Mantoux skin test) should be performed for all at-risk patients to identify any old infection or active disease.

Group B Streptococcus Screening

All pregnant women should be screened for group B-streptococcus between 35 and 37 weeks of gestation (CDC, 2002) (see Chapter 25).

Maternal Serum Markers Screen

Optimally, second trimester maternal serum markers or the quadruple marker screen—which includes unconjugated estriol, human chorionic gonadotropin (the free beta subunit), inhibin-A, and alpha fetoprotein—should be measured between 14 and 22 weeks of gestation. Such serum markers may be measured to assess for developmental defects such as neurotube defects, ventral abdominal wall defects, and esophageal and duodenal atresia. These markers also detect such trisomies as Down syndrome and trisomy 18. There is a 5% false positive rate that produces anxiety for the expectant couple (Wald, Huttly, and Hackshaw, 2003).

First-trimester ultrasound nuchal translucency (NT) combined with HCG and pregnancy-associated plasma protein-A (PAPP-A) can be measured between 9 and 13 weeks to screen for Down syndrome, trisomy 18, or major heart defects but not spina bifida (Wapner and others, 2003). See Chapter 4 for greater detail regarding these screens.

Antepartum Ultrasound

Ultrasound has become commonplace in obstetric care. However, according to the Cochrane Review (Bricker and Neilson, 2000) and ACOG (2004), evidence exists that routine ultrasound in low risk women does not reduce perinatal morbidity and mortality or lower the rate of unnecessary interventions. They concluded that ultrasound should be performed only for specific indications in low risk pregnancies:

- To verify gestational age
- To evaluate fetal growth
- To diagnose fetal malformation
- To confirm cardiac activity
- To count fetuses
- To determine placenta location
- To diagnose uterine anomaly
- To rule out ectopic pregnancy, spontaneous abortion, hydatidiform mole, or fetal demise
- To determine fetal presentation
- As a special procedure adjunct for tests such as amniocentesis or chorionic villus sampling, biophysical profile, amniotic fluid index, and external version. However, if the family requests the test, it is reasonable to grant their request (ACOG, 2004).

ANTEPARTUM PHYSICAL ASSESSMENT

Ongoing assessment of a high risk pregnancy demands more frequent prenatal visits. An in-depth physical assessment should be done at each prenatal visit, along with an evaluation of complication-related parameters. Various parameters to evaluate follow.

Maternal Weight

See the section on nutrition (Chapter 1).

Fundus Height

Fundus height should be measured each visit after the 20 weeks of gestation. It is measured in centimeters from the top of the symphysis pubis to the top of the fundus of the uterus. It is roughly equal in centimeters to the number of weeks of gestation. Thus at 28 weeks, fundal height would be expected to be 28 cm. Because care providers have varying techniques, it is important to use a consistent method and to know how each staff member takes this measurement. It is acceptable to find variations of 1 to 3 cm. Variations more than 3 cm should prompt further investigation of possible estimated date of delivery inaccuracies or growth abnormalities.

Blood Pressure

Blood pressure should be taken at each visit in the same arm and in the same position. The diastolic blood pressure normally drops 7 to 10 mm Hg during the first and second trimesters, followed by a return to nonpregnant baseline during the third trimester. A blood pressure of 140/90 or greater may warn of a hypertensive disorder of pregnancy and should be evaluated.

Physiologic/Pathologic Edema

Because edema has a low specificity and sensitivity in predicting the development of preeclampsia, the Institute for Clinical Systems Improvement (ICSI, 2004) recommended discontinuing routine evaluation for edema.

Urine Dipstick Test

Because a urine dipstick test gives unreliable protein and glucose readings, the ICSI (2004) recommended discontinuing its use as a diagnostic tool for pathologic condition. Its value lies only in screening and then, if positive, in using it as diagnostic evaluation specific to the concern.

Fetal Heart Rate

Doppler readings begin at 10 to 12 weeks of gestation and continue at each visit. They enable the practitioner to auscultate the fetal heart rate (FHR). The technique for calculating heart rate is to listen for a full 60 seconds. The FHR is usually not detectable by fetoscope until 16 to 18 weeks. FHR documentation helps to confirm early dating and document fetal life.

Fetal Movement

After 18 weeks of gestation, the woman is asked about fetal movement. After 24 weeks, she is instructed to count movements at least once daily as a simple way of creating a dependable report of expected fetal well-being. See Chapter 3 for further discussion.

Risk Evaluation (ICSI, 2004)

The following assessments help evaluate fetal and maternal risks:
- Prescription and over-the-counter medication use
- Domestic violence screen (see Chapter 24)
- Personal or family history of psychiatric disease, including depression (see Chapter 6)
- Occupational hazards
- Genetic anomalies
- Preterm labor risk factors (see Chapter 22)
- Gestational diabetes risk factors (see Chapter 10)
- Modifiable infection risk factors: rubella/varicella immunity, tuberculosis, HIV, and other sexually transmitted diseases (see Chapter 25)
- Nutritional insufficiency (see Chapter 1)
- Substance use (see Chapter 26)

HIGH RISK FACTORS

Factors that significantly influence the pregnancy's outcome may be divided into categories.

Genetic Risk

There is a 5% risk for a congenital abnormality in the general population (Lemyre, Infante-Rivard, and Dallaire, 1999). To determine the family's heritable risk, conduct a genetic risk assessment. A sample prenatal genetic risk assessment form can be found in the Institute for Clinical Systems Improvement (ICSI) Health Care Guidelines for Routine Prenatal Care (http://www.icsi.org).

Demographic Characteristics

Geographic Location

Factors such as altitude, unsafe soil conditions, environmental exposure to pollutants, and water contamination are indigenous to certain regions of the United States and should be considered.

Socioeconomic Status

Factors such as substandard living conditions, poor hygiene, inadequate nutritional status, limited income, and limited educational level are interrelated in adverse perinatal outcomes.

Educational Attainment

The risk for adverse prenatal outcome decreases as the length of education increases, probably related to the socioeconomic index, improved nutrition, and decreased substance use (Hays and others, 2000).

Marital Status

An unmarried mother or a mother from a broken marriage has twice the risk for an adverse perinatal outcome, which is usually related to a low birth weight and inadequate prenatal care (McIntosh, Roumayah, and Bottoms, 1995).

Maternal Age

The ideal childbearing age range is 20 to 34 years, with a slightly increased adverse perinatal outcome for mothers younger than 20 years and those older than 34 years (Cogswell and Yip, 1995).

Racial and Ethnic Origins

In different countries, the ethnic groups at risk vary. In the United States, African Americans are at increased risk (USDHHS, 2000). As reported in the *Healthy People 2010* report, overall maternal mortality was 5.1/100,000 in the United States in the year 2000 (USDHHS, 2000). For African American women, maternal mortality was 20.3/100,000. The reasons for the disparity in maternal mortality are unclear, but suppositions include lack of access to or use of early prenatal care and differences in pregnancy-related morbidity. American Indians or Alaska natives have a 5.2/1000 risk for fetal alcohol syndrome, compared with a 0.4/1000 risk in the general population (USDHHS, 2000).

Occupational Hazards

Because a broad range of adverse perinatal risks are related to various occupational health hazards, the perinatal nurse has an important role in screening women for these hazards. Occupational hazards can be grouped into three categories. Table 2-1 lists potential hazards and possible effects. The risk to the growing fetus depends primarily on dose, timing of exposure, and maternal and fetal susceptibility.

The greatest risk for a congenital abnormality occurs during embryogenesis (the first 60 days). However, brain development can be affected significantly between 8 and 15 weeks of gestation and even up through 25 weeks (Lidstrom,

Table 2-1   Occupational Hazards and Possible Reproductive Risk

Occupational Hazards	Possible Reproductive Risk
Chemical Hazards	
Mercury	Spontaneous abortion, low birth weight, cognitive impairment (MOD, 2005)
Lead	Spontaneous abortion, low birth weight, fetal death, impaired neurologic development, cognitive impairment (MOD, 2005)
Passive smoking	Low birth weight (Dejin-Karlsson and others, 1998)
Pesticide	Decreased fertility, congenital anomalies (Keleher, 1991)
Organic solvents	Congenital defects (Khattak and others, 1999)
Anesthetic agents	Spontaneous abortion, congenital defect (ICSI, 2004)
Physical Hazards	
Physically demanding work such as heavy and/or repetitive lifting or load carrying and manual work	Preterm birth, SGA, preeclampsia (Mozurkewick and others, 2000)
Severe fatigue caused by standing more than 4-6 hours or by working long shifts (more than 10 hours) or double shifts	Prematurity, low birth weight (ICSI, 2004; Mozurkewich and others, 2000)
Extreme heat (core temp 38.9° C or higher)	Spontaneous abortion; birth defects (Paul, 1993)
Noise	Decreased fertility, congenital anomalies, preterm labor, and small for gestational age (ICSI, 2004; Lidstrom, 1990)
Vibration	Decreased fertility, spontaneous abortion, preterm labor, and hyperemesis gravidarum (Lidstrom, 1990; Pelmear, 1990)
Radiation such as x-ray	Reduced fertility, childhood leukemia, and central nervous system congenital anomalies, especially microcephaly and mental retardation related to doses over 10 rads (Toppenberg, Hill, and Miller, 1999)
Biologic Hazards	
Contact in crowded places or with a group at higher risk such as school children and the sick	If the woman contracts an infectious disease, congenital anomalies and premature rupture of membranes (Chamberlain, 1991)
Psychologic Hazards	
Stress	Spontaneous abortion, prematurity, pregnancy-induced hypertension (Copper and others, 1996; Hedegaard, 1999; Hobel and others, 1999)

1990). Exposure to occupational hazards later in pregnancy most frequently restricts fetal growth. According to Stapleton (1996), the most common hazardous occupational exposure encountered during pregnancy is lead. People most at risk for lead exposure are stained glass artists and automotive and aircraft painters. Computer monitors do not appear to pose any reproductive risk (Lidstrom, 1990; Bentur and Koren, 1991; Paul, 1993; Keleher, 1995).

Behavioral Characteristics

Substance Abuse

Smoking is the cause of 20% to 30% of all low-birth-weight infants in the United States, related to intrauterine growth restriction (USDHHS, 2000). The uses of licit and illicit drugs increase the risk for spontaneous abortion, preterm delivery, and infectious diseases (USDHHS, 2000). See Chapter 26 for specific factors.

Failure to Seek Prenatal Care

Failure to seek prenatal care is one of the factors that most negatively influences pregnancy outcome. It may reflect an unintended pregnancy or a lifestyle less likely to promote health, especially regarding nutrition and exposure to fetal toxins such as alcohol, nicotine, and other drugs (Warner and others, 1996; Hulsey, 2001).

Nutritional Status

Inadequate nutritional intake and inadequate prenatal care are the two most significant factors influencing pregnancy outcome. A low prepregnancy weight and an inadequate pregnancy weight gain are important indicators of poor nutritional status. An inadequate pregnancy weight gain, especially during the second trimester, may negatively affect the maternal plasma value, reducing the transfer of nutrients to support appropriate growth (Abrams and Selvin, 1995).

Dental Hygiene

Periodontal disease increases the risk for preterm birth and low birth weight. This is probably because the endotoxins from the periodontal infection cause fetotoxic substances (Offenbacher and others, 1998; Carl, Roux, and Matacale, 2000).

Psychosocial Stressors

Extreme maternal stress and anxiety can negatively influence pregnancy outcome. They can affect the mother's health by compromising her immune state and comprise the baby's health by increasing the risk for preterm labor and decreasing birth weight (Hedegaard, 1999; Hobel and others, 1999).

Abuse and Violence

Domestic violence is a serious problem, and the risk increases during pregnancy (FVPF, 2005). Physical abuse during pregnancy increases the risk for abruptio placenta, preterm delivery, and low-birth-weight infants, possibly related to abdominal trauma and subsequent placental damage, infection from forced sex, or stress (Furniss, 1997). There is also an increased risk for child abuse once the baby is born (Lemmey and others, 2001).

Multiples

The incidence of multiple births continues to rise. There are associated physiologic and psychologic risks related to multiple births. Risk factors identified by Watson-Blasioli (2001) include:

- Preterm labor
- Pregnancy-induced hypertension (PIH)
- Fetal growth restriction and low birth weight
- Maternal anemia
- Discomfort
- Parental stress (related to health outcomes, pregnancy progress, and care issues)
- Child abuse
- Marital breakdown
- Substance abuse
- Postpartum depression

CONCLUSION

Meticulous, ongoing prenatal assessment is essential in order to achieve an optimal perinatal outcome. In a thorough nursing assessment, the nurse focuses on (1) health-promoting activities that can prevent complications and (2) recognizing developing complications early, when treatment is most effective.

BIBLIOGRAPHY

Abrams B, Selvin S: Maternal weight gain pattern and birth weight, *Obstet Gynecol* 86(2):163–169, 1995.

American College of Obstetricians and Gynecologists (ACOG): Ultrasonography in pregnancy, *Clinical Management Guidelines for Obstetrician-Gynecologists*, No. 58, Washington, DC, 2004, ACOG.

American Nurses Association: *Nursing's social policy statement*, ed 2, Kansas City, Mo, 2003, ANA.

Bentur Y, Koren G: The three most common occupational exposures reported by pregnant women: an update, *Am J Obstet Gynecol* 165(2):429–437, 1991.

Bricker L, Neilson J: Routine Doppler ultrasound in pregnancy, *Cochrane Database Syst Rev*, Issue 2, 2000.

Carl D, Roux G, and Matacale R: Exploring dental hygiene and perinatal outcomes: oral health implications for pregnancy and early childhood, *AWHONN Lifelines* 4(1):22–27, 2000.

Carpenito L: *Nursing diagnosis: application to clinical practice*, ed 11, Philadelphia, 2005, Lippincott Williams & Wilkins.

Centers for Disease Control and Prevention: Prevention of perinatal group B streptococcal disease, *MMWR Morb Mortal Wkly Rep* 51:1–22, 2002.

Chamberlain G: ABCs of antenatal care: work in pregnancy, *BMJ* 302(6784):1070–1073, 1991.

Cogswell M, Yip R: The influence of fetal and maternal factors on the distribution of birthweight, *Semin Perinatol* 19(3):222–240, 1995.

Copper R and others: The preterm prediction study: maternal stress is associated with spontaneous preterm birth at less than thirty-five weeks' gestation. National Institute of Child Health and Human Development Maternal-Fetal Medicine Units Network, *Am J Obstet Gynecol* 175(5):1286–1292, 1996.

Dejin-Karlsson E and others: Does passive smoking in early pregnancy increase the risk of small-for-gestational-age-infants? *Am J Public Health* 88(10):1523–1527, 1998.

Family Violence Prevention Fund's National Health Resource Center on Domestic Violence (FVPF): *Domestic violence risk measurement tool online*, San Francisco, 2005, FVPF. Retrieved from *http://endabuse.org/programs/healthcare*

Furniss K: Battered women: how nurses can help, *AWHONN Lifelines* 1(4):12–14, 1997.

Gordon M: *Nursing diagnosis: process and application,* ed 3, St Louis, 1994, Mosby.

Hays B and others: Public health nursing data: building the knowledge base for high-risk prenatal clients, *MCN Am J Matern Child Nurs* 25(3):151–158, 2000.

Hedegaard M: Life style, work and stress, and pregnancy outcome, *Curr Opin Obstet Gynecol* 11(6):553–556, 1999.

Hobel C and others: Maternal plasma corticotropin-releasing hormone associated with stress at 20 weeks' gestation in pregnancies ending in preterm delivery, *Am J Obstet Gynecol* 180(1 Pt 3):5257–5263, 1999.

Hulsey T: Association between early prenatal care and mother's intention of and desire for the pregnancy, *J Obstet Gynecol Neonatal Nurs* 30(3):275–282, 2001.

Institute for Clinical Systems Improvement (ICSI): *Health care guidelines: routine prenatal care,* Bloomington, Minn, 2004, ICSI. Retrieved from *http://www.icsi.org*

Keleher K: Occupational health: how work environments can affect reproductive capacity and outcome, *Nurse Pract* 16(1):23–30, 1991.

Keleher K: Primary care for women: environmental assessment of the home, community, and workplace, *J Nurse Midwifery* 40(2):88–96, 1995.

Khattak S and others: Pregnancy outcome following gestational exposure to organic solvents: a prospective controlled study, *JAMA* 281(12):1106–1109, 1999.

Lemyre E, Infante-Rivard C, and Dallaire L: Prevalence of congenital anomalies at birth among offspring of women at risk for a genetic disorder and with a normal second trimester ultrasound, *Teratology* 60(4):240–244, 1999.

Lemmey D and others: Intimate partner violence: mothers' perspectives on effects on their children, *MCN Am J Matern Child Nurs* 26(2):98–103, 2001.

Lidstrom I: Pregnant women in the workplace, *Semin Perinatol* 14(4):329–333, 1990.

March of Dimes (MOD): *Environmental risks and pregnancy,* White Plains, NY, 2005, March of Dimes Birth Defects Foundation. Retrieved from *http://www.marchofdimes.com/printableArticles/14332_9146.asp?printable=true*

McIntosh L, Roumayah N, and Bottoms S: Perinatal outcome of broken marriage in the inner city, *Obstet Gynecol* 85(2):233–236, 1995.

Mozurkewich E and others: Working conditions and adverse pregnancy outcome: a meta-analysis, *Obstet Gynecol* 95(4):623–635, 2000.

Offenbacher S and others: Potential pathogenic mechanisms of periodontitis associated pregnancy complications, *Ann Periodontol* 3(1):233–250, 1998.

Paul M: Physical agents in the workplace, *Semin Perinatol* 17(1):5–17, 1993.

Pelmear P: Low frequency noise and vibration: role of government in occupational disease, *Semin Perinatol* 14(4):322–328, 1990.

Stapleton R: Silent hazard: lead poisoning in utero, *Childbirth Instruct Mag* 6(3):12, 1996.

Toppenberg K, Hill D, and Miller D: Safety of radiographic imaging during pregnancy, *Am Fam Physician* 59(7):1813–1818, 1999.

US Department of Health and Human Services (USDHHS): *Healthy People 2010: understanding and improving health,* Washington, DC, 2000, USDHHS. Retrieved from *http://www.healthypeople.gov/document*

Wald N, Huttly W, and Hackshaw A: Antenatal screening for Down's syndrome with the quadruple test, *Lancet* 361(9360):835–836, 2003.

Wapner R and others: First trimester screening for trisomies 21 and 18, *N Engl J Med* 349(15):1405–1413, 2003.

Warner R and others: Demographic and obstetric risk factors for postnatal psychiatric morbidity, *Br J Psychiatry* 168(5):607–611, 1996.

Watson-Blasioli J: Double-take: defining the need for specialized prenatal care for women expecting twins: a Canadian perspective, *AWHONN Lifelines* 5(2):34–42, 2001.

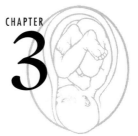

Assessment of Fetal Well-Being

A ntepartum and intrapartum assessments of the fetus have continued to gain momentum, although not solely with conventional fetal heart rate (FHR) monitors. In the past, it was assumed that if the mother was well, the fetus was well. More recently, it is assumed that if the FHR tracing is normal, the fetus will be a normal healthy newborn. Several studies since 1999 refute that assumption (Thacker, Stroup, and Chang, 2001; ACOG, 2005). Several means of fetal surveillance are now available, and both patients—mother and fetus—can be assessed. Our understanding of the limitations of fetal surveillance, as well as the benefits, has changed dramatically since the 1990s. Intermittent auscultation in the care of low risk women needs to be considered by all childbirth practitioners, especially midwives (Albers, 2001).

Sophisticated technology and biochemical analyses aid in the care of both patients. Nurses working in modern obstetric units must understand a myriad of technologic and laboratory data to effectively care for the mother and fetus and to educate women regarding their choices in fetal heart monitoring (Wood, 2003). Differentiation of maternal heart rate (MHR) and FHR must be provided to nursing staff since MHR may mimic FHR, leading to misdiagnosis of fetal compromise or death (Murray, 2004). A critical issue is to select one set of definitions for fetal heart rate patterns and communicate it consistently to avoid confusion with health care providers (Simpson, 2004). At the same time, family-centered concepts of care must be integrated into the care plan.

FETAL HEART RATE MONITORING
Electronic Monitoring

Electronic FHR monitoring (EFM) provides a current and continuous observation of indirect, subjective information about fetal oxygenation at the time the monitoring is being done. Of approximately 4 million live births in 2002, 85% were assessed with EFM in the United States (ACOG, 2005). It does not explain oxygenation in the past or predict the future oxygenation during fetal life in the same way we once expected. Continuous or intermittent FHR tracings provide a convenient and reasonably predictable way of assessing fetal well-being. EFM, although controversial, is suggested as a way to reduce perinatal morbidity and mortality.

U.S. health statistics from 2003 indicated that overall infant mortality (deaths per 1000 live births through first year of life) is at 6.9 in 1000 births (Kochanek and Martin, 2005), ranking the United States 28th among industrialized nations (United Health Foundation, APHA, and Partnership for Prevention, 2005). Perinatal deaths (20 weeks of gestation through first 30 days after birth) are 6.8 in 1000, with morbidity still estimated much higher (Kochanek and Martin, 2005).

In the United States, continuous EFM is still routine in most hospital perinatal/maternity centers. This is true despite the recommendation by the American College of Obstetrics and Gynecology (ACOG, 2005) to limit continuous use of EFM. Feinstein, Sprague, and Trepanier (2000) compared intermittent auscultation with EFM and reported that research still supported intermittent auscultation as an equivalent alternative to EFM when practitioners were experienced in recognizing the sound of significant FHR changes.

Perinatal mortality has improved since 1990, and EFM is one reason for the improvement. However, morbidity statistics have not improved, raising three main concerns regarding routine use of EFM (Thacker, Stroup, and Chang, 2001; ACOG, 2005):

• Effects of EFM on the incidence of cerebral palsy (CP)
• Effects of routine continuous EFM on cesarean birth rates
• Legal implications of FHR assessment (Mahlmeister, 2000)

With improved neonatal care, especially for extremely premature infants, the actual rate of CP has risen slightly since 1985 (Phelan and Kim, 2000). In fact, because more premature infants are surviving and because they have an associated increased risk for congenitally acquired neurologic damage, CP rates are unlikely to improve (Phelan and Kim, 2000; Freeman, Garite, and Nageotte, 2003). There is also some suggestion in the literature that CP actually may start with the development of an abnormal fetal brain (Phelan and Kim, 2000). A large percentage of asphyxial damage occurs before labor and thus would not benefit from electronic FHR monitoring-prompted interventions offered during labor (Freeman, 2002; Freeman, Garite, and Nageotte, 2003).

The most discussed risk of EFM is the rise of cesarean birth rates. In the United States, the current cesarean birth rate is 22% or higher in most centers (ACOG, 2000; Thacker, Stroup, and Chang, 2001). One study examined the cesarean birth rate in more than 7000 births at a large Southwestern tertiary perinatal center in a more divided manner (Radin, Harmon, and Hanson, 1993). In this study, term primiparas, regardless of demographic data, physician practice, complications, induction, regional anesthesia, or stage of labor when admitted, had an 18% cesarean birth rate. Excluded from the study were those with multiple gestations, those with intrauterine fetal death, and those who were less than 35 weeks' pregnant.

The variables of assigned nurse (there is little to no opportunity for self-assignment) and phases of labor during care were examined. Three discrete groups of nurses were identified, regardless of other variables. The low cesarean birth rate group had a cesarean birth rate lower than 5%. The middle cesarean birth group had an overall 18% cesarean birth rate. The highest cesarean birth rate group had a rate as high as 35% to 49%. No significant differences existed in neonatal Apgar scores.

This study suggested that some nurses may manage technologic data from EFM to provide expert nursing care and manage patients with epidurals differently, whereas other nurses may use the data solely to report fetal assessment data to the physician to alter medical management. This study warrants further investigation of specific differences in nursing care practices and effects on cesarean birth rates.

Intermittent Auscultation

When done at prescribed intervals and for 60 seconds, especially during and immediately after contractions, intermittent auscultation has been supported by research to be equally valuable as electronic fetal monitoring in predicting fetal outcomes (ACOG, 1999; Thacker, Stroup, and Chang, 2001). The value of EFM may, in fact, be that we now better understand what we hear, realizing that we know only the present state of the fetus. It therefore should not be discarded but, rather, used differently by nurses than by physicians for the management of intrapartum care. These studies also used a 1:1 ratio of nurse midwife to patient, with continuous bedside care.

With research findings supporting the use of both EFM and intermittent auscultation, it is apparent that perinatal nurses must understand how to use FHR monitoring. To do this, perinatal nurses must be fully acquainted with the following (Trepanier and others, 1996; Haggerty and Nuttall, 2000; Schmidt, 2000):

- Physiology and pathophysiology of fetal oxygenation
- Physiologic basis of FHR control
- Instrumentation and the application of external and internal fetal monitoring methods
- Baseline FHR, variability patterns, periodic rate changes, arrhythmias, and artifacts, which describe effects of maternal contractions on FHR control
- Nursing management related to EFM
- Skills and techniques for antepartum evaluation of fetal well-being through auscultation, EFM testing, and fetal movement counts
- Advanced methods of fetal evaluation, such as biophysical profile and Doppler flow studies

Physiology and Pathophysiology of Fetal Oxygenation
Maternal Circulatory and Cardiovascular Adaptation

One of the most dramatic adaptations to pregnancy is the increase in maternal blood volume by 20% to 100% over prepregnant volume. Plasma increases

plateau around 32 to 34 weeks of gestation. The number of red blood cells increases in response to the plasma volume. Both volume and blood cell increases are in response to cell proliferation and growth of the uterus, placenta, and fetus.

Under physiologically nonstressful conditions, the vascular system in the maternal pelvic region remains widely dilated. In the presence of stressors, it is capable of marked constriction and reduction of uteroplacental blood supply. The most common and easily preventable stressor is mechanical obstruction of the maternal inferior vena cava and aorta by the gravid uterus when in a supine position. Activation of the maternal autonomic nervous system (ANS) in response to other hemodynamic changes may also trigger marked constriction of the pelvic vasculature, which is physiologically expendable to general maternal circulatory needs.

The usual state of the uterine vasculature is one of low resistance to blood flow. This occurs in part because of new vascularization of the uterus and in response to the systemic influence of estrogens, which increase overall vasodilation. It is now estimated that uterine blood increases from 50 ml/min in early pregnancy to 700 ml/min by term.

Because of vasodilation and increased volume, cardiac output (Stroke Volume × Heart Rate) is greater during pregnancy. The heart rate is generally 10 to 15 bpm faster than prepregnant rates, and stroke volume is increased by approximately 15% because of increased blood volume. The increase in cardiac output helps circulate more blood to the uterus during pregnancy.

Uteroplacental-Fetal Exchange*

The placenta performs several major organ functions for the fetus. It acts as the following:
- Lung for respiratory functions of exchanging oxygen (O_2) and carbon dioxide (CO_2)
- Gastrointestinal tract for nutritive functions and exchange of waste products and electrolytes
- Skin for thermoregulation
- Kidney for renal functions of acid-base balance and electrolyte homeostasis
- Endocrine organ for production of hormones that promote placental perpetuation
- Barrier to maternal blood and bacteria

After implantation, the placenta begins to form the chorionic tissues. By 14 weeks, the placenta is a discrete organ with independent functions and purpose. It is at this point that segments of the placenta, called *cotyledons*, form and connect by vascular channels to the umbilical cord. The surface of the placenta then thins to a membranous, single layer of cells. Maternal blood and fetal blood, although not mixing, are exposed to one another across this membrane. By this exposure, fetal respiration, acid-base and electrolyte

---

*Meschia, 2004.

homeostasis, nutrition, and excretion take place. The space in which these functions take place is the intervillous space, which contains maternal blood. The fetus, therefore, totally depends on its mother for most homeostatic mechanisms.

Transfer and exchange of molecules occur in the intervillous space. Molecules enter through the epithelial cells on the surface of the villi and move through the villous stroma and into the fetal capillary vessels within the villi. Molecules pass back and forth between maternal and fetal tissues. Exchange processes are accomplished by means of simple or selective diffusion.

Simple diffusion is a relatively uncomplicated process responsible for the rapid exchange of small molecules, such as O_2, CO_2, water, electrolytes, creatinine, and uric acid, across the placental membrane. Simple diffusion also allows potentially harmful drugs—antibiotics, narcotics, barbiturates, and anesthetic agents, to name a few—to cross quickly to the fetus. Simple diffusion depends totally on the adequacy of uterine blood flow and on the concentration gradient of the molecules.

Selective transfer is a complex process and therefore occurs more slowly than simple diffusion. It can occur against a concentration gradient by an energy-dependent process. Glucose, for instance, is transported in this manner from stores in the placenta.

Selective transfer can also be actively facilitated by specific enzyme systems. For example, amino acids and buffering substances are transferred using specific enzyme groups to facilitate the process. Selective transfer, by energy-dependent or enzyme-dependent processes, depends on the sufficiency of the placental surface area and placental thickness rather than on uterine blood flow.

Because simple diffusion is faster (taking only minutes), O_2, CO_2, and water can be transported and exchanged rapidly to correct fetal hypoxia if uterine and umbilical blood flow and maternal O_2 are sufficient. On the other hand, the more complex processes of selective transfer, which take hours, cannot correct an acid-base imbalance from hypoxia.

Fetal Capabilities for Maintaining Health

The fetus has certain remarkable capabilities that enable it to withstand stressors. Fetal stressors may be caused by physiologic maternal adaptation failures, disease, or mechanical or physiologic obstruction of maternal blood flow through the uterus and into the intravillous space. The fetus is equipped with a high concentration of hemoglobin in plasma (60% hematocrit). Each hemoglobin molecule, because of its unique shape, can be supersaturated with O_2. This is fortunate and necessary because by the time maternal O_2 is transferred to the fetus, the O_2 partial pressure (P_{O_2}) is at best 35 to 40 mm Hg. Compared with an adult P_{O_2} of 90 to 96 mm Hg, the fetal P_{O_2} would be inadequate were it not for different fetal hemoglobin. The low fetal P_{O_2} causes the diffusion gradient to facilitate O_2 delivery from mother to fetus (Gilstrap III, 2004).

The fetal heart must be significantly hypoxic before myocardial depression occurs. It is only after fetal myocardial depression that significant fetal central nervous system (CNS) hypoxia occurs. Protection from myocardial hypoxia exists, in part, because of the well-supplied and unimpeded blood supply from the coronary vessels. Impulses travel through the heart, originating at the sinoatrial node and traveling across the atrioventricular junction, down the bundle branches, and out the Purkinje fibers in the ventricles. When myocardial depression occurs from hypoxia, cardiac arrhythmias may occur. The fetus can effectively compensate only by increasing FHR; it cannot increase output by changing cardiac output.

Function of Amniotic Fluid Related to Evaluation of Fetal Heart Rate

Amniotic fluid is produced primarily by maternal blood, although the fetus contributes to the volume through urinary excretion and diuresis. Amniotic fluid has a number of functions. It is a buoyant medium, allowing the umbilical cord to float and preventing it from becoming entrapped between the wall of the uterus and the fetal body, especially during contractions. This function is imperfect but, for the most part, effective.

When the amniotic fluid is filled with fetal meconium, the meconium promotes stiffening and loss of flexibility of the cord with extended exposure. This is one reason why it is dangerous for meconium to be passed before the baby is born.

Physiologic Basis of Fetal Heart Rate Control
Central Nervous System Control

Regulation of the FHR originates in the fetal CNS. By week 10 of gestation, both the CNS and the cardiac system are developed enough to begin and maintain the FHR.

Sympathetic. Initially, the sympathetic portion of the rudimentary ANS is functionally active. The sympathetic branch is responsible for establishing and sustaining FHR. The normal rate throughout fetal life ranges from 110 to 160 bpm for most, tending toward the upper range of 150 to 160 in early fetal life and the middle to lower range of 110 to 140 by term. The sympathetic branch of the ANS also serves as a reserve throughout intrauterine life, accelerating the FHR in response to various stimuli, as needed for fetal circulation, and supporting compensatory responses to physical insults.

Parasympathetic. Early in fetal life, the parasympathetic branch of the ANS begins to influence the FHR. The parasympathetic branch serves as an opposing force against the steady beat sustained by the dominant sympathetic branch. This opposition exerts a differing strength of opposing force on each beat. Three effects of this opposing force are observed on the FHR (Parer and Nageotte, 2004):

- It gradually slows the intrinsic rate from early gestation through term.
- It causes beat-to-beat differences in rate per minute of 2 to 3 bpm, referred to as *short-term variability* (STV).
- It results in two or more cyclic fluctuations per minute of 6 to 25 beats amplitude, referred to as *long-term variability* (LTV).

Instrumentation and Application of Fetal Monitoring Methods

Although still indirect and somewhat subjective, EFM gives data slightly more objective than intermittent auscultation and infers information about current and ongoing fetal oxygenation. It does this by calculating and recording an average FHR per minute, indicating STV and LTV, and by providing a continuous graphic printout of rate patterns and periodic changes.

To fully appreciate patterns, it is helpful to have a continuous record for interpretation. Correct application of monitor methods and an understanding of the way to properly operate the monitor help the user obtain accurate information. Fetal monitors are made by a variety of manufacturers and may have capabilities for external (indirect) monitoring only or for both external and internal (direct) monitoring of FHR and maternal contractions (Fig. 3-1). Other features, such as fetal electrocardiogram (ECG) monitoring, twin monitoring, amnioinfusion, ambulatory monitoring, transmission of strips from one location to another (usually by telephone), central displays, and computer record storage are available from most manufacturers.

External (Indirect) Monitoring

The external monitor parts are the tocotransducer (Fig. 3-2, *A*) for assessing contractions and the ultrasound transducer (Fig. 3-2, *B*) for assessing FHR. To place the transducers properly, it is important to ascertain by abdominal palpation how the baby is positioned.

External contraction monitoring. Near term, the tocotransducer should be placed over the fundus of the uterus, two to three fingers below the top and slightly off center from the umbilicus on the side where the fetal back is palpated. A good rule of thumb for placement of the tocotransducer for preterm contractions is to palpate the uterus for firmness and place the tocotransducer where this is best felt. The placement may be in any quadrant, including those lower than the umbilicus. There is a pressure-sensitive area on the underside of the tocotransducer that must respond to changes in the abdominal wall when the uterus contracts against it. The tocotransducer is secured in place with a belt that is tightened only enough to keep it from slipping or it is secured with a stretchy band. The monitor has an indicated dial or button to artificially set the reference for uterine resting tone, usually between 5 and 15 mm Hg on the graph paper. Box 3-1 presents the advantages and limitations of external contraction monitoring.

External fetal heart rate monitoring. The ultrasound transducer has sending and receiving crystals encased in a disk. If possible, it should be placed over the fetal chest wall for detection of the best signal. The signal is detected from the motion of the heart valves closing between the atria and ventricles.

The ultrasound transducer selects the complex of two sound waves from the motion of the two atrioventricular valve closures, or it selects the one sound wave that is timed within the logical sequence of events; then it calculates the

A

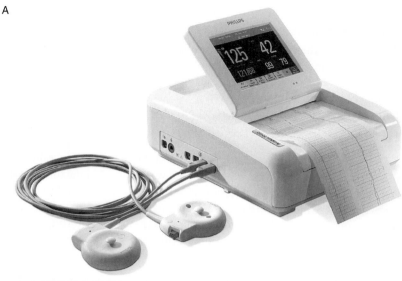

B

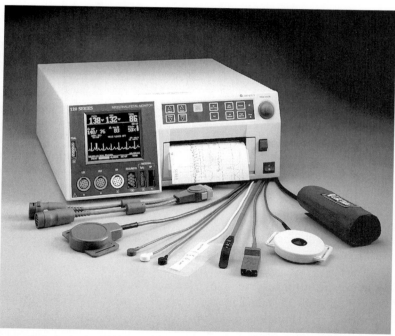

Figure 3-1 A, Avalon FM30 transducer. **B,** Corometrics Model 129 maternal/fetal monitor provides measurement of FHR, fetal oxygen saturation, UA, and maternal parameters, including SpO_2, ECG, FHR, and noninvasive BP. The audible and visual "spectra alert" option may be added to this monitor. (**A,** Courtesy Philips Medical Systems, Andover, Mass. **B,** Courtesy GE Medical Systems Information Technologies, Milwaukee, Wisc.)

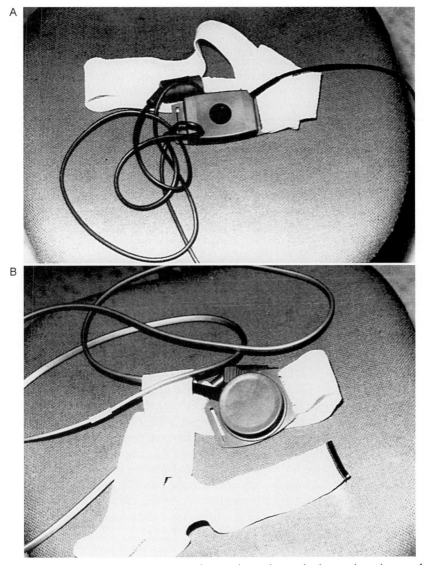

Figure 3-2 A, Corometrics tocotransducer is located over the best palpated area of the uterus, usually near the umbilicus near term. **B,** Corometrics ultrasound transducer is located over the fetal chest wall facing the fetal heart.

Box 3-1   Advantages and Limitations of External Contraction Monitoring

Advantages
- Noninvasive
- Convenient
- Provides continuous record of frequency and duration of contractions

Limitations
- Cannot accurately measure strength
- Loses some information at beginning and end of each contraction
- Restricts patient movement or must be adjusted frequently with position change

---

Modified from Tucker S: *Pocket guide to fetal monitoring and assessment*, ed 5, St Louis, 2004, Mosby.

Box 3-2   Advantages and Limitations of External Fetal Heart Rate Monitoring

Advantages
- Noninvasive
- Does not require dilation or membrane rupture
- Convenient
- Continuous recording of FHR
- Can assess presence of cyclic fluctuations (LTV) and absence of both LTV and STV

Limitations
- Tracing quality affected by maternal position, obesity, and fetal movement

---

Modified from Tucker S: *Pocket guide to fetal monitoring and assessment*, ed 5, St Louis, 2004, Mosby.
FHR, Fetal heart rate; *LTV,* long-term variability; *STV,* short-term variability.

rate per minute. Through a system of logic, it samples a set number of valve closures, compares the previous intervals, and decides which to count. The logic system tends to give the appearance of slightly greater rate differences than are truly present. This causes the appearance of "roughness" or a "jiggle" to the line (Freeman, Garite, and Nageotte, 2003). Because there are still different generations and models of equipment in use, it is important to recognize the parameters and to know from which era the monitor in use comes. If the rate differences are not logical compared with the previous calculated rates, blanks will appear in the tracing. Blanks also occur when the signal is lost from fetal movement or shift in maternal position. Box 3-2 presents the advantages and limitations of external FHR monitoring.

Internal (Direct) Monitoring

Internal monitoring uses different components: an intrauterine pressure catheter (IUPC) (Fig. 3-3, *A*) and a fetal spiral electrode (FSE) (Fig. 3-3, *B*).

Intrauterine pressure catheter. The IUPC may be inserted by qualified, registered nurses (RNs) (Tucker, 2004). It is inserted before the spiral electrode, in an aseptic manner, into the uterine cavity. According to licensing board regulations, a qualified RN has earned the credentials, has been approved by the institution, and is licensed in a state that allows insertion.

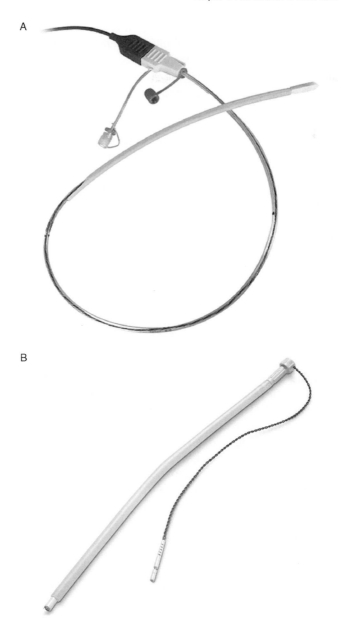

Figure 3-3 A, Intrauterine pressure catheter. **B,** Fetal spiral electrode for attachment to leg plate. (Courtesy Kendall-LTP, Chicopee, Mass.)

The two types of IUPCs are a fluid-filled system, which is not commonly used, and a solid catheter. The fluid-filled catheter must first be flushed with sterile water; a syringe is left attached to a three-way stopcock at the distal end. The catheter is a flexible, narrow-gauge tube with holes along a short distance and at the proximal end. It is partially enclosed in a firmer plastic catheter introducer.

The examiner's hand carefully lifts the presenting part and inserts the introducer with the catheter just through the dilated cervix. Then the fluid-filled catheter is carefully advanced to a specific marker visualized on the outside of the perineum. The introducer is drawn back toward the distal end, and the catheter remains behind. The catheter is then taped to the patient's abdomen or thigh.

As the uterus contracts and relaxes, the intercavitary pressure is reflected against the fluid-filled catheter. The distal end is connected to a strain gauge and to the monitor. The three-way stopcock and transducer with dome allow the catheter to be referenced to the atmosphere by zeroing, flushing with additional fluid as necessary, and directing the reflected pressure from contractions to the strain gauge. Pressure of contractions is measured in millimeters of mercury (mm Hg).

Another type of IUPC is the closed, or solid, catheter with the transducer at or near the tip. Some are single-lumen catheters, which measure pressure only, whereas others have a triple lumen, allowing pressure monitoring, amnioinfusion, and fluid sampling. The solid catheters must be connected to the monitor by a cable and zeroed before placement into the uterine cavity. The triple-lumen catheter allows the IUPC to be re-zeroed after being disconnected—without replacing it with a new catheter. The single-lumen catheter does not allow this option.

Fetal spiral electrode. The FSE may also be placed by qualified RNs. It is attached to the presenting part of the fetus, avoiding such potentially dangerous areas as the fontanels, facial features, or genitalia, if breech. The FSE has two color-coded wires attached to it. These are twisted together, and all are encased in an introducer. The examiner identifies the area of the presenting part and then inserts the introducer between the fingers and flush against the presenting part. The distal ends of the wires are rotated counterclockwise and attached to the presenting part. A leg plate is strapped to the patient's thigh, and the leg plate cord is plugged into the fetal ECG receiver on the monitor.

The monitor, in this way, directly counts from the fetal R wave (the highest amplitude electrical impulse from the fetal heart). It does not need to respond to or disregard other fetal impulses but may count maternal R-R intervals if the fetus is dead. What is plotted on the graph paper is each rate from every R-R interval calculated, as it is, for 1 minute. Thus the FSE can accurately assess the beat-to-beat rate differences known as STV. Box 3-3 presents advantages and limitations of internal monitoring.

Box 3-3 Advantages and Limitations of Internal Monitoring

Advantages
Contractions are measured accurately for
- Strength
- Duration
- Frequency
- Resting tone
- More comfortable than external monitoring

Limitations
- Requires ruptured membranes and dilation
- If prolonged, ruptured membranes may carry a small increase in infection
- Possible injury to uterine wall or fetus if forcefully introduced

Modified from Tucker S: *Pocket guide to fetal monitoring and assessment*, ed 5, St Louis, 2004, Mosby.

Other Features on Monitors

The newer models of electronic monitors sometimes have other features for monitoring the mother. It is possible to monitor the pulse oxygenation and maternal blood pressure and print these out on the monitor strips. Intrapartum monitors are equipped with these capabilities. In addition, there are remote devices for charting from a handheld keyboard to such things as physician visits, vaginal examinations, position changes, oxytocin (Pitocin) changes, and intravenous (IV) fluids given, and this information prints onto the monitor strip.

Baseline Fetal Heart Rate

The fetal CNS, specifically the ANS, controls the FHR. Because the autonomic nervous system (ANS) of the fetal brain is developed first, it is the most rudimentary. It requires a significant degree of hypoxia before FHR control shows the effects. Observation of entirely reassuring FHR and patterns predicts adequate CNS oxygenation. However, nonreassuring features are considerably more subjective and of less predictive value for fetal oxygenation. In other words, little is known about how long it takes for what degree of hypoxia (Freeman, Garite, and Nageotte, 2003).

Each examination of a fetal monitor strip should follow the same systematic steps:
- Evaluate patient history and status.
- Evaluate contraction frequency, duration, and if IUPC is used, intensity and resting tone.
- Determine the average baseline rate rounded to the nearest increment of 5.
- Describe baseline FHR and presence or absence of variability.
- Identify, if present, accelerations.
- Describe or, when possible, name patterns of periodic or episodic decelerations in the FHR.
- Describe changes in trends of the FHR pattern over 10 minutes or more.
- Diagnose fetal response to stimuli, initiate independent nursing interventions, and collaborate with the physician for medical management.

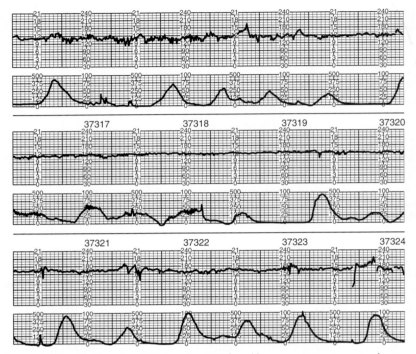

Figure 3-4 Normal baseline FHR. Baseline FHR found between contractions, in absence of periodic changes, and observed in 10-minute segments (*panels 37317 through 37319 in center*) is 150 to 155. This is normal range. *FHR,* Fetal heart rate.

Rate

Baseline FHR is the average rate lasting at least 10 consecutive minutes, observed as occurring between contractions and in the absence of other stimuli. If contractions are occurring quite close together, the usual place to observe is just before each contraction (Fig. 3-4). The baseline FHR is normally 110 to 160 bpm, although rates from 90 to 110 and 160 to 180 may also be normal if all other features are reassuring and if that rate is appropriate for gestation—that is, faster in early pregnancy and slower in later pregnancy. Rates above the 160s for more than 10 minutes are termed tachycardia, and those below 110 for more than 10 minutes are termed bradycardia. Table 3-1 summarizes baseline FHR abnormalities.

Variability

Variability is the most important FHR characteristic. It is the most important indicator of normal fetal pH or acidosis and reflects a healthy nervous system, chemoreceptors, baroreceptors, and cardiac responsiveness (Sweha, Hacker, and Nuovo, 1999). According to the National Institute of Child Health and Human Development (NICHD, 1997), variability is defined as fluctuations

Table 3-1   Summary of Baseline Fetal Heart Rate Abnormalities

Tachycardia (Fig. 3-5)

Description	Rate higher than 160 bpm for at least 10 consecutive minutes
Etiology	Acute, short-term hypoxia
	Drugs given to mother such as betasympathomimetics (terbutaline, ritodrine)
	Stress
	Arrhythmia
	Fetal infection
	Maternal fever (may be due to epidural analgesia)
	Maternal hyperthyroid disease
Mechanism	Sympathetic response
Significance	Serious when higher than 180 bpm
Nursing interventions	Look for cause
	Turn patient to left side
	Hydrate to improve circulating volume
	O_2 at 8–10 L/min by tight facemask
	Reduce stressors: turn off oxytocin (Pitocin); treat maternal fever

Bradycardia (Fig. 3-6)

Description	Rate lower than 100 bpm for at least 10 consecutive minutes
Etiology	Chronic long-term hypoxia
	Drugs such as beta-blockers (propranolol [Inderal])
	Arrhythmia
	Terminal event after severe stress
	Prolapsed cord
Mechanism	Parasympathetic response
Significance	Serious when lower than 80 bpm or lasting more than 10 minutes
Nursing interventions	Turn side to side or to knee-chest position
	O_2 at 8–10 L/min by tight face mask
	Correct maternal hypotension
	Look for cause such as prolapsed cord
	Prepare for delivery by most expeditious means

Modified from Freeman R, Garite R, and Nageotte M: *Fetal heart rate monitoring*, ed 3, Baltimore, 2003, Lippincott Williams & Wilkins.

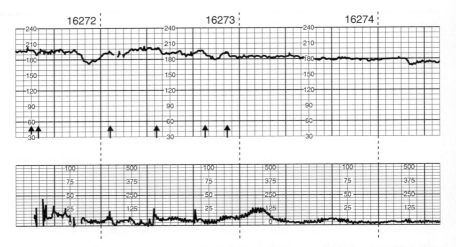

Figure 3-5 Tachycardia. Baseline fetal heart rate *between panels 16272 and 16274* is 180 to 200 bpm. Long-term variability is present. Arrows are result of maternal use of remote marker to indicate fetal movement.

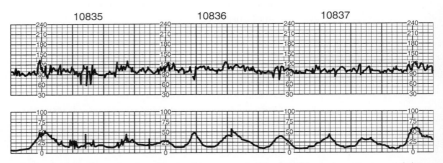

Figure 3-6 Bradycardia. Baseline fetal heart rate is 95 to 105 bpm. Long-term variability is present.

in the baseline FHR of greater than two cycles per minute. Grades of fluctuation are based on amplitude range (ACOG, 2005) as follows:

- Absence: amplitude range undetectable
- Minimal: fewer than 5 bpm amplitude range
- Moderate (average): 6 to 25 bpm amplitude range
- Marked: more than 25 bpm amplitude

There are two characteristics of FHR variability: short-term and long-term. Short-term variability (STV) is considered to be the beat-to-beat changes in the baseline FHR from one heart beat to the next. Long-term variability (LTV) is considered the rhythmic rise and fall that occupies a 1-minute cycle of the baseline FHR. With latest technology, the only benefit of recognizing these as separate from each other is to understand the preterminal patterns: a sinusoidal pattern, a saltatory pattern, and a wandering baseline. With these patterns, STV is absent and LTV is aberrant (Table 3-2). According to the

Table 3-2 Abnormalities of Baseline Variability*

Marked Variability (see Fig. 3-7, *panel 4*)

Description	Persistent cyclic fluctuations, of amplitude higher than 25 bpm
Etiology	Recovery from previous insult
	Response to sudden stimuli
	Stimulant drugs such as cocaine or methamphetamines
	Sympathomimetic drugs such as terbutaline
	Sudden hypoxia often following nonreassuring variable decelerations (Tables 3-5 and 3-7 and Fig. 3-11, *B*)
Mechanism	Increased interplay between sympathetic and parasympathetic branches of ANS or loss of ANS control
Significance	If episodic and less than 2–3 min in duration: benign
	If persistent: nonreassuring and should be treated
Nursing interventions	Look for cause and treat by repositioning laterally
	Start and/or increase IV
	Give O$_2$ at 8–10 L/min by face mask

Minimal Variability (see Fig. 3-7, *panel 2*)

Description	Baseline FHR fluctuations less than 5-beat amplitude
Uncomplicated causes	Sleep, narcotic, barbiturate, or other CNS depressant; usually does not persist after 20–40 min or length of initial medication effect
Nonreassuring causes	Early hypoxia, congenital anomalies, fetal cardiac arrhythmias, extreme prematurity
Mechanism	CNS depression during sleep or after medication
Significance	Usually benign
Nursing interventions	Continued observation
	Acoustic stimulations

Absent Variability (see Fig. 3-7, *panel 1*)

Description	Undetectable fluctuations in FHR
Etiology	Severe degree of hypoxia
Mechanism	Loss of interplay between branches of ANS
Significance	Nonreassuring and indicative of fetal acidemia (pH less than 7.1)
Nursing interventions	Same as for marked variability

*See Figure 3-7.
ANS, Autonomic nervous system; *CNS,* central nervous system; *FHR,* fetal heart rate; *IV,* intravenous; *LTV,* long-term variability.

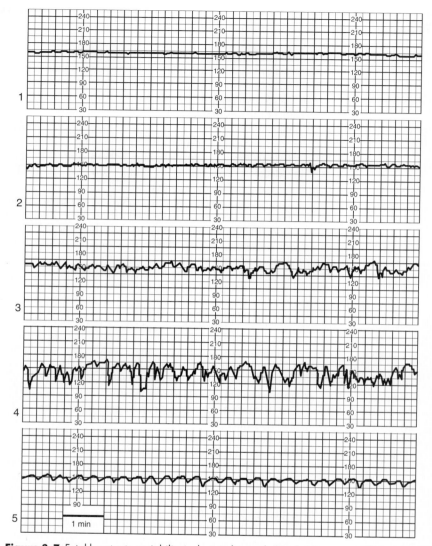

Figure 3-7 Fetal heart rate variability is depicted in each panel. All are traced from a spiral electrode. *1,* Undetectable. *2,* Minimal. *3,* Moderate. *4,* Marked. *5,* Sinusoidal pattern. Original scaling, 30 bpm per cm vertical axis, and paper speed 3 cm/min⁻1 horizontal axis.

National Institute of Child Health and Human Development, no distinction is made between short-term and long-term variability for other purposes. The two are now assessed as a single unit of the FHR baseline (NICHD, 1997).

Fetal Arrhythmia and Artifact

Fetal arrhythmias occur as a result of abnormalities in the automatic origination of impulses throughout the myocardium, a disruption of the normal impulse conduction pathway, or both. Some are benign, whereas others are pathologic.

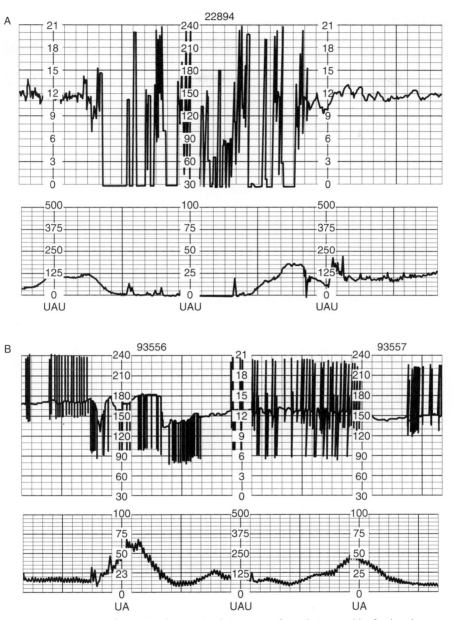

Figure 3-8 A, Artifact. Note disorganized scattering of impulses traced by fetal scalp electrode. **B,** Arrhythmia. Note organized distribution of impulses traced by fetal spiral electrode.

To determine benign from pathologic fetal arrhythmias, features of both must be kept in mind. Those that are benign tend to appear in labor and disappear shortly after delivery. These neonates tend to have no heart abnormalities—neither anatomic nor functional. Pathologic fetal arrhythmias tend to

Table 3-3   Artifact versus Arrhythmia

Instrument	Artifact	Arrhythmia
Auscultation device	Regular rate and rhythm	Abnormal rate or rhythm
Fetal spiral electrode	Perpendicular excursions irregular and baseline completely obscured	Baseline can be read despite perpendicular excursions

be associated with certain maternal conditions such as lupus, illicit drug use, infection, and hyperthyroidism or fetal cardiac abnormalities; they also tend to be present and detected prenatally and to be present during labor and persist into the neonatal period (Kleinman, Nehgme, and Copel, 2004; Snyder and Copel, 2005).

Fetal arrhythmias usually can be detected as vertical lines through the baseline. Although these lines are sometimes so close together that they almost appear as solid blocks, the baseline can be found through them. There are rarely other nonreassuring features about the baseline (Fig. 3-8). They are also generally audible (Tucker, 2004).

Artifact is a disruption of the normal logic system in the machine, which typically calculates the FHR by counting intervals of R wave to R wave. When it is unable to function in this way, the tracing appears as a garbled mess of vertical lines, through which one cannot identify a baseline rate or patterns. Table 3-3 describes and summarizes artifact versus dysrhythmia, and Table 3-4 describes and summarizes dysrhythmias and their significance.

If a fetal arrhythmia is suspected, M-mode or spectral Doppler fetal echocardiography is most commonly used to diagnosis and monitor the arrhythmia (Snyder and Copel, 2005). Of all possible fetal arrhythmias, supraventricular tachycardia (SVT) and congenital heart block are serious. SVT may be treated in utero, whereas heart block is not treatable. Medical management of SVT consists of pharmacologic fetal cardioversion. The pharmacologic agents used are such drugs as digoxin, beta-blockers, procainamide, and quinidine.

Fetal Heart Rate Patterns and Periodic Rate Changes

FHR patterns or periodic rate changes express the mechanism of insult to the fetus. Knowing the mechanism facilitates appropriate nursing response and intervention. It also helps predict whether a change can be made and how long it might take. Periodic changes are also in response to certain stimuli. When reassuring changes are observed, they are usually explained by fetal movement or healthy response to contractions. The FHR can demonstrate patterns of acceleration or deceleration in response to most stimuli (Tables 3-5 to 3-7). (Progressive FHR changes in response to gestation, oxygenation, and certain stimuli are shown in Fig. 3-9.)   *Text continued on p. 70*

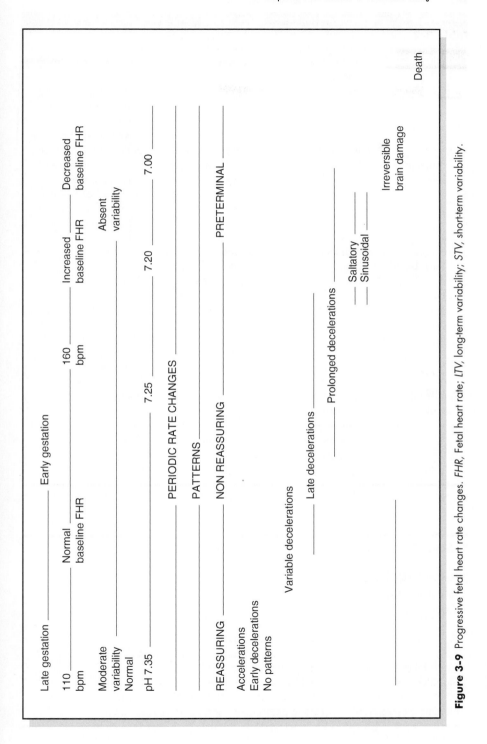

Figure 3-9 Progressive fetal heart rate changes. *FHR*, Fetal heart rate; *LTV*, long-term variability; *STV*, short-term variability.

Table 3-4   Dysrhythmias: Appearances, Audible Features, and Significance

Dysrhythmia	Appearance	Audible Features	Significance
PACs	Excursions above and below baseline	Compensatory pauses	Benign
PVCs	Same	Same	Usually benign unless superimposed on preterminal rate or wandering baseline
PAT or continuous SVT	Rate too fast to trace	Rate higher than 240 bpm; irregular	Serious and treatable; can be converted while in utero Fetal hydrops (similar to adult congestive heart failure) may be fatal
Congenital heart block	Suddenly drops by half	Fetoscope rate same as slowed rate Doppler rates 2 × fetoscope rate = 2:1 block	May result in fetal death Associated with maternal connective tissue disease Newborn will need immediate placement of pacemaker
Sinoatrial arrest	In lowest point of variable deceleration, rectangular deflection appears	Absent audible impulse	Benign

PAC, Premature atrial contraction; *PAT*, paroxysmal atrial tachycardia; *PVC*, premature ventricular contraction; *SVT*, supraventricular tachycardia.

Table 3-5   Summary of Accelerations and Decelerations

Reassuring Rate Changes
Uniform Accelerations (Fig. 3-10, *A*)

Description	Uniform shape Begin when contraction begins and ends when contraction ends Often mirror intensity of contractions
Mechanism of insult	Sympathetic response to stimuli
Significance	Healthy CNS response Often associated with breech presentations
Nursing intervention	Totally benign, so none needed; document

Modified from Freeman R, Garite R, and Nageotte M: *Fetal heart rate monitoring*, ed 3, Baltimore, 2003, Lippincott Williams & Wilkins; American College of Obstetricians and Gynecologists, *ACOG Technical Bulletin*, No. 9, 1999.
CNS, Central nervous system; *IV*, intravenous; O_2, oxygen.

Table 3-5   Summary of Accelerations and Decelerations—cont'd

Nonuniform Accelerations (Fig. 3-10, *B*)

Description	Nonuniform in shape
	Usually occur in response to fetal movement so they vary in contraction cycle
Mechanism of insult	Sympathetic response to stimuli
Significance	Healthy CNS response; reassuring
Nursing intervention	None

Early Decelerations (Fig. 3-11, *A*)

Description	Uniform in shape
	Frequently mirror contraction intensity
	Begin when contraction begins and end when contraction ends
	When noted, usually occur between 4- and 7-cm dilation of cervix, but can occur at any time
Mechanism of insult	Head compression
	Parasympathetic (vagal) reflex caused by pressure on fontanels against resisting cervix
Significance	Reassuring, although not normal because they do not occur in all fetuses
Nursing interventions	Differentiate these from late decelerations
	No action necessary or helpful; document

Variable Decelerations

Description	Variable in shape, often V- or W-shaped
	Variable placement in relationship to contractions; may occur between or with contractions
	Heart rate falls abruptly and rises abruptly
Mechanism of insult	Cord compression
Significance	Reassuring if:
	Infrequent
	Low point is within normal heart rate range
	Last less than 45 sec
Nursing intervention	Change maternal position

Nonreassuring Rate Changes
Variable Decelerations (Fig. 3-11, *B*)

Significance	Nonreassuring if:
	Repetitive
	Fall to lower than 90 bpm
	Last more than 50 sec
	Followed by tachycardia
	Slow return to baseline
	Loss of variability between decelerations
Nursing interventions	Turn side to side or to knee-chest position
	Give O_2 at 8–10 L/min by tight face mask
	Improve circulating volume
	Expect expeditious delivery if ominous; document

Continued

Table 3-5   Summary of Accelerations and Decelerations—cont'd

Late Decelerations (Fig. 3-11, *C*)

Description	Uniform in shape
	Sometimes reflect intensity of contractions
	Begin anywhere in contraction cycle, although common near peak
	End after contraction has ended with slow, sloping return to baseline
Mechanism of insult	Uteroplacental insufficiency, leading to CNS hypoxia or myocardial depression
Significance	Always nonreassuring, regardless of depth of deceleration or degree of variability
	Acute episodes usually demonstrate good variability and are more likely to be correctable
	Chronic episodes usually are accompanied by decreased or absent variability and are less likely to be correctable; usually associated with fetal acidosis
Nursing interventions	Turn patient to left side
	Administer O_2 at 8–10 L/min by tight face mask
	Rapidly infuse IV fluid
	Correct hypotension
	If oxytocin (Pitocin) used, turn it off
	Expect expeditious delivery if not corrected in 30 min; document

Table 3-6   Summary of Nonreassuring or Preterminal Rate Changes

Prolonged Deceleration (Fig. 3-11, *D*)

Description	Abrupt deceleration of at least 15 bpm, lasting 2–10 minutes
	Usually falls to less than 90 bpm
Mechanism of insult	Prolonged cord compression
Significance	If lasts longer than 10 minutes, fetus may become acidemic, followed by myocardial depression, which is a preterminal event
Nursing interventions	Notify physician or midwife of first occurrence
	Check for cord prolapse
	Turn patient side to side or to knee-chest position until change is affected
	Give O_2 at 8–10 L/min by tight face mask
	Correct maternal hypotension; increase IV fluids
	Continually observe until delivery; document
	Be prepared for emergency delivery
Significance	If lasts more than 10 minutes, fetus may become acidemic, myocardial depression occurs, and is then a preterminal event.

Modified from Freeman R, Garite R, and Nageotte M: *Fetal heart rate monitoring*, ed 3, Baltimore, 2003, Williams & Wilkins.
IV, Intravenous, *O_2,* oxygen.

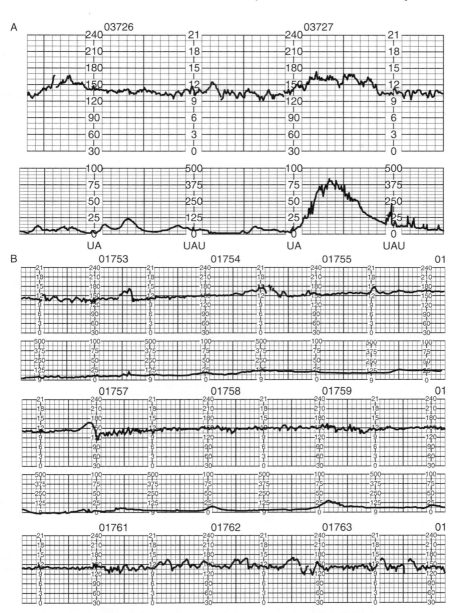

Figure 3-10 A, Uniform acceleration is noted beginning in *panel 03727* in response to contraction beneath. **B,** Nonuniform accelerations can be seen between contractions. Baseline fetal heart rate of 150 to 155 bpm with accelerations to 170 bpm.

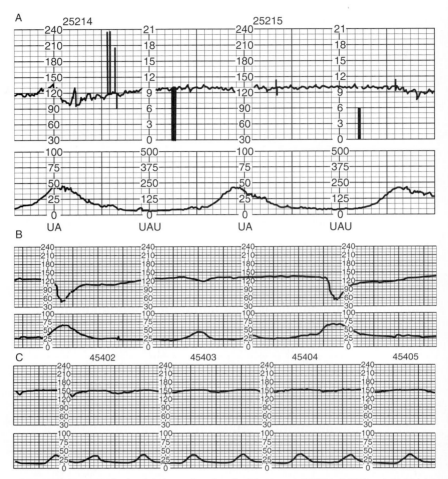

Figure 3-11 A, Early decelerations. Baseline fetal heart rate (FHR) is 130 bpm. Gradual decelerations to 120 bpm are seen in *panel 25215*. The rate has returned to baseline FHR of 130 bpm by end of contraction. **B,** Severe nonreassuring variable decelerations. Note abrupt fall in heart rate from baseline of 130 bpm. Also note depth of deceleration to 55 to 60 bpm, sloping return to baseline and absent variability. Those features make these severe decelerations, and prognosis for the fetal outcome is poor. **C,** Late decelerations. Baseline FHR is 150 bpm. Subtle decelerations are seen with each contraction beginning near or just after peak and not returning to baseline until 30 to 40 seconds after contraction has ended. Note poor to absent variability that accompanies baseline and is transmitted by external ultrasound. **D,** Prolonged deceleration in *panels 43786 and 43787*. This deceleration follows initiation of epidural anesthesia and frequently can be avoided with intravenous fluid preload. Note occurrence of late decelerations with good baseline variability following recovery period.

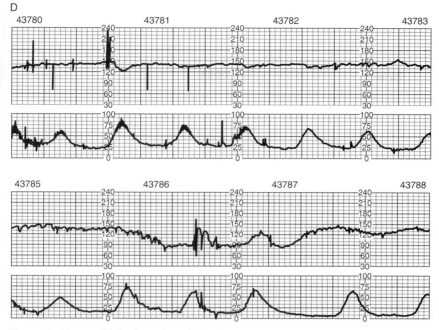

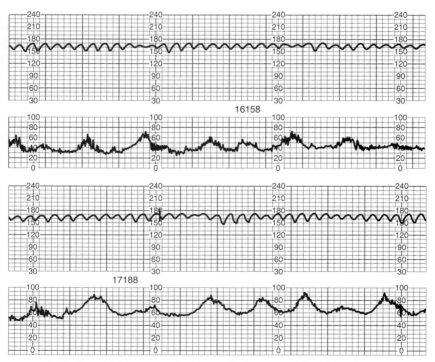

Figure 3-11, cont'd For legend see facing page.

Figure 3-12 Sinusoidal heart rate. Regular oscillations around baseline reflect present long-term variability and absent short-term variability. This unusual rate disturbance is a preterminal occurrence.

Table 3-7   Usual Rate Changes

Sinusoidal (Fig. 3-12)	
Description	Smooth, undulating baseline with regular (2–5) oscillations per minute without long- or short- term variability
Mechanism of insult	Derangement of CNS control of FHR secondary to increased arginine vasopressin
	When severe degree of hypoxia from fetal anemia is coupled with fetal hypovolemia, this unusual rate change occurs
Significance	Categorized as a preterminal event that precedes fetal death if not immediately treated
	Only way to treat successfully in utero is by fetal intrauterine transfusion
Nursing interventions	Prepare for emergent delivery
	Prepare for intrauterine transfusion
	Position patient laterally
	Infuse IV fluids rapidly
	Administer O_2 at 6–10 L/min by face mask; document

Modified from Freeman R, Garite R, and Nageotte M: *Fetal heart rate monitoring*, ed 3, Baltimore, 2003, Lippincott Williams & Wilkins.
ANS, Autonomic nervous system; *CNS,* central nervous system; *FHR,* fetal heart rate; *IV,* intravenous; O_2, oxygen.

ANTEPARTUM AND INTRAPARTUM FETAL SURVEILLANCE

The latest census statistics estimate that more than two thirds of fetal deaths occur in the antepartum period (ACOG, 1999). Certainly, a means of surveillance that allows detection of that risk before damage occurs could greatly benefit those pregnancies. Antepartum monitoring provides a means of doing just that. When fetal compromise takes place, fetal activities are lost in reverse order of their development. FHR decelerations occur first, followed by loss of, in order, accelerations, breathing movements, body movements, and muscle tone and then death (Harman, 2004; Tucker, 2004). Decreased amniotic fluid can also indicate fetal compromise because decreased renal blood flow lowers fetal urinary output, resulting in decreased amniotic fluid volume. Decreased amniotic fluid, on the other hand, can cause fetal compromise because of the increased risk for cord compression (ACOG, 1999).

The most common maternal conditions associated with fetal compromise follow:
- Intrauterine growth restriction
- Hypertensive disorders of pregnancy
- Chronic hypertension
- Diabetes
- Postterm pregnancy
- Connective tissue disease
- Renal disease
- Hemolytic incompatibility
- Multiple gestation
- Placental abnormalities

The decision as to when to test is usually made based on viability (not before 26–28 weeks of gestation), severity of the condition, and when the condition is recognized. With the availability of regionalized centers, transportation capabilities, and long-distance telemetry, early detection of fetal compromise is possible and desirable for optimal treatment and outcome. The most frequently used tests to detect early fetal compromise are presented in Boxes 3-4 through 3-10, which may serve as useful guides for nursing policies and procedures (ACOG, 1999). *Text continued on p. 80*

Box 3-4   Nonstress Test

Definition
An NST is a widely accepted method of evaluating fetal status by observing accelerations of the FHR following a stimulus such as fetal activity, indicating normal fetal pH and neurologic status.

Procedure
- Explain the testing procedure to the patient.
- Have the patient empty her bladder and then position herself in a semi-Fowler's, lateral tilt position. Sitting or walking may stimulate fetal reactivity (Cito and others, 2005).
- Place the ultrasound transducer and tocotransducer.
- Document the date and time the test is started, the make and model of the monitor, the external modes used, the patient's name, the reason for the test, and the maternal vital signs.
- Record maternal blood pressure at least once in 20 minutes.
- Run a 10- to 20-minute FHR contraction strip.
- If, at the end of the first 20 minutes, reactive criteria have not been met, stimulate the fetus acoustically and then wait an additional 20 minutes for reaction that meets the criteria.
- At the end of the test, interpret the results and report them to the physician, midwife, or provider.

Interpretation
Reactive
- There are at least two accelerations of peak amplitude of at least 15 bpm above the baseline lasting 15 or more seconds within a 20-minute period. Other reassuring features such as presence of variability and absence of nonreassuring periodic changes with any spontaneous contractions or fetal movement are described and expected for a test to read as reactive (Fig. 3-13).

Nonreactive
- There are no accelerations over a 40-minute period or they fail to meet reactive criteria (Fig. 3-14).

Management
- A reactive NST should be repeated every 3 or 4 days for continued prediction of fetal well-being.
- If the NST remains nonreactive after the second 20 minutes or if any nonreassuring periodic change is present, another more definitive evaluation of the fetus, such as ultrasound for a biophysical profile, is indicated (Harman, 2004).

CST, Contraction stress test; *FHR,* fetal heart rate; *NST,* nonstress test.   *Continued*

Box 3-4   Nonstress Test—cont'd

Advantages
- It is a noninvasive test requiring no initiation of contractions.
- It is quick to perform.
- There are no known side effects.
- It has a low false-negative rate (less than 1%) (ACOG, 1999).

Disadvantages
- It is not as sensitive to fetal oxygen reserves as CST.
- It has a high false-positive rate, 80% to 90% (ACOG, 1999).

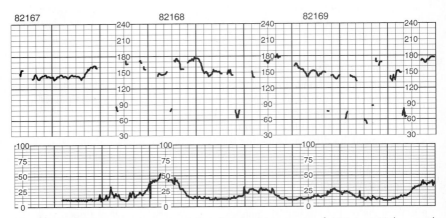

Figure 3-13 Reactive nonstress test. Baseline fetal heart rate of 130 to 140 bpm with numerous accelerations of greater than 15 beats lasting for more than 15 seconds. Small spikes in tocotransducer tracing represent fetal activity.

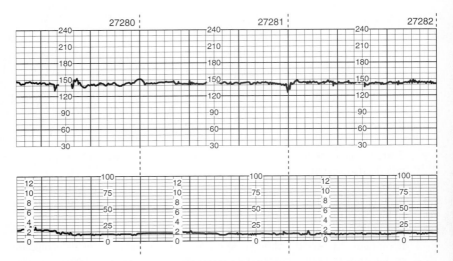

Figure 3-14 Nonreactive nonstress test. Although there is apparent adequate beat-to-beat variability, no accelerations are seen that can be described as meeting criterion of 15 beats more than baseline for 15 seconds.

Box 3-5   Vibroacoustic Stimulation Test

Definition

This test is a method of evaluating fetal status by observing accelerations of the FHR following vibroacoustic stimulation.

Procedure

- Explain the testing procedure to the patient and the reasons for its use; assure her it is not harmful to the fetus.
- Have the patient empty her bladder and then position herself in a semi-Fowler's position. A wedge may be placed under her right hip to prevent supine hypotension, if needed.
- Place the ultrasound transducer and tocotransducer.
- Document the date and time the test is started, the make and model of the monitor, the external modes used, the patient's name, the reason for the test, and the maternal vital signs.
- Obtain a 20-minute FHR tracing to establish a baseline.
- Record maternal blood pressure once during the first 20 minutes of the test.
- If no fetal movements are observed, use an acoustic stimulation device or an electrolarynx to produce a vibratory sound stimulus.
- Apply stimulus to the maternal abdomen over the fetus' head for 1 second; wait 1 minute.
- If no acceleration occurs after the first stimulus, apply a second stimulus for 1 second; wait 1 minute.
- If no acceleration occurs after the second stimulus, apply for 2 seconds; wait 1 minute.

Interpretation

Reactive

- Two FHR accelerations in 10 minutes: A duration of a minimum of 15 seconds and a peak of at least 15 bpm above the baseline should characterize acceleration.

Advantages

- It decreases NST length (Tan and Smyth, 2001).
- It decreases the incidence of nonreactive NST (Tan and Smyth, 2001).
- It reduces the need for fetal scalp pH during labor by as much as 50%.
- In labor, there is a false-negative rate of approximately 2.5% and a false-positive rate of approximately 60% (Richardson and Gagnon, 2004).
- There are no known risks if the protocol outlined is followed.

Limitations

- Influence of gestational age: For example, before 30 weeks of gestation, FHR response to vibroacoustic stimulation may be absent or fewer than 10 bpm over baseline FHR.
- Influence of prestimulation basal FHR: In the presence of fetal tachycardia, the FHR response can be absent in 50% of healthy fetuses after 30 weeks of gestation; therefore FHR may be of limited value in predicting fetal outcome if absent.
- There is insufficient evidence at present regarding the effect, if any, on fetal hearing or on neurologic development (Tan and Smyth, 2001).

FHR, Fetal heart rate; *NST*, nonstress test.

Box 3-6 Fetal Movement Monitoring

Definition
The fetus reduces movement or stops moving in response to chronic hypoxia in an attempt to reduce oxygen consumption and conserve energy.

Procedure
- Teach patient the significance of fetal movements.
- Teach patient a fetal assessment method.
- *Count fetal movements* for a fixed period of time. Instruct the patient to lie down on her side and count all the fetal movements felt in 1 hour.
- *Record time* taken to count a fixed number of fetal movements. Instruct the patient to start counting at 9 a.m. and stop counting for the day and record the time when 10 fetal movements have been noted.
- Demonstrate how to record movements on a daily fetal movement record.

Interpretation
- Report decreased fetal movement compared with the previous day's counts or fewer than 10 fetal movements in any 2 hours (ACOG, 1999).

Management
- If decreased fetal movement is reported, evaluate fetal status with an NST or a biophysical profile immediately and manage according to the results.

Gestational Influences
- Gestational age: Fetal movements show a maturational decrease in number but increase in duration.
- Diurnal rhythm: Normally fetal movement is increased in the late evening.

Fetal Behavior
- State: There is usually no fetal movement during quiet sleep—20-min sleep cycle at 28 weeks of gestation to approximately 60-minute sleep cycles at term (Harman, 2004).
- Drugs: Depressant drugs such as barbiturates, narcotics, and alcohol can reduce fetal movement. In therapeutic doses, most drugs do not reduce fetal movement.
- Fetal malformation: A fetus with a malformation is more likely to have reduced activity.

NST, Nonstress test.

Box 3-7 Contraction Stress Test

Definition
A CST is a fetal well-being test that is infrequently used to determine how the fetus responds to relative hypoxia during a contraction. A compromised fetus, with a limited ability to compensate for mild hypoxia because of limited oxygen reserves, demonstrates a consistent pattern of late decelerations during the test.

Procedure
- Explain the testing procedure to the patient.
- Have the patient empty her bladder and then position herself in a semi-Fowler's position. A wedge may be placed under her left hip to prevent supine hypotension if needed.

Box 3-7   Contraction Stress Test—cont'd

- Place the ultrasound transducer and tocotransducer.
- Document the date and time the test is started, make and model of monitor, the external modes used, the patient's name, the reason for the test, and the maternal vital signs.
- Run a 20-minute NST for baseline information regarding FHR and uterine contractions.
- Stimulate contractions either by nipple stimulation of endogenous oxytocin or with intravenous oxytocin.
- Observe for uterine hyperstimulation.
- Assess maternal blood pressure every 10 to 15 minutes during the test and when the test is completed.
- Discontinue contraction stimulation when three or more contractions of more than 40 seconds' duration within a 10-minute period occur.
- Interpret the test results and report findings to the physician or midwife.
- Continue monitoring until uterine and FHR activity have returned to prestimulation state.

Initiation of Contractions with Nipple Stimulation
- Have the patient begin, on one side, nipple brushing through clothing. Have her continue until a contraction begins or for 10 minutes.
- If no contraction occurs in 10 minutes of brushing, have her change sides and continue for 10 minutes. If still not effective, have her brush both nipples simultaneously.
- Have the patient continue nipple brushing on effective side or sides until a contraction occurs. Stop until the contraction is over, and then begin again until three contractions occur in 10 minutes.

Stimulation of Contractions with Oxytocin
- Start mainline intravenous normal saline or Ringer's lactate.
- Piggyback oxytocin diluted so that increments of 0.5 mU/min can be delivered.
- Start at 0.5 mU/min; double amount every 15 to 20 minutes until 4 mU and then increase by 2 mU until three contractions occur in 10 minutes or maximum dose of 16 mU is reached.

Interpretation
Negative (Fig. 3-15)
- No decelerations are noted on the entire strip. LTV is present, and there is an absence of any nonreassuring changes.

Equivocal
- A test may be equivocal for one of three reasons:
  1 Suspicious. Less than 50% of the contractions on the entire strip have late decelerations. Variability is usually good (Fig. 3-16, A).
  2 Hyperstimulation. A contraction frequency of more than four in 10 minutes, fewer than 60 seconds between contractions, or a contraction lasting longer than 90 seconds with a late deceleration occurring (Fig. 3-16, B).
  3 Unsatisfactory. The quality of the tracing is too poor to accurately interpret FHR with contractions; or the frequency of three contractions in 10 minutes cannot be obtained for an endpoint of the test (Fig. 3-16, C).

Continued

Box 3-7 Contraction Stress Test—cont'd

Positive (Fig. 3-17)
- Fifty percent or more of the contractions on the strip have late decelerations associated with them even if the endpoint of three contractions in 10 minutes is not obtained. If associated with decreased variability, the prognosis is poor.

Management
- A negative CST predicts continued fetal well-being for 7 days and needs only to be repeated weekly provided maternal well-being is the same (Freedman, Garite, and Nageotte, 2003).
- An equivocal CST should be repeated in 24 hours. If a test remains equivocal for 3 consecutive days, another form of fetal assessment is usually used from then on instead of CSTs (Freeman, Garite, and Nageotte, 2003).
- A positive CST necessitates more vigorous management. If the variability is good and the fetus is mature by the proper dates and in a vertex position, a very carefully monitored induction can be attempted. If the fetus is immature, treating the maternal condition that might have precipitated the problem may be the best treatment to give the baby a chance.
- With a positive CST when variability is poor, delivery by an emergency cesarean is the only chance for optimal outcome for the baby regardless of maturity.
- Regardless of test results, if variable decelerations are noted, an amniotic fluid index is recommended.

Advantages
- It is more sensitive to fetal oxygen reserves than NST.
- It has a low false-negative rate (less than 1%) (ACOG, 1999).

Disadvantages
- CST is contraindicated in such high risk conditions as preterm labor and placenta previa.
- It must be administered in a birthing setting.
- It has a false-positive rate greater than 50% (ACOG, 1999).

CST, Contraction stress test; *FHR,* fetal heart rate; *LTV,* long-term variability; *NST,* nonstress test.

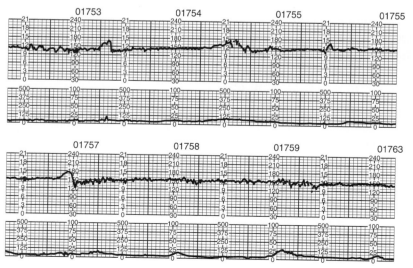

Figure 3-15 For legend see facing page.

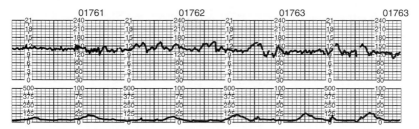

Figure 3-15 cont'd. Negative and reactive contraction stress test obtained with breast stimulation. No late decelerations are noted in any panel. Good apparent beat-to-beat variability is present, and fetal heart rate accelerates periodically. Three contractions are present in 10 minutes (*panels 01761 through 01763*).

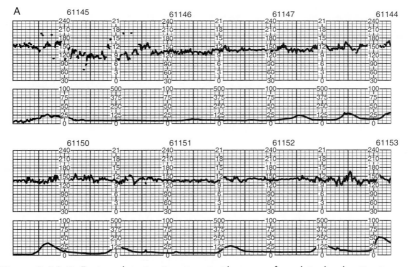

Figure 3-16 A, Equivocal contraction stress test because of one late deceleration in *panel 61145*. Breast stimulation was started to further challenge placental function and determine whether late deceleration would persist. Because remainder of test was negative for late decelerations and reactive, test was repeated the following day.

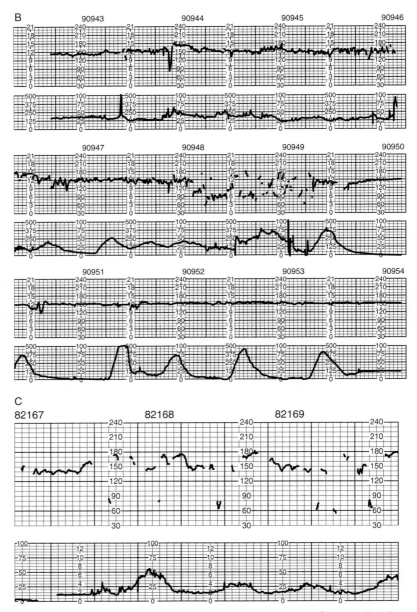

Figure 3-16 Cont'd. **B,** Equivocal contraction stress test because of later and prolonged deceleration with excessive and hyperstimulated uterine activity in *panels 90948 and 90949.* Previous portion of strip had good apparent variability and reactivity, although remaining portion, during recovery, demonstrates poor variability. Tracing was continued until adequate recovery was evidenced. Then test was repeated the following day. **C,** Equivocal contraction stress test, because tracing immediately following each contraction is unsatisfactory for accurate interpretation of fetal heart rate response.

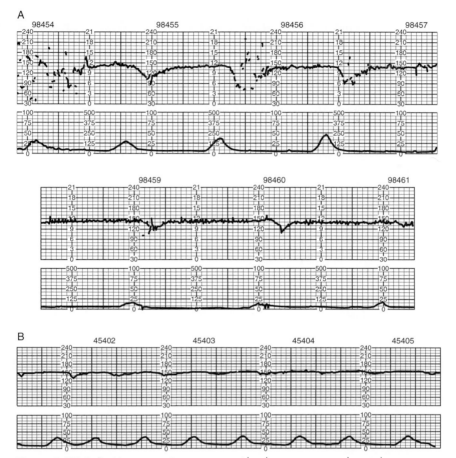

Figure 3-17 A, Positive contraction stress test with adequate apparent beat-to-beat variability. Baseline fetal heart rate is 140 to 150 bpm. Tracing was continued, and reactivity was also noted while decisions were made for delivery in postterm pregnancy. **B,** Positive nonreactive contraction stress test with poor to absent variability. Baby was delivered by emergent cesarean birth with Apgar scores below 6. Mother was stable with preeclampsia.

Box 3-8   Biophysical Profile

Definition

A biophysical profile is an evaluation of fetal well-being through the use of various reflex activities that are CNS-controlled and sensitive to hypoxia, as well as the fetal environment that can affect fetal well-being.

Procedure

Scan the abdomen and assess fetal tone, movement, breathing, fetal reactivity, and amniotic fluid.

AFV, Amniotic fluid volume; *BPP,* biophysical profile; *CNS,* central nervous system; *CST,* contraction stress test; *FHR,* fetal heart rate; *NST,* nonstress test.   *Continued*

Box 3-8   Biophysical Profile—cont'd

Interpretation (Harman, 2004)

The biophysical activities that are the first to develop are the last to disappear when asphyxia occurs.

- *Fetal tone:* One or more episodes of extension of a fetal extremity with return to flexion
  - Starts to function at 7.5 to 8.5 weeks of gestation
  - Is abolished at a pH less than 7.0
- *Fetal movement:* Three or more body or limb movements within 30 minutes
  - Starts to function at 9 weeks of gestation
  - Is abolished when the pH is between 7.1 and 7.2
- *Fetal breathing:* One or more episodes of rhythmic fetal breathing movements of at least 30 seconds duration
  - Starts to function at approximately 20 to 21 weeks of gestation
  - Is abolished at a pH of 7.2
- *Fetal reactivity:* Two or more FHR accelerations of a least 15 bpm for at least 15 seconds within 20 minutes
  - Starts to function at 26 to 28 weeks of gestation
  - Is abolished at a pH of less than 7.19
- *Amniotic fluid:* Decreased amniotic fluid can be the result of chronic hypoxia or can cause hypoxia. Normal amniotic fluid is recognized as largest pocket of amniotic fluid exceeding 2 cm (Manning, 2004).

Scoring

- Assign 0 or 2 points each for fetal tone, movement, breathing, reactivity, and amniotic fluid volume.
- A BPP of 8 to 10 is reassuring if AF is normal. The test needs be repeated in 3 to 4 days.
- A BPP of 6 is considered equivocal. The test should be repeated. A persistent score of 6 indicates delivery of a mature fetus; if fetus is immature repeat the test in 24 hours.
- A BPP score of 4 is nonreassuring. If fetal pulmonary maturity is assured and the cervix is favorable, deliver; otherwise, repeat in 24 hours. If score persists, deliver if fetal pulmonary maturity is certain. Otherwise, treat with steroids and deliver in 48 hours.
- A BPP score of 0 to 2 means immediate delivery.
- Oligohydramnios constitutes an abnormal biophysical assessment regardless of the overall score (ACOG, 1999).

Advantages

- It permits conservative therapy and prevents premature intervention.
- BPP evaluates multiple fetal variables.

Fetal Oxygen Saturation Monitoring with Fetal Pulse Oximetry Assessment During Labor

Simpson and Porter (2001) and Garite and colleagues (2000) described the benefits of taking fetal O_2 saturation measurements during labor and compared them with the benefits of EFM. In a few studies, assessing fetal status with fetal O_2 saturation measurements was found to be as accurate as with EFM. Fetal O_2 saturation measurements can also be used as an adjunctive method to prevent unnecessary procedures such as fetal blood sampling, operative vaginal birth,

Box 3-9   Amniotic Fluid Volume Index (Manning, 2004; Tucker, 2004)

Definition

AFI is the evaluation of the quantity of amniotic fluid. Amniotic fluid is the result of fetal urine production. Adequate placental blood flow usually promotes adequate fetal renal blood flow and therefore adequate urine output. Thus amniotic fluid volume reflects long-term uteroplacental function.

Procedure

Scan each of the four quadrants of the abdomen. Measure one pocket of fluid in each quadrant. The pockets that are selected are free of fetal small parts. The centimeters of each measurement are added together.

Interpretation

- From 0 to 5 cm of amniotic fluid or no vertical pocket of AF is abnormally low and indicates need for delivery or close maternal and fetal surveillance.
- 5.1 to 9.9 cm: low normal
- 10 to 24 cm: normal
- More than 24 cm: increased

AF, Amniotic fluid; *AFI*, amniotic fluid volume index.

Box 3-10   Doppler Flow Studies

Definition

Doppler flow studies are noninvasive methods for studying intrauterine environment, specifically the uteroplacental blood flow in the umbilical arteries. Doppler flow studies can facilitate the decision-making process regarding delivery time in pregnancies complicated by intrauterine growth restriction.

Procedure

- The nurse should help the patient position herself in a supine position and place a wedge under her right side to facilitate adequate blood flow and to reduce maternal positional side effects.
- A pulsed Doppler device is positioned over the fetus. The umbilical artery blood flow is distinguished from other blood flow by its characteristic waveform.
- The directed blood flow within the umbilical arteries is calculated using the difference between the systolic and the diastolic flow. Measurements are averaged from at least five waveforms.

Interpretation

- Elevations of the systolic/diastolic (S/D) ratio above 3.0 are considered abnormal.
- Elevations of the S/D ratio are seen in hypertensive disorders of pregnancy, fetal growth retardation, or other causes of uteroplacental insufficiency.

and even cesarean birth. Fetal pulse oximetry added to cardiotocography showed reduced caesarean section rates for nonreassuring fetal status in a single trial, although no difference was found in the overall caesarean section rate or the mother's or newborn's health (East, 2004). The Food and Drug Administration approved fetal O_2 saturation in May 2000 after careful consideration of the results of a multicenter randomized clinical study (Garite and others, 2000).

However the American College of Obstetricians and Gynecologists did not endorse this device because of the cost without improving clinical outcomes (ACOG, 2001).

This represents the first major technological breakthrough in fetal intrapartum assessment since EFM was introduced in the 1960s. Therefore all practitioners involved in caring for laboring women will eventually need to know how to use this technology and how to interpret the results and their effect on continuing labor or on altering the plan and opting for a surgical approach (Garite and others, 2000; Simpson and Porter, 2001).

The system uses a single-use disposable sensor that is inserted into the uterus via the cervix and rests against the fetal temple, cheek, or forehead and is held in place by the uterine wall. The sensor usually rotates and descends with the fetus as labor progresses, although infrequent adjustments may be needed. Its measurements are based on the same premise as pulse oximetry in that the major light sensors in the blood are oxyhemoglobin (with O_2) and deoxyhemoglobin (without O_2). The fetal temple, cheek, and forehead were found to be the most favorable areas for the sensor to work.

The normal range for fetal O_2 saturation during labor is 30% to 70%. If it remains greater or equal to 30% between uterine contractions, the provider can be assured that the fetus is adequately oxygenated even if the FHR tracing is less than reassuring. The findings are displayed on the monitor, along with the FHR and uterine contractions on a graph. Meconium in the fluid is not thought to affect the sensors. The readings on the monitor may or may not be continuous (as is the FHR); they may be intermittent instead. Either way, fetal O_2 saturation monitoring provides a sampling over time. Trends can then be taken into consideration, along with clinical judgment about the FHR tracing, the general progress of labor, and the estimated time to delivery. The potential effects of time can thus be used to factor into a decision of whether to continue labor or proceed with surgical, vaginal, or cesarean birth (Garite and others, 2000; Simpson and Porter, 2001).

Inserting the sensor is relatively easy and can be taught to practitioners with preceptored experiences until proficiency is attained. Generally, nurses and physicians who have mastered the FSE, the IUPC, or both can apply the similar technique and learn this procedure readily. It is generally found to be easier to insert the sensor posteriorly at either the 5 o'clock or 7 o'clock position. The sagittal suture line and one or both fontanels should be identified for accurate placement. If the cervix is minimally dilated (i.e., 2 to 4 cm), it may be more difficult to determine fetal position. In this case, insertion is usually more successful if an occiput anterior position of the fetus is assumed. Leopold's maneuvers or ultrasound may be helpful. The sensor should be inserted between contractions and only in the presence of a normal heart rate (Simpson and Porter, 2001).

If the 30% measurement begins to trend lower or dramatically fall, the nurse should have immediate access to the physician or midwife and be prepared for an emergent response. Because the sensor is generally used only on selected patients with questionable heart rate tracings, it is presumed that close communication between nurse and provider has already been established (Simpson and Porter, 2001).

NURSING MANAGEMENT

Assessments

Assessments for fetal health can be categorized as follows:

- Assess for fetal intolerance to labor by EFM, by fetal oxygenation sampling in labor, and through the use of ultrasonography for biophysical profiles and other evaluations for fetal health.
- Assess the acid-base balance immediately after delivery.

Antepartum

- Auscultate FHR with fetoscope or Doppler for 60 seconds and record at appropriate intervals.
- In the presence of a high risk condition, be prepared to explain the reasons for testing and the procedure and to assist in antepartum surveillance using such tests as the nonstress test, contraction stress test, biophysical profile, or Doppler studies as ordered.
- Explain the significance of and the procedure for monitoring fetal movement at home on a daily basis. Teach the patient when to notify her health care provider.
- Explain the importance of follow-up care.
- Refer to the social office for financial concerns if the family is without health benefits.

Intrapartum

Low risk patients
- When the patient is admitted in labor, apply external EFM for 20 minutes. Then assess FHR by intermittent auscultation during and after contractions or by continuous fetal monitoring.
- During latent phase of labor, assess and record FHR every 30 to 60 minutes (AAP/ACOG, 2002; AWHONN, 2003).
- During active labor, assess and record FHR every 30 minutes (AWHONN, 2000; AAP/ACOG, 2002).
- During second-stage labor, assess and record FHR every 15 minutes (AAP/ACOG, 2002; AWHONN, 2003).
- Assess maternal blood pressure, pulse, and respirations every 1 to 2 hours before the onset of active labor and every hour during active labor.
- Assess maternal temperature every 1 to 4 hours, depending on the stage of labor and the status of membranes.

High risk patients
- When the woman is admitted in labor, apply external EFM for 20 minutes. Then assess FHR by intermittent auscultation during and after contractions or by continuous fetal monitoring.
- During latent-phase labor, assess and record FHR pattern every 30 minutes (AWHONN, 2003; AAP/ACOG, 2002).
- During active-phase labor, assess and record FHR pattern every 15 minutes (AWHONN, 2000; AAP/ACOG, 2002).

- During second-stage labor, assess and record FHR pattern every 5 minutes (AWHONN, 2000; AAP/ACOG, 2002).
- FHR pattern assessment should include baseline heart rate, variability, and FHR changes over time.
- Assess maternal blood pressure, pulse, and respirations every 1 to 2 hours before the onset of active labor and every hour in active labor.
- Assess maternal temperature every 1 to 4 hours, depending on the stage of labor and status of membranes.

Interventions

On identification of a nonreassuring pattern, (1) reposition the patient laterally, turn her from side to side, or have her get in a hands-and-knees position or modified Trendelenburg position, depending on pattern and fetal response; (2) start and/or infuse IV fluids (lactated Ringer's) rapidly; (3) discontinue labor stimulant if being administered or, if not, obtain an order for 0.25 mg subcutaneous terbutaline; (4) administer O_2 at 8 to 10 L/min by mask; (5) notify physician or midwife; and (6) vibroacoustic or fetal scalp stimulation to assess fetal response may be used.

- Treat by position change, fluids, and medications such as terbutaline for cessation of contractions if intolerance to labor is detected and there are more than 15 to 30 minutes before delivery set up.
- Monitor maternal contractions every 30 minutes, and maintain a safe and effective labor pattern with maternal positioning (of choice and therapeutic), fluids, and comfort measures as appropriate (see Chapters 28 and 29).
- Record fetal and maternal responses to nursing interventions. Notify physician or midwife of any adverse effects on fetal response (ACOG, 1999; AWHONN, 2003).

CONCLUSION

Assessment of fetal well-being throughout pregnancy and intrapartum is paramount in order to achieve an optimal perinatal outcome. Nurses need skill in fetal assessment to accurately assess, develop, implement, evaluate, and document effective care to promote optimal outcomes.

BIBLIOGRAPHY
Electronic Fetal Monitoring

American Academy of Pediatrics (AAP) and American College of Obstetricians and Gynecologists (ACOG): *Guidelines for perinatal care,* ed 5, Elk Grove Village, Ill, and Washington, DC, 2002, AAP/ACOG.

American College of Obstetricians and Gynecologists (ACOG): *Evaluation of cesarean deliveries: executive summary,* Washington, DC, 2000, ACOG. Retrieved from *http://www.ACOG.org*

American College of Obstetricians and Gynecologists (ACOG): Antepartum fetal surveillance, *Practice Bulletin,* No. 9, Washington, DC, 1999, ACOG.

American College of Obstetricians and Gynecologists (ACOG): Intrapartum Fetal Heart Rate Monitoring, *Practice Bulletin,* No. 62, Washington, DC, 2005, ACOG.

Association of Women's Health, Obstetric, and Neonatal Nurses (AWHONN): *Fetal heart rate monitoring: principles and practices,* Washington, DC, 2003, AWHONN.

Association of Women's Health, Obstetric, and Neonatal Nurses (AWHONN): *Issue: fetal assessment,* Position Statement, Washington, DC, 2000, AWHONN.

Feinstein N, Sprague A, and Trepanier M: Fetal heart rate auscultation. Comparing auscultation to electronic fetal monitoring, *AWHONN Lifelines* 4(3):35–44, 2000.

Freeman K: Problems with intrapartum fetal heart rate monitoring interpretation and patient management, *Obstet Gynecol* 100(4):813–826, 2002.

Freeman R, Garite R, and Nageotte M: *Fetal heart rate monitoring,* ed 3, Baltimore, 2003, Lippincott Williams & Wilkins.

Gilstrap L III: Fetal acid-base balance. In Creasy R, Resnik R, and Iams J, editors: *Maternal-fetal medicine: principles and practice,* ed 5, Philadelphia, 2004, Saunders.

Goldenberg R: Cerebral palsy. In Creasy R, Resnik R, and Iams J, editors: *Maternal-fetal medicine: principles and practice,* ed 5, Philadelphia, 2004, Saunders.

Haggerty L, Nuttall R: Experienced obstetric nurses' decision-making in fetal risk situations, *J Obstet Gynecol Neonatal Nurs* 29(5):480–490, 2000.

Inturrisi M: Perioperative assessment of fetal heart rate and uterine activity, *J Obstet Gynecol Neonatal Nurs* 29(3):331–336, 2000.

Kleinman C, Nehgme R, and Copel J: Fetal cardiac arrhythmias: diagnosis and therapy. In Creasy R, Resnik R, and Iams J, editors: *Maternal-fetal medicine: principles and practice,* ed 5, Philadelphia, 2004, Saunders.

Kochanek K, Martin J: *Supplemental analyses of recent trends in infant mortality,* Hyattsville, Md, 2005, National Center for Health Statistics (NCHS).

Mahlmeister L: Legal implications of fetal heart assessment, *J Obstet Gynecol Neonatal Nurs* 29(5):517–526, 2000.

McCartney P: Computer analysis of the fetal heart rate, *J Obstet Gynecol Neonatal Nurs* 29(5):527–536, 2000.

Meschia G: Placental respiratory gas exchange and fetal oxygenation. In Creasy R, Resnik R, and Iams J, editors: *Maternal-fetal medicine: principles and practice,* ed 5, Philadelphia, 2004, Saunders.

Murray M: Maternal or fetal heart rate? Avoiding intrapartum misidentification, *J Obstet Gynecol Neonatal Nurs* 33(1):93–104, 2004.

National Institute of Child Health and Human Development Research Planning Workshop (NICHD): Electronic fetal heart rate monitoring: research guidelines for interpretation, *J Obstet Gynecol Neonatal Nurs* 26(6):635–640, 1997.

Parer J, Nageotte M: Intrapartum fetal surveillance. In Creasy R, Resnik R, and Iams J, editors: *Maternal-fetal medicine: principles and practice,* ed 5, Philadelphia, 2004, Saunders.

Phelan J, Kim J: Fetal heart rate observations in the brain-damaged infant, *Semin Perinatol* 24(3):221–229, 2000.

Porter M: Fetal pulse oximetry: an adjunct to electronic fetal heart rate monitoring, *J Obstet Gynecol Neonatal Nurs* 29(5):537–548, 2000.

Radin T, Harmon J, and Hanson D: Nurses' care during labor: its effect on the cesarean birth rate of healthy, nulliparous women, *Birth* 20(1):14–21, 1993.

Schmidt J: The development of AWHONN's fetal heart monitoring principles and practices workshop, *J Obstet Gynecol Neonatal Nurs* 29(5):509, 2000.

Schmidt J, McCartney P: History and development of fetal heart assessment: a composite, *J Obstet Gynecol Neonatal Nurs* 29(3):295–305, 2000.

Snyder C, Copel J: Fetal cardiac arrhythmias: diagnosis and therapy. In James D and others, editors: *High risk pregnancy: management options,* ed 3, Philadelphia, 2005, Saunders.

Society of Obstetricians and Gynecologists of Canada (SOGC): *Clinical practice guidelines: fetal health surveillance in labour,* No 112, 2002.

Simpson K: Standardized language for electronic fetal heart monitoring, *MCN Am J Matern Child Nurs* 29(5):336, 2004.

Sweha A, Hacker TW, and Nuovo J: Interpretation of the electronic fetal heart rate during labor, *Am Fam Physician* 59(9):2487–2500, 1999.

Thacker SB, Stroup D, and Chang M: Continuous electronic heart rate monitoring for fetal assessment during labor, *Cochrane Database Syst Rev,* Issue 2, 2001. Art. No.: CD000063. DOI: 10.1002/14651858.CD000063.

Trepanier M and others: Evaluation of a fetal monitoring education program, *J Obstet Gynecol Neonatal Nurs* 25(2):137–144, 1996.

Tucker S: *Pocket guide to fetal monitoring and assessment,* ed 5, St Louis, 2004, Mosby.

Antepartum Fetal Surveillance

Albers L: Monitoring the fetus in labor: evidence to support the methods, *J Midwifery Womens Health* 46(6):366–373, 2001.

American College of Obstetricians and Gynecologists (ACOG): Antepartum fetal surveillance, *Practice Bulletin,* No. 9, Washington, DC, 1999, ACOG.

Baser I, Johnson T, and Paine L: Coupling of fetal movement and fetal heart rate accelerations as an indicator of fetal health, *Obstet Gynecol* 80(1):62–66, 1992.

Cito G and others: Maternal position during non-stress test and fetal heart rate patterns, *Acta Obstet Gynecol Scand* 84(4):335–338, 2005.

Freda M and others: Fetal movement counting: which method? *MCN Am J Matern Child Nurs* 18(6):314–321, 1993.

Freeman R, Garite R, and Nageotte M: *Fetal heart rate monitoring,* ed 3, Baltimore, 2003, Lippincott Williams & Wilkins.

Harman C: Assessment of fetal health. In Creasy R, Resnik R, and Iams J, editors: *Maternal-fetal medicine: principles and practice,* ed 5, Philadelphia, 2004, Saunders.

Kisilevsky B, Kilpatrick K, and Low J: Vibroacoustic induced fetal movement: two stimuli and two methods of scoring, *Obstet Gynecol* 81(2):174–177, 1994.

Manning F: General principles and applications of ultrasonography. In Creasy R, Resnik R, and Iams J, editors: *Maternal-fetal medicine: principles and practice,* ed 5, Philadelphia, 2004, Saunders.

Manning F and others: Fetal assessment based on fetal biophysical profile scoring, *Am J Obstet Gynecol* 178(4):696–706, 1998.

Richardson B, Gagnon R: Fetal breathing and body movements. In Creasy R, Resnik R, and Iams J, editors: *Maternal-fetal medicine: principles and practice,* ed 5, Philadelphia, 2004, Saunders.

Tan KH, Smyth R: Fetal vibroacoustic stimulation for facilitation of tests of fetal well being, *Cochrane Database Syst Rev,* Issue 1, 2001. Art. No.: CD002963. DOI: 10.1002/14651858. CD002963.

Tempkin B: *Pocket protocols for ultrasound screening,* St Louis, 1999, Mosby.

United Health Foundation, American Public Health Association (APHA), and Partnership for Prevention: *America's health ranking, 2005,* Minnetonka, Minn, 2005, United Health Foundation.

Wood S: Choices about fetal assessment in labor, *MCN Am J Matern Child Nurs* 28(5): 293–298, 2003.

Zimmer E and others: Vibroacoustic stimulation evokes human fetal maturation, *Obstet Gynecol* 81(2):178–180, 1993.

Fetal Oxygenation Saturation

American College of Obstetricians and Gynecologists (ACOG): Fetal pulse oximetry, Committee Opinion, No. 258. *Obstet Gynecol* 98(3):523–524, 2001.

East CE, Chan FY, and Colditz PB: Fetal pulse oximetry for fetal assessment in labour, *Cochrane Database Syst Rev,* Issue 2, 2004. Art. No.: CD004075. DOI: 10.1002/14651858.CD004075. pub2.

Garite T and others: A multicenter controlled trial of fetal pulse oximetry in the intrapartum management of non-reassuring fetal heart rate patterns, *Am J Obstet Gynecol* 183(5): 1049–1058, 2000.

Simpson K, Porter M: Fetal oxygen saturation monitoring: using this new technology for fetal assessment during labor, *AWHONN Lifelines* 5(2):26–33, 2001.

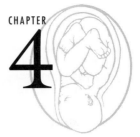

Perinatal Screening, Diagnoses, and Fetal Therapies

A dvances have been made in antepartum fetal surveillance, diagnosis, and medical therapies. These advances include the following:
- Prenatal genetic screening
- Prenatal diagnostic tests
- Prenatal therapies such as transfusion, stem cell transplantation, surgery, and multifetal pregnancy reduction

PRENATAL GENETIC SCREENING

Chromosomal abnormalities occur in 0.1% to 0.2% of all live births. Down syndrome is the most common clinically significant chromosomal abnormality (Smith-Bindman and others, 2001). This meiotic abnormality occurs most often in women over age 35. Prenatal care includes various prenatal screening and diagnostic tests to evaluate for congenital abnormalities and genetic disorders and should be offered to women considered at significant risk.

Purpose

Prenatal genetic screening is used to detect or define risk for fetal congenital malformations and inherited disorders.

Indications

Prenatal genetic screening starts with a risk assessment that includes maternal age, a family history, and ethnicity. Table 4-1 identifies the at-risk population group that should be offered screening for certain high risk genetic conditions. Other indications for prenatal genetic screening:
- Abnormal genetic history of mother or father
- Previous child with genetic defect
- Maternal phenylketonuria (PKU) or congestive heart disease
- Maternal history of two or more miscarriages
- Extreme parental anxiety/concern about potential for genetic abnormalities

Table 4-1   Population Groups at High Risk for a Genetic Condition

Population Group	Genetic Condition
Maternal age over 35	Down syndrome
Positive family history	Positive disease found in the history
Ashkenazi Jewish descent	Tay-Sachs disease
	Cystic fibrosis
	Canavan disease
French Canadian or Cajun descent	Tay-Sachs disease
	Cystic fibrosis
Southeast Asian descent	α-Thalassemia
Middle Eastern/Mediterranean descent	β-Thalassemia
African-American descent	Sickle cell disease
Hispanic descent	Sickle cell disease

Modified from March of Dimes Defects Foundation: Integrating genetics into your practice. *Contemporary OB/GYN* Nov. 1, 2003; ACOG Committee on Genetics: Opinion Number 298, Prenatal and preconceptional carrier screening for genetic diseases in individuals of Eastern European Jewish descent, *Obstet Gynecol* 104(2):425–428, 2004.

Resources

Informative online resources:

- ACOG—*http://www.acog.net*
- GeneTests—*http://www.genetests.org*
- March of Dimes—*http://www.marchofdimes.com/gyponline*
- National Society of Genetic Counselors—*http://www.nsgc.org*

SCREENING METHODS

Since most genetically abnormal children are born at varying ages to parents without a history of abnormality, routine screening is recommended and is cost-effective. Traditionally, routine prenatal genetic screening has been performed during the second trimester of pregnancy. To facilitate detection of fetal abnormalities earlier, first trimester screening is being conducted in two large studies: the FASTER trial and the 1-stop clinic for first trimester assessment of risk (OSCAR) trial (Bindra and others, 2002; Avgidou and others, 2005).

Second Trimester Screening

Definition

One marker is maternal serum alpha-fetoprotein (MSAFP), a protein produced by the fetal liver. MSAFP screening is useful in identifying certain developmental defects in the fetus. High levels may indicate neural tube defects with 80% to 90% accuracy, ventral abdominal wall defects with 50% accuracy, esophageal and duodenal atresia, some renal or urinary tract anomalies, and sudden infant death syndrome (SIDS) (Koos, 2005). Abnormally low levels have been noted in some cases of Down syndrome.

Other serum markers are also measured. *Triple marker screening* is another method of screening that can be performed in the second trimester. The triple screen detects the AFP, human chorionic gonadotropin (hCG), and unconjugated estriol (uEST). Combining all three chemical markers with the mother's age allows a detection rate of some trisomies of 60% to 75%, or two to three times the detection rate with MSAFP alone. Low MSAFP, low uEST, and high hCG are associated with Down syndrome with approximately 60% accuracy in women under 35 years of age and with 75% accuracy in women 35 years of age and older (ACOG, 2001). Low values in all three markers is associated with trisomy 18 with 60% to 75% accuracy. However, there is a high false-positive rate of 7% (Haddow and others, 1998). In addition to the trisomies, triple marker screening detects 85% to 90% of open neural tube defects (Jorde and others, 2000; Wilson, 2000).

The *quad-screen* adds a fourth marker, inhibin A (a placental hormone), to enhance the accuracy of screening for Down syndrome in women younger than 35 years of age. It has a lower false-positive rate of 5% or less (ACOG, 2001; Wald, Huttly, and Hackshaw, 2003). Low inhibin A levels indicate the possibility of Down syndrome.

Timing

The optimal time for AFP, triple marker screening, or quad-screen is 16 to 18 weeks of gestation (Jorde and others, 2000; ACOG, 2001).

Method

Maternal serum is routinely drawn as a screen between 16 and 18 weeks of gestation. It is necessary to have accurate information about gestational dating, maternal weight, race, number of fetuses, and insulin dependency.

The following can cause falsely elevated levels of MSAFP:
- Low birth weight
- Oligohydramnios
- Multifetal gestation
- Decreased maternal weight
- Underestimated fetal gestational age

The following can cause false low levels of MSAFP:
- Fetal death
- Increased maternal weight
- Overestimated fetal gestational age

Physiology

AFP is similar to serum albumin in chemical structure and is the major fetal serum protein (Jorde and others, 2000). It is produced in the yolk sac for the first 6 weeks and then by the fetal liver and gastrointestinal tract (Jorde and others, 2000).

Although its biologic function is unknown, AFP may have an immunoregulatory role, protecting the fetus against maternal immunologic attack

(Jenkins and Wapner, 2004). It is normally present in amniotic fluid, presumably by way of fetal urinary excretion.

AFP reaches its peak amniotic fluid concentration between 10 and 14 weeks of gestation, and it decreases steadily thereafter. It diffuses across the membranes and is detectable in maternal serum beginning at approximately 12 to 14 weeks of gestation.

Interpretation of Results

Second trimester maternal serum marker levels are not diagnostic; instead, they serve as a screen for fetal risk factors. Elevated or low levels indicate a need to follow up with other diagnostic studies, such as ultrasound, chorionic villus sampling, or amniocentesis, to help make specific diagnoses. Normal maternal serum markers indicate that there is a low risk for specific abnormalities, but they do not ensure a perfect, normal baby.

First Trimester Screening

Definition

First trimester screening uses ultrasound for measuring the nuchal translucency (NT), a fluid collection at the nape of the fetus' neck, and two serum protein markers: plasma protein-A (PAPP-A) and free beta subunit of human chorionic gonadotropin (B-hCG). Increased nuchal translucency, greater than 3 mm between 10 and 14 weeks of gestation, with decreased serum PAPP-A and B-hCG levels indicates a possible increased risk for certain trisomies such as 21 (Down syndrome), 18 (Edwards syndrome), and 13 (Patau syndrome). Increased nuchal translucency alone indicates a 10% to 15% risk for fetal cardiac disease (ACOG, 2004a).

Timing

The optimal time for first trimester screening is 10 to 14 weeks of gestation (ACOG, 2004a).

Interpretation of Results

First trimester maternal serum marker levels and nuchal translucency are not diagnostic, but rather serve as a screen for fetal risk factors. Elevated or low levels indicate a need to follow up with other diagnostic studies, such as ultrasound, chorionic villus sampling, or amniocentesis. Normal maternal serum markers indicate that there is a low risk for specific abnormalities, but they do not ensure a perfect, normal baby.

Combining First and Second Trimester Screening

Combining first and second trimester screening lowers false-positive rates as indicated by the preliminary results of the FASTER trial (Malone and others, 2003).

ULTRASOUND EVALUATION FOR FETAL ABNORMALITIES

Ultrasound has been used to evaluate the fetus since the early 1980s. As equipment has become more technologically accurate, so have the technicians and the reading radiologists and perinatologists. Many practices use ultrasound routinely in the first two trimesters. First, it is used to validate or establish the estimated date of delivery. It is particularly useful for this purpose when done before 20 weeks. Second, it is used between 16 and 18 weeks of gestation (as a level II ultrasound) to evaluate the fetal anatomy and to check for certain markers of chromosomal abnormalities (Menihan, 2000; Tempkin, 2000).

In a level II ultrasound, the anatomy is evaluated from head to extremities. Evaluations include the following (Tempkin, 2000):

- Ventricles of the head for size—the middle cerebral artery may be evaluated for blood flow after 24 weeks of gestation
- Face, profile and full-on views
- Nuchal translucency—a fluid collection at the nape of the fetus' neck is associated with increase incidence of Down syndrome between 10 and 14 weeks of gestation (ACOG, 2001; Beamer, 2001)
- Heart and its four chambers—blood flow through valves may be evaluated with a fetal echocardiogram after 20 to 22 weeks of gestation
- Abdominal contents, including the intestines, liver, spleen, and kidneys
- All four extremities, including hands and feet

Much controversy surrounds the use of ultrasound level II evaluations and markers for genetic abnormalities (Tempkin, 2000; Bindman and others, 2001). Some believe, there is a greater degree of predictability when level 11 ultrasound is combined with other factors such as maternal age or the presence of abnormal markers.

Ultrasound is useful in other stages of pregnancy to evaluate growth parameters, cerebral artery blood flow, and already known abnormalities for progressive or worsening trends. It also may be useful for the opposite, that is, to evaluate for therapeutic procedures or treatment effects that help confirm reasons to continue the pregnancy (Tempkin, 2000; Finberg, 2001).

PRENATAL DIAGNOSTIC TESTS

When a screening test is positive, the diagnosis is confirmed or ruled out by a diagnostic procedure of chorionic villus sampling (CVS) or amniocentesis.

Chorionic Villus Sampling

Definition

In CVS, a portion of the chorion is aspirated and analyzed for evidence of genetic, chromosomal, or biochemical abnormalities.

Routes

CVS is done by transabdominal aspiration (needle) or transcervical aspiration (catheter).

Risks

The benefit of diagnosing fetal disorders earlier must be weighed against the risks. Transabdominal CVS is equally as safe as second trimester amniocentesis (Brambati and Tului, 2005). According to the Cochrane review by Alfirevic, Sundberg, and Brigham (2003), transcervical CVS is more difficult to perform and carries a significantly higher risk for spontaneous abortion and fetal loss. The transcervical CVS approach is contraindicated in the presence of a cervical infection such as chlamydia or herpes.

Timing

Transabdominal CVS needle aspiration is done in the first or second trimester. Transcervical CVS catheter aspiration is done at 10 to 12 weeks of gestation.

Procedure for Abdominal Route

The woman drinks 300 to 400 ml of water before the transabdominal CVS. With ultrasonographic guidance, an 18-gauge spinal needle with stylet is inserted through the maternal abdominal wall and myometrium into the chorion. The stylet is withdrawn, and a 20-ml syringe is attached to an aspiration device. Chorionic villi are obtained by repeated (15 to 20) rapid aspirations of the syringe plunger to 20-ml negative pressure. Simultaneously, the needle tip is redirected several times within the placenta. The needle is withdrawn under continuous 20-ml negative pressure. The specimen is then transferred to a Petri dish for inspection under a microscope to judge quantity of tissue. After the specimen is transferred to a genetics laboratory, cells are harvested at 5 to 8 days (Hunter and Soothill, 2006; Jorde and others, 2000).

Procedure for Transcervical Route

In the transcervical approach, a speculum is placed in the vagina under ultrasonic guidance. The vagina is cleansed, and the cervix is secured with a tenaculum. A 20-mm catheter with a pliable stainless steel obturator is then passed through the cervix and into the chorion. The obturator is removed, and a 10-ml syringe is attached to the catheter. Chorionic villi are obtained by applying 2 to 5 ml of negative pressure at several sites on the chorion. The specimen is then transferred to a Petri dish for inspection under a microscope to judge quantity of tissue. Then the specimen is sent to the genetics laboratory, where cells are harvested in 5 to 8 days (Hunter and Soothill, 2006; Wilson, 2000). Because no fluid is collected, a maternal serum markers screen cannot be done.

Postprocedure Care

The fetal heart rate (FHR) is auscultated twice in 30 minutes. Unsensitized Rh D-negative patients are given 300 mg of anti-D immune globulin. A repeat ultrasound is scheduled to be performed at 16 weeks of gestation.

Amniocentesis

Definition

Amniocentesis is the transabdominal needle aspiration of 10 to 20 ml of amniotic fluid for laboratory analysis.

Timing

There are two types of amniocentesis, early and second trimester (sometimes called conventional). The second trimester/conventional amniocentesis is preferred for genetic screening and is performed between 15 and 20 weeks of gestation (ACOG, 2001). Early amniocentesis, performed between 11 and 14 weeks, results in significantly higher rate of pregnancy loss (2.5% compared with 1%), other complications such as talipes equinovarus (1.6% compared with 3.1%), and postprocedural amniotic fluid leakage of 3.5% compared with 1.7% (CEMAT, 1998; Brambeti, Tului, 2005). According to the Cochrane review (Alfirevic, Sundberg, and Brigham 2003), early amniocentesis is associated with a greater risk for spontaneous abortion and neonatal talipes compared with transabdominal CVS.

Risks

Risks with amniocentesis include the following:
- Spontaneous abortion
- Trauma to the fetus or placenta
- Bleeding
- Preterm labor
- Maternal infection
- Rh sensitization from fetal bleed into maternal side of circulation

Preparation

In preparation for amniocentesis, the nurse explains the procedure to the patient. The patient is encouraged to urinate just before the procedure to avoid the risk for bladder puncture. Usually, a 20-minute electronic fetal monitoring (EFM) strip is run or an ultrasound evaluation is made before the procedure to explore the potential site for probability of obtaining the fluid.

Procedure

First, a detailed ultrasound is performed to take fetal measurements, obtain an anatomic survey of the fetus, locate the placenta, and choose an amniocentesis site. Then the abdomen is prepped with an antiseptic such as povidone-iodine (Betadine). Most practitioners do not use lidocaine (Xylocaine). A spinal-gauge needle is then inserted into the site selected under ultrasound guidance. Approximately 20 to 30 ml of fluid is withdrawn for a genetic analysis and alpha-fetoprotein (AFP) screen. If the procedure is being used as a method of draining excess amniotic fluid, the needle is anchored, tubing is attached, and the necessary amount of fluid is removed by gravity (Jorde and others, 2000; Wilson, 2000; Hunter and Soothill, 2006).

After amniocentesis, if performed after 24 weeks, an EFM strip is run, primarily to detect contractile patterns suggestive of preterm labor or abruption. The FHR is monitored and evaluated as appropriate for the gestational age (Hunter and Soothill, 2006; Jorde and others, 2000; Wilson, 2000). The Rh D-negative woman should receive anti-D immune globulin (300 mg) because there is potential for a procedure-associated fetal-maternal hemorrhage.

The woman should be advised not to lift anything heavy for 2 days and to report any amniotic fluid leakage, fever, severe cramps, or vaginal bleeding. Slight cramping for the first day or two is normal.

Percutaneous Umbilical Blood Sampling

Purpose

Percutaneous umbilical blood sampling is done to obtain fetal blood samples for rapid chromosomal analysis if there is no alternative to achieve a timely diagnosis, to measure fetal hemoglobin in case of erythroblastosis fetalis, to take a fetal platelet count in alloimmune thrombocytopenia or thrombocytopenia purpura, or to assess for a fetal infection (Jenkins and Wapner, 2004).

Risks

There is a 3% to 7% risk for fetal loss with percutaneous umbilical blood sampling. Morbidity is high also. Associated complications of this procedure are bleeding, cord hematomas, transient fetal bradycardia, infection, and fetal-maternal hemorrhage (Mountain States Regional Genetic Services Network, 2001).

Timing

The blood sample may be drawn as early as an early amniocentesis but is generally done late in the second trimester when such diagnoses may change options and recommendations for medical management (Jorde and others, 2000).

Method

With concurrent ultrasonographic visualization, a 23- or 25-gauge spinal needle is directed into the umbilical vein about 1 cm from the site of cord insertion into the placenta (Jorde and others, 2000).

Postprocedure Care

External fetal monitoring is done for 1 to 2 hours after the procedure. Also, the nurse should instruct the mother how to count fetal movements so that she can count them when she is discharged home.

PRENATAL THERAPY

Fetal Intrauterine Transfusion

Definition

Fetal intrauterine transfusion is a relatively newly accepted procedure that is now associated with increased success, new clinical applications, and more common use; however, it is not a new concept. In the 1970s, fetal intrauterine transfusions were being done experimentally only as a last resort in the most technologically sophisticated level III facilities. The procedure at that time was done by placing a parenteral catheter through the maternal abdominal wall and, by ultrasound guidance, placing it in proximity to the fetal diaphragmatic lymph system. The transfused blood was then indirectly absorbed through the lymphatics into the fetal circulation. The procedure was fraught with risks of maternal infection, fetal injury, and poor success. As a result, it was seldom used. At the time, ultrasound technology made placement difficult, and a safe procedure for fetal direct intravenous transfusion was improbable. Now, the direct route through intravascular umbilical venous placement has reduced risks and improved success (Jorde and others 2000; Flake, 2004; Weiner, 2005).

Purpose

Direct intrauterine fetal transfusion is indicated for the severely hydropic infant before 33 weeks of gestation in an Rh D-negative sensitized pregnant woman. It is also indicated when intravascular sampled umbilical venous blood demonstrates a significant lowering of fetal hemoglobin or hematocrit or if amniotic fluid samples indicate a rising bilirubin level and delta optical density increase.

Risks

Risks associated with intrauterine fetal transfusion surgery include the following:
- Maternal infection
- Overtransfusion
- Fetal vascular trauma
- Onset of preterm labor
- Fetal bradycardia (Weiner, 2000; Flake, 2004)

Method

Careful aseptic preparation of the maternal abdomen is necessary. The nurse should premedicate the mother with enough narcotic and tranquilizer to render the fetus quiet. The fetal vein is located using ultrasound. A 22-gauge long spinal needle is guided toward the vessel. Once the tip is placed correctly, blood—20 to 50 ml/kg (depending on gestation), cross-matched to the mother, and spun down tightly packed to a hematocrit greater than 70%—is then instilled slowly. EFM is used for 1 to 2 hours after the procedure. The mother is instructed to continue fetal movement counts and other fetal testing (Jorde and others, 2000).

Fetal Intrauterine Surgery
Definition

Therapeutic advances in technology that led to fetal intrauterine surgical corrections evolved from interventions for Rh D sensitization and for effects on the fetus (Weiner, 2000; Flake, 2004). Initially, therapy was directed at disease acquired in utero. In the early 1980s, therapies for congenital disorders began to be attempted (Flake, 2004).

All forms of fetal surgery remain experimental, although some trends are becoming evident:

- Surgical correction of obstructive uropathies: the rationale for such therapy is to bypass the site of the obstruction and thereby prevent progressive renal damage.
- Surgical placement of shunts for pleural effusions.
- Surgical correction of obstructive hydrocephalus: the rationale is to reduce ventricular size and expansion to minimize compression damage to the cerebral cortex.
- Repair of a myelomeningocele prior to neuronal damage.
- Repair of fetal diaphragmatic hernia: presumably, repair of the hernia provides release of compressive forces and restores normal lung development. The following fetal surgery has not proved very successful:
- In utero plastic repair of such abnormalities as cleft palate and lip: theoretically, plastic repairs before birth would heal with less scarring.

All but the last three surgical procedures are performed without incision into abdomen or uterus. They involve the use of a fiberoptic scope and ultrasonic guidance for placement.

Methods

Surgical corrections may be accomplished by ultrasound-guided percutaneous placement of catheter shunts or by hysterotomy with direct visualization and surgical repair. The type of congenital malformation, as well as the skill and training of the perinatologist, determine the exact method (Jorde and others, 2000; Weiner, 2000; Bindman and others, 2001; Kleinman, Nehgme, and Copel, 2004).

Risks

Problems arise when assessing the success and benefit of fetal intrauterine surgical corrections, not the least of which are ethical dilemmas. Because of increased fetal and neonatal survival and the nature of accompanying disabilities, with surgical corrections of some disorders, more fetuses survive as infants with disabilities. Without fetal surgery, many of these fetuses would not survive. Therefore it appears that increased survival will increase the societal problems of caring for infants with disabilities.

Some repairs corrected with intrauterine fetal surgery have higher success than others. Infants with diaphragmatic hernia repair have the lowest survival rate. Those with repair of uropathologic conditions have the highest survival, although the best is with posterior urethral valve syndrome and the worst is with urethral atresia.

Hydrocephalic disorders are generally well screened for the amount of adequate cerebral cortical tissue before attempting the repair. If other associated neurotube defects accompany hydrocephalus, the degree of handicap in surviving infants also varies (Weiner, 2000; Flake, 2004).

When hysterotomy is the chosen route for accomplishing the repair, there are other attendant problems. First, the incision into the uterus generally is as risky as, and requires similar treatment to, the uterine incision of a classic cesarean. Second, as the procedure is being carried out, loss of amniotic fluid and interruption of the integrity of the amnion occur. Stapling the amnion to the uterine wall as the incision is being made compensates for interruption of the integrity of the amnion. Loss of amniotic fluid is restored by warmed normal saline as the cavity is closed. Third, keeping the head and upper respiratory system of the fetus out of the fluid during the procedure is essential to prevent stimulating the switch from fetal cardiopulmonary circulation to neonatal circulation.

The number and type of fetal therapies for congenital disorders probably are limited by the difference in the relative size of the fetus and the available technology and surgical instruments. Those problems can be expected to be overcome as innovative and creative solutions are found to manage them.

Multifetal Pregnancy Reduction
Definition
Multifetal pregnancy reduction is a procedure to reduce the number of multiple embryos conceived usually by one of the fertility modalities. It is done by injecting high doses of potassium chloride into the fetuses that are easiest to reach after carefully evaluating a complete fetal survey to determine that healthy fetuses, those most likely to survive, have remained. The procedure carries a risk for causing preterm labor, previable delivery, and infection.

Fertility procedures are fraught with multiple concerns. Through manipulation outside the uterus, they more often result in monoamniotic twins and thus carry a higher risk for twin-to-twin transfusion. Other concerns are generally related to the ethical dilemmas presented to the family and care providers. Because of their decision to selectively terminate or to carry multiple embryos and risk losing all, parents are at high risk for complicated grief, potentially requiring referral for therapeutic psychologic support.

NURSING MANAGEMENT
Prevention
The main functions of nursing care are to prevent uninformed decisions by parents, fetal compromise after intrauterine therapies, and unnecessary distress of the human spirit because of decisions for fetal testing or therapy.

Counselors and teachers are of prime importance. The ultimate goal is to empower families to make difficult decisions considering their ability to parent and the quality of life for their unborn child.

Assessment
Assessment of stressors, coping styles, general knowledge, and locus of control related to physical and emotional health helps in formulating nursing diagnoses. The nurse must articulate diagnoses and collaborative problems related

to alterations in, risks to, complicating factors in, and strengths and deficiencies of the individuals and the family as a unit as follows:

- Assess for coping styles.
- Assess parents' need for comforting spiritual rituals (see Chapter 7).

Intervention

The nurse should help the parents come to an understanding of the potential risks and benefits of the various methods of prenatal genetic screening and of essential fetal therapy. The nurse should help them cope in the event of an unanticipated fetal outcome as follows:

- Prepare for potential unexpected result.
- Establish a trusting relationship.
- Encourage and foster open communication with health providers.
- Coordinate a multidisciplinary conference with parents in attendance.
- Assist with preparations for extended family visitation while the patient is hospitalized.
- Encourage questions.
- Give anticipatory guidance.
- Be prepared to repeat information more than once.
- Provide more than one viewpoint or opinion.
- Provide accurate information about fetal tests and therapy.
- Encourage and facilitate close family contact; eliminate separation.
- Refer to parents' spiritual or psychologic support person(s).
- Communicate acceptance of expressed spiritual pain.
- Encourage expression and exploration of feelings.
- Support parents' decisions without expressing personal conflict and attitudes that may be in opposition to parents' attitudes.

CONCLUSION

The continued rapid growth in technologic and innovative advances in fetal evaluation and therapies has exceeded considerations of physical, psychologic, and social consequences. It has become increasingly difficult for parents with a high risk pregnancy to obtain adequate information about expected benefits and negative consequences of fetal evaluation and therapies. The rapid growth also contributes to difficulty in keeping current with information needed to counsel and guide parents in making thoroughly informed decisions about fetal evaluation or therapy. Nurses have a professional responsibility to seek, be receptive to, and be intelligently critical of information that is on the cutting edge of the future.

BIBLIOGRAPHY

Alfirevic Z, Sundberg K, and Brigham S: Amniocentesis and transabdominal chorion villus sampling for prenatal diagnosis, *Cochrane Database Syst Rev,* Issue 1, 2003.

American College of Obstetricians and Gynecologists (ACOG): *First-trimester screening for fetal aneuploidy,* Committee Opinion, No. 296, Washington, DC, 2004a, ACOG.

American College of Obstetricians and Gynecologists (ACOG): *Prenatal and preconception carrier screening for genetic diseases in individuals of Eastern European Jewish descent,* Committee Opinion, No. 298, Washington, DC, 2004b, ACOG.

American College of Obstetricians and Gynecologists (ACOG): *Prenatal diagnosis of fetal chromosomal abnormalities,* Practice Bulletin, No. 27, Washington, DC, 2001, ACOG.

Avgidou K and others: Prospective first-trimester screening for trisomy 21 in 30,564 pregnancies, *Am J Obstet Gynecol* 192(6):1761–1767, 2005.

Beamer L: Fetal nuchal translucency: a prenatal screening tool, *J Obstet Gynecol Neonatal Nurs* 30(4):376–385, 2001.

Bindman R and others: Second-trimester ultrasound to detect fetuses with Down syndrome: a meta-analysis, *JAMA* 285(8):1044–1055, 2001.

Bindra R and others: One-stop clinic for assessment of risk for trisomy 21 at 11–14 weeks: a prospective study of 15,030 pregnancies, *Ultrasound Obstet Gynecol* 20(3):219–225, 2002.

Brambati B, Tului L: Chorionic villus sampling and amniocentesis, *Curr Opin Obstet Gynecol* 17(2):197–201, 2005.

Canadian Early and Mid-Trimester Amniocentesis Trial (CEMAT): Randomised trial to assess safety and fetal outcome of early and midtrimester amniocentesis, *Lancet* 351(9098): 242–247, 1998.

Finberg H: *Assessing the risk of aneuploidy in pregnancy.* Presentation at Obstetrical Challenges of the New Millennium Conference, Phoenix, Ariz, March, 2001.

Flake A: Fetal therapies, medical surgical approaches. In Creasy R, Resnik R, and Iams J, editors: *Maternal-fetal medicine: principles and practice,* ed 5, Philadelphia, 2004, Saunders.

Haddow J and others: Second trimester screening for Down's syndrome using maternal serum dimeric inhibin A, *J Med Screen* 5(3):115–119, 1998.

Hunter A and Soothill P: Invasive procedure for antenatal diagnosis. In James D and others, editors: *High risk pregnancy: management options,* ed 3, Philadelphia, 2006, Elsevier Saunders.

Jenkins T, Wapner R: Prenatal diagnosis of congenital disorders. In Creasy R, Resnik R, and Iams J, editors: *Maternal-fetal medicine: principles and practice,* ed 5, Philadelphia, 2004, Saunders.

Jorde L and others: Medical genetics, St Louis, 2000, Mosby. In Creasy R, Resnik R, and Iams J, editors: *Maternal-fetal medicine: principles and practice,* ed 5, Philadelphia, 2004, Saunders.

Kleinman C, Nehgme R, and Copel J: Fetal cardiac arrhythmias: diagnosis therapy. In Creasy R, Resnik R, and Iams J, editors: *Maternal-fetal medicine: principles and practice,* ed 5, Philadelphia, 2004, Saunders.

Koos B: Too much information or not enough? *Curr Opin Obstet Gynecol* 17(2):161–162, 2005.

Lemon B: Nuchal translucency for prenatal screening? What nurses need to know about their tool, *AWHONN Lifelines* 8(6):520–526, 2005.

Malone F and others: First- and second-trimester evaluation of risk (FASTER) trail: principal results of the NICHD Multicenter Down Syndrome Screening Study, *Am J Obstet Gynecol* 189:S56, 2003.

Menihan C: Limited obstetric ultrasound in nursing practice, *J Obstet Gynecol Neonatal Nurs* 29(3):325–330, 2000.

Mountain States Regional Genetic Services Network: Percutaneous umbilical blood sampling (PUBS), 2001. Retrieved from *http://www.obgyn.net/fm/umbilical_blood.htm*

Simpson J: Choosing the best prenatal screening protocol, *N Engl J Med* 353(19):2068–2070, 2005.

Smith-Bindman R and others: Second-trimester ultrasound to detect fetuses with Down syndrome: a meta-analysis, *JAMA* 285(8):1044–1055, 2001.

Tempkin B: *Pocket protocols for ultrasound scanning,* Philadelphia, 2000, Saunders.

Wald N, Huttly W, and Hackshaw A: Antenatal screening for Down syndrome with the quadruple test, *Lancet* 361(9360):835–836, 2003.

Wapner R and others: First-trimester screening for trisomies 21 and 18, *N Engl J Med* 349(15):1405–1413, 2003.

Weiner C: Fetal hemolytic disease. In James D and others, editors: *High risk pregnancy: management options,* ed 3, Philadelphia, 2005, Saunders.

Wilson R: Amniocentesis and chorionic villus sampling, *Curr Opin Obstet Gynecol* 12(2):81–86, 2000.

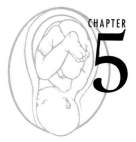

Integrative Therapies in Pregnancy and Childbirth

Since the 1990s, complementary and alternative medicine has been rapidly gaining in popularity for both consumers and health care practitioners. This chapter is intended to acquaint nurses with some of the alternative and complementary therapies that are frequently requested by families experiencing high risk pregnancies. Surveys indicate that patients find complementary and alternative therapies congruent with their own values, beliefs, and philosophical orientation toward health and life. Each year more people are using these services (Petrie and Peck, 2000).

This chapter is simply an introduction to these therapies; readers are strongly encouraged to refer patients to a complementary and alternative medical specialist for treatment. The listed therapies are safe and effective during pregnancy when administered by a person who is properly trained. Although complementary and alternative therapies are generally not supported by solid scientific research, most are based on empirical use and have been practiced for hundreds or even thousands of years. In the case of traditional Chinese medicine (TCM), Chinese herbs and acupuncture have been used for more than a thousand years, and the applications, cautions, and contraindications are well known but only now being scientifically proven.

Therefore these therapies should not be discarded based on the lack of solid scientific evidence. To set such a standard would be disadvantageous; for instance, although much of conventional allopathic medicine is also unsupported by solid, evidence-based literature, it still produces desired results.

When conventional medical treatment is combined with alternative or complementary therapies, the term *integrative medicine* is commonly used. In 1992, the Office of Alternative Medicine was established by the National Institutes of Health to begin to investigate the safety and efficacy of integrative medicine. In 1999, this office was renamed the National Center for Complementary and Alternative Medicine (NCCAM). According to the NCCAM (2006), there are five complementary and alternative fields of practice:

- *Alternative medical systems.* Alternative medical systems are complete systems of medical theory and practice. They include TCM, ayurvedic medicine (India's traditional medicine), homeopathy, naturopathy, and Native American healing.
- *Mind-body interventions.* Mind-body interventions are various techniques designed to enhance the capacity of the mind. Examples are biofeedback, yoga, meditation, hypnotherapy, dance, music and art therapy, relaxation therapy, integrated guided imagery, aromatherapy, spirituality and prayer, humor, journaling, and dream work.
- *Biologic based therapies.* These therapies include herbal, dietary, and nutritional therapies, including vitamin, mineral, and other supplements, as well as exercise and other lifestyle changes.
- *Manipulative and body-based methods.* These include various hands-on healing techniques such as acupressure, massage, osteopathy, chiropractic, reflexology, and kinesiology.
- *Energy therapies.* Energy therapies include acupuncture, healing touch, therapeutic touch, polarity, Reiki, jin shin jyutsu, external qi gong, touch for health, and reflexology.

BRIEF OVERVIEW OF SELECTED INTEGRATIVE THERAPIES IN PREGNANCY

Alternative Medical Systems

Traditional Chinese Medicine (TCM) and Acupuncture

TCM is a complete medical system that originated in China more than 4000 years ago to diagnose and treat illness, prevent disease, and improve well-being. TCM developed independently from the Western view of anatomy, physiology, and pathology. Qualified practitioners observe, diagnose, and treat illness using a different set of principles and vocabulary than those commonly used in conventional Western medicine.

TCM, on the most fundamental level, is the harmony and balance of qi (pronounced *chee*) in the body. *Qi* can be defined as the essence and the basis of all life, or the vital energy. It warms the body, keeps the mind active, creates breath, expels a baby during birth, and gives us each a distinct personality. Qi is not only part of the human body but also part of the surrounding environment. The general category of qi can be broken down into *yin* and *yang*, which represent the dualistic poles of nature. The sign of the *tai ji* is used to illustrate the nature of yin and yang. Yin and yang maintain the homeostasis of the body. *Yin* represents the dark, inclusive, night, material, cold, inactive, and interior pole. *Yang,* in contrast, is the bright, exclusive, day, immaterial, warm, active, and exterior pole.

TCM is based on the theory of the normal functioning of the human body and its relationship to the environment. The environment includes weather (cold, hot, arid, humid), lifestyle (type of work and hours, exercise, diet), pathogens (viruses, bacteria, fungi, pollens), and relationships (married, single, death of close family), all which affect health and balance. Any aberration is considered a disharmony, which is ultimately a precursor to disease. Once an imbalance or disease has arisen, the TCM methods of diagnosis such as pulse and tongue assessments are used to identify the pattern of disharmony. The treatment principle is formed, and the appropriate modalities are applied.

The most recognized TCM treatment modality in the United States is *acupuncture*. Acupuncture is the insertion of fine (32- to 38-gauge) solid needles into the skin at acupuncture points, which are located along and independent of the meridian system. There are more than 2000 different acupuncture points on the body, situated along the limbs, chest, abdomen, back, spine, ears, face, and scalp. There are 12 major *meridians* (channels of energy flow), each connecting to an organ and running distally throughout the body. The energy that flows through the meridians is qi. The depth of puncture varies, depending on the location and treatment effect desired. Once placed, the needles are retained for a varied length of time, most commonly between 15 and 45 minutes. The number of acupuncture treatments in a course of therapy varies based on the disease being treated and the overall health of the individual. Certain points are contraindicated for use in pregnancy because they can stimulate uterine contractions and result in premature labor.

Chinese herbal medicine is an integral part of TCM. In China, herbal prescriptions are used more frequently and for a wider range of conditions than acupuncture. The theories of Chinese herbal medicine are identical to those of acupuncture. The practitioner obtains a TCM diagnosis using the techniques of observation, auscultation and olfaction, interrogation, and palpation. A treatment plan is then devised, and an herbal prescription is constructed that is very specific to the state of the individual.

Herbal prescriptions usually contain between 2 and 14 individual herbs selected from a pharmacopoeia of thousands. Over hundreds of years of prescribing herbs, the Chinese have empirically and, more recently, scientifically studied the effects of herbs on the human body. Information has been obtained regarding the toxicity levels, preparation procedures, contraindications, and cautions of using Chinese herbs. Chinese herbal medicine is advanced and traditionally used with many disorders. It is complementary to acupuncture therapy, as well as to most prescription drugs.

Other TCM therapies include (Fontaine, 2005):

- *Tuina.* This manipulative or therapeutic bodywork uses massage techniques to treat physical problems.
- *Cupping.* This is a treatment technique whereby suction is applied to the skin surface using small jars in which a vacuum is created. The cups are commonly retained for 1 to 15 minutes. Cupping is frequently used to treat disorders of the musculoskeletal system.
- *Moxibustion.* This is a common adjunctive technique used in TCM. The name refers to the technique with which heat is applied to the acupuncture points by igniting products made from the dried leaves of the mugwort

plant (*Artemisia vulgaris*). There are many ways to warm the "moxa" on the acupuncture point. Sometimes the moxa pole can be used to warm acupuncture needles that have already been inserted. This method is commonly used to turn a baby from the breech position.

- *Chinese nutritional therapy.* In this system, foods are categorized by their energetic properties and their effect on organ systems. A diet of beneficial foods is prescribed to treat disease, and recommendations are given about foods that should be avoided or eaten in moderation.
- *Gua sha.* This is a manual technique that uses a coin or spoon to scrape the surface of the skin. It promotes the circulation of qi and blood and is also used to treat musculoskeletal pain syndromes.
- *Plum blossom needling.* This is a form of cutaneous needle therapy. The acupuncture points are stimulated by lightly tapping an instrument that has a head composed of a bundle of five or seven small, short needles attached to a handle. This tapping causes a reddening of the skin and promotes circulation. It is most applicable for disorders of the skin and nervous system.
- *Electrical stimulation.* The most common form of electrical stimulation uses a machine similar to a TENS unit with clips attached to the end of retained needles. Therapy is used in conjunction with acupuncture and lasts from 10 to 30 minutes; the presence of the current may or may not be felt by the patient. Electroacupuncture is most often used as analgesia and is applicable during labor and delivery.

Homeopathy

Homeopathy is an energy-based, pharmacologic system of medicine that uses a set of principles and laws for prescribing specifically prepared medicines to correct disease. Developed by Dr. Samuel Hahnemann (1755–1843) of Germany, the basic theory of homeopathy is "like cures like" or the "Law of Similars." For example, for constipation, a homeopathic remedy that in crude form is known to *produce* constipation can actually treat the same condition when used in minute doses.

Homeopathic remedies are prepared from almost anything that can be used to help relieve disease. The process of preparing homeopathic remedies is complex and includes the process of dilution in a solution of water and alcohol. Frequently, the remedy dilution is so great that no trace of the original substance remains. The process of dilution imprints the energetic pattern of the material into the solution.

The homeopathic approach toward disease is different from the allopathic approach. Homeopaths take into consideration all aspects of health, including the physical, mental, emotional, and spiritual life. Every occurrence that is connected with the onset of the ailment is considered. The information gathered during case taking is extensive. Once a treatment plan is made, a single remedy or a combination remedy is administered, most often in the form of a liquid or small pills that are placed sublingually.

Mind-Body Interventions

Aromatherapy

Aromatherapy is described as the therapeutic application of essential oils through the skin using the mediums of lotions, creams, or baths or the methods of inhalation or massage. Essential oils are highly concentrated complex essences obtained from flowers, leaves, stems, barks, fruits, seeds, and resins. Each of the hundreds of oils has specific effects and different properties. As the oils are absorbed into the body, there are pharmacologic, physiologic, and psychologic reactions. The ancient practice of aromatherapy has been found in Chinese and Greek literature, and it has experienced a revival in Europe, the United States, and Canada.

Only a trained aromatherapist should administer aromatherapy; many essential oils should be avoided during pregnancy because they have uterine-stimulating and emmenagogic effects (Box 5-1).

Hypnotherapy

Hypnotherapy is a form of deep relaxation with an alert mind producing alpha waves. In this state, critical faculties are suspended and the subconscious mind can be more easily accessed (Tiran and Mack, 2000). Hypnotherapy can be likened to deep relaxation, daydreaming, or meditation in which a similar state is experienced. This state of mind is a naturally occurring phenomenon that we have all experienced; therefore it can be assumed that there is no intrinsic danger when administered by a highly trained professional.

Spiritual Healing and Prayer

Spiritual healing and *prayer* are terms that define a wide range of different belief systems and the power that these beliefs have to heal the body and spirit.

Box 5-1   Aromatherapy Oils That Are Completely Contraindicated During Pregnancy

Arnica	Deertongue	Rue
Bitter almond	Dwarf pine	Sassafras
Boldo leaf	Elecampane	Savin
Broom	Exotic basil	Summer savory
Buchu	Fennel (bitter)	Tansy
Calamus	Horseradish	Thuja
Camphor	Jaborand leaf	Tonki
Cassia	Mubwort (armoise)	Vanilla
Chervil	Mustard	Wintergreen
Cinnamon Bark	Origanum	Wormseed
Clove	Pennyroyal	Wormwood
Costus		

From Tiran D, Mack S: *Complementary therapies for pregnancy and childbirth*, ed 2, London, 2000, Bailliere Tindall.

Spirituality is a basic human need. Although spirituality is believed to be associated with religion, the concept of spirituality goes beyond religion. Conventional medicine has traditionally ignored the mind-body connection and its impact on health and healing; prayer and spiritual healing are avenues to incorporate this type of healing system into the mainstream. It is important for health care professionals to be sensitive to all the belief systems that exist.

Benefits of spiritual healing and prayer include availability of an increased support system and community, increased self-esteem and self-love, and increased connectedness to the divine. Increased spirituality has been associated with decreased maternal complications in labor and delivery and fewer neonatal intensive care unit admissions (Petrie and Peck, 2000).

Yoga

Yoga is a mind-body exercise based on East Indian philosophy, and it has been practiced for nearly 6000 years. It has been said that the highest level of yoga is the recognition of the true self. There are many types of yoga, each including a vast repertoire of asanas (postures, positions, or connections) that establish a relationship to the earth. These are performed while standing, sitting, or lying on the floor. Prenatal yoga is a subspecialty.

Benefits of yoga include increased flexibility, increased muscle strength and cardiorespiratory endurance, improved mental attitude, increased self-esteem, better sleep, healthier eating habits, and better communication pathways between body, mind, and spirit. As with any new exercise program, there are basic guidelines to keep in mind: go slowly, listen to the body, pay attention to warning signals, and, most important, keep at it.

Biologic-Based Therapies
Herbal Medicine

Herbal medicine is defined as the use of crude plant-based products to treat, prevent, or cure a disease. It is undoubtedly the earliest form of medicine. In the United States there are two main systems used for prescribing botanical medicine: TCM and Western herbalism. This section focuses on the application of herbs according to the system developed in the West. Chinese herbs are covered in the Traditional Chinese Medicine section.

In the United States, herbs are not classified as drugs by the Food and Drug Administration, but they can be considered drugs from the medical perspective because many provoke a pharmacologic response within the body. This dispels the myth that because herbs are natural, they are always safe. When used by a trained practitioner, herbal therapy can provide effective treatment with low risk for side effects. Herbal medicine is health-oriented rather than disease-oriented and can be administered by infusions, decoctions, tinctures, and oils.

Box 5-2 lists herbs that should be avoided or used only with caution by a trained herbalist. Many of the herbs listed are abortifacients and are used to induce labor. For more specific and exhaustive lists of components and

Box 5-2	Herbal Remedies That Are Contraindicated or to be Used with Caution During Pregnancy

Common Name	Latin Name
Arbor vitae	*Thuja occidentalis*
Barberry	*Berris vulgaris*
Beth root	*Trillium erectum*
Black cohosh	*Cimicifuga racemosa*
Blue cohosh	*Caulophyllum thalictroides*
Cinchona bark	*Chichona spp*
Cotton root bark	*Gossypium hebaceum*
Goldenseal	*Hydrastis canadensis*
Juniper	*Juniperus communis*
Motherwort	*Leonurus cardiaca*
Mugwort	*Artemisia vulgaris*
Pennyroyal	*Mentha pulegium*
Poke root	*Phytolacca americana*
Rue	*Ruta graveolens*
Sage	*Salvia officinalis*
Squaw vine	*Mitchella repens*
Tansy	*Tanacetum vulgare*
Wormwood	*Artemisia absinthium*

From Tiran D, Mack S: *Complementary therapies for pregnancy and childbirth*, ed 2, London, 2000, Bailliere Tindall.

properties of herbs produced in Western medicine and their effects on pregnancy, refer to the book *Natural Medicines: Comprehensive Database, 2000* (Pharmacist's Letter, 2000). Herbal remedies can be used during pregnancy to treat many ailments, such as hypertension, dysglycemia, nausea and vomiting, threatened miscarriage, varicose veins, hemorrhoids, constipation, anemia, heartburn, cystitis, herpes, fatigue, mood changes, and bacterial, fungal and yeast infections.

Nutritional Therapy

Nutritional therapy includes the use of vitamins, minerals, amino acids, enzymes, and natural food supplements to maintain health or treat disease. Vitamins are essential to all life and contribute to good health by regulating the metabolism and assisting the biochemical processes that release energy from digested food.

Minerals are needed by every living cell to ensure proper function and structure. They are needed for proper composition of body fluids, formation of blood and bone, maintenance of healthy nerve function, and regulation of muscle tone, including that of the muscles of the cardiovascular system. Amino acids are the chemical units or building blocks that make up protein. Protein is a necessary part of every living cell in the body, including the muscles, ligaments, tendons, organs, glands, nails, hair, bones, and many vital body fluids. Enzymes are energized protein molecules that act as catalysts to hundreds of thousands of biochemical reactions that control life's processes. They are essential for digesting food, stimulating the brain, providing cellular energy, and repairing all tissues, organs, and cells. Natural food supplements include a wide variety of products. In general, they can be high in certain nutrients, contain active ingredients that aid in the digestive or metabolic processes, or provide a combination of nutrients and active ingredients.

Manipulative and Body-Based Methods
Chiropractic

The science of *chiropractic* focuses on the relationship of the nervous system to the mechanical framework of the body. Chiropractors generally manipulate only the protruding parts of the spinal vertebrae, but the focus is on attaining a holistic balance of the body.

The following are the aims of chiropractic treatment during pregnancy (Tiran and Mack, 2000):
- Improve spinal alignment and stability of the pelvis
- Minimize musculoskeletal and related discomforts
- Optimize neurologic function
- Improve posture
- Provide a better space and environment for the baby
- Reduce stress
- Enhance self-image and feelings of well-being
- Enable the body to work at its optimum during and after labor
- Accelerate postpartum recovery

Massage Therapy

Therapeutic massage is defined as follows:

> [T]he scientific art and system of the assessment of and the manual application to the superficial soft tissue of skin, muscles, tendons, ligaments, fascia, and the structure that lie within the superficial tissue by using the hand, foot, knee, arm, elbow, forearm through the systematic external application of touch, stroking (effleurage), friction, vibration, percussion, kneading [pétrissage], stretching, compression, or passive and active joint movements within the normal physiologic range of motion. Also included are adjunctive external applications of water, heat, and cold for the purposes of establishing and maintaining good physical condition and health through normalizing and improving muscle tone, promoting relaxation, stimulating circulation, and producing therapeutic effects on the respiratory and nervous systems, and the subtle interactions between all body systems. These intended effects are accomplished through the energetic and mind-body connections in a safe, nonsexual environment that respects the client's self-determined outcome for the session (Fritz, 2004).

The benefits of therapeutic massage therapy are vast and include physical, emotional, and mental effects. Gentle massage can be especially beneficial for the woman with a high risk pregnancy complicated by multiple gestation, preterm labor, or both (see Chapters 22 and 23). Massage and manual therapies are safe during pregnancy when administered gently, avoiding pressure on the abdomen and uterus and prolonged supine positioning during therapy sessions.

Physically, massage can reduce cortisol levels and blood pressure, increase the flow of lymph through the body, and increase immunity. It can also stretch and loosen muscles, improve blood flow, facilitate the removal of metabolic waste, and increase the flow of oxygen and nutrients to cells and tissue. Most important, massage stimulates the release of endorphins and decreases pain. On a mental level, massage therapy increases relaxation, reduces mental stress, and enhances clarity and creative thinking. Emotionally, massage satisfies the need for human touch and caring, which increases the sense of well-being and reduces anxiety levels.

Osteopathy

Osteopathy focuses on restoring and maintaining balance in the neuromusculoskeletal systems of the body. In comparison with chiropractors, osteopaths use arms and legs as fulcrums to bend and twist the body; this is called *long-lever manipulation*. The osteopath aims to preserve the balance between joints, muscles, ligamentous structures, and nerves, which allows the body to function at its most optimal capability. Osteopathic treatment is safe, gentle, and noninvasive and therefore appropriate for pregnant women. There are a few side effects and a few contraindications to treatment, including (Tiran and Mack, 2000) any history of or threatened miscarriage, active pathology, inflammatory conditions, and some cases of joint hypermobility. Conditions that can benefit from osteopathy include sciatica, carpal tunnel syndrome, neuralgia paraesthetica, diabetes, symphysis pubis pain, coccydynia, edematous ankles, indigestion and heartburn, and round ligament pain.

Energy Therapies
Cranial Sacral Therapy

The osteopathic physician John Upledger pioneered cranial sacral therapy in the United States. *Cranial sacral therapy* is a gentle, hands-on method of evaluating and enhancing the functioning of a physiologic body system called the *craniosacral system*, which is comprised of the membranes and cerebrospinal fluid that surround and protect the brain and spinal cord.

By complementing the body's natural healing process, cranial sacral therapy is increasingly used as a preventative health measure for its ability to bolster resistance to disease, and it is effective for a wide range of medical problems associated with pain and dysfunction.

Polarity

Polarity is a holistic, natural health care system, founded by Dr. Randolph Stone, combining the discoveries of quantum physics with the wisdom of the ancients. It is based on the premise that we are fields of pulsating life-force energy made up of specific frequencies known as the five elements: ether, air, fire, water, and earth. Each element relates and flows in a balance of positive and negative attractions arising from a neutral center. Imbalances and blockages can arise when our thoughts, emotions, and physical body are out of alignment. Polarity teaches that pain and discomfort are signals for us to learn, change, and realign our lives.

A polarity practitioner works together with the client using the tools of bodywork, exercise, nutrition, and verbal guidance to evaluate and balance life-force energy. Polarity bodywork involves gentle rocking, stretching, and pressure-sensitive touching based on energy flow. Polarity exercises are easy yoga-type stretching postures that combine sound, breath, and self-massage. Polarity nutrition views food as energy and develops an ongoing, ever-changing, and creative nutritional awareness rather than a rigid set of rules. Polarity verbal guidance is based on the assumption that "right thinking" is the cornerstone of good health. Verbal processes involve understanding and feeling our emotions, taking responsibility for our lives, and creating life-enhancing thoughts.

Benefits of polarity therapy include release of pain and stiffness, increased relaxation, clearer thinking, greater flexibility, amplified energy levels, enhanced ability to cope with stress, improved communication and relationships, healthier lifestyle, and elevated levels of self-acceptance.

MANAGEMENT OF ALTERNATIVE AND COMPLEMENTARY THERAPIES IN PREGNANCY

Only those people who are trained in specific certified programs of study should apply the therapies and treatment modalities described in this section. No traditional providers should experiment with the use of therapies that are unfamiliar; they could cause harm if they do. It is essential that all providers of traditional therapies are aware of when to refer and to whom they should refer for certain conditions in high risk pregnancies.

Hyperemesis
Traditional Chinese Medicine

In TCM, hyperemesis occurs when there is a relative imbalance in the organ systems and meridians associated with digestion. The aim of treatment is to restore proper balance and stop nausea and vomiting. As with any TCM treatment, a collection of points is selected according to the individual pattern of disharmony.

Stimulation of the acupuncture point P6 (Neiguan) has been shown in multiple trials to be effective in reducing nausea and vomiting. This point is therefore added to almost all acupuncture protocols. The number of acupuncture treatments varies greatly according to the individual patient and severity of illness. In most cases, there is improvement after the first treatment. Three to five points are usually chosen. The intensity and duration of the sickness has a direct relationship to the state of the woman's digestive system (spleen and stomach meridians) before conception. The effects of the acupuncture calm the digestive system, decrease fatigue, expel phlegm, and decrease nausea and vomiting. To prevent hyperemesis in future pregnancies, it is recommended to start acupuncture treatments a couple of months before conception to balance and build the digestion and the spleen-stomach organ system.

In a study conducted in China of a formula consisting of 11 herbs, about 90% of patients with nausea and vomiting showed improvement within 2 days. Most symptoms disappeared within 10 days (Jin, 2003).

Homeopathic Approaches

Homeopathy can be an excellent choice for treatment of hyperemesis because small tasteless pills are dissolved under the tongue with little chance of inducing nausea and vomiting. *Sepia* is the remedy most helpful for ordinary nausea and vomiting of pregnancy. It is indicated when nausea is intensified by the smell or thought of foods, and/or when the woman is regarded as irritable, emotional, and selfish because of her need to be alone and quiet. *Pulsatilla* is another excellent remedy that should be used when symptoms include intolerance of warm rooms, improvement in the open air, and sensitivity to fatty or rich foods, bread, milk, or fruit. *Nux Vomica* is the remedy of choice when the patient exhibits nervous hyperstimulation with a history of drug abuse or intolerance, constipation, insomnia or ailments from lack of sleep or emotional excitement. *Ignatia* is given when there is evidence of acute grief, sorrow or disappointment. *Phosphorus* is very effective for ailments of pregnancy and is recommended when there are complaints related to an overactive imagination with exaggerated fears, burning pains, and thirst for cold drinks. Homeopathic *Ipecac* is most likely to be helpful when the condition is characterized by severe and constant nausea unrelieved by vomiting; undiluted ipecac is a very strong purgative and should never be used in pregnancy (Moskowitz, 1992). These remedies can be used alone or in combination, but caution needs to be used to ensure the homeopathic preparations of these substances are not confused with herbal products.

Hypnotherapy

When emotional factors are implicated in the cause of hyperemesis, the use of hypnosis with positive suggestions can be helpful. One approach involves the removal of any fears of hypnosis, along with an explanation of the role of the vomiting center in the brain and how it works, coupled with a general discussion about the value of good nutrition in pregnancy. Guided imagery can also be used with the mother imagining herself eating, enjoying, and retaining familiar foods in a relaxed environment where she feels safe and secure.

Herbal Therapy

The cutaneous application of wild yam cream has been anecdotally reported to reduce nausea and vomiting (Petrie and Peck, 2000). Dandelion root tea calms and strengthens the stomach, improves the appetite, and supports the liver. An infusion of ginger (in small amounts), chamomile, peppermint, catnip, fennel, red raspberry, or lemon balm can also help.

Nutritional Therapy

Food therapy includes recommendation of eating small portions of bland cooked foods frequently. Eating protein can help sustain blood sugar levels. Avoiding greasy, fatty, and sugary foods can be beneficial. Carbonated or noncarbonated water with a squeeze of lemon, grape, grapefruit, or orange juice can be a palatable way to replenish fluids. It is best to avoid coffee, soda, and other caffeine- or sugar-laden drinks. Herbal formulas also can be administered.

Common nutritional deficiencies include too little iron, vitamin B (specifically B_6, pyridoxine) (Petrie and Peck, 2000), magnesium, calcium, and protein. It can be difficult for a woman with hyperemesis to take vitamins. It is best for her to take vitamins with food because they are easier to digest and less likely to induce nausea and vomiting (see Chapter 1 for more specific traditional nutritional approaches).

Cranial Sacral and Polarity Therapy

Cranial sacral and polarity therapies can be used together energetically to normalize the adaptational processes of the body. If anxiety or any other emotional issues are at the root of the sickness, these therapies allow the body, mind, and spirit to integrate and relax in a nurturing environment.

Breech Presentation

Traditional Chinese Medicine

The use of acupuncture and TCM to correct breech presentation has attracted much attention. The technique involves stimulation of acupuncture point UB 67, located on the lateral edge of the small toe, with laser, acupuncture, electroacupuncture, or moxibustion. The technique using moxibustion involves gently heating UB 67 for 15 minutes once a day for 10 days total. It is recommended to pause after the fifth day for a couple of days and to check for change in fetal positioning. If the fetal position has not corrected, the treatment can be resumed for another 5 days (Maciocia, 2005).

It is believed that this technique increases corticoadrenal secretion through the increase of placental estrogens and changes in prostaglandin levels. This, in turn, raises the basal tone and enhances uterine contractility, thus stimulating fetal activity (Maciocia, 2005). Studies conducted in China report varying success ranging from 80.9% to 90.3% (Tiran and Mack, 2000). Studies conducted in Italy reported success rates of 66.6% (Cardini and Marcolongo, 1993) and 75.4% (Cardini and Weixin, 1998). Most research papers on moxibustion show the highest rate of success to occur at 34 weeks of gestation, making this the optimal time to administer the technique (Yelland, 2004).

Auricular stimulation therapy using a seed of *Vaccaria segetalis* on seven acupuncture points located on the ear was shown to increase the rotation to a cephalic position (Petrie and Peck, 2000).

Homeopathy

The homeopathic remedy *Pulsatilla* may potentially be successful in encouraging babies to turn.

Hypnotherapy

Hypnotherapy techniques using imagery can be helpful. It has been demonstrated that patients may experience successful turning of the baby when they attend weekly office hypnosis sessions providing suggestions for general relaxation and release of anxiety and fear in addition to listening to relaxation tapes at home. Hypnosis has been used to facilitate both spontaneous and external versions (Petrie and Peck, 2000).

Constipation

Traditional Chinese Medicine

There is a physiologic disposition for constipation during pregnancy. From the TCM point of view, it can be caused by an insufficient amount of qi and nutrients or an excess of stagnated qi. It is difficult to treat constipation during pregnancy, whether by acupuncture or herbs, because the basic treatment principle of moving qi downward is absolutely forbidden during pregnancy. Treatment is further complicated because no acupuncture points on the abdomen can be used. A skilled TCM practitioner will make dietary recommendations, prescribe safe herbal formulas, and manipulate approved points with gentle acupuncture.

Aromatherapy

The use of essential oils during pregnancy is controversial. Some aromatherapy schools condone the use of essential oils throughout pregnancy, even during the critical first three months, whereas others question the safety of their use during pregnancy at all. Citrus oils, including mandarin orange and grapefruit, used in conjunction with the massage technique described in the following text can help relieve constipation.

Yoga and Exercise

Lifestyle changes, such as adding a brisk walk each morning, can be a great boost to the digestion as well as promoting regular bowel movements. Many yoga exercises may also be beneficial. It is helpful to set aside time each day to sit on the toilet to encourage regularity. During this time, relaxation methods focusing on releasing the abdominal and pelvic floor muscles may help.

Herbal Therapy

Herbal medicine offers a variety of herbs to aid in the relief of constipation. It is important to avoid botanicals that act as strong laxatives, purgatives, and cathartics. Herbs such as dandelion root, yellow dock, flax or psyllium seeds, catnip, or crampbark can all be used.

Nutritional Therapy

Nutritional therapies can play an important part in relieving constipation. Eating an abundance of fresh vegetables and two pieces of fresh fruit a day can add bulk to the stool. It may also help to add a fiber supplement for this purpose. Congesting foods such as cheese, meat, and greasy foods should be avoided or eliminated. Water is also very important; a half to a whole gallon of water should be consumed daily.

Massage Therapy

Massage, especially gentle abdominal massage following the route of the large intestine in a clockwise direction, can help stimulate peristaltic movement.

Mental and Emotional Problems

Traditional Chinese Medicine

In Chinese medical theory, mental and emotional problems have a connection to the organ systems. Energetic disharmonies on the physical level can give rise to mental and emotional disharmonies, just as long-standing mental and emotional problems can give rise to physical problems.

Depression during pregnancy and the postpartum period are common, but it is imperative to refer a patient with severe symptoms to a qualified health care professional for immediate evaluation and care. Both acupuncture and Chinese herbs are generally effective for the treatment of minor mental and emotional problems. Acupuncture is preferred during the first 3 months of pregnancy. Prognosis depends on the TCM diagnosis. Depression related to pregnancy responds better to treatment than long-standing clinical depression and inherited chemical imbalances. The University of Arizona is conducting a study on acupuncture and the treatment of depression. So far, the results have been favorable. Stanford University is also beginning to research the efficacy of acupuncture treatment for depression during pregnancy.

Homeopathy

There are many different remedies that can treat mental and emotional problems; this is one of the biggest strengths of homeopathy. The diagnosis and treatment is intricate and individualized. Many factors are taken into account when a remedy is prescribed. Because of this, specific remedies will not be listed.

Aromatherapy

Neroli essential oil works as an antidepressant and is effective in alleviating nervousness, tension, and anxiety. *Chamomile* has a soothing and calming nature and helps promote sleep and rest. *Geranium* and *lavender essential oils* can also be used for their antidepressant qualities during the third trimester.

Hypnotherapy

Hypnotherapy promotes deep relaxation and offers a way to get in touch with deeper emotions in a safe atmosphere. Many techniques may promote the reduction of stress and anxiety.

Spiritual Healing and Prayer

Getting in touch with the divine and acknowledging a higher purpose in life can promote a general sense of stability and well-being. Counseling within the patient's religion or spirituality of choice can also be beneficial.

Yoga

Practicing yoga fosters an improvement in self-awareness and self-image. It also promotes physical health that is interconnected with mental-emotional health.

Herbal Therapy

Western herbs that can help promote relaxation include chamomile, oatstraw, lemon balm, lavender flowers, skullcap, dandelion, and valerian. All of these herbs are commonly prescribed by trained practitioners.

Cranial Sacral and Polarity Therapy

Both cranial sacral and polarity therapies work on integrating the mind, body, and spirit while promoting relaxation and stimulating the body to heal itself.

Nutritional Therapy

Nutritional deficiencies, dehydration, and lack of exercise can also contribute to mental and emotional problems. Maintaining a nutritious diet with adequate fruits, vegetables, whole grains, and lean meats can prevent mood swings caused by low blood sugar levels. Daily intake of six to eight glasses of water along with daily walking or other exercise can promote mental and physical health. Holistic theory believes that mental health is congruent with physical health and vice versa.

Low Back Pain

Traditional Chinese Medicine

Low back pain is a common problem in the last trimester of pregnancy. Acupuncture is recognized for its success in treating musculoskeletal pain, including low back problems. Low back pain is often improved within a few treatments and usually has lasting effects. The etiology of the pain is diagnosed primarily through assessments of pulse and tongue characteristics, and sensitivity of acupuncture points, which are chosen to alleviate discomfort. Both distal and local points are selected.

Yoga and Exercise

Yoga is also beneficial in balancing and strengthening the musculoskeletal system. For the best results, yoga should be started before conception or at the beginning of the pregnancy to strengthen the body in preparation for the increased weight of the baby in the third trimester. Yoga can promote good posture, which can help prevent sciatic nerve discomfort as well as back pain.

Swimming can also help relieve back pain and is quite refreshing toward the end of pregnancy. It is a great way to become weightless and provides an effective low-impact exercise. Exercise in general is a good way to relieve muscular and emotional tension and can significantly improve back problems.

Herbal Medicine

Topically, arnica can be used to relieve low back pain. A warm bath with Epsom salt and aromatherapy oils such as lavender, rosemary, chamomile, and lemon balm can help relax the muscles. Some Western herbs that can help relieve low back pain during labor are skullcap, St. John's wort, black haw, and crampbark (Petrie and Peck, 2000).

Nutritional Therapy

Nutritional deficiencies such as insufficient calcium and magnesium can lead to muscle aches and lowered threshold of discomfort. Food sources of calcium include milk, hard cheeses, yogurt, leafy green vegetables, almonds, sea vegetables, salmon, and blackstrap molasses. It is best to avoid coffee, chocolate, cola, cocoa, and red meats.

Chiropractic

Chiropractic care has been proven to be effective in the treatment of acute low back pain and can be safely administered during pregnancy (Petrie and Peck, 2000).

Massage and Bodywork

Massage and bodywork can also treat low back pain. Most pregnancy bodyworkers have special pillows that can accommodate comfortable positions for the end of the pregnancy. Benefits of massage and bodywork are twofold: massage can not only reduce pain and increase circulation, but also relax and promote well-being.

Osteopathy

Osteopathy is excellent at correcting sacroiliac problems and sciatica. Manipulations are used based on an accurate diagnosis and mostly involve long-leverage techniques.

Hypertensive Disorders

Traditional Chinese Medicine

There is no TCM category that encompasses pregnancy-induced hypertension, preeclampsia, and eclampsia. In the book *Obstetrics and Gynecology in Chinese Medicine*, Maciocia (2005) categorized these diseases according to their symptoms in pregnancy, which include edema, dizziness, headache, and convulsions.

Hospital admission and careful evaluation may be necessary. Acupuncture should be used only as an adjunctive therapy to enhance the effects of conventional medical treatment.

Nutritional Therapy

Diet and food therapy have a role in the treatment of hypertension, and a thorough dietary evaluation should be included in the initial assessment of all patients. General recommendations are increased consumption of whole grains, high-quality protein (100 g/day), calcium, and potassium-rich foods such as beets, greens, and bananas with the avoidance of refined foods. Specific foods for reducing high blood pressure include cheese, yogurt, nuts, seeds, fish, watermelon, cucumbers, parsley, buckwheat, raw onions, and garlic. It is also important to drink at least eight cups of liquid daily.

Yoga and Exercise

Daily exercise helps to improve circulation. Yoga, walking, swimming, or any exercise that stimulates circulation is excellent for prevention of high blood pressure. Yoga gives the added benefit of incorporating relaxation therapy, which in turn also reduces the risk for increased blood pressure. For more benefit, add 20 minutes of relaxation therapy to daily exercise.

Herbal Therapy

If a rise in blood pressure is due to stress and anxiety, herbs can help. Western herbs for the treatment of hypertension include dandelion leaf and root, nettles, red raspberry, hawthorn berry, lemon balm, chamomile, lavender, hops, oat straw, lime blossom, skullcap, valerian, passion flower, lady's slipper, and wood betony.

Massage Therapy

Massage therapy can promote deep relaxation and stimulate the removal of fluids from the body. Massage therapy is applicable for mild hypertensive disorders.

Preterm Labor

Traditional Chinese Medicine

Premature labor is generally considered a deficiency condition; the body does not have enough qi to "hold" the baby in position. Acupuncture and Chinese herbal therapy are aimed at tonifying the qi of the body, thus stopping premature contractions. The stimulation of the acupuncture point Spleen 4 has been shown to help the body carry the baby to term (Petrie and Peck, 2000).

Hypnotherapy

Audio-guided relaxation sessions combined with pharmacologic treatments have been demonstrated to postpone labor better than pharmacologic therapies alone (Petrie and Peck, 2000).

Induction of Labor
Traditional Chinese Medicine

Acupuncture, acupressure, and Chinese herbs have been found to be effective in the induction of labor. Women choose to be induced for various reasons, ranging from elective to mandatory. In approximately 12 separate clinical studies of the induction of labor with acupuncture, no negative side effects have been reported or identified (Tiran and Mack, 2000). One to three acupuncture treatments in conjunction with Chinese herbs can induce labor within 2 to 72 hours. Elective induction is not recommended prior to 38 weeks of gestation because success rates are higher closer to term.

Induction of labor by acupuncture involves using electroacupuncture equipment to intensely stimulate the "forbidden" points of pregnancy. Contractions are usually felt immediately and most often have lasting effects. There are specific acupuncture points for cervical dilation and for production of uterine contractions. If uterine contractions do not persist after the first treatment, another treatment is recommended within the next 48 hours, followed by ingestion of a Chinese herbal prescription. Acupuncture can be used to complement conventional medical induction techniques.

Homeopathy

Remedies such as *Pulsatilla*, *Secale cornutum*, *Caulophyllum thalictroides*, *Cimicifuga*, and *Arnica montana* can be used daily for 1 to 2 weeks before the due date. These can limit false labor, protracted first stages, and postpartum blood loss. Homeopathy remedies such as blue cohosh and *Pulsatilla* can be given during labor to stimulate progress.

Herbal Therapy

Blue cohosh and black cohosh are Western herbs often used to stimulate the uterus, ripen the cervix, and induce or augment labor. These herbs should **never** be used in conjunction with Pitocin. Evening primrose oil, taken orally or applied locally to the cervix, can also augment labor.

Analgesia in Labor
Traditional Chinese Medicine

The use of acupuncture as analgesia began in the 1950s in China with the integration of TCM and conventional medical care. *Acupuncture analgesia* refers to the pain-relieving effects and the physiologic regulatory effects obtained after stimulation of specific acupuncture points on the patient (Tureanu and Tureanu, 1999).

Both distal and local points are used, including points on the ear, limbs, and lower back. The amount of pain relief is subjective and therefore hard to ascertain precisely and objectively. Study results vary tremendously. In most cases, pain relief is significant.

Hydrotherapy

Water and baths offer a soothing and relaxing form of pain relief, which also help soften the perineal tissues. Women have been using water therapy for as long as they have had access to baths and hot water. Most women find water to be comforting and once immersed, they have an easier time letting go and allowing labor to take its course. Access to a water bath may be easier to attain at a birth center than in the hospital. If a water birth is an option, it is important to plan ahead. Some considerations follow (Wesson, 2000):

- Hospital or birth center policy
- Birth attendant's clinical experience with water births
- Cost
- Type of pool
- Floor strength, space requirements, heating and electrical safety issues

Herbal Therapy

Some Western herbs help decrease pain and tone the uterus for labor and delivery. Raspberry leaf tea has been consumed to help women have an easier labor. It tones the uterus and is a source of iron and vitamin C. Most women drink three cups a day during the last trimester. Skullcap is an antispasmodic that relaxes muscles and acts as a tonic to the nervous system. Motherwort is an herb that can be used for pain relief in the early part of a regular labor. St. John's wort can be useful for controlling anxiety and spasms. The practitioner must always obtain a thorough medication history and be aware of potential drug and herb interactions during labor and childbirth.

Aromatherapy

There are essential oils that can tone the uterus, encourage contractions, reduce pain, relieve tension and spasms, diminish fear and anxiety, and enhance the feeling of well-being. Clove bud oil can help reduce pain and is a stimulant and antispasmodic. Rose oil acts as an antidepressant, sedative, and uterine tonic. Clary sage is a specific pain reliever for labor and also acts as an antidepressant and sedative. It should not be used during pregnancy, but it is valuable during labor. Neroli oil helps to reduce fear, anxiety, and inhibitions. Jasmine oil strengthens contractions and reduces feelings of pain and panic.

Homeopathy

Homeopathy can be used to help relieve pain in labor. *Caulophyllum* may help when contractions are ineffective or when the cervix is too rigid. It can also be used during the last trimester of pregnancy to prepare for childbirth. *Pulsatilla* promotes irregular contractions and has also been used to turn a malpositioned baby. *Kali carbonicum* decreases pain in the back, buttocks, and thighs. *Cimicifuga* is effective in reducing feelings of fear and despair, as well as alleviating the pain of contractions that improve when the mother lies on her left side.

Massage Therapy

Massage and counterpressure techniques can be applied during contractions to reduce lumbar and sacroiliac pain. A variety of massage techniques have been shown to be safe and effective during labor (Petrie and Peck, 2000).

Addictions

Traditional Chinese Medicine

In 1985, substance abuse counselors and acupuncturists formed the National Acupuncture Detoxification Association to support treatment of addictions. A treatment protocol was developed at the Lincoln Hospital Substance Abuse Clinic and is being used in hundreds of settings across the country. Acupuncture detoxification can assist recovery in many ways. Biochemical effects include increased endorphin production, which results in an improved ability to cope with stress, withdrawal symptoms, and cravings. The body's natural detoxification process is strengthened. Psychologically, acupuncture enhances the sense of vitality and well-being and reinforces the ability to stay clean. Benefits include reduced cravings and stress, increased ability to solve the problems of daily living, and increased feelings of relaxation and self-confidence.

The treatment protocol consists of bilateral insertion of needles into five ear points. The duration of the treatment can be 25 to 45 minutes, depending on the need of the patient. In the acute withdrawal phase, which can last from 1 to 30 days, acupuncture is recommended five times a week or more. During the postacute withdrawal phase, which may last 6 months or longer, treatment is recommended for a minimum of three times a week. Follow-up treatments are assessed on an individual basis to prevent relapse. As with any other addiction therapy, support groups and counseling are recommended.

Hypnotherapy

Hypnotherapy and other relaxation techniques can be used in conjunction with conventional therapies to increase the success of addiction recovery.

Postpartum Bleeding

Traditional Chinese Medicine

There are acupuncture points that specifically stop bleeding, in particular Spleen 1, which can be used in conjunction with conventional methods to increase effectiveness.

Herbal Therapy

The Western herb Shepherd's purse can be administered in tea or tincture form to help control postpartum bleeding. Yarrow is also regarded as an excellent homeostatic agent and is often used with Shepherd's purse. Cinnamon and cayenne have also been used effectively.

Table 5-1   Evidence-Based Databases

Database	Description	Web Address
CHID	Easy retrieval of journal citations for professionals, patients, and the general population about different health topics	http://chid.nih.gov/
CRISP	Searchable database of federally funded biomedical research projects	http://crisp.cit.nih.gov
IBIDS Database	Database of published, international, scientific literature on dietary supplements, including vitamins, minerals, and botanicals	http://grande.nal.usda.gov/ibids/index.php
Consumer Lab	Reports of product reviews	http://consumerlab.com/
Clinical Trial	Reports of clinical trials	http://clinicaltrials.gov

CHID, Combined health information database; *CRISP,* computer retrieval of information on scientific projects; *IBIDS,* international bibliographic information on dietary supplements.

CONCLUSION

Nurses and other health care practitioners should be aware of this growing body of knowledge and recognize when to refer patients for complementary or alternative treatment. When making a referral, the health care practitioner needs information about the education, training, credentialing, and licensing of the practitioner to whom they are referring the patient. In order to keep abreast to this ever-changing body of medicine, refer to Table 5-1 for evidence-based databases.

BIBLIOGRAPHY
General

Fontaine K: *Complementary and alternative therapies for nursing practice,* ed 2, Upper Saddle River, NJ, 2005, Prentice Hall.

National Center for Complementary and Alternative Medicine (NCCAM): *What is complementary and alternative medicine,* Gaithersburg, Md, 2006, National Institutes of Health. Retrieved from *http://nccam.nih.gov*

Petrie P, Peck M: Alternative medicine in maternity care, *Prim Care* 27(1):117–136, 2000.

Tiran D, Mack S: *Complementary therapies for pregnancy and childbirth,* ed 2, London, 2000, Bailliere Tindall.

Wesson N: *Labor pain: a natural approach to easing delivery,* Rochester, Vt, 2000, Healing Arts Press.

Traditional Chinese Medicine

Abouleish E, Depp R: Acupuncture in obstetrics, *Anesth Analg* 54(1):82–88, 1975.

al-Sadi M, Newman B, and Julious S: Acupuncture in the prevention of postoperative nausea and vomiting, *Anaesthesia* 52(7):658–661, 1997.

Cardini F, Marcolongo A: Moxibustion for correction of breech presentation: a clinical study with retrospective control, *Am J Chin Med* 21(2):133–138, 1993.

Cardini F, Weixin H: Moxibustion for correction of breech presentation: a randomized controlled trial, *JAMA* 280(18):1580–1584, 1998.

de Aloysio D, Penacchioni P: Morning sickness control in early pregnancy by Neiguan point acupressure, *Obstet Gynecol* 80(5):852–854, 1992.

Holland A: *Voices of qi: an introductory guide to traditional Chinese medicine,* Seattle, 1997, Northwest Institute of Acupuncture and Oriental Medicine.

Jin Y: *Handbook of obstetrics and gynecology in Chinese medicine: an integrated approach,* Seattle, 2003, Eastland Press.

Li Q, Wang L: Clinical observation on correcting malposition of fetus by electro acupuncture, *J Tradit Chin Med* 16(4):260–262, 1996.

Maciocia G: *Obstetrics and gynecology in Chinese medicine,* ed 2, New York, 2005, Churchill Livingstone.

Martoudis S, Christofides K: Electroacupuncture for pain relief during labor, *Acupunct Med* 8(2):51, 1990.

Moskowitz, R: *Homeopathic medicines for pregnancy and childbirth,* 1992, North Atlantic Books.

Tureanu V, Tureanu L: *Acupuncture in obstetrics and gynecology,* St Louis, 1999, Warren H. Green.

West Z: *Acupuncture in pregnancy and childbirth,* London, 2001, Churchill Livingstone.

Yelland S: *Acupuncture in midwifery,* ed 2, Cheshire, England, 2004, Books for Midwives Press.

Zhao CX: Acupuncture treatment of morning sickness, *J Tradit Chin Med* 8(3):228–229, 1988.

Relaxation Therapy

Benson H, Stuart E: *The wellness book: the comprehensive guide to maintaining health and treating stress-related illness,* Boston, 1992, Mind Body Institute, New England Deaconess Hospital at Harvard Medical School.

Kolkmeier L: Relaxation: opening the door to change. In Dossey B and others, editors: *Holistic nursing: a handbook for practice,* ed 2, Gaithersburg, Md, 1995, Aspen.

Massage and Bodywork

Fritz S: *Fundamentals of therapeutic massage,* St Louis, 2004, Mosby.

Yoga

Baker JP: *Prenatal yoga and natural birth,* ed 3, Monroe, Utah, 2002, Freeston Publishing Co.

Balaskas J: *Preparing for birth with yoga,* London, 2003, Thorsons Publishers.

Homeopathy

Jacobs J, Moskowitz R: Homeopathy. In Micozzi M, editor: *Fundamentals of complementary and alternative medicine,* New York, 1996, Churchill Livingstone.

Lockie A, Geddes N: *Homeopathy: the principles and practice of treatment,* London, 2000, Dorling Kindersley.

Aromatherapy

Tiran D, Mack S: *Complementary therapies for pregnancy and childbirth,* ed 2, London, 2000, Bailliere Tindall.

Tiran D: *Clinical aromatherapy for pregnancy and childbirth,* London, 2000, Bailliere Tindall.

United States Essential Science Publishing: *People's desk reference for essential oils,* 2005, Essential Science Publishing.

Western Herbs

McIntyre A: *The herbal for mother and child,* Rockport, Mass, 2003, Elements Books.

Mills S, Bone K: *The essential guide to herbal safety,* New York, 2005, Churchill Livingstone.

Pharmacist's Letter and Prescriber's Letter: *Natural medicines: comprehensive database,* Stockton, Calif, 2000, Therapeutic Research Faculty.

Psychologic Implications of a High Risk Pregnancy

N ursing and the behavioral sciences point to the need to consider the high risk mother as a unique person who must cope with a complex group of psychologic and physiologic problems. In addition to undergoing the normal maturational process of childbearing, the high risk mother must cope with a great emotional burden and psychologic adjustment to a childbearing experience that may not culminate in a happy, healthy mother-infant dyad.

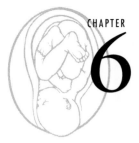

Psychologic Adaptations

To understand the emotional work and psychologic adjustments a high risk mother and her family must accomplish, certain concepts should be examined. Understanding concepts of attachment, the tasks of pregnancy, and the concept of adaptation in relation to crisis, anxiety, and frustration can be helpful when developing a plan of care for a high risk pregnant family.

ATTACHMENT

Attachment is a process influenced by many complex factors and is a permanent, interactional, emotional bond that exists for life. Parent-infant attachment usually begins at the time the pregnancy is planned or during the pregnancy, even in many high risk pregnancies (Klaus and Kennell, 1982; Kemp and Page, 1987a).

Maternal

For the mother, attachment to the fetus is enhanced when the baby begins to move, the mother's body begins to change shape, and the uterus grows. Her focus is usually turned to the baby and its well-being, at which time she establishes a relationship with the fetus (Rubin, 1970; Gay, Edgil, and Douglas, 1988). If the mother is afraid the fetus may die, this attachment may not take place because she is too fearful to establish a relationship. If family relationships are strained, it is more difficult for an expectant mother to form a positive attachment with her baby (Gupton, Heaman, and Cheung, 2001).

Paternal

The father's attachment to the fetus differs from that of the mother's. Most of his attachment centers on acceptance and support of the mother's changing physical and emotional state. When a threat to maternal or fetal health develops, the father may feel guilty for his inability to protect the mother and the fetus and to ensure a safe passage for them (Wohlreich, 1987). This may affect his attachment.

Influencing Factors

Parental attachment to the fetus and newborn depends on the following factors:

- Emotional maturity
- Experience in being nurtured
- Interpersonal relationships with significant others
- Ability to cope with physiologic and psychologic stressors
- Desire for pregnancy and self-concept of parenthood
- Fears and fantasies during the pregnancy

There is a sensitive period, immediately after birth, when attachment is enhanced through the interactions of parents with their infant. These interactions are categorized into observable sensory levels (Rubin, 1984; Sherwen, 1987).

Tactile

When given the opportunity, most parents will make immediate tactile contact with their infant. The initial contact is exploratory and is made with the fingertips. Progression of tactile contact follows an orderly pattern but can vary in its length of time. After the fingertips, the palms of the hands are used to stroke and massage the baby. Then the baby is drawn into close contact with the mother and encompassed (Tulman, 1985).

Verbal

Some parents make early verbal contact by carrying on a continual stream of soft, high-pitched verbalization (Tomlinson, 1990). The context usually involves relating how the infant resembles other family members.

Visual

Early eye-to-eye contact is sought even when the infant is not being held. The parents usually try to position themselves so that they and the infant are en face. If the infant does not open his or her eyes, they implore him or her to do so.

Entrainment

The speech pattern of either parent has a powerful influence on the infant's activity. The infant very soon forms activity patterns in a reciprocal relationship that resembles a dance. The infant's response in this manner seems to lock the parent into repeating speech over and over.

Synchrony

The first act of synchrony occurs in the feeding process. The mother responds to the infant's sucking bursts and pauses for breath. Mothers learn to respond in the cycles of sucking and pausing at the appropriate points to stimulate or discourage sucking.

If the neonate is sick and the parents' interactions and caregiving opportunities are limited, attachment may lag behind. However, according to Klaus and Kennell (1984), these parents become attached to their babies, but the attachment might be delayed.

MATERNAL TASKS

A series of developmental tasks must be accomplished in pregnancy for the mothering attachment behaviors to occur (Rubin, 1975; Gay, Edgil, and Douglas, 1988; Patterson, Freese, and Goldenberg, 1990).

Pregnancy Acceptance

Pregnancy validation or acceptance usually takes place during the first trimester when the woman determines that she is pregnant and begins securing acceptance of the pregnancy from significant others. During this time, she is concerned about herself and seeking "safe passage" for herself.

Establishing a Relationship with the Fetus

The pregnant woman begins to establish a relationship with the fetus when she can look beyond her concern about herself and focus on the fetus being part of her (fetal embodiment). This is when she becomes more dependent and wants to socialize with other pregnant women. As her relationship with her fetus grows, she begins to view the fetus as a separate individual from her (fetal distinction). The focus of safe passage at this time is for the fetus as well as for herself through prenatal care and making lifestyle changes.

Role Transition

Role transition involves preparing for the birth and early motherhood. Now the mother is seeking safe passage for herself and her baby during the delivery process.

PATERNAL TASKS

The expectant father's unconscious feelings and early memories of childhood play an important part in his emotional adjustment to the pregnancy. His involvement in the birth promotes and enhances nurturing behavior (Colman and Colman, 1971; Sherwen, 1987). The father's involvement and accomplishment of paternal tasks can be divided into three phases: the announcement phase, moratorium phase, and focusing phase (May, 1982; Diamond, 1986).

Announcement Phase

The announcement phase is the period when the pregnancy is first recognized and the father informs others of the pregnancy. This period varies in length from a few hours to a few weeks. It may be characterized by strong feelings of elation or shock, depending on the desire for the pregnancy. However, the father's response is usually mixed with pride, joy, concern, and conflict.

Moratorium Phase

The moratorium phase also varies in length but typically spans from the 12th week to the 25th week of gestation. The pregnancy does not seem real to the father during this time and is characterized by emotional distancing. Distancing allows the man to work through any ambivalence about what he will give up because of the pregnancy, such as an exclusive relationship with the mother-to-be, privacy, quiet home, and social freedom. He often spends more time at work because of his financial concerns. Marital tension and disrupted communication are common during this phase.

Focusing Phase

The focusing phase begins around the 25th to the 30th week of gestation and extends to the onset of labor. The expectant father focuses on his experience, begins to feel more in tune with the mother, and redefines his world in terms of his future fatherhood role.

HIGH RISK STRESSORS

Stress is defined as any real or perceived difficulty that results in the release of stress hormones. Recent studies (Wadhwa and others, 1998; Teixeira, Fisk, and Glover, 1999) reconfirm a correlation between maternal stress during pregnancy and increased risk for a small-for-gestational-age baby and preterm delivery. It appears that it is the woman's perception of stress that affects her and her fetus' overall health (Adler and others, 2000).

Situational and Maturational Stressors

Pregnancy itself is a situational stressor. The cognitive process of pregnancy is one of questioning and uncertainty (Rubin, 1970; Affonso and Sheptak, 1989). When a pregnancy becomes high risk and the expectant mother or her fetus is at risk for illness or death, the family is faced with a far greater situational stressor. At the same time, the family is also faced with maturational stressors.

The development of a high risk condition may disrupt the accomplishment of maternal or paternal tasks, and added stressors may result. Fears for the mother's well-being can cause heightened ambivalence about the pregnancy. Previous pregnancy losses may be recalled. This may complicate acceptance of the reality of a current pregnancy and increase the risk for prenatal and postpartum depression (PPD) (Hughes and others, 1999). If signs of bleeding or other ominous physical signs occur, it might be difficult to validate the pregnancy. Preparations for the baby may be halted. Prenatal education for self and partner also might not be an option offered to an ill or hospitalized mother. Unmet expectations for the pregnancy may be a source of frustration at a time when activities would otherwise be directed at preparation for parenthood.

Preparation for the birth process might be totally out of the parents' control if the mother's well-being is in question. Fears about procedures and care may take precedence over the usual plans. The growth rate of the mother's body may be a great concern. Choices for infant feeding, the birth process, or the coach's support might differ from what were desired.

When all or any of the developmental tasks are thwarted or interfered with, bonding can be slow in the neonatal period. If either the neonate or mother is ill immediately after delivery, early contact may not occur. When the neonate is premature or is connected to machinery, the parents might fear touching the infant. The appearance and behavior of the neonate can be so new to the parents that their visual inspection finds nothing to identify with. Finally, if the pregnancy was thought to be in jeopardy, efforts might have been devoted to "letting go" rather than "attaching to." If this is so, the parents must resolve these feelings before they can begin to attach. The depth of emotion surrounding the possible death of the baby can be so strong as to permanently interfere with attachment if feelings are not explored.

Hospitalization Stressors

Antepartal hospitalization can cause added stressors for the family of a high risk pregnancy. These stressors include separation from home, family, and other support persons, which can cause increased loneliness. Other stressors are feelings of added loss of control or powerlessness, boredom, changes in family circumstances causing stress on family functioning, and concern for the family members at home (Mercer and others, 1988; Loos and Julius, 1989; Gupton, Heaman, and Cheung, 2001). Dependency needs may not be fulfilled. Socialization with other pregnant women can be limited.

PSYCHOLOGIC RESPONSES TO A HIGH RISK PREGNANCY

A high risk pregnancy affects the whole family (Coffman and Ray, 2002). The family may react in a variety of ways to the diagnosis of a high risk pregnancy. It depends on what significance they place on the condition, their experience with coping skills, their ability to effectively problem solve, and available situational supports (Aguilera, 1997).

Anxiety

Anxiety can arise when expectations are not met. In a high risk pregnancy, the expectation of a normal pregnancy culminating in delivery of a healthy baby is threatened. The strength of the unmet needs and degree of awareness about them determine the extent of anxiety.

Threat to Self-Esteem

If the expectant mother feels the diagnosis is a blow to her self-confidence, she may experience a sense of low self-esteem (Kemp and Page, 1987b). This may cause her to feel she has failed as a woman (loss of a perfect pregnancy) and as a mother (fear of loss of a perfect baby), lowering her confidence in her ability to be a mother.

Self-Blaming

The parents may react by blaming themselves for real or imagined wrongdoing, or one parent may blame the other.

Frustration

Frustration occurs when obstacles prevent the achievement of a goal. The behavioral effects of frustration include anger, aggression, withdrawal, fixation, or finally, even learning. Frustration occurs in a high risk pregnancy when goals such as a healthy pregnancy, having a perfect baby, or having the perfect birth experience are impeded by the obstacles of illness, separation, and rigid rules.

Conflict

Conflict results when there are simultaneous, opposing goals of equal strength. If the desired pregnancy causes physical restrictions requiring financial strains or imposes difficulty in mothering tasks with other children, conflict can result. The choices offered to the mother might all be unappealing. If her goal is to have a vaginal delivery and a cesarean delivery is the only safe option for her, conflict occurs.

Crisis

A crisis occurs when an important life goal is threatened and no immediate solution is apparent (Aguilera, 1997). Inability to function results, and a state of disequilibrium ensues.

HORMONAL RESPONSE TO A HIGH RISK PREGNANCY

Placental corticotrophin-releasing hormones blunt the hypothalamic-pituitary-adrenal (HPA) axis. Suppression of the HPA axis can affect mood and increase the risk for postpartum depression. Skin-to-skin mother-infant contact stimulates hormonal production that promotes the return of normal HPA axis functioning, minimizing risk for PPD (Dombrowski, 2001). If mother-infant skin-to-skin contact is not possible because there are maternal or infant health problems, the risk for PPD is increased.

High Risk Adaptation

The ability to restore equilibrium depends on three balancing factors. First, an individual must have a realistic perception of an event resulting in psychologic crisis. Second, there must be adequate support from significant others. Third, an individual must have developed adequate coping mechanisms in the past or the ability to problem-solve (Aguilera, 1997).

To deal with the multiple crises a high risk pregnancy imposes, the mother and her family must call on past coping mechanisms and also must learn new ones. The nurse should discuss with parents ways they have responded in the past and encourage the use of tactics that have previously worked. Prior pregnancy loss should be discussed early in a current pregnancy to assess for coping strategies.

Information must be provided repeatedly about the disease or condition the woman is facing and should be explained thoroughly to provide autonomy and choices where possible. Information facilitates a realistic appraisal of the events and prepares the couple for potential future events. Significant people, especially the partner, should accompany the mother when information is given. Hospitalization should include flexible rules to allow for the father's presence whenever he can be there, and separations should be minimized whenever possible.

When both the woman and her partner can be given choices in care, personal strategies for coping are less limited and thus more effective. Skill in encouraging these coping mechanisms is necessary in a high risk obstetric setting because of the psychologic impact on the entire family. To maintain the unity of the family when the pregnancy is over, it is important to facilitate the sharing of events. Interventions in a crisis should be aimed at restructuring the present by suppressing negative uses of energy and supporting positive efforts.

Sittner, DeFrain, and Hudson (2005) found that similar themes emerge from their descriptive narratives related to the psychosocial impact of a high risk pregnancy on the family. These themes are mixed emotions, adjustments and support, and information care. From their research, Sittner, Defrain, and Hudson (2005) identified five characteristics that facilitate family coping: positive communication, enjoyable time together, appreciation and affection for each other, spiritual well-being, and commitment to the family.

NURSING MANAGEMENT DURING A HIGH RISK PREGNANCY

Prevention

A high risk pregnancy carries with it a threat not only to the physical well-being of the mother and fetus but also to the emotional well-being of the entire family unit. Therefore serious consideration must be given to assisting all family members. The nurse must assess and assist the high risk family in the use of previously learned, effective coping styles and in the development of new coping skills. To do this, the focus of nursing care must be on identifying and exploring feelings of fear, anxiety, and frustration and the resolution of conflicts in needs. Maintaining the family as a unit as much as possible, especially the mother and her partner, is paramount. Except for situations when the mother's life may be in jeopardy, the father should be encouraged to spend normal family time with the hospitalized woman. Other children should be brought in for frequent supervised visits. Socialization needs and nesting preparations should be encouraged in creative and innovative ways.

Assessment

An initial and ongoing assessment to determine the individual's and family's functioning response to the actual threat to optimal physical and emotional pregnancy outcome is paramount. This is the basis for formulating appropriate nursing diagnoses and an individualized plan of care. This eliminates making assumptions regarding how the expectant parents are feeling and how they are coping. A prenatal psychologic assessment guide, using the functional health patterns, has been developed (Box 6-1).

Nursing Interventions to Allay Fear and Facilitate Coping During a High Risk Pregnancy

- Provide time for the patient and her family to express their concerns regarding the possible outcome for the baby and to discuss the inconvenience to the mother and family of the treatment. Encourage them to vent any apprehension, uncertainty, fear, anger, and worry they may be experiencing. Talking can help them identify, analyze, and understand the events

Box 6-1   Psychologic Assessment for High Risk Pregnancy

Health-Perception and Health-Management Pattern
- What choices in your birth plan have been limited, such as attendance at childbirth education classes, type of delivery, need for anesthesia, or other medical interventions, because of the development of a high risk condition?
- Do you feel your control has been affected?

Nutritional and Metabolic Pattern
- What dietary changes need to be made because of your high risk condition?
- Why do you need to make these dietary changes?

Elimination Pattern
- What kinds of elimination changes, if any, have developed because of your high risk condition or treatment?

Activity and Exercise Pattern
- What activity changes have been necessary because of your high risk condition?
- Why do you need to make these activity changes?
- What does bedrest or limited activity, if ordered, mean to you and your family?

Sleep and Rest Pattern
- Have you had any disturbing dreams?
- How do you feel after sleeping or resting at night?
- Does this high risk condition affect your normal sleeping pattern? If so, how?

Cognitive and Perceptual Pattern
- What is your understanding of the high risk condition, proposed plan of treatment, and possible effects on self, fetus, and neonate?

Self-Perception and Self-Concept Pattern
- What does this high risk condition mean to you and your family?
- Are you or your family experiencing any guilt feelings, or asking questions such as "What did we do to cause this"?
- Is anyone upset at you or blaming you for this high risk condition?
- How do you feel it has affected your self-confidence, maternal role, and acceptance of the pregnancy?

Role and Relationship Pattern
- What are the family stressors?
- Who lives in the home?
- How has this high risk condition affected your home, work, and other responsibilities?
- How can the nurse help you and your family plan any needed restructuring of roles and activities?
- What are your financial concerns because of this high risk condition such as medical bills, child care expenses, traveling and lodging expenses for out-of-town family?

Sexuality and Reproductive Pattern
- Assess the patient and her significant other of the need to modify or restrict sexual activity.
- How does the modified or restricted sexual activity affect you and your significant other?

Continued

Box 6-1   Psychologic Assessment for High Risk Pregnancy—cont'd

Coping and Stress-Tolerance Pattern
- What are you most worried or fearful about?
- Identify stressors that are affecting you and your family because of this high risk condition.
- How is this hospitalization affecting your life?
- How supportive is the baby's father and your family and friends?
- What coping techniques have been effective for you in the past?
- What resources are available to you?
- What referral services would be helpful?

Value and Belief Pattern
- Which values, if any, are being affected or threatened by this high risk condition?

causing the fear. Beginning such discussion with a mother can be facilitated with statements such as "Many women in your situation feel . . . ."

- Encourage the father to release his fear and anxiety in a positive way instead of keeping it to himself. Couples who do not receive help together might otherwise increase each other's fear and anxiety.
- Help parents discuss their feelings with the other children in the family so that the siblings can understand why their parents are upset. Allow the children to express any guilt they may be experiencing. If they wished that the fetus would "go away," provide reassurance that they did not cause the situation and that the parents still love them.
- Encourage the expectant family to express feelings and concerns about the anticipated labor and delivery experience.
- Explain the high risk condition, all treatment modalities, and reasons for each.
- Define terms that health professionals use in talking to the family.
- Clarify misconceptions. Explain causes of the condition and, if causes are unknown, any associations or lack of association with patient activities.
- Keep the patient informed of her health status, results of tests, and fetal well-being.
- Encourage bedrest exercises.
- Help the family obtain needed social support (Logsdon and Davis, 1998).
- Refer the family to a community support group such as Sidelines (*http://www.sidelines.org*).
- Refer the family to a perinatal clinical nurse specialist, counselor, social worker, or pastoral care, whichever they desire.

Nursing Interventions to Enhance Self-Esteem During a High Risk Pregnancy

- Encourage verbalization of feelings by "active listening."
- Provide emotional support as needed.

- Help the patient identify strategies for accomplishing pregnancy acceptance, fetal embodiment, fetal distinction, and role transition.
- Encourage the patient to participate in her own care and decision making as much as possible. For example, allow her to self-administer medications and encourage her and her partner's involvement in the treatment plan.
- Support, encourage, and enhance information gathering for childbirth preparation and acquisition of parenting skills. Special childbirth education classes designed to meet the unique needs of the high risk pregnant couple are clearly beneficial (Soeffner and Hart, 1998).
- Alter the environment to enable the mother and father to meet their needs for acquiring parenting skills and for parent-child interaction.
- Allow the mother to choose her own foods within the restrictions, and encourage foods to be brought from home.
- Develop flexible visiting policies for the high risk unit. Provide extra beds for fathers-to-be to feel welcome to spend the night. Encourage siblings-to-be to visit.
- Make needed referrals, such as to social service and mental health specialists, if problems are identified.

Nursing Interventions to Promote Family Processes During a High Risk Pregnancy

- Assess the patient's responsibilities to determine difficulties she will face in implementing prescribed bedrest or limited activity.
- Teach the patient and her significant others about the importance of bedrest or limited activity for her high risk condition.
- Help the family problem-solve difficulties in implementing maternal bedrest or limited activity.
- Make needed referrals, such as to the social worker, if problems are identified that the family cannot work out.
- Provide and encourage extended and private visiting time.
- Encourage couple closeness.
- Promote spiritual well-being as the family defines spirituality.
- Involve appropriate family members in decisions.

Diversional Activity Interventions During a High Risk Pregnancy

- Assess patient's interest in various diversional activities within the activity limit.
- Provide crafts, reading, games, and puzzles that can be done in bed, or encourage the patient to have these things brought in.
- Provide classes in preparation for childbirth by way of video, a hospital television, or group classes that can be attended while reclining.
- Encourage writing in a journal.
- Refer to a divisional therapist or volunteer to provide reading materials, handicrafts, or other interesting things.

POSTPARTUM DEPRESSION (PPD)

Definition

High risk pregnant women are at risk for PPD, one of the postpartum mood disorders. PPD can occur in the antenatal or postpartum period. Understanding this, the provider and nurses should assess for predictors in the antenatal or postpartum period by the 6-week check-up and intervene early with appropriate referrals. It is also important to be able to recognize the difference between the normal "blues" and one of the four postpartum mood disorders: PPD, postpartum panic disorder, obsessive-compulsive disorder, and postpartum psychosis (Beck, 1999; Mills, 2001; Currid, 2004).

Types

The blues affect 50% to 80% of postpartum women (ICEA, 2003; Suri and Altshuler, 2004). The onset is within the first week and lasts up to 6 weeks. Symptoms include dysphoria, mood lability, irritability, tearfulness, anxiety, and insomnia.

PPD affects 10% to 15% of postpartum women (Suri and Altshuler, 2004), and the risk is higher for women with a history of previous mood disorder. According to two meta-analyses (Beck, 1996; O'Hara and Swain, 1996) and summarized by Beck (1999), the most common predictors follow:

- Prenatal depression
- Child care stress related to health problems, difficult temperament, difficulty sleeping, or difficulty feeding the infant
- Life stress factors such as divorce, job change, death of a loved one, and hospitalization
- Lack of social support
- Prenatal anxiety
- Ambivalence about the pregnancy
- Maternity blues
- Marital dissatisfaction
- History of previous depression

The onset of PPD is usually insidious, and it may take 2 to 3 months to fully manifest itself. Symptoms include depressed mood, excessive anxiety, irritability, fatigue, changes in appetite, somatic complaints, insomnia, feelings of worthlessness or guilt, and difficulty making decisions or concentrating lasting well beyond the first 1 to 2 weeks (Rice and others, 2001; Bozoky and Corwin, 2002). Ambivalent or negative feelings toward the infant are often reported, as is suicidal ideation. The sooner the identification, the earlier the referral and treatment can begin. Earlier treatment has a better prognosis than later treatment (Mills, 2001).

Metz and colleagues first described postpartum onset panic disorder in 1988. Symptoms include extreme anxiety, fear, and sense of doom accompanied by the physical manifestations of difficulty breathing, heart palpitations, dizziness, or shaking.

Sichel and associates identified postpartum obsessive compulsive disorder in 1993. Symptoms include repetitive thoughts of harming the baby leading to compulsive overprotection of the child.

Postpartum psychosis may result from unrecognized and untreated depression or independent of it. It affects 0.1% to 2.0% of postpartum women. The onset is usually within the first 2 to 4 weeks, but in acute onset, it may occur as early as 48 to 72 hours postpartum. Symptoms include agitation, irritability, depressed mood or excessive euphoria, delusions, depersonalization, inability to sleep, and disorganized behavior. Infanticide can be as high as 4%, and suicide is also very high in this group (Scottish Intercollegiate Guidelines Network, 2002; Cantwell and Cox, 2003).

Differential Diagnoses of Postpartum Depression

Differential diagnoses include the following:
- Hypothyroidism
- Anemia
- Preexisting psychiatric illness
- Sheehan's syndrome
- Autoimmune disorders
- Human immunodeficiency virus (HIV)
- Intoxication or withdrawal states
- Intracranial mass

Neonatal Effects

Untreated PPD may influence mother-infant attachment, mothering role, and family functioning. According to Beck (2002), Currid (2004), and Suri and Altshuler (2004), adverse effects on the infant include problems such as:
- Cognitive and emotional development
- Infant attachment
- Infant behavior
- Cognitive development

USUAL MEDICAL MANAGEMENT AND PROTOCOLS FOR NURSE PRACTITIONERS

Management of Baby Blues

Provide reassurance and validation of what the mother describes as her feelings. Problem-solve for support in caring for herself, the home, and the baby. This is usually sufficient to facilitate resolution in 80% of the patients (Suri and Altshuler, 2004).

Screening for Postpartum Depression

Antenatal

The first step is to identify who is at risk for developing PPD. Assess for precursors or risk factors in the antenatal period (Beck, 1999; Mills, 2001).
- History of previous depression, including PPD

- Stressful life events occurring presently, such as divorce, job change, or death of a loved one
- Lack of spousal or partner support
- Lack of adequate social support system
- Previous pregnancy loss through miscarriage, stillbirth, or neonatal death
- Previous pregnancy complicated by an unexpected or unintended outcome
- Current pregnancy, which is complicated with or without potential unintended outcomes

The next step in the management of postpartum depression is early detection. Several screening tools are available to health care providers to screen for PPD, such as the Postpartum Depression Predictors Inventory (PDPI), Postpartum Depression Screening Scale (PDSS), Beck Depression Inventory-II (BDI-II), and Edinburgh Postnatal Depression Scale (EPDS) (Beck, 1999, 2002; Beck and Gable, 2001a, 2001b; Clemmens, Driscoll, and Beck, 2004; Hanna and others, 2004) (Box 6-2). Screening is imperative and should be carried out by all health care providers managing the woman's health during the first year following childbirth. It can start as early as 2 to 3 days postpartum (Dennis, Janssen, and Singer, 2004). Assessment can also be carried out during well-child visits (Chaudron and others, 2004).

Diagnosis of Postpartum Depression

It is also important to identify timing of onset of symptoms in relation to the delivery, and providers must recognize their own limitations. Providers of women's health care and nurses caring for women in these areas are gatekeepers. We are there to know how to identify the problem and to make the appropriate referrals in a timely manner. Depression After Delivery Inc. *(http://www. depressionafterdelivery.com)* provides a current list of health care providers, such as psychiatrists, psychologists, psychologist and psychiatric nurse practitioners, licensed professional counselors, and clinical social workers, who specialize in postpartum depression. Use the ICD–9 code definition for a major episode of depression with the postpartum onset specifier (Box 6-3) when the diagnosis is determined.

Treatment of Postpartum Depression

Treatment for PPD should be evidence-based, utilizing national clinical guidelines. The Scottish Intercollegiate Guideline Network (SIGN) (2002) guideline on Postnatal Depression and Puerperal Psychosis is one such guideline and can be accessed by way of the Internet *(http://www.sign.ac.uk/guidelines/fulltext/60/ index/html)*. Treatment includes:

- Medical workup to rule out a physiologic cause such as thyroid or anemia
- Psychiatric evaluation
- Counseling and psychotherapy
- Involvement in a PPD support group for social support and coaching (Maley, 2002)
- Family-focused interventions
- Possibly, pharmacologic supplementation

Box 6-2   Edinburgh Postnatal Depression Scale

Instructions to the Provider or Nurse Administering the Screen:

- The mother is asked to underline the response that comes closest to how she has been feeling the last 7 days.
- All 10 items must be completed.
- Care should be taken to avoid the possibility of the mother discussing her answers with others.
- The mother should complete the scale herself, unless she has limited English skills or has difficulty with reading.
- The EPDS may be used at 6 to 8 weeks to screen postnatal women.

Scoring

Response categories are scored 0, 1, 2, and 3, according to increased severity of the symptom. Items marked with a bullet are reverse-scored (e.g., 3, 2, 1, and 0). The total score is calculated by adding together the scores for each of the 10 items. Users may reproduce the scale without further permission providing they respect copyright (which remains with the *British Journal of Psychiatry*) by quoting the names of the authors, the title, and the source in all reproduced copies.

> EDINBURGH POSTNATAL DEPRESSION SCALE TOOL
> J.L. Cox, J.M. Holden, R. Sagovsky
> Department of Psychiatry, University of Edinburgh
> From *Br J Psych* 150(6):782, 1987
> Name _____
> Your date of birth _____
> Address _____
> Phone _____
> Insurance _____
> Baby's(ies') age(s) _____

Instructions to the Patient:

You have recently had a baby, and we are interested in how you are feeling. Please underline the answer that comes closest to how you have felt in the past 7 days, not just how you are feeling today. Here is an example, already completed:

- I have felt happy:
  - Yes, all of the time
  - Yes, most of the time
  - No, not very often
  - No, not at all

This means: "I have felt happy most of the time" during the past week.
Please complete the other questions in the same way.
In the past 7 days:

- I have been able to laugh and see the funny side of things:
  - As much as I always could
  - Not quite so much now
  - Definitely not so much now
  - Not at all

Continued

Box 6-2   Edinburgh Postnatal Depression Scale—cont'd

- I have looked forward with enjoyment to things:
  - As much as I ever did
  - Rather less than I used to
  - Definitely less than I used to
  - Hardly at all
- I have blamed myself unnecessarily when things go wrong:
  - Yes, most of the time
  - Yes, some of the time
  - Not very often
  - No, never
- I have been anxious and worried for no good reason:
  - No, not at all
  - Hardly ever
  - Yes, sometimes
  - Yes, very often
- I have felt scared or panicky for no very good reason:
  - Yes, quite a lot
  - Yes, sometimes
  - No, not much
  - No, not at all
- Things have been getting on top of me:
  - Yes, most of the time I haven't been able to cope at all
  - Yes, some of the time I haven't been coping as well as usual
  - No, most of the time I have coped quite well
  - No, I have been coping as well as ever
- I have been so unhappy that I have had difficulty sleeping:
  - Yes, most of the time
  - Yes, sometimes
  - Not very often
  - No, not at all
- I have felt sad or miserable:
  - Yes, most of the time
  - Yes, quite often
  - Not very often
  - No, not at all
- I have been so unhappy that I have been crying:
  - Yes, most of the time
  - Yes, quite often
  - Only occasionally
- The thought of harming myself has occurred to me:
  - Yes, quite often
  - Sometimes
  - Hardly ever
  - Never

From Cox J, Holden J, Sagovsky R: Detection of postnatal depression: development of the 10 item Edinburgh Postnatal Depression Scale, *Br J Psychiatry* 150:782–786, 1987.

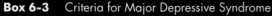

Box 6-3   Criteria for Major Depressive Syndrome

The patient must have at least five of the symptoms listed below during one 2-week
  period:
Dysphoria
Useful Question for Screening
• "Have you been feeling sad . . . down in the dumps?"
Anhedonia
Useful Questions for Screening
• "What do you do to enjoy yourself?"
• "Have your interests in these things changed recently?"
Insomnia or Hypersomnia
Fatigue or Loss of Energy
Psychomotor Agitation or Retardation
Change in Appetite or Weight
Low Self-Esteem or Guilt
Useful Question for Screening
• "Have you been really down on yourself recently?"
Poor Concentration or Indecisiveness
Thoughts of Death/Suicidal Ideation
Useful Questions for Screening
• "How does the future look to you?"
• "Do you sometimes feel life is not worth living?"
• "Do you ever wish you were dead?"
• "Do you have thoughts of hurting yourself?"
• "Do you have a plan?"

Modified from American Psychiatric Association: *Diagnostic and statistical manual of mental disorders,*
ed 4, Washington, DC, 1994, APA.

Pharmacologic Considerations During Pregnancy and Lactation

General prescribing principles during pregnancy or breastfeeding include the
need to establish a clear indication for the drug treatment, to use the lowest
effective dose for the shortest period necessary, and to use drugs with a better
evidence base of least harm. Assess the benefit/risk ratio of depression and
pharmacological risk for both mother and fetus/breastfed infant (SIGN, 2002).
Both maternal depression and pharmacotherapy have risks. When pharmacologic therapy is deemed necessary, consider the following pharmacologic principles
according to SIGN's (2002) evidence-based review of prescribing in pregnancy
and during the breastfeeding period:
• Avoid lithium, antiepileptic drugs such as valporate sodium, and benzo-
  diazepines during pregnancy and lactation, if possible.
• Selective serotonin reuptake inhibitors (SSRIs) and tricyclic (TCAs) antidepressants, except doxepin, are usually considered first-line agents if
  antidepressants are necessary. The dose may need to be increased to

maintain efficacy during pregnancy (Weiner and Buhimnschi, 2004). A systematic review of randomized controlled trials by Lewis-Hall and others (1997) conclude that SSRIs appear to have fewer side effects than do TCAs. Studies have indicated no increased teratogenic risk (Epling, 2004; Gentile, 2005); however, increased motor activity and decreased deep sleep time in the infant has been noted (Zeskind, 2004). Preferred choices of a SSRI are fluoxetine (Prozac), sertraline (Zoloft), or paroxetine (Paxil). Preferred choices of a TCA are nortriptyline (Pamelor) or desipramine (Norpramin).

- When prescribing antidepressants during breastfeeding, it is best to prescribe a single dose to be taken before the baby's longest sleep period.
- All women of childbearing age on an antiepileptic drug should take a daily dose of 5 mg folic acid. These drugs are folic acid antagonists.
- According to the Cochrane Review by Webb, Howard, and Abel (2004), the risk for continued use of antipsychotic drugs during pregnancy and lactation to the fetus/infant is unknown. Therefore use of antipsychotic drugs raises serious clinical and ethical concern without sound evidence.
- Postpartum hormonal treatment with transdermal estrogen patch has been used to treat PPD with some success (Albert, 2002).

Nursing Management

Prevention

To reduce mental illness and complications as outlined in *Health People 2010*, prevention and early recognition of postpartum depression are imperative.

Assessment and Interventions for Postpartum Depression

- Institute formal screening using the EPDS (Cox, Holden, and Sagovsky, 1987) (see Box 6-2) or another appropriate screening tool such as Postpartum Depression Predictors Inventory (PDPI), Postpartum Depression Screening Scale (PDSS), or Beck Depression Inventory-II (BDI-II).
- Provide educational materials about signs and symptoms of PPD to let patients know that you are concerned about their emotional as well as physical health.
- Refer to support groups such as Depression After Delivery (800-944-4PPD; *http://www.depressionafterdelivery.com*), Postpartum Support International (805-967-7636; *http://www.postpartum.net*), Postpartum Education for Parents (*http://www.sbpep.org*).
- If there are signs of clinical depression or PPD, make referrals for individual or family counseling.
- Assess for suicidal ideation or plans to harm self or another to determine whether referral is emergent or can wait for an opening in a schedule. It is most helpful to have interviewed prospective referral sources to determine their comfort and competencies in these two highly specialized areas of depression.
- Provide family support since PPD affects the entire family.

CONCLUSION

A high risk pregnancy imposes a myriad of psychologic stressors on individuals and the family unit. Supportive care that considers the needs of the family is a must. Without adequate support, families experiencing a high risk pregnancy are also at high risk for permanent separation, divorce, substance abuse, and physically and emotionally abusive situations. With adequate support, family members can achieve a sense of accomplishment in the face of adversity and become emotionally closer to one another.

BIBLIOGRAPHY

Adler N and others: Perspective on life can affect women's health, according to new studies, *Health Psychol* 19:544, 2000.

Affonso D, Sheptak S: Maternal cognitive themes during pregnancy, *MCN Am J Matern Child Nurs* 18:147, 1989.

Aguilera D: *Crisis intervention: theory and methodology,* ed 8, St Louis, 1997, Mosby.

Albert C: The dark days of postpartum depression, *Adv Nurse Pract* 6:67, 2002. Retrieved from *http://www.advanceforNP.com*

American Psychiatric Association: *Diagnostic and statistical manual of mental disorders: DSM-IV,* ed 4, Washington, DC, 1994, APA.

Beck C: Perceptions of nurses' caring by mothers experiencing postpartum depression, *J Obstet Gynecol Neonatal Nurs* 24(9):814–825, 1995.

Beck C: A meta-analysis of predictors of postpartum depression, *Nurs Res* 45:297, 1996.

Beck C: *Postpartum depression: case studies, research, nursing care,* Washington, DC, 1999, Association of Women's Health, Obstetric, and Neonatal Nurses.

Beck C, Gable R: Postpartum Depression Screening Scale: development and psychometric testing, *Nurs Res* 49(5):272–282, 2000.

Beck C: Revision of the postpartum depression predictors inventory, *J Obstet Gynecol Neonatal Nurs* 31(4):394–402, 2002.

Beck C, Gable R: Comparative analysis of the performance of the postpartum depression screening scale with two other depression instruments, *Nurs Res* 50(4):242–250, 2001a.

Beck C, Gable R: Further validation of the Postpartum Depression Screening Scale, *Nurs Res* 50(3):155–164, 2001b.

Bozoky I, Corwin E: Fatigue as a predictor of postpartum depression, *J Obstet Gynecol Neonatal Nurs* 31(4):436–443, 2002.

Cantwell R, Cox J: Psychiatric disorders in pregnancy and the puerperium, *Curr Obstet Gynaecol* 13:7, 2003.

Chaudron L and others: Detection of postpartum depression symptoms by screening at well-child visits, *Pediatrics* 113(3):551–558, 2004.

Clemmens D, Driscoll J, and Beck C: Postpartum depression as profiled through the depression screening scale, *MCN Am J Matern Child Nurs* 29(3):180–185, 2004.

Coffman S, Ray M: African American women describe support processes during high-risk pregnancy and postpartum, *J Obstet Gynecol Neonatal Nurs* 31(5):536–544, 2002.

Colman A, Colman L: *Pregnancy: the psychological experience,* New York, 1971, Herder & Herder.

Cox JL, Holden JM, and Sagovsky R: Detection of postnatal depression: development of the 10-item Edinburgh Postnatal Depression Scale, *Br J Psychiatry* 150:782–786, 1987.

Currid T: Improving perinatal mental health care, *Nurs Stand* 19(3):40–43, 2004.

Dennis C, Janssen P, and Singer J: Identifying women at-risk for postpartum depression in the immediate postpartum period, *Acta Psychiatr Scand* 110(5):338–346, 2004.

Diamond M: Becoming a father: a psychoanalytic perspective on the forgotten parent, *Psychoanal Rev* 73(4):445–468, 1986.

Dombrowski M: Kangaroo (skin-to-skin) care with a postpartum woman who felt depressed, *MCN Am J Matern Child Nurs* 26(4):214–216, 2001.

Epling J: FPIN's clinical inquiries: antidepressant medications in pregnancy, *American Family Physician* 70(11):2195, 2004. Retrieved from *http://www.aafp.org/afp/20041201/fpin.html*

Gay J, Edgil A, and Douglas A: Reva Rubin revisited, *J Obstet Gynecol Neonatal Nurs* 17(6):394–399, 1988.

Gentile S: The safety of newer antidepressants in pregnancy and breastfeeding, *Drug Saf* 28(2):137–152, 2005.

Gupton A: Bed rest from the perspective of the high-risk pregnant woman, *J Obstet Gynecol Neonatal Nurs* 26(4):423–430, 1997.

Gupton A, Heaman M, and Cheung L: Complicated and uncomplicated pregnancies: women's perception of risk, *J Obstet Gynecol Neonatal Nurs* 30(2):192–201, 2001.

Hanna B and others: The early detection of postpartum depression: midwives and nurses trial a checklist, *J Obstet Gynecol Neonatal Nurs* 33(2):191–197, 2004.

Hughes P, Turton P, and Evans C: Stillbirth as risk factor for depression and anxiety in the subsequent pregnancy: cohort study, *BMJ* 318(7200):1721–1724, 1999.

International Childbirth Education Association (ICEA): ICEA position statement and review of postpartum emotional disorders, *IJCE* 18(3):35, 2003.

Kemp V, Page C: Maternal prenatal attachment in normal high-risk pregnancies, *J Obstet Gynecol Neonatal Nurs* 16(3):179–184, 1987a.

Kemp V, Page C: Maternal self-esteem prenatal attachment in high-risk pregnancy, *Matern Child Nurs J* 16:195, 1987b.

Klaus M, Kennell J: *Parent-infant bonding*, ed 2, St Louis, 1982, Mosby.

Klaus M, Kennell J: Bonding: another view, *Perinatol Neonatol* 8(2):72, 1984.

Lamberg I: Safety of antidepressant use in pregnancy and nursing women, *JAMA* 282(3):222–223, 1999.

Lewis-Hall F: Fluoxetine versus tricyclic antidepressants in women with major depressive disorder, *J Womens Health* 6(3):337–343, 1997.

Logsdon M, Davis D: Guiding mothers of high-risk infants in obtaining social support, *MCN Am J Matern Child Nurs* 23(4):195–199, 1998.

Loos C, Julius L: The client's view of hospitalization during pregnancy, *J Obstet Gynecol Neonatal Nurs* 18(1):52–56, 1989.

Maley B: Out of the blue: creating a postpartum depression support group, *AWHONN Lifelines* 6(1):62–65, 2002.

May K: Three phases of father involvement in pregnancy, *Nurs Res* 31(6):337–342, 1982.

Mercer R and others: Effect of stress on family functioning during pregnancy, *Nurs Res* 37(5):268–275, 1988.

Metz A, Sichel D, and Goff D: Postpartum panic disorder, *J Clin Psychiatry* 49(7):278–279, 1988.

Mills M: In *The moody blues: mood disorders in pregnancy*, Presentation at Obstetrical Challenges of the New Millennium, Phoenix, Az, April 2001.

O'Hara M, Swain A: Rates and risk of postpartum depression: a meta-analysis, *Int Rev Psychiatry* 8:37, 1996.

Patterson E, Freese M, and Goldenberg R: Seeking safe passage: utilizing health care during pregnancy, *Image J Nurs Sch* 22(1):27–31, 1990.

Rice M and others: Postpartum depression: identification, treatment, and prevention in primary care, *Clin Lett Nurse Pract* 5(4):1, 2001.

Rubin R: Cognitive style in pregnancy, *Am J Nurs* 70(3):502–508, 1970.

Rubin R: *Maternal identity and the maternal experience*, New York, 1984, Springer.

Rubin R: Maternal tasks in pregnancy, *MCN Am J Matern Child Nurs* 4:143, 1975.

Scottish Intercollegiate Guidelines Network (SIGN): *Postnatal depression and puerperal psychosis: a national clinical guideline*, Edinburgh (Scotland): Scottish Intercollegiate Guideline Network (SIGN), 2002, June 28 (SIGN publication; No. 60). Retrieved from *http://www.sign.ac.uk/guidelines/fulltext/60/index/html*

Sherwen L: Maternal role attainment. InSherwen L, editors: *Psychosocial dimensions of the pregnant family*, New York, 1987, Springer.

Sichel D and others: Postpartum obsessive compulsive disorder: a case series, *J Clin Psychiatry* 54(4):156–159, 1993.

Sittner B, DeFrain J, and Hudson D: Effects of high-risk pregnancies on families, *MCN Am J Matern Child Nurs* 30(2):121–126, 2005.

Soeffner M, Hart MA: Back to class: helping high-risk moms cope with hospitalization, *AWHONN Lifelines* 2(3):47–51, 1998.

Suri R, Altshuler L: Postpartum depression: risk factors and treatment options, *Psychiatric Times* XXI(11): 2004. Retrieved from *http://www.psychiatrictimes.com/p041064.html*

Teixeira J, Fisk N, and Glover V: Association between maternal anxiety in pregnancy and increased uterine artery resistance index: cohort based study, *BMJ* 318(7177):153–157, 1999.

Tomlinson P: Verbal behavior associated with indicators of maternal attachment with the neonate, *J Obstet Gynecol Neonatal Nurs* 19(1):76–77, 1990.

Tulman L: Mothers and unrelated persons' initial handling of newborn infants, *Nurs Res* 34(4):205–210, 1985.

Wadhwa P and others: Maternal corticotrophin-releasing hormone levels in the early trimester predict length of gestation in human pregnancy, *Am J Obstet Gynecol* 179(4):1079–1085, 1998.

Webb R, Howard L, and Abel K: Antipsychotic drug for non-affective psychosis during pregnancy and postpartum, *Cochrane Database Syst Rev* Issue 2, 2004.

Weiner C, Buhimschi C: *Drugs for pregnant and lactating women,* Philadelphia, 2004, Churchill Livingstone.

Weissman A and others: Pooled analysis of antidepressant levels in lactating mothers, breast milk, and nursing infants, *Am J Psychiatry* 161(6):1066–1078, 2004.

Wohlreich M: Psychiatric aspects of high-risk pregnancy, *Psychiatr Clin North Am* 10(1): 53–68, 1987.

Zeskind P: Depression during pregnancy: are antidepressants safe for the fetus?, *Women's Health in Primary Care* 7(3):142, 2004.

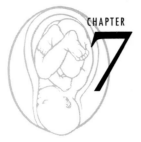

7

Pregnancy Loss and Perinatal Grief

There is a growing awareness of the significance a fetal or newborn death has on parents. This parental crisis not only involves the actual death of the baby but also shatters dreams and hopes for the future. Despite the fact that grief is a universal feeling at some time in life, the scientific study of the psychology of grief is only 54 years old, beginning with Lindemann's classic study of the survivors of the Coconut Grove fire in 1944. Although psychologic symptomatology associated with the death of a child, spouse, parent, or sibling has been widely accepted, only recently has the impact of pregnancy loss and infant death been acknowledged by society.

If one examines the incidence of miscarriage, including spontaneous events, induced abortions, and ectopic pregnancy, it is estimated that 15% to 50% of all pregnancies end very early in gestation (Brown, 1992). Taking the lowest of these estimates and adding it to the 15% incidence of stillbirth, newborn death, and sudden infant death syndrome that occur in the first year of life, approximately one third of all pregnancies, by the end of the expected first year of life, do not culminate in the healthy, bouncing baby of societal dreams (Kenner, Lott, and Flandermeyer, 2003).

Death is rarely predicted at any but the final stages of the life cycle. During gestation and shortly after birth, death seems a remote possibility. Uniformly recognized social rituals associated with death in later life are well known, whereas pregnancy loss has few accepted societal rituals. It is often said that fetal and neonatal deaths are celebrated only in the tears of the parents, yet the experience is common among people during their childbearing years. Women often tell their stories when they gather together to describe their childbearing experiences, or they tell their stories with self-imposed control during a routine gynecologic or obstetric history. Often, many details of the events surrounding pregnancy loss or infant death are told with great clarity and poignancy.

It is imperative that health care professionals in the field of maternity and family care acknowledge and learn about helpful and comforting responses needed by families at the time of perinatal loss and help them acquire support in the following 1 to 2 years. To understand the dynamics of grief work and the mourning that takes place, it is necessary to do the following:

- Explore the concepts of loss and grief as defined in the classic literature (Bowlby, 1982; Davidson, 1984; Rando, 1991).
- Describe the different types of loss experienced at various stages of gestation and at early death of a newborn.
- Identify and analyze the feelings expressed by individual family members (mothers, fathers, and siblings), as well as other support people.
- List strategies for care and follow-up that have been acknowledged by parents to be most helpful and comforting.
- Explore the potential roles of various members of the health care team in providing support and comfort.
- Describe and practice therapeutic communication skills relevant to grief support.

LOSS*

Loss occurs when something or someone valued by a person is denied to him or her or taken away after acquisition. Although the definition appears relatively simple, the feelings surrounding the loss or losses are complex.

As pregnancy and infant loss become better understood and described, it is best not to compare losses at different times in gestation or in the postnatal period but rather to identify those losses most significant to the individual. Some of the losses described by parents are the following:

- **Loss of a loved and valued person or relationship.** This loss includes adults, elderly people, children, and infants.
- **Loss of some aspect of self.** Loss of self may include loss of self-worth, of a special quality or position within society that provides "safe passage," of attractiveness, of body image, of feeling special, or of a visible or invisible body part.
- **Developmental losses.** Developmental losses include loss of parental status, of social interaction with other parents, and of sharing in firsts, such as holding one's infant for the first time, celebrating a first birthday, and sending a child to kindergarten.
- **Loss of material or external objects.** Material objects may include nursery items, layette, toys, memorabilia such as photographs, baby book, handprints and footprints, and other tangible evidence of the baby's existence.

Grief Terms

Three terms—*grief, bereavement*, and *mourning*—are commonly used, sometimes interchangeably. It is helpful to know the meanings of these terms before discussing the phases of psychologic work (Rando, 1991).

Grief is the total system response to and feelings about loss. Grieving is the process of assimilating the changes into a new sense or definition of reality.

---

*Bowlby, 1982.

Bereavement is the entire dynamic process precipitated by loss. *Mourning* is the process through which the reality of loss is integrated and assimilated. The four tasks of mourning (Worden, 1991) are as follows:

1   To accept the reality of the loss
2   To experience the pain of grief
3   To adjust to life without this baby
4   To withdraw emotional energy from grief for this baby and reinvest it in other relationships

Phases

There are four interwoven phases of bereavement (Table 7-1) (Davidson, 1984). Phases, unlike stages, do not have sharp lines of demarcation. It is not possible to move from one phase into another without retaining a sense of those phases that came before or will come to be. Phases are dynamic, symbolically likened to interweaving a tapestry of life. Kübler-Ross (1969) contributed much to our understanding of a person facing his or her own death. Bowlby (1982) and Peppers and Knapp (1985) laid the foundation for us to understand parental grieving for the death of a wished for or expected child. Davidson (1984) contributed to the understanding of the amount of time involved in the progression of grief work or mourning. Finally, grieving parents provide the most important lessons in the tremendous effort involved in grief work.

Provided with time and support to grieve, parents may take 6 to 24 months to begin to feel renewed, reorganized, and generally okay. The time it takes does not depend on the length of the gestation. Rather, it depends more on the individual's strengths, coping strategies, and ability to seek and accept support, as well as other stressors in life at the time (Davidson, 1984; Rando, 1986; Woods and Esposito, 1987).

Types of Grief

Wheeler and Pike (1991) described the following five distinct types of grief.

Anticipatory Grief

Anticipatory grief occurs when a perceived life-threatening diagnosis is given or a pregnancy is threatened. Anticipatory grief is somewhat different from conventional grief in the work the person does to adapt and the feelings expressed. Feelings of ambivalence often exist in relation to hastening the end or the actual death so that the parent can "get on with life" versus doing "everything possible" to reverse the inevitable. With anticipatory grief work, the phases must be hastened to prepare for the inevitable; thus shock is less, and a sense of finality predominates.

Inhibited Grief

Inhibited grief is kept inward and private. Outward expressions of feelings are not acceptable to the individual. Commonly, there is incongruence in feelings and expressions of them. Inhibited grief retards the ability to reach out for support and often leads to later manifestations of grief feelings and psychologic pain than would otherwise be expected.

Table 7-1   Phases of Bereavement

Phases and Times	Definition	Physical Manifestations	Feelings	Psychologic Characteristics
Phase 1: Shock and numbness Highest peak at 1–2 wk and at 12 mo	Shock and numbness protect human spirit, although temporarily; these feelings allow a person time to sort through multitude of intense feelings surrounding event; this phase permits parents an opportunity to take one thing at a time and thus make initial events more manageable and controllable	Pain in various body parts, especially constriction of throat and heaviness in chest "Heavy" heart Empty arms or emptiness in abdomen Tears, weeping, screaming Dry mouth Sighing Loss of muscle power, uncontrolled trembling, startle response Sleep disturbance Loss of appetite	Disbelief Confusion Restlessness Feelings of unreality or instability Regression or helplessness	Egocentric phenomena Preoccupation with thoughts of deceased Psychologic distancing of self; feeling as though looking at self from outside
Phase 2: Searching and yearning Highest peak at 2 wk to 4 mo	During this phase, bereaved parents have enormous energy; they have a need to look for information and find answers; there are often repeated descriptions of events leading up to and during time of death; awareness of reality of loss is beginning to be integrated into life	Crying Acting out feelings of anger Sleeplessness Change in eating habits	Separation anxiety Conflict Prolonged stress Sense of something sinister	Oversensitive Searching Disbelief and denial Anger and frustration Sense of presence or phantom crying Dreaming or nightmares Fear Guilt or shame

Continued

Table 7-1   Phases of Bereavement—cont'd

Phases and Times	Definition	Physical Manifestations	Feelings	Psychologic Characteristics
Phase 3: **Disorganization and depression** Highest peak at 4–5 mo	In this phase, parents are struck by their keen sense of reality of their baby's death and the fact that nothing can be done to turn back time and change what has occurred; they have identified some of what they miss most and can never have with their child; depression is most predominant feature of this phase	Weakness Fatigue Need for a great deal of sleep Weakened immune system	Withdrawal, social isolation, loneliness Despair or depression Helplessness or powerlessness Sick or ailing	Hibernation or holding pattern Obsessional review Working at grieving, seeking to explain sense in experience Turning point; conscious decision to go forward with life or not Most dangerous time; three choices: move forward, status quo, or not survive Forgiving oneself and others
Phase 4: **Reorganization** Highest peak begins at 1 yr and from then on	In this phase, parent has faced decision to survive, chosen survival, and taken control of life; as healing of heart and mind begins, physical well-being also returns	Physical healing or immune restoration Increased energy Sleep restoration Appetite returns	Control Sense of restructured identity Responsible Can live with knowledge of baby's death	Forgetting intense pain for longer periods of time Searching for meaning; may reach out to help others experiencing similar loss Closing circle/having a place to go Has hope for future Lives for oneself and others Takes needed time to grieve Expects and prepares for anniversary reactions

Delayed Grief

When grief is delayed, someone else must make decisions for care of the baby after death. Preferably, the person designated to make these decisions is the one most sensitive to the grieving person's desires and needs, such as the family's spiritual advisor or close, reasonably objective friend. However, in situations in which grief is delayed because of the physical status of the mother, the duty of care of the baby after death often falls to the father. Caught in his own grief at the time, he may see it as his duty to protect the mother's feelings. He may do this by delaying his grief so that he can tend to the business at hand.

Absent Grief

Absent grief may occur because of unresolved grief from a previous loss, death of one or more multiples with one or more survivors, or a concurrent mental disorder. Grief that is delayed or absent will, in all likelihood, assault the individual at a later, unanticipated time.

Long-Term Grief or Sorrow

Mourning persists in any one of the first three phases of grief, and movement through or into another phase is seemingly impossible. When chronic sorrow is evidenced, life basically stops and simple activities are impossible. In a family, chronic grief on the part of one individual disables all members.

Complicated Grief

When progress in grief work halts and the parents are emotionally incapable of continuing to work through their grief, it is called *complicated grief*. Complicated grief requires referral to a professional psychologist or crisis intervention counselor. Signs of complicated grief, according to the *Bereavement Services Manual* (Midland, 2001), include the following:

- *Persistent thoughts of self-destruction.* The person focuses on self-destructive thoughts and develops a plan of self-destruction.
- *Failure to provide for basic needs for survival.* Indications of this include social isolation; weight gain or loss in excess of 24 pounds; increased or abusive use of alcohol, nicotine, or illegal drugs; sleep deprivation; inability to care for basic needs of children in the home; or inability to maintain or initiate basic activities of daily life.
- *Persistent mourning or long-term depression.* This is characterized by being stuck in a phase of mourning for more than several months; no expression of grief after the loss; flat affect, with no demonstration of real feelings about anything; preoccupation with the image of the baby; expression of real guilt rather than imagined guilt; or hostile reactions out of proportion to the situation.
- *Substance abuse.* Use of substances such as alcohol or illegal drugs on a regular basis or talking about using to dull feelings indicates abuse.

- *Occurrence or recurrence of mental illness.* The manifesting mental illness is usually clinical or manic depression.
- *Lack of balance in life.* This may be evidenced by workaholic activity, spending increasing time away from home, or religious fanaticism.
- *Interpersonal relationship problems.* Relationship problems often are apparent when a great deal of blaming or hostility occurs.

EARLY PREGNANCY LOSS
Definition

Early pregnancy loss may be spontaneous or elective, induced events. By definition, a *miscarriage* is a pregnancy loss that occurs before 20 weeks of gestation. In the United States, state laws often stipulate that, in addition, the weight of the fetus is less than 350 g and signs of life are absent. *Abortion* is the medical term used for both spontaneous and elective, induced events occurring before 20 weeks of gestation (see Chapter 15).

Elective, induced abortions are generally performed in the first or second trimester before 20 weeks of gestation. Those done in the first trimester are usually performed by dilation and curettage or evacuation, using general anesthesia, regional anesthesia, or a paracervical block. First trimester abortions are typically done for birth control reasons, although some may be done for maternal indications, such as end-stage renal disease, life-threatening cardiac disease, vascular malformations in any area of the body that are life-threatening, or any other underlying unstable medical condition. First trimester abortions also may be done for fetal reasons, such as known teratogenic exposure.

Second trimester abortions are most frequently done for maternal medical or fetal indications. Second trimester abortions are generally induced with prostaglandin vaginal suppositories or misoprostol (Cytotec) or oxytocin (Pitocin) drips. Frequently, the procedure may be started by introducing laminaria into the cervix 12 to 18 hours before the start of any medication to induce labor contractions. The woman labors and delivers a fetus that may be born with signs of life. Some of the common fetal indications for second trimester abortion include diagnoses of abnormalities such as Down syndrome, Potter syndrome, neural tube defects, and other lethal and nonlethal fetal conditions. Maternal indications are less well defined because many maternal contraindications for pregnancy are often worsened during labor and immediately postpartum, regardless of gestation at the time of delivery. (See individual chapters on specific maternal medical complications and chapters about abortion and ectopic pregnancy.)

Feelings

Feelings Surrounding a First Trimester Spontaneous Abortion

In a first trimester spontaneous abortion, a wide spectrum of feelings may be expressed. These feelings vary from expressed relief to extreme sadness and despair.

Relief. The mother may express relief because she did not desire a pregnancy at this time. She may genuinely want this threat to herself and the embryo or fetus to end because she has been bleeding profusely off and on. Another reason may stem from her view of early pregnancy as the loss of a process, not the loss of a baby.

Sadness, grief, or despair. The mother may express sadness, grief, or despair if she has a high emotional investment in this pregnancy secondary to previous pregnancy loss and has announced her pregnancy to family and friends. She may feel the need to "untell" and to acknowledge (1) her perception of herself as a failure, (2) the sight of the baby and the beating heart on a prior ultrasound, (3) her spiritual beliefs and values surrounding life, (4) the futility of perfect planning for this pregnancy, or (5) the incongruence of feelings between herself and her significant other or other people important to her.

Neutral or unsure feelings. The mother may feel neutral or be unsure of her feelings if she finds out she is pregnant simultaneously with the time of miscarriage. She may have neutral feelings if she has had no previous experience with loss of a loved one. These feelings may also occur if this pregnancy was not planned, or if there was a physical threat to the mother from excess bleeding or pain. Many women experience feelings of being alone or concern for other family members, especially small children.

Feelings Surrounding a Second Trimester Spontaneous Abortion

It is important to understand that most women, by the time they are 12 weeks' pregnant, have made some preparations for having a baby, even if it is no more than seeking obstetric care (Swanson-Kauffman, 1986; Allen and Marks, 1993). Sometimes, at an early prenatal visit, an ultrasound is performed and the woman can see the baby and its heartbeat. This validation of pregnancy, along with ultrasound confirmation of delivery date, often changes the perception of pregnancy from being only a process to being a pregnancy that will result in a baby.

This means that the feelings of loss may be great. When discussing the loss with a woman but being unsure of her feelings, it is best to start by referring to the pregnancy and listening for her use of either the terms *pregnancy* or *baby* when referring to the loss. The nurse's neutrality encourages the woman to express her feelings without being encumbered by what she "should" do and what she "should" feel and eliminates the perceived expectations negatively influencing the woman.

Feelings Surrounding an Ectopic or Tubal Pregnancy

Ectopic or tubal pregnancy has some unique features in relation to the woman's feelings. Clouding the initial feelings may be pain or fear for one's own safety. Body image disturbance may confuse feelings, as may loss or potential loss of future fertility. Unfamiliar and invasive procedures may increase the woman's sense of vulnerability. The knowledge that there is an increased chance of ectopic pregnancy in women with sexually transmitted disease may also complicate her grief with feelings of shame or guilt if she understands that past sexual behaviors and practices contributed to the cause of her loss.

Feelings Surrounding an Elective, Induced Abortion

Elective, induced abortion adds some dimensions to grief work. Some parents have grief work complicated by strong feelings of guilt. This complication is particularly true for women who have referred to the *baby* in the first trimester and for women who have early second trimester elective, induced abortions. Some of the feelings expressed include descriptions of having decided the time of death for the baby, choosing one's own or the family's convenience over a helpless baby, feeling pressured to do what someone else advised without seeking adequate information about alternatives, or believing that the baby suffered during the procedure.

Rillstone and Hutchison (2001) reported that many parents suffer prolonged grief secondary to the stigma that surrounded their difficult decision. Often, they find it difficult or impossible to discuss this with family and friends. As a result, if there are subsequent pregnancies, they find their feelings of guilt and shame resurface. Thus they experience complicated bereavement for extended periods of time and often never come to terms with their loss. It is not surprising that this may lead to lifelong problems with reinvestment in living and relating. For most families, psychotherapy can be beneficial, especially when referrals are made early in the decision making and loss. In fact, the earlier the referral, the less likely the process becomes mired in prolonged grief.

Other feelings sometimes expressed are those centered around having extreme conflicts with beliefs and values and the need to do what is right for the family. Some women express surprise at feelings of guilt instead of sadness. Other feelings frequently expressed include feelings of abandonment by staff, physician, and even family and friends. The mother's feelings of guilt may lead to anger at those who cared for her or at those who encouraged and supported her in the decision. Although a certain amount of guilt and anger can be expected, getting stuck in these feelings or finding them totally unacceptable can adversely affect moving to another phase of bereavement. These feelings may necessitate referral for professional psychologic therapy.

Terminology

Terms used to identify the diagnosis should also be carefully chosen. Many women find the term *abortion* harsh and unkind when referring to spontaneous events. Some may feel insulted or misunderstood, believing that abortion refers only to an elective procedure. The term *miscarriage* is more neutral.

Some terms are too clinical and convey a lack of sincere feeling on the part of the caregiver. Products of conception are better referred to as *tissue* and the embryo or fetus as *baby*. *Habitual abortion*, which may be caused by an incompetent cervix, may also be offensive and prevent meaningful communication. Many women respond best to *consecutive* or *repeated* miscarriage caused by a weakened cervix.

Therapeutic Interventions*

During and after early pregnancy loss, the following aspects are what parents say meant the most to them:

- Being supported by a significant person during the experience
- Seeing the tissue
- Holding the baby
- Saving mementos
- Using symbolic mementos (When other mementos are not possible, symbolic mementos can be very important.)
- Being allowed time to grieve
- Being allowed choices (Allow time to make informed decisions about care of mother and baby.)
- Having sensitive caretakers (Assign caretakers who are educated and sensitive to feelings regarding early pregnancy loss.)
- Being allowed options (Allow the option to bury or cremate the baby even though not required by state laws. If this method is chosen, most parents feel comforted when the baby's body is sent to the morgue rather than the pathology department.)

STILLBIRTH LOSS

The diagnosis of stillbirth causes grief at any gestational stage and regardless of personal situation. *Stillbirth* by definition is birth of a baby more than 19 weeks of gestation without signs of life at the time of birth. Etiology of stillbirth varies from unexplained to severe maternal medical complications such as diabetes, renal disease, cardiovascular disease, connective tissue disease, autoimmune disease, placental abruption, labor with a fetus less than 24 weeks of gestation, malnutrition, maternal trauma, or postterm pregnancy beyond the estimated date of delivery by 2 or more weeks. Many unexplained stillbirths are attributed to possible cord accidents. Stillbirth related to the fetus is usually attributable to either extreme prematurity or congenital or genetic abnormalities incompatible with life.

In a stillbirth, often there has been little or no advance warning for the mother, despite concurrent medical problems. Frequently, the diagnosis is made immediately before the onset or induction of labor. On questioning, many women report decreased or absent fetal movement for several hours or a day or more before the stillbirth.

Feelings

At the time the diagnosis is made and the family is told, parents report a variety of feelings:

- *Shock.* They may report feeling overwhelmed.
- *Denial of reality.* They may wish that time could be reversed.
- *Confusion.* They may be confused by medical information and anticipatory information aimed at assisting them with decisions that need to be made.

---

*Worden, 1991; AWHONN, 1993, 1998; ACOG/AAP, 1997.

- *Fear.* They may fear that losing the baby to intrauterine death is equated with doing something very bad in a place where only good things should happen.
- *Anger.* They may be angry with God or with their physicians and the medical staff.
- *Guilt.* They may experience imagined guilt from inconsequential departures from perfect self-care, such as not taking prenatal vitamins regularly, not resting enough, or working during the pregnancy. They may experience real guilt about possible contributing factors such as substance abuse, including smoking cigarettes and using alcohol and crack cocaine.

Therapeutic Interventions*

Some of the things parents remember as most helpful follow:
- *Being together.* Parents appreciated being together when the diagnosis was discussed with them.
- *Having simple explanations.* Parents appreciated being given simple explanations in nonclinical terms.
- *Being talked to directly.* Parents wanted to be talked to directly when confirmatory information was given, such as during the ultrasonic examination.
- *Receiving anticipatory guidance.* When anticipatory guidance was given, it was best done slowly and in small increments.
- *Being allowed to grieve.* Unrushed time to grieve should be provided.
- *Receiving mementos.* The ultrasound picture or tape, as well as photographs after delivery, should be offered to the parents.
- *Being touched.* Parents were comforted by touch from each other and from the staff caring for them.
- *Receiving empathy from staff.* It was comforting to feel that the staff was grieving too or crying with them.

The time for labor and delivery does not usually need to be determined immediately, except when the mother's physical well-being is in jeopardy. In fact, most parents can use additional time to begin to make plans for the labor and delivery experience, as well as for the care of the infant after the delivery. Except when the mother is ill herself, she is usually able to participate in making better decisions for burial and services before the onset of labor fatigue.

During labor and immediately postpartum, what parents appreciate and remember is summarized according to Limbo and Wheeler (1986, 1995):
- *Closeness and touch.* Parents appreciated being close to each other and to family, important friends, and staff. Touch was especially appreciated.
- *Independent decisions.* Parents appreciated the encouragement and support of educated and sensitive staff in making their own decisions about care.
- *Praise.* Liberal praise for a job well done during labor and delivery was therapeutic.

---

*Rando, 1991; Worden, 1991; AWHONN, 1993, 1998; Rybarik, 1996.

- *Shielding from unnecessary questioning.* There is a need to be shielded from the necessity of telling their story or giving their health history to people not essential to the team.
- *Continuity in care.* Allowing the same nurse to continue to care for the parents during a shift and preventing unnecessary moves from the labor room to delivery room to recovery room are helpful.
- *Unlimited time with the infant after delivery.* Parents benefit from being encouraged and allowed to spend as much time as desired with the infant immediately following delivery. If the parents desire, they should be allowed additional opportunities to see the baby again. There are few rules or laws surrounding the seeing and holding of infants following death (Table 7-2).
- *Mementos.* Take many photographs and poses of the baby. Include poses with the baby clothed and unclothed, and include family members in the photographs. Collect as many mementos as possible. Mementos may include such things as a measuring tape, baby comb, blanket, clothing, footprints or handprints, blessing or baptismal certificate, shell or other special receptacle used for blessing water, other special memory certificates, and identification bracelets.
- *Referral services.* Visits and supportive help from social service, from hospital pastoral care, or from the parents' own spiritual advisor, assistance with burial or cremation decisions, and follow-up from hospital staff involved in the care may be beneficial.

NEWBORN LOSS

Two unique features of grief are present when a newborn dies. First, parents experience anticipatory grief when a newborn is predicted to die. With that anticipatory grief comes ambivalence in expectations and hopes. On the one hand, parents want the baby to survive against all odds. On the other hand, parents want the baby not to suffer or go through extraordinary treatments. In addition, the grief work needed to prepare for the inevitable is greatly accelerated. Second, often tremendous differences exist between parents' reality and caregivers' reality. Parents usually believe the baby ought to survive, whereas staff may know the baby cannot.

Parents' Feelings

Parents' feelings that need to be considered include the following:
- Parents may feel abandoned, lose hope, and have a sense of futility if given no choice as to location or route of delivery.
- Parents may fear high technology in the nursery.
- Parents may be jealous or angry at other parents whose babies are likely to survive.
- Parents may wish that the baby would just die and get it all over with.
- Parents may experience guilt about their wish for the baby to die and fear that their wish, if spoken aloud, may come true.

Table 7-2   Myths and Truths Related to Parents Seeing and Holding Their Baby After Death

Common Myths	Truths
Body must be embalmed or refrigerated as soon as possible.	Some states do not require embalming for any body, and refrigeration can be postponed for up to 24 hr. However, because of the high percentage of water in a baby, the longer the baby is out of refrigeration, the sooner the loss of moisture will hasten visual deterioration.
Parents cannot have the baby returned for additional visits related to risk for infection.	There is no risk for infection to parents, since the baby has not come into direct contact with any other body while being held in a morgue, as long as handled safely and properly.
A baby who looks macerated or clearly abnormal should not be viewed by the parents.	Studies have shown that parents who do not hold or see their infant after death regret it the most and often attribute that decision to the fact that staff actively discouraged them from doing do or gave no encouragement (Woods and Esposito, 1987).
Once the parents have decided not to see or hold their stillborn baby, it would be cruel to suggest it later.	The first decision made by parents not to hold or see the baby is often made because of fear of the dead body and not knowing what to expect. It is a decision made when the feelings of shock and numbness take hold before the mind is ready to consider consequences and when denial is in full force.
One visit with the baby is enough and should be for a limited time.	One visit with the baby is not enough for most parents. Visits are a part of searching and yearning and testing what is real.
The father or close family member knows best what each parent needs.	Whenever possible, each parent should be encouraged to make his or her own decisions about contact with the baby, making personal memories. Respecting the individuality of family members and accommodating their need to grieve in their own way are integral to mutual support.
Once the autopsy is done, it is no longer possible for parents to view or hold the baby.	Once the autopsy is done, hospital pathologists do not generally return anything to the body cavities or suture their incisions. As a result, the infant's body may be less cosmetically acceptable than before the autopsy. Certain cosmetic treatments may be performed to make the body more acceptable for viewing. Parents need to be made aware of the alterations in the infant's appearance even after cosmetic treatment. Some parents will still desire viewing. In that event, the nurse, social worker, or chaplain assisting in this should be adequately educated in the best way to support the parents. It is rarely recommended that the request be refused.

- Parents may feel guilty about minor or major departures from self-care during pregnancy.
- Parents may be angry at each other if their opinions differ about needed care for the baby, about decisions for removal of life support, or about self-care or care of each other.
- Parents may feel guilt about having "bad genes."
- Parents may feel helpless about their ability to care for their baby while he or she is so sick and dependent on technology. They may be detached from their idea of parental love for the baby.

Issues and Concerns of Parents*

Issues and concerns facing parents when a newborn dies include confusion regarding the following:
- Doing everything reasonable for their baby versus extraordinary resuscitation
- How emotionally close to get to the baby
- How often to visit the baby
- Concern that the baby will die in pain, cold, or alone

Therapeutic Interventions
Unified Plan

It is important for the health care team to create a unified plan, and parents should participate to whatever degree they are able and desire. This unified plan entails a combined approach between the obstetrician and pediatrician. Frequently, the nurse and social worker act as liaisons among the obstetrician, pediatrician, and parents.

Three important elements are needed for a successful unified approach: (1) agreement among all parties; (2) continuum of care; and (3) provision of information to the parents that presents both the pediatrician's and the obstetrician's view of the plan. The plan should not catch parents in the middle of two opposing or conflicting plans.

Documentation of this plan should include the following:
- Plans for the birth and the anticipated outcome
- Brief summary of the clinical situation
- Description of the alternatives open for discussion with the parents
- Input from the parents
- Actual decisions made and parents' responses

Helpful Strategies for Parents Experiencing a Newborn Death

- Parents are given the opportunity to be close to each other and the baby.
- Parents know they can help with some care or comforting of the baby. For some mothers, it is important to pump breast milk, even if the baby never receives the milk.

---

*Swanson, 1990; Davis, 1993; Calhoun, 1994.

- Parents know that when the baby dies, the baby was not alone, cold, or in pain. They trust and hope the nurse will take care of these things in their absence.
- Some parents want to hold the baby while it dies, whereas others prefer for someone else to do this. See Table 7-2 regarding myths and truths related to parents seeing and holding their baby after death.
- After death, parents participate in care, such as bathing, dressing, and holding after technologic equipment has been removed.
- Parents are given advance information about the baby's chances for survival.
- Parents are informed and encouraged to participate in decisions about continuing or discontinuing life support as desired or not desired by them.
- The baby is kept alive long enough that parents can get to the hospital if absent when the baby's condition worsens.
- Parents can have the baby blessed or baptized before death.
- Parents have privacy at the time of death.
- Parents are being cared for by people who are educated in death and dying and sensitive to their needs.
- When parents arrive at the hospital after the baby has died or taken a turn for the worse, the nurse, physician, or social worker meets with them as soon as possible.
- Parents have relatives or close friends included when desired.
- Parents take photographs of the baby before and after death.
- Parents collect all possible mementos, such as blanket, clothes, blood pressure cuff, comb, and remaining diapers.
- Parents make footprints and handprints.
- Parents assist with funeral arrangements and selection of a mortuary.
- Creative arrangements are made for letting the baby hear special music, breathe fresh air, and so on before death.
- A primary nurse cares for the mother before birth, and the primary nursery nurse attends the funeral.

Photographic Mementos*

Perhaps the most important mementos made or collected for the parents when a baby of any gestational age dies are photographs of their infant. Some hints for creating good photographs follow:

- Take at least one roll of 12 photographs with a 35 mm or similar quality immediate-processing camera. The immediate photographs give parents something to keep and hold onto while awaiting quality photographs to be processed. Generally, the clarity and color are truer with the latter.
- Take photographs of the baby clothed and unclothed whenever possible. Even a severely macerated baby usually has some acceptable unclothed pose.

---

*Brown, Kozich, 1994; Johnson and Johnson, 1985.

- Take each photograph as a separate pose. For multiples, take one roll of each baby separately and one roll of all babies together.
- When taking pictures with the infant on its back, prop the nape of the neck with a small rolled towel. This helps keep the baby's mouth partially closed. It also poses the baby so that the features are fully visible (Fig. 7-1).
- Use various lighting, such as some with room light on, dimmed, and off.
- Remove technologic equipment and supplies from surrounding environment.
- Select background colors carefully. Pink rarely works well, whereas royal blue, purple, and lavender are effective backgrounds.
- Use toys smaller and larger than baby and soft and fuzzy to create an environment with texture and size (Fig. 7-2).
- Include parents in some pictures, or include the nurse's arms or hands to communicate caring.
- Create a family portrait, if desired. Include siblings if they are prepared for the experience.
- Very tiny babies, younger than 20 weeks of gestation, often look best when a small-print blanket is used as a background (Fig. 7-3).
- Suggest inclusion of a religious medal or parents' wedding bands.

Picture taking is a standard of care. It is not necessary or often advised to ask permission to take photographs or to have a permit signed (AAP/ACOG, 1997; AWHONN, 1998). Parents risk saying "no" to something they later regret and cannot retrieve. Be aware, however, that for some Native Americans

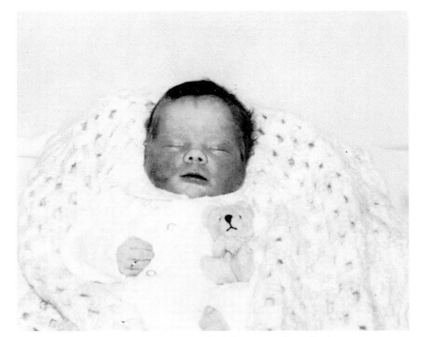

Figure 7-1 Miranda, full-term, newborn death.

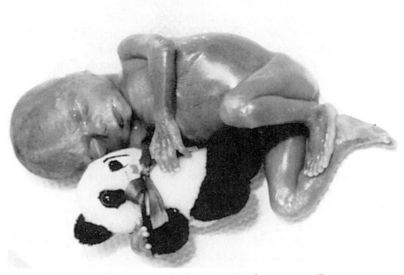

Figure 7-2 Kimberly, 23 weeks of gestation, stillborn.

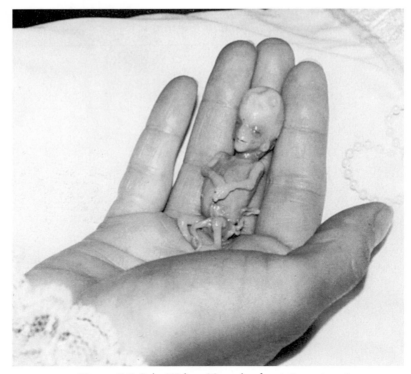

Figure 7-3 Baby Weber, 12 weeks of gestation, miscarriage.

and those of other cultures, photographs may be considered offensive or violate their spiritual beliefs. All parents should be included, informed, and consulted first.

Other Keepsakes to Make or Collect

- Footprints and handprints can be made with ink. Plaster of Paris can be used to make a mold of the shell used for the blessing, or a felt-tipped pen can be used to ink the foot or hand of a very premature baby who has no creases.
- Give a baby ring or other symbolic keepsake to the parents.
- Collect or write a special poem or message for this baby.
- Suggest the mother and father make a diary of their thoughts while their baby was alive.
- Encourage the parents to make a baby book.
- Collect a lock of hair with parents' permission.
- Powder the baby's blanket before use. Give parents only the blanket used, even if soiled. Put blanket into a sealed plastic bag, and the powder scent will remain for several years.

Morgue or Pathology Preparation*

- Use a soft wrap, without nap, next to the baby's skin.
- Position the baby's arms up alongside the head.
- Use soft rolls of towels at either side of the baby's head and body and under the chin, if needed.
- Wrap the outer cover snugly around the baby and leave its head out. Use a third wrap to cover the entire baby.
- Babies going to the pathology departments whose parents wish to see them again should be put into saline, not formalin.

OTHER LOSSES

The unexpected nature of infant death and the relative lack of societal rituals make the loss of the wished-for baby especially sad. Infant loss may also occur in ways other than death. Some such situations include the less than perfect baby with anomalies or early prematurity problems. Loss may also occur through the decision to put a baby up for adoption. Feelings discussed in this chapter may not be solely limited to loss of a baby through death.

EFFECT OF GRIEF ON INDIVIDUAL FAMILY MEMBERS AND FRIENDS

Mother's Grief

A woman has a strong sense of both physical and emotional attachment to an unborn baby from the moment she begins to think of the concept of *baby* resulting from the process of pregnancy or when she first sees the baby on the

---

*Morgan, 1993.

ultrasound. Therefore fetal distinction may develop before fetal movement is felt. The woman may feel a distinct sense of failure when she gives birth to a baby who has died or will die. In addition, she may feel blamed by her partner. Women tend to find it easier to express feelings of sadness with tears and crying. As a result, it tends to be comparatively easier for them to reach out for understanding and empathy than it is for men.

Father's Grief

The father, on the other hand, often has less emotional attachment until the woman's body begins to take on a noticeably pregnant shape. Even then he does not have the almost constant physical reminder of the reality of the baby and pregnancy. As a result, the father generally lags behind the mother in his accomplishment of the pregnancy tasks of validation, fetal distinction, and embodiment. Often, it is only at the time of birth, when caretaking activities are assumed by both, that the father's attachment feelings merge. Therefore when the baby is lost before term or born too premature for normal caretaking activities by the parents, the father's and mother's grieving experiences are incongruent.

The father also experiences a learned role expectation of protector. This assumed and imposed role often prevents the father from expressing grief as sadness. Sometimes he is, in fact, more comfortable expressing it as anger at the situation, at those caring for the mother and baby, at the mother, and at himself for not protecting the family sufficiently.

Impact on Marital Stability

The father often feels forgotten because of his calm exterior and the frequent inquiries of family and friends as to the mother's well-being. At the same time, the mother feels misunderstood by him and alone in her grief, which she expected to share. If these troublesome feelings and misunderstandings are not discussed openly, tremendous resentment can result. When the mother becomes preoccupied with her grief and the father feels forgotten, the emotional distance between them widens. Absence of mutual support and sharing can be a significant contributor to complicated grief (DeFrain, 1991).

Teen's Grief*

Every year, approximately 500,000 pregnancies end in abortion or miscarriage. Little is known about the response of adolescents to such loss or the effect it may have on their subsequent pregnancies. Wheeler and Austin (2001) studied 164 females, aged 13 to 19 years, who were sexually active, never married, and of low socioeconomic status. Those who experienced early pregnancy loss or early pregnancy loss and a subsequent pregnancy had significantly poorer scores on tools measuring depression, self-esteem, family relationships, grief responses, and perceptions of life changes. This may imply that teens who experience early pregnancy loss are at high risk for lifelong major depressive

---

*Wheeler and Austin, 2001.

symptoms. Nurses caring for them should be very sensitive to adolescent responses to early pregnancy loss and provide teen-sensitive care. Discharge planning needs to include age-appropriate literature and discussion about grief, emotions, and referrals.

Children's Grief*

According to Wass and Corr (1984), childhood concepts of death occur in four stages.

Infancy

A baby has no real concept of death, although babies form internal images of people or things in their immediate environment.

Early Childhood

Children in early childhood are governed by their own experiences and believe that everything in their world is alive, even inanimate object. They believe that wishes are made possible and events happen for personal reasons. Thus if a child wished that a new baby would not enter the family, the child may believe that this wish has come true. Children at this age also have difficulty comprehending things as final.

Late Childhood and Preadolescence

Death is understood as a final and permanent event. The child, however, feels it is an event that cannot happen to him or her. The child finds the process of dying and the dead body to be a source of curiosity and interest.

Mature Stage

Understanding death as an adult begins in adolescence. Death is finally understood to be irreversible and inevitable. By this stage, adolescents can develop abstract views about death.

Siblings have varying degrees of attachment to an expected new baby in the family. When pregnancy loss occurs in a family, siblings may develop symptoms of depression, aggression, sleep disturbances, and anxiety. Children are vulnerable and very dependent on the adults in their world. When parents are perceived as withdrawn from the child because of grief over their loss, the other children feel threatened and unsafe.

It is advisable for parents to call on trusted extended family members or friends to be available to children, especially in the beginning. Siblings should be included in age-appropriate discussions and expressions of grief and sadness. Although it normally takes adults at least 1 to 2 years to work through their grief, a child may accomplish this in 3 to 6 months. This rapid progression may be distressing to parents. Parents with other children should receive education and assistance in providing support to their children.

---

*AAP, 1992; Silverman, Worden, 1992a; Wolfelt, 1992.

Responses of Grandparents

Often, grandparents of the baby who died find it very difficult to help their children, the parents. The inability to console and support is caused by their involvement in their own grief. Grandparents have grief for the death of their grandchild and are, at the same time, hurting from the pain their own child, the parent, must experience. These feelings may lead to an understandable although unhelpful overprotectiveness. Feeling this way may cause them to avoid the more desired approach of assisting the couple in making their own decisions. Instead, they may make decisions for them and hasten the process, heedless of the parents' need to participate.

Later, grandparents may avoid future references to the baby and fail to acknowledge the grief in the misguided belief that it is kinder to their child, the parent. This chasm in expression of feelings leads to anger and loss of shared feelings at an important time. Therapeutic guidance and counseling of families during follow-up calls or visits should address this sensitive area of potential misunderstanding.

Responses of Friends

Friends and acquaintances may not know what to say or do to support the couple. This may cause them to avoid the parents or make insensitive or moralizing remarks.

Avoidance

Friends may avoid talking about the baby at all or avoid the parents. Usually, they truly believe this is kinder. Occasionally, in ignorance, they believe that it is or should be finished business. Without a similar experience of their own with loss, they are not self-educated in appropriate responses.

Insensitive or Moralizing Responses

Frequently used insensitive or moralizing statements include the following:
- "At least you never knew the baby."
- "You can always have another."
- "You should get pregnant right away, and then you can put this behind you."
- "It was for the best. The baby would probably have been abnormal anyway."
- "God must have wanted a little angel in heaven."
- "If you had eaten better, stopped working, and so on, this wouldn't have happened to you."
- "I don't understand why you want to keep talking about the baby. If you'd get busy with other things, you'd feel better."
- "I understand just how you feel. My friend lost a baby from SIDS."

These responses may all be well intended but they belittle the loss experienced by the parents. Statements such as "I'm sorry. What can I do to help?" or "I'm here for you if you need to talk or tell me about it" are more therapeutic.

Self-disclosure of a personal loss that was truly similar may also be appropriate and give parents a sense of having a kindred spirit to share some of the troubled thoughts of being slightly crazy, falling apart, or not being able to make it because it hurts so much.

Supportive Responses

Remembering the baby on important anniversaries, calling the baby by name, and acknowledging the fact of the parents' parenthood also help to support the family. Expressed grief is healthy. Discussion of feelings helps the family get in touch with the reality of the experience and begin to move on to another phase of grief work. It also gives an underlying message of belief in the inner strength of the individual's ability to find solutions from within (Worden, 1991).

The following have been reported by parents to be helpful (Midland, 2001):

- Qualities of a good listener
- Silence
- Noncommittal acknowledgement, such as "uh huh," "um," "I see," "really"
- Door openers, that is, open-ended questions, such as:
  - "Could you tell me more?"
  - "When did you notice this change in your emotions?"
  - "How are you and your partner getting along?"
  - "How are things going at work? With your family?"
  - "Tell me about . . ."
  - "What helps you get through the days?"
- *Content paraphrasing.* Repeat what has been said in your own words, check accuracy, and clarify statements. For example, "What I hear you saying is . . ."
- *Reflective listening.* Partially restate what the person has said. For example, if the person says, "I can't sleep at night," respond with "You can't sleep?"
- *Active listening.* Reflect the parents' feelings relative to the content by validating what you think you heard and naming the feeling. For example, "You're sounding pretty angry about . . . . Is that right?"
- Other phrases that are helpful include the following:
  - "Could it be that . . . ?"
  - "As I hear it, you . . ."
  - "I wonder if . . ."
  - "Is this what you mean?"
  - "I'm not sure if I'm with you, but . . ."
  - "Is that the way it is?"
  - "Would you buy this idea?"
  - "Is that the way you feel?"
  - "What I guess I'm hearing is . . ."
  - "Correct me if I'm wrong . . ."
  - "Does it sound reasonable to you that . . . ?"
  - "You appear to be feeling . . ."
  - "Could this be what's going on with you? You . . ."

- "Is it possible that . . .?"
- "You appear to be feeling . . ."
- "I somehow sense that you might be feeling . . ."
- "I get the impression that . . ."

Cultural Differences in Grief*

There is probably a biologic basis to grief. If this is true, grief is universal. Tears are thought to be the one common expression of grief and are believed to contain a chemical that has a cathartic effect when expressed. Another commonality is that the greater the personal crisis or stress, the greater the need to consider issues of personal space and touching expressions.

Although many similarities exist in the way various cultures deal with the death of a baby, it is important to become aware of some important distinctions. To work with different cultures effectively, the nurse must learn to be sensitive to what parents are saying they need and want when the family's cultural beliefs are unfamiliar. A broad understanding of generalities for that culture can be learned through study, but the unique needs of that family must be gathered through an assessment. Areas to consider follow:

1   What does death mean?
2   How are various family members expected to show their grief?
3   What are the parents saying they need and want?

The grief counselor should address predetermined cultural and ethnic needs, develop a cultural and ethnic sensitivity about grief issues, and provide caring that reflects cultural sensitivity to every person. It should be kept in mind that even members of the white American majority have intercultural differences.

Cultural differences of some groups in the United States are summarized in Box 7-1.

COUNSELING PRINCIPLES

According to Worden (1991), there are 10 principles of counseling to prevent complicated grief:

1   Help the parents actualize the loss. This can be done by helping them tell their story by asking specific questions about the baby and their responses to the death.
2   Interpret "normal" behavior. To interpret behavior, the health professional must understand what is normal. Then he or she can explain responses of family and friends to the parents.
3   Allow for individual differences. Each person grieves differently.
4   Provide time to grieve. People need privacy and options. The health professional should use a nonjudgmental attitude in delivery of care and allow the grieving family time for decision making. An important question that requires a decision should be asked at least three times.
5   Examine defenses and coping styles.

---

*Corrine and others, 1992; Doka and Morgan, 1993; Beeman, 1995.

Box 7-1   Cultural Differences in Grieving

African Americans
- More than 50% are matriarchal households.
- Extended family holds very special value.
- Highest infant mortality (14.1/1000 live births) in the United States (Giger and Davidhizar, 2004).
- Illness beliefs
  - Secondary to impaired social relationships
  - Divine punishment
  - Everything has an opposite, for example, birth-death
  - Health is a gift from God
  - Some continued reliance on folk medicine secondary to frequent humiliation in health care system

Hispanics
- This group comprises Mexicans, Puerto Ricans, and Cubans.
- Father makes decisions; mother directs home.
- Children are essential; loss of a child is the loss of the future.
- From caregivers, they want an understanding of the importance of family members' presence, the ability to speak Spanish, the need for touch, incorporation of home remedies, and folk beliefs.

Native Americans
- It is difficult to generalize their cultural values because there are many tribal groups, each with unique beliefs and customs.
- Their culture is in a state of flux.
- Navajos are the largest subcultural group.
- Most are agricultural.
- The individual and nature, which are closely tied and interact, are highly valued.
- Illness is the result of being out of harmony.
- The infant is more susceptible to death while the fontanels are still open; the spirit leaves the child through the fontanels.
- Taking photographs and naming the child steal the spirit; if the infant dies and the spirit is stolen, grieving must move the infant back to the spirit world, and it is therefore more difficult than if no photographs and no naming have taken place.
- Healing and religion are inseparable; pregnant women often see both the medicine man and the doctor.
- Eye contact is rude, but close proximity at a 45-degree angle is a must.

Chinese
- There are good and bad deaths; yin and yang are belief in a balance of opposites.
- Death ensures that the spirit will begin its next stage of existence in the best way.
- There is a public sphere of self, which includes friends and acquaintances, and a private sphere, where only feelings and thoughts are explored.
- They will discuss perception of causes of death with family.
- They believe in communications with the dead.

Continued

Box 7-1   Cultural Differences in Grieving—cont'd

Southeast Asians
- This group includes Vietnamese, Cambodians, Laotians, and others.
- Family is the basis for society; large families are valued.
- Society is patriarchal.
- They are proud of children, and their high value leads to deep mourning when death occurs.
- They have a history of survival of recent horrible tragedies and loss.
- They are often Buddhist and are warned against expression of strong emotion; if angry or distressed, they will respond with increased smiling.
- Smiling shows both agreement and respect.

Reference: Yanda J: *Cultural issues in perinatal grief,* Valley Forge, Pa, 1996, Presentation.

6   Help the parents live without the baby.

7   Facilitate emotional withdrawal from the baby.

8   Help the parents identify and express their feelings. Parents should be helped to understand the importance of expressing anger, guilt, and sadness.

9   Provide continuing support. Continued support should be provided through follow-up telephone calls or visits after discharge, a sympathy card, and referral to self-help support groups.

10 Identify complicated (pathologic) grief and refer for counseling. The various family members' movement through phases of bereavement should be assessed, ineffective coping and defense mechanisms recognized, and appropriate referrals for therapy made when needed.

STRATEGIES OF CARING

It is important for caregivers to understand the nature of caring before offering support for healthy grieving. Swanson (1993) described caring strategies as follows:

Knowing. Knowing includes avoiding assumptions and centers on the patient. The nurse thoroughly assesses the patient, seeks clues, engages the patient in self, recognizes shock, and keeps in mind that parents might not hear what is being said; the parents are feeling terror.

Being with. Being with means conveying availability, sharing feelings that are not burdening, keeping promises, slowing the system down if necessary, and being with the parents after death through follow-up calls and sympathy notes.

Doing for. Doing for includes comforting, anticipating needs, performing competently, and setting up a plan of help.

Enabling. Enabling means informing and explaining, supporting and allowing, focusing, generating alternatives, and validating and giving feedback by teaching and encouraging, providing time to make difficult decisions, and asking questions at least three times if a decision must be made.

Maintaining belief. Belief can be maintained by manifesting belief in the individual, maintaining a hope-filled attitude about the individual's ability to cope, offering realistic optimism, and being willing to go the distance with the parents. This includes respecting them. The nurse must respect the parents' knowledge of the baby as a person and their knowledge of what they need.

ROLES OF VARIOUS TEAM MEMBERS*
Nurse
The nurse has many functions in providing support and comfort:
- Communication with other hospital personnel and support services
- Provide consistent responses
- Serve as patient advocate
- Provide support
- Provide continuity of care
- Assess each individual's needs
- Identify pathologic responses
- Be willing to bend the rules
- Provide privacy

Social Worker
The social worker is usually the advocate for the immediate and extended family. The social worker, as advocate, has several responsibilities (Woods and Esposito, 1987):
- Assesses family dynamics after the loss
- Responds to individual needs
- Interacts with the family after discharge
- Provides education about other children's needs
- Counsels extended family, such as grandparents
- Makes needed referrals

Chaplain
The hospital chaplain is an important team member. It is generally best to involve him or her as early as possible. It is wise to let the chaplain explain his or her role to the parents. The major functions of the chaplain (Woods and Esposito, 1987) are listed below:
- Acts as a nonmedical friend and companion who has been educated in the skills of therapeutic listening
- Helps the family to define faith
- Allows the family to express negative feelings, especially anger
- Acknowledges parents' hopes and dreams
- Provides a personalized approach to assisting with plans for memorial or funeral services as needed

*Woods and Esposito, 1987; Rybarik, 1994.

Funeral Director

The funeral director is integral in assisting with the creation of a moment to acknowledge grief. The main role of the funeral director is to facilitate a special remembrance of the significance of this baby. According to Woods and Esposito (1987), the funeral director does this in the following manner:

- Provides choices
- Assists in selection of casket, vault, or urn
- Can suggest low-cost options for parents who have no funds (may include assuming the cost of honoraria, cemetery charges, newspaper notices, and flowers)
- Performs embalming procedures, dressing, and casketing
- Communicates with pathologists to preserve the integrity of the body
- Guides parents as they dress, hold, and photograph their baby
- Comforts the extended family
- Provides visitation privacy if desired
- Assembles the family
- Conducts the service
- Offers a post funeral reception
- Supplements extended support through education and referrals

Obstetrician, Pediatrician, Perinatologist, Neonatologist, or Primary Care Provider (Physician, Midwife, or Nurse Practitioner)

This provider has both inpatient and outpatient roles.

Inpatient Roles

- Discusses maternal and fetal conditions with parents
- Provides alternatives to the medical plan from which parents have a right to choose
- Works with the grief support team, that is, nurse, social worker, and chaplain
- Communicates important considerations to the pathologist
- Plans with the pediatric or neonatal team when baby is or may be under his or her care

Outpatient Roles

- Discusses events and repeats explanations for events leading up to the delivery
- Assesses psychologic need for short-term or long-term counseling
- Makes psychologic referrals appropriate to the parents' needs as a couple or as individuals
- Refrains from assuming the role of professional counselor when this would be inappropriate but distinguishes between healthy grief and complicated grief
- Provides 1-week follow-up postpartum care

The care providers and nursing team for the newborn should be involved in contributing to the treatment plan and communicating with the family as soon as potential or probable problems are evident. Either the obstetrician or the pediatrician should discuss autopsy or genetic study results with the parents. This should be done at a scheduled conference and preferably in person (see Bibliography).

Geneticist

A geneticist should be involved when structural or genetic abnormalities are possible or obviously apparent. The geneticist provides information at the earliest possible time before the loss. The two main functions of the geneticist are to provide information and to provide counseling relative to the genetic results.

Peer Support

Peer support may be nationally affiliated or locally affiliated with such sources as a church or voluntary agency. These groups may have several purposes:
- Education
- Professional facilitation
- Self-help support
  Box 7-2 summarizes resources for dealing with perinatal loss.

NURSING MANAGEMENT

Prevention

Nursing care is directed at care of the immediate family and prevention of the following:
- Complicated grief
- Ineffective coping
- Individual reactive depression
- Ineffective individual or family coping
- Spiritual distress

Nursing Interventions

- Assess for expressions of normal grieving through the four phases of bereavement (see Table 7-1).
- Assess the mother for postpartum depression using the Edinburgh Postnatal Depression Scale. Refer her to a knowledgeable grief counselor if the score is higher than 15 points. Urgent referral is required if the score is higher than 24.
- Evaluate normal family coping mechanisms and relationships among family members. Evaluate effectiveness of coping with the stress.
- Observe for signs of change, signs of conflict, denial of role responsibilities, or inability to perform role responsibilities as culturally appropriate.
- Assess the family's support system.
- Screen for effective or ineffective management of adaptive tasks.

Box 7-2 °Resources for Dealing with Perinatal Loss

The Compassionate Friends
P.O. Box 3696
Oak Brook, IL 60522-3696
Phone: 630-990-0010
www.compassionatefriends.org
  This nondenominational self-help organization offers friendship and support to parents who have suffered the death of a child of any age. Support and friendship are provided in the forms of monthly meetings, telephone friends, and resource material. Any bereaved parent can become a member by simply requesting assistance from the local chapter. There are no dues or membership fees. Because families who have experienced the death of a baby through miscarriage, stillbirth, or newborn death often do not feel comfortable in such a diverse group, The Compassionate Friends provides umbrella support through education for groups who want to focus on infant loss.

Pregnancy and Infant Loss Network
1421 East Wayzata Boulevard
Suite #30
Wayzata, MN 55391
Phone: 612-473-9372
  Founded in 1983 by a group of bereaved parents, this national organization promotes an environment in which families can participate in healthy grieving, helps families find and use their own support networks, provides information and education to professionals, and serves as parent advocate after the death of a high risk neonate. PILC makes referrals to local support groups, publishes a quarterly newsletter, distributes literature on perinatal bereavement, and gives workshops and in-service programs.

RTS Bereavement Services
Gundersen Lutheran Medical Foundation
1900 South Avenue
La Crosse, WI 54601
Phone: 800-362-9567/608-775-4747
www.bereavementservices.org
  This comprehensive hospital-based perinatal bereavement program provides guidelines for professionals caring for families who have experienced miscarriage, ectopic pregnancy, stillbirth, or neonatal death. It aims to ensure consistent, sensitive care for grieving family members. Its activities include nationwide educational and certification programs for perinatal nurses and childbirth educators.

SHARE Pregnancy and Infant Loss Support
St. Joseph Health Center
300 First Capitol Drive
St. Charles, MO 63301-2893
Phone: 800-821-6819/314-947-6164
www.nationalshareoffice.com

Box 7-2   Resources for Dealing with Perinatal Loss—cont'd

This organization aims to ensure support for parents from the time they anticipate a problem by helping them express grief and related emotions. It maintains a national listing of relevant resources and helps parents contact local support groups and other resources, such as fertility specialists and printed materials. SHARE publishes a bimonthly newsletter for caregivers and families and presents workshops throughout the United States and abroad.

- Assess each grieving member of the family for persistent social withdrawal, immobilizing emotional pain that results in incapacity to care for basic needs, chronic low self-esteem, or signs of substance abuse.
- Assess the patient's and family's spiritual beliefs, needs, and practices.
- Assess the patient's and family's faith; energize them by fostering whatever type of faith they wish to exhibit (Kennison, 1987).
- Assess for persistent distress of the human spirit and anger at God.
- Take note of expressions of inner conflict with meaning of life.
- Assess for inability of family members to deal with death constructively, to meet basic needs of individual members, to accept and receive needed help, or to express and accept various family members' individualized expressions of feelings.
- Encourage expression of feelings through the establishment of rapport. Bring up the subject and make references to the baby.
- Allow an adequate amount of time for the family to become acquainted with and say goodbye to the baby or to acknowledge the pregnancy loss.
- Slow down the system when institutional time frames interfere with the amount of time needed by the family. Be a parent advocate.
- Give simple explanations initially.
- Answer only those questions that truly ask for answers. Understand that many times, initial questions are a lament of emotional pain.
- Give anticipatory guidance for what is to come next regarding physical responses, responses of family and friends, and grief work.
- Make mementos and collect keepsakes that will provide comfort in the future.
- Provide follow-up support for healthy, functional, adaptive grief work (see Box 7-2).
- Refer to pastoral care, if the family desires.
- Refer to social worker for assistance with funeral or other ritual memorial.
- Refer to self-support group or psychotherapy as appropriate.
- Encourage both parents to experience the event together while supporting individual differences in expression of grief.
- Educate parents regarding individual responses.
- Help parents recognize signs of ineffective coping in siblings; for example, interpersonal problems at school or in the home, excessive quarreling, or regressive behaviors.
- Provide information regarding cause or lack of cause of pregnancy loss or infant death.

- Promote reliance on previously learned coping skills.
- Refer to supportive therapy when reliance on maladaptive behaviors is diagnosed.
- Promote acceptance of outside support and assistance for the first 2 years.
- Provide a resource for follow-up.
- Refer for psychotherapy when powerlessness or hopelessness threatens the individual or family safety.
- Help to prevent considerable distress for parents who are of the Catholic, Eastern Orthodox, Episcopalian, or Lutheran religions by facilitating infant baptism before death. Some members of these religions believe the unbaptized soul cannot go to heaven (Eich, 1987). If a priest or minister is not available, any nurse who believes in God can perform the baptism. Sprinkle water on the head or body while saying the words "I baptize you in the name of the Father, and of the Son, and of the Holy Spirit." For a stillborn, prefix the statement with "If this be valid." It is sometimes possible to baptize the baby through the mother's abdomen to meet the parents' desire to baptize the baby while he or she is still alive before birth but is expected to die during or immediately after birth or when a pregnancy termination has been chosen for lethal conditions in the baby.
- Encourage the various family members to express their beliefs, anger, and any perceptions of unfairness they are experiencing.
- Listen and maintain a nonjudgmental attitude.
- Refer to hospital chaplain, rabbi, or appropriate religious specialist.
- Provide follow-up therapeutic listening and communication for a minimum of 3 months.
- Explain responses of others and incongruent grief of mothers and fathers.
- Follow the principles of counseling when making these follow-up contacts.
- Refer to appropriate therapy when the family unit is identified as dysfunctional.

CONCLUSION

The primary goals of the nurse in providing nursing care at the time of pregnancy loss or infant death are to maintain the integrity of the family unit and promote healthy, uncomplicated grief. This is best accomplished through compassionate, sensitive caring at the time of the death and by referring for appropriate follow-up during the first year after the loss.

BIBLIOGRAPHY
Bereavement

American Academy of Pediatrics and American College of Obstetrics and Gynecology: *Guidelines for perinatal care,* ed 4, Elk Grove, Ill, 1997, AAP/ACOG.

American College of Obstetrics and Gynecology: Grief related to perinatal death, *Technical Bulletin,* No. 86, Washington, DC, 1985, ACOG.

Appleton R, Gibson B, and Hey E: The loss of a baby at birth: the role of the bereavement officer, *Br J Obstet Gynaecol* 100(1):51–54, 1993.

Association of Women's Health, Obstetric, and Neonatal Nurses: *AWHONN standards and guidelines for professional nursing practice in the care of women and newborns,* ed 5, Washington, DC, 1998, AWHONN.

Association of Women's Health, Obstetric, and Neonatal Nurses: *Competencies and guidelines for nurse providers of perinatal education,* Washington, DC, 1993, AWHONN.

Backer B, Hannon N, and Russel N: *Death and dying: understanding and care,* ed 2, Albany, NY, 1994, Delmar.

Bhattacharjee C: Improving the care of bereaved parents, *Nurs Stand* 4(22):18–20, 1990.

Black K, Ecker M, and Librizzi R: Prevention of recurrent fetal loss caused by antiphospholipid syndrome, *J Perinatol* 16(3 Pt 1):181–185, 1996.

Borg S, Lasker J: *When pregnancy fails: families coping with miscarriage, stillbirth and infant death,* New York, 1989, Bantam Books.

Bowlby J: *Attachment and loss,* vol 1, ed 2, New York, 1982, Basic Books.

Bridwell D: *The ache for a child,* Wheaton, Ill, 1994, Victor Books.

Brown Y: The crisis of pregnancy loss: a team approach to support, *Birth* 19(2):82–89, 1992.

Buckman R: *How to break bad news: a guide for health care professionals,* Baltimore, 1992, Johns Hopkins University Press.

Calabrese J, Kling M, and Gold P: Alterations in immunocompetence during stress, bereavement and depression: focus on neuroendocrine regulation, *Am J Psychiatry* 144(9): 1123–1134, 1987.

Carr D, Knupp S: Grief and perinatal loss: a community hospital approach to support, *J Obstet Gynecol Neonatal Nurs* 14(2):130–139, 1985.

Cohen M, editor: *The limits of miracles: poems about the loss of babies,* South Hadley, Mass, 1984, Bergin & Garvey.

Conley B: *Handling the holidays,* Elburn, Ill, 1993, Conley Outreach.

Corr C, Morgan J, and Wass H: *Statements on death, dying and bereavement,* London, Ontario, 1994, King's College.

Costello A, Gardner S, and Merenstein G: State of the art: perinatal grief and loss, *J Perinatol* 8(4):361–370, 1988.

Davidson G: *Understanding the death of the wished-for child,* Springfield, Ill, 1979, OGR.

Davidson G: *Understanding mourning,* Minneapolis, 1984, Augsburg.

Davis D: *Empty cradle, broken heart,* ed 2, Golden, Colo, 1996, Fulcrum.

Davis D, Stewart M, and Harmon R: Perinatal loss: providing emotional support for bereaved parents, *Birth* 15(4):242–246, 1988.

DeFrain J: Learning about grief from normal families: SIDS, stillbirth and miscarriage, *J Marital Fam Ther* 17:215, 1991.

Ewy D, Ewy R: *Death of a dream: miscarriage, stillbirth, and newborn loss,* New York, 1984, Dutton.

Fretts R and others: The changing pattern of fetal death, 1961–1989, *Obstet Gynecol* 79(1):35–39, 1992.

Friedman R, Gradstein B: *Surviving pregnancy loss,* Boston, 1996, Little, Brown.

Galinsky E: *Between generations: the six stages of parenthood,* New York, 1987, Addison Wesley.

Graves S, Williams S: *Holiday help: hope and healing for those who grieve,* Louisville, Ky, 1992, Accord.

Harrigan R and others: Perinatal grief: response to the loss of an infant, *Neonatal Netw* 12(5):25–31, 1993.

Ilse S: *Empty arms: coping with miscarriage, stillbirth and infant death,* Maple Plain, Minn, 1990, Wintergreen Press.

Irwin M, Daniels M, and Weiner H: Immune and neuroendocrine changes during bereavement, *Psychiatr Clin North Am* 10(3):449–465, 1987.

Klaus M, Kennel J: *Parent-infant bonding,* St Louis, 1982, Mosby.

Kohn I, Moffit PL: *A silent sorrow,* New York, 1992, Bantam Doubleday Dell.

Kowalski K: Loss bereavement: psychological, sociological, spiritual and ontological perspectives, In Simpson KR, Creehan PA, editors: *AWHONN's perinatal nursing,* Philadelphia, 1996, Lippincott-Raven.

Kübler-Ross E: *On death and dying,* New York, 1969, MacMillan.

Lasker J, Toedter L: Acute versus chronic grief: the case of pregnancy loss, *Am J Orthopsychiatry* 61(4):510–522, 1991.

Lederman R: *Psychosocial adaptation in pregnancy,* Englewood Cliffs, NJ, 1984, Prentice Hall.

Leon I: The psychoanalytic conceptualization of perinatal loss: a multidimensional model, *Am J Psychiatry* 149(11):1464–1472, 1992.

Leon I: Understanding and coping with reproductive losses, *Womens Psychiatr Health* 3(1):1, 1994.

Limbo R, Wheeler S: Coping with unexpected outcomes, *NAACOG Update Series* 5(3):1, 1986.

Limbo R, Wheeler S: *When a baby dies: a handbook for healing and helping,* La Crosse, Wisc, 1995, Bereavement Services/RTS.

Lindemann E: Symptomatology and management of acute grief, *Am J Psychiatry* 101:141, 1944.

Locke SA: *Coping with loss: a guide for caregivers,* Springfield, Ill, 1994, Charles C Thomas.

Manning D: *Don't take my grief away from me,* San Francisco, 1984, Harper & Row for Insight Books.

Meier P and others: Perinatal autopsy: its clinical value, *Obstet Gynecol* 67(3):349–351, 1986.

Midland D, editor: *Bereavement services RTS bereavement training manual,* ed 4, La Crosse, Wisc, 2001, Bereavement Services, La Crosse Lutheran Hospital/Gundersen Medical Foundation.

Nelson C, Niederberger J: Patient satisfaction surveys: an opportunity for total quality management, *Hosp Health Serv Adm* 35(3):409–427, 1990.

Oaks J, Ezell G: *Dying and death: coping, caring and understanding,* ed 2, Scottsdale, Ariz, 1993, Gorsuch Scaresbrich.

Peppers L, Knapp R: *How to go on living after the death of a baby,* Atlanta, 1985, Peachtree.

Rando T: *Grief, dying and death,* Champaign, Ill, 1984, Research Press.

Rando T: *How to go on living when someone you love dies,* 1991, Bantam Books.

Rando T: *Parental loss of a child,* Champaign, Ill, 1986, Research Press.

Rillstone P: Not all babies live, *J Childbirth Educ* 8(4):27, 1993.

Rillstone P, Hutchison S: Managing the reemergence of anguish: pregnancy after loss due to anomalies, *J Obstet Gynecol Neonatal Nurs* 30(3):291–298, 2001.

Rubin R: Maternal tasks in pregnancy, *Matern Child Nurs J* 4(3):143–153, 1975.

Schwiebert P, Kirk P: *When hello means goodbye,* Portland, Ore, 1985, Perinatal Loss.

Shively P: *Reaching out: a guide for developing or enhancing a comprehensive bereavement program for hospitals, clinics, and other healthcare centers,* La Crosse, Wisc, 1995, Bereavement Services/RTS.

Simonds W, Rothman B: *Centuries of solace: expressions of maternal grief in popular literature,* Philadelphia, 1992, Temple University Press.

Swanson K: Nursing as informed caring for the well-being of others, *Image J Nurs Sch* 25(4):352–357, 1993.

Swanson-Kauffman K: Caring in the instance of unexpected early pregnancy loss, *Top Clin Nurs* 8(2):37–46, 1986.

Swanson-Kauffman K: There should have been two: nursing care of parents experiencing the perinatal death of a twin, *J Perinat Neonatal Nurs* 2(2):78–86, 1988.

Theut S and others: Resolution of parental bereavement after perinatal loss, *J Am Acad Child Adolesc Psychiatry* 29(4):521–525, 1990.

Van der Zalm J: The perinatal death of a twin: Karla's story of attaching and detaching, *J Nurse Midwifery* 40(4):335–341, 1995.

Wallerstedt C, Higgins P: Perinatal circumstances that evoke differences in the grieving response, *J Perinatol Educ* 3(2):35, 1994.

Wheeler S, Limbo R, and Gensch B: Loss grief. In Bobak I, Jensen M: *Maternity and gynecologic care: the nurse and the family,* ed 5, St Louis, 1992, Mosby.

Witter D, Tolle S, and Moseley J: A bereavement program: good care, quality assurance, and risk management, *Hosp Health Serv Adm* 35(2):263–275, 1990.

Care for Caregiver

Arlen S: Good selfishness, *Bereavement Magazine,* p 10, June 1990.

Borysenko J: *Minding the body, mending the mind,* New York, 1987, Bantam Books.

Callanan M, Kelly P: *Final gifts,* New York, 1992, Poseidon Press.

Cameron J: *The artist's way,* New York, 1992, Putnam.

Carter R, Golant S: *Helping yourself help others: a book for caregivers,* New York, 1994, Time Books.

Deits B: *Life after loss: a personal guide to dealing with death, divorce, job change and relocation,* Tucson, 1988, Fisher Books.

Feldstein M, Gemma P: Oncology nurses and chronic compounded grief, *Cancer Nurs* 18(3):228–236, 1995.

Figley C, editor: *Compassion fatigue: secondary traumatic stress disorders from treating the traumatized,* New York, 1995, Brunner/Mazel.

Heinrich K, Killeen M: The gentle art of nurturing yourself, *Am J Nurs* 93(10):41–44, 1993.

Katherine A: *Boundaries: where you end and I begin,* Park Ridge, Ill, 1991, Parkside.

Kenner C, Lott J, and Flandermeyer A: *Comprehensive neonatal nursing: a physiologic perspective,* ed 3, St Louis, 2003, Saunders.

Klein A: *The healing power of humor,* Los Angeles, 1989, Jeremy P Tarcher.

Larson D: *The helper's journey: working with people facing grief, loss and life-threatening illness,* Champaign, Ill, 1993, Research Press.

Osmont K: *More than surviving: caring for yourself while you grieve,* Omaha, 1990, Centering.

Smith D: *The Tao of dying,* Washington, DC, 1994, Caring Press.

Springer L: Caregiver characteristics as seen by patients, family, and caregivers, *The Forum,* p 7, 1992.

Taigman M: Can empathy and compassion be taught? *JEMS* 21(6):42–43, 1996.

Travis J, Callander M: *Wellness for helping professionals,* Mill Valley, Calif, 1990, Wellness Associates.

Wolfelt A: *Self-care for the bereavement caregiver: the codependent syndrome,* Fort Collins, Colo, 1992, Companion Press (training videotape).

Wolfelt A: *Understanding grief: helping yourself heal,* Muncie, Ind, 1992, Accelerated Development.

Children and Grief

American Academy of Pediatrics Committee on Psychosocial Aspects of Child and Family Health: The pediatrician and childhood bereavement, *Pediatrics* 89(3):516–518, 1992.

Arnold J, Gemma P: *A child dies: a portrait of family grief,* Philadelphia, 1994, Charles Press.

Baker J, Sedney M, and Gross E: Psychological tasks for bereaved children, *Am J Orthopsychiatry* 62(1):105–116, 1992.

Bowden V: Children's literature: the death experience, *Pediatr Nurs* 19(1):17–21, 1993.

Cohn J: *Molly's rosebush,* Morton Grove, Ill, 1994, Whitman & Co.

Dodge N: *Thumpy's story,* Springfield, Ill, 1983, Prairie Lark Press.

Goldman L: *Life and loss: a guide to help grieving children,* Bristol, Pa, 1994, Accelerated Development.

Grollman E: *Talking about death: a dialogue between parent and child,* Boston, 1990, Beacon Press.

Haasl B, Marnocha J: *Bereavement support group program for children,* Muncie, Ind, 1990, Accelerated Development.

Heiney S: Sibling grief: a case report, *Arch Psychiatr Nurs* 5(3):121–127, 1991.

Johnson PP, Williams DR: *Morgan's baby sister,* San Jose, Calif, 1993, Resource Publications.

Kübler-Ross E: *On children and death,* New York, 1983, MacMillan.

O'Toole D: *Aarvy aardvark finds hope: a read-aloud story for people of all ages about loving and losing, friendship and hope,* Burnsville, NC, 1988, Rainbow Connection.

Overbeck B, Overbeck J: *Helping children cope with grief,* Dallas, 1992, TLC Group.

Resler R: *Remembering you: a book for children and teenagers who experience the loss of a brother or sister,* Cleveland, 1996, Rainbow Babies' and Children's Hospital.

Sanders C: *How to survive the loss of a child,* Rocklin, Calif, 1992, Prima.

Schaefer D, Lyons C: *How do we tell the children?* New York, 1993, Newmarket Press.

Schonfeld D: Talking with children about death, *J Pediatr Health Care* 7(6):269–274, 1993.

Silverman P, Worden J: Children's reactions in the early months after the death of a parent, *Am J Orthopsychiatry* 62(1):93–104, 1992a.

Van-Si L, Powers L: *Helping children heal from loss: a keepsake book of special memories,* Portland, Ore, 1994, Portland State University.

Wass H, Corr C: *Helping children cope with death: guidelines and resources,* Washington, DC, 1984, Hemisphere.

Wheeler S, Austin J: The impact of early pregnancy loss on adolescents, *MCN Am J Matern Child Nurs* 26(3):154–159, 2001.

Wolfelt A: *Healing the bereaved child,* Fort Collins, Colo, 1995, Companion Press.

Clergy/Spiritual Issues

Carpenito-Moyet L: *Nursing diagnosis: application to clinical practice*, Philadelphia, 2006, Lippincott Williams & Wilkins.

Coleman G: Baptizing dying infants not always required, *Health Progr* 67(8):46–49, 1986.

Corrine L and others: The unheard voices of women: spiritual interventions in maternal-child health, *MCN Am J Matern Child Nurs* 17(3):141–145, 1992.

Cox G, Fundis R: *Spiritual, ethical and pastoral aspects of death and bereavement*, Amityville, NY, 1993, Baywood.

Di Meo E: Rx for spiritual distress, *RN* 54(3):22–24, 1991.

Doka K, Morgan J, editors: *Death and spirituality*, Amityville, NY, 1993, Baywood.

Eich W: When is emergency baptism appropriate? *Am J Nurs* 87(12):1680–1681, 1987.

Feinstein D, Mayo P: *Mortal acts: eighteen empowering rituals for confronting death*, San Francisco, 1993, Harper.

Fickling K: Stillborn studies: ministering to bereaved parents, *J Pastoral Care* 47(3): 217–227, 1993.

Fish S, Shelly J: *Spiritual care: the nurse's role*, ed 3, Downer's Grove, Ill, 1988, Intervarsity Press.

Haase J and others: Simultaneous concept analysis of spiritual perspective, hope acceptance and self-transcendence, *Image J Nurs Sch* 24(2):141–147, 1992.

Kennison M: Faith: an untapped health resource, *J Psychosoc Nurs Ment Health Serv* 25(10):28–30, 1987.

Meyer C: *Surviving death*, Mystic, Conn, 1991, Twenty-Third Publications.

Parrott C: *Parent's grief: help and understanding after the death of a baby*, Redmond, Wash, 1992, Medic.

Rybarik F: What are the roles of pastoral caregivers and funeral directors in dealing with perinatal loss? *AWHONN Voice* 3(8):8, 1995.

Thearle M and others: Church attendance, religious affiliation and parental responses to sudden infant death, neonatal death and stillbirth, *Omega* 31(1):51, 1995.

VandeCreek L and others: Patient and family perceptions of hospital chaplains, *Hosp Health Serv Adm* 36(3):455–467, 1991.

Wolfelt AD: *Death and grief: a guide for clergy*, Muncie, Ind, 1988, Accelerated Development.

Communication

Black R: Women's voices after pregnancy loss: couple's patterns of communication and support, *Soc Work Health Care* 16(2):19, 1991.

Burley-Allen M: *Listening: the forgotten skill*, ed 2, New York, 1995, Wiley & Sons.

Crowther M: Communication following a stillbirth or neonatal death: room for improvement, *Br J Obstet Gynaecol* 102(12):952–956, 1995.

Davis H, Hallowfield L, editors: *Counseling and communication in health care*, New York, 1991, Wiley.

Gerken K: What (and what not) to say after pregnancy loss, *Bereavement Magazine*, p 24, July/Aug 1993.

Nance T: Intercultural communication: finding common ground, *J Obstet Gynecol Neonat Nurs* 24(3):249–255, 1995.

Range L, Walston A, and Pollard P: Helpful and unhelpful comments after suicide, homicide, accident or natural death, *Omega* 25(1):25, 1992.

Rybarik F: What communication skills are most helpful with families grieving a perinatal loss? *AWHONN Voice* 4(6):4, 1996.

Tannen D: *You just don't understand: women and men in conversation*, New York, 1990, Morrow.

Wolfeldt A: *What does a good listener do?* (MS 20-13), Boulder, Colo, Career Track Tapes.

Cultural Issues

Beeman P: Cultural concepts in clinical care, *J Obstet Gynecol Neonatal Nurs* 24:327, 1995.

Counts D, Counts D: *Coping with the final tragedy: cultural variation in dying and grieving*, Amityville, NY, 1993, Baywood.

DeSpelder L, Strickland A: *The last dance: encountering death and dying*, Palo Alto, Calif, 1992, Mayfield.

Geissler E: *Pocket guide to cultural assessment,* ed 2, St Louis, 1998, Mosby.

Giger J, Davidhizar R: *Transcultural nursing: assessment and intervention,* ed 4, St Louis, 2004, Mosby.

Henry-Jenkins W: The Muslim way of death, *Bereavement Magazine,* p 33, Jan 1993.

Hutchinson M, Baqi-Aziz M: Nursing care of the childbearing Muslim family, *J Obstet Gynecol Neonatal Nurs* 23(9):767–771, 1994.

Irish D, Lundquist K, Nelsen V, editors: *Ethnic variations in dying, death and grief: diversity in universality,* Washington, DC, 1993, Taylor & Francis.

Layne L: Motherhood lost: cultural dimensions of miscarriage and stillbirth in America, *Women Health* 16(3–4):69–98, 1990.

Mehta L, Verna IC: Helping parents to face perinatal loss, *Indian J Pediatr* 57:607, 1990.

Randall E: *Strategies for working with culturally diverse communities and clients,* Washington, DC, 1994, Association for Care of Children's Health.

Shuzman E: Facing stillbirth or neonatal death: providing culturally appropriate care for Jewish families, *AWHONN Lifelines* 7(6):537–543, 2003.

Stroebe W, Stroebe M: Is grief universal? Cultural variations in emotional reaction to loss. In Rulton R, Bendiksen R, editors: *Death and identity,* ed 3, Philadelphia, 1994, Charles Press.

Yanda J: *Cultural issues in perinatal grief, presentation,* Valley Forge, Pa, 1996.

York C, Stichler J: Cultural grief expressions following infant death, *Dimens Crit Care Nurs* 4(2):120–127, 1985.

Depression

Agency for Health Care Policy and Research: *Depression in primary care: detection, diagnosis and treatment,* Silver Spring, Md, 1993, AHCPR Publications.

American Psychiatric Association: *Diagnostic and statistical manual of mental disorders,* ed 4, Washington, DC, 1994, APA.

Armstrong D: Impact of prior perinatal loss on subsequent pregnancies, *J Obstet Gynecol Neonatal Nurs* 33(6):765–773, 2004.

Bowlby J: *Attachment and loss,* vol 2, ed 2, New York, 1982, Basic Books.

Horowitz J: Postpartum depression: issues in clinical assessment, *J Perinatol* 15(4):268–278, 1995.

Leahy J: A comparison of depression in women bereaved of a spouse, child, or parent, *Omega* 26:207, 1993.

Neugebauer R and others: Depressive symptoms in women in the six months after miscarriage, *Am J Obstet Gynecol* 166(1 Pt 1):104–109, 1992.

Ectopic Pregnancy

Breault C: Ectopic pregnancy is also a perinatal loss, *J Emerg Nurs* 15(3):217, 1989.

Grainger D, Seifer D: Laparoscopic management of ectopic pregnancy, *Curr Opin Obstet Gynecol* 7(4):277–282, 1995.

Maiolatesi C, Peddicord K: Methotrexate for nonsurgical treatment of ectopic pregnancy: nursing implications, *J Obstet Gynecol Neonatal Nurs* 25(3):205–208, 1996.

Powell M, Spellman J: Medical management of the patient with an ectopic pregnancy, *J Perinat Neonatal Nurs* 9(4):31–43, 1996.

Rolnick S and others: Decrease in the rate of ruptured ectopic pregnancies: a successful team approach, *HMO Pract* 8(3):105–109, 1994.

Ethics

Cox G, Fundis R: *Spiritual, ethical and pastoral aspects of death and bereavement,* Amityville, NY, 1993, Baywood.

McFadden E: Moral development and reproductive health decisions, *J Obstet Gynecol Neonatal Nurs* 25(6):507–512, 1996.

Miya P and others: Ethical perceptions of parents and nurses in NICU: the case of baby Michael, *J Obstet Gynecol Neonatal Nurs* 24(2):125–130, 1995.

Monagle J, Thomasma DC: *Medical ethics: policies, protocols, guidelines and programs,* Gaithersburg, Md, 1992, Aspen.

Family Relationships/Gender Issues

DeFrain J: Learning about grief from normal families: SIDS, stillbirth and miscarriage, *J Marital Family Ther* 17:215, 1991.

Doerr M: *For better or worse: for couples whose child has died,* Omaha, 1992, Centering.

Gilbert K: Interactive grief and coping in the marital dyad, *Death Stud* 13:605, 1989.

Gilbert K: "We've had the same loss, why don't we have the same grief?" Loss and differential grief in families, *Death Stud* 20:269, 1996.

Goldbach K and others: The effects of gestational age and gender on grief after pregnancy loss, *Am J Orthopsychiatry* 61(3):461–467, 1991.

Kissane D, Bloch S: Family grief, *Br J Psychiatry* 164(6):728–740, 1994.

Lang A, Gottlieb L, and Amsel R: Predictors of husbands' and wives' grief reactions following infant death: the role of marital intimacy, *Death Stud* 20(1):33–57, 1996.

Lister M, Lovell S: Healing together: helping couples cope with miscarriage, stillbirth or early infant loss, *Bereavement Magazine,* p 12, Oct 1990.

Rosof B: *The worst loss: how families heal from the death of a child,* New York, 1994, Holt.

Wallerstedt C, Higgins P: Facilitating perinatal grieving between the mother and the father, *J Obstet Gynecol Neonatal Nurs* 25(3):389–394, 1996.

Wheeler S, Pike M: *Seasons of a woman's grief.* Presentation at the National NAACOG Convention, Orlando, June 1991.

Follow-Up

Ewton D: A perinatal loss follow-up guide for primary care, *Nurse Pract* 18(12):30, 1993.

Piper W, McCallum M, and Azim HFA: *Adaptation to loss through short term group psychotherapy,* New York, 1993, Guilford.

Worden J: *Grief counseling and grief therapy,* ed 2, New York, 1991, Springer.

Funerals

Lamb J, editor: *Bittersweet ... hello goodbye: a resource in planning farewell rituals when a baby dies,* St Charles, Mo, 1989, SHARE.

Manning D: *A minister speaks about funerals,* Springfield, Ill, 1992, Human Services Press.

Morgan E: *Dealing creatively with death: a manual of death education simple burial,* ed 13, Bayside, NY, 1993, Zinn Communications.

Silverman P, Worden J: Children's understanding of funeral ritual, *Omega* 25:319, 1992b.

Wolfelt A: *Interpersonal skills training: a handbook for funeral home staffs,* Muncie, Ind, 1990, Accelerated Development.

Interventions and Supportive Care

Brost L, Kenney J: Pregnancy after perinatal loss: parental reactions and nursing interventions, *J Obstet Gynecol Neonatal Nurs* 21(6):457–463, 1992.

Calhoun L: Parents' perceptions of nursing support following neonatal loss, *J Perinat Neonatal Nurs* 8(2):57–66, 1994.

Catlin A: Emotional support for early pregnancy loss: how you can do it, *Matern Child Health Educ Resources* 7(2):1, 1992.

Conrad B: *When a child dies: ways you can help a bereaved parent,* Santa Barbara, Calif, 1995, Fithian Press.

Courtney S, Thomas N, and Predmore B: Reverse transport of the deceased neonate: an aid to mourning, *Am J Perinatol* 2(3):217–220, 1985.

Limbo R, Wheeler S: *When a baby dies: a handbook for healing and helping,* La Crosse, Wisc, 1995, Bereavement Services/RTS.

Maloni J and others: Transforming prenatal care: reflections on the past and present with implications for the future, *J Obstet Gynecol Neonatal Nurs* 25(1):17–23, 1996.

Neumann M, Hudson P: Solution-oriented therapy techniques for women's health nurses, *J Obstet Gynecol Neonatal Nurs* 23(1):16–20, 1994.

Rybarik F: Coping with perinatal loss: the role of a perinatal bereavement team, *Adv Nurse Pract* 2(12):21, 32, 1994.

Scott M, Grzybowski M, and Webb S: Perceptions and practices of registered nurses regarding pastoral care and the spiritual needs of hospital patients, *J Pastoral Care* 48(2):171–179, 1994.

Sexton P, Stephen S: Postpartum mothers' perceptions of nursing interventions for perinatal grief, *Neonatal Netw* 9(5):47–51, 1991.

Thearle M, Gregory H: Evolution of bereavement counselling in sudden infant death syndrome, neonatal death and stillbirth, *J Paediatr Child Health* 28(3):204–209, 1992.

Welch I: Miscarriage, stillbirth or newborn death: starting a healthy grieving process, *Neonatal Netw* 9(8):53–57, 1991.

Wolfelt A: *Growth-oriented grief counseling: therapeutic interventions for caregivers,* Muncie, Ind, 1992, Accelerated Development.

Men and Fathers

Hughes C, Page-Lieberman J: Fathers experiencing a perinatal loss, *Death Stud* 13:537, 1989.

Merrill S: *Miscarriage and the fathers: the need for an availability of social support,* master's thesis, Eau Claire, Wisc, 1986, University of Wisconsin-Eau Claire School of Nursing.

Nelson J, editor: *The rocking horse is lonely: and other stories of fathers' grief,* Wayzata, Mich, 1994, Pregnancy and Infant Loss Center.

Page-Lieberman J, Hughes C: How fathers perceive perinatal death, *MCN Am J Matern Child Nurs* 15(5):320–323, 1994.

Staudacher C: *Men and grief,* Oakland, Calif, 1991, New Harbinger.

Wheat R: *Miscarriage: a man's book,* Omaha, 1995, Centering.

Wolfelt A: *Gender roles and grief: why men's grief is naturally complicated,* p 20, 1990, Thanatos.

Young-Mason J: Baby Susan, *Clin Nurs Spec* 6(2):104, 1992.

Miscarriage

Allen M, Marks S: *Miscarriage: women sharing from the heart,* New York, 1993, John Wiley & Sons.

Easterwood B: Silent lullabies: helping parents cope with early pregnancy loss, *AWHONN Lifelines* 8(4):356–360, 2004.

Flagler S, Nicoll L: A framework for the psychological aspects of pregnancy, *NAACOG's Clin Issu Perinat Womens Health Nurs* 1(3):267–278, 1990.

Friedman R, Gradstein B: Miscarriage: an unrecognized loss. In Friedman R, Gradstein B: *Surviving pregnancy loss,* Boston, 1992, Little, Brown.

Frost M, Condon J: The psychological sequels of miscarriage: a critical review of the literature, *Aust N Z J Psychiatry* 30(1):54–62, 1996.

Harris B, Sandelowski M, and Holditch-Davis D: Infertility … and new interpretations of pregnancy loss, *MCN Am J Matern Child Nurs* 16(4):217–220, 1991.

Hutti M: Parents' perceptions of the miscarriage experience, *Death Stud* 16:401, 1992.

Lefkof J, Glazer G: Grief after miscarriage: practical interventions can assist with far-reaching loss, *Adv Nurse Pract* 10(10):79–82, 2002.

Ramsden C: Miscarriage counselling: an accident and emergency perspective, *Accid Emerg Nurs* 3(2):68–73, 1995.

Reed K: The effects of gestational age and pregnancy planning status on obstetrical nurses' perceptions of giving emotional care to women experiencing miscarriage, *Image J Nurs Sch* 24(2):107–110, 1992.

Roberts H: Managing miscarriage: the management of the emotional sequelae of miscarriage in training practices in the west of Scotland, *Fam Pract* 8(2):117–120, 1991.

Winslow S: Miscarriage, the unrecognized tragedy, *Bereavement Magazine* 25, March/April 1991.

Zaccardi R, Abbott J, and Kosiol-McLain J: Loss and grief reactions after spontaneous miscarriage in the emergency department, *Ann Emerg Med* 22(5):799–804, 1993.

Newborn Death/Neonatal Intensive Care Unit

Davis D: *Loving and letting go,* Omaha, 1993, Centering.

Downey V and others: Dying babies and associated stress in NICU nurses, *Neonatal Netw* 14(1):41–46, 1995.

Frey D: "Does anyone here think this baby can live?" *New York Times Sunday Magazine,* p 22, July 9, 1995.

Gustaitis R, Young E: *A time to be born, a time to die: conflicts and ethics in an intensive care nursery,* Reading, Mass, 1986, Gustaitis and EWD Young.

Miya P and others: Ethical perceptions of parents and nurses in NICU: the case of Baby Michael, *J Obstet Gynecol Neonatal Nurs* 24(2):125–130, 1995.

Swanson K: Providing care in the NICU: sometimes an act of love, *ANS Adv Nurs Sci* 13(1):60–73, 1990.

Todd A: *Journey of the heart,* Nashville, Tenn, 1995, Medical Center North.

Photography

Brown C, Kozich P: Reconstructing reality: reserving memories through the creation of impressions, *Int J Childbirth Educ* 9(1):38, 1994.

For K: *Tips for picture taking,* Beech Grove, Ind, 1991, St Francis Hospital Center.

Griesbach S: A medical photographer's role on a perinatal bereavement team, *J Biol Photogr* 56(4):149–153, 1988.

Johnson J, Johnson S: *A most important picture: a tender manual for taking pictures of stillborn babies and infants who die,* Omaha, 1985, Centering.

McGhie J: Portraiture of the stillborn ... should we or should we not? *J Audiov Media Med* 12(1):9–10, 1989.

Primeau M, Recht C: Professional bereavement photographs: one aspect of a perinatal bereavement program, *J Obstet Gynecol Neonatal Nurs* 23(1):22–25, 1994.

Ruby J: Portraying the dead, *Omega* 19(1):1, 1988–1989.

Schweibert P: *When hello means goodbye,* Portland, Ore, 1985, Perinatal Loss.

Wright J: What's wrong with this picture? *American Baby,* p 32, Feb 1991.

Physician Articles

American Academy of Pediatrics Committee on Psychosocial Aspects of Child and Family Health: The pediatrician and childhood bereavement, *Pediatrics* 89(3):516–518, 1992.

Buckman R: *How to break bad news: a guide for health care professionals,* Baltimore, 1992, Johns Hopkins University Press.

Chez R, Davidson G: Helping patients and doctors cope with perinatal death, *Obstet Gynecol* 85:1059, 1995.

Curry C: Pregnancy loss, stillbirth and neonatal death: a guide for the pediatrician, *Pediatr Clin North Am* 39(1):157–192, 1992.

Forrest G, Standish E, and Baum J: Support after perinatal death: a study of support and counseling after perinatal bereavement, *Br Med J* 285:1475, 1982.

Freeman R, Poland R, editors: *Guidelines for perinatal care,* ed 3, New York, 1990, AAP and ACOG with March of Dimes.

Lake M, Knuppel R, and Angel J: The rationale for supportive care after perinatal death, *J Perinatol* 7(2):85–89, 1987.

Leash R: *Death notification: a mutual guide to the process,* Hinesburg, Vt, 1994, Upper Access.

Lemmer CM: Parental perceptions of caring following perinatal bereavement, *West J Nurs Res* 13(4):475–489, 1991.

Leon I: Perinatal loss: a critique of current hospital practices, *Gen Pediatr* 31:366, 1992.

Newman L, Williams J: The family physician's role following a neonatal death, *J Fam Pract* 29(5):521–525, 1989.

Schmidt T, Tolle S: Emergency physicians' responses to families following patient death, *Ann Emerg Med* 19(2):125–128, 1990.

Statham H, Dimavicius J: Commentary: how do you give the bad news to parents? *Birth* 19(2):103–104, 1992.

Wiseman B: Death of a child: a bereaved doctor's perspective, *Bereavement Magazine,* May/June 1994.

Woods J, Esposito J: *Pregnancy loss: medical therapeutics and practical considerations,* Baltimore, 1987, Williams & Wilkins.

Prenatal Diagnosis and Decision Making

Blasco P, Blasco P: Prenatal diagnosis: current procedures and implications for early interventionists working with families, *Infants Young Child* 7(2):33, 1994.

Dallaire L and others: Parental reaction and adaptability to the prenatal diagnosis of fetal defect or genetic disease leading to pregnancy interruption, *Prenatal Diagn* 15(3):249–259, 1995.

Delp K, Minnick M: *Support group manual: a training manual for conducting support programs for parents who have interrupted pregnancies secondary to fetal anomalies,* St John's, Mich, 1995, Pineapple Press.

Green J: Obstetricians' views on prenatal diagnosis termination of pregnancy: 1980 compared with 1993, *Br J Obstet Gynaecol* 102(3):228–232, 1995.

Isle S: *Precious lives, painful choices,* Maple Plain, Mich, 1993, Wintergreen Press.

Kolker A, Burke B: Grieving the wanted child: ramifications of abortion after prenatal diagnosis of abnormality, *Health Care Women Int* 14(6):513–526, 1993.

Lyon W: *A mother's dilemma,* St John's, Mich, 1992, Pineapple Press.

Minnick M, editor: *Yesterday, I dreamed of dreams,* St John's, Mich, 1991, Pineapple Press.

Seller M and others: Grief and midtrimester fetal loss, *Prenat Diagn* 13(5):341–348, 1993.

Zeanah C and others: Do women grieve after terminating pregnancies because of fetal anomalies? A controlled investigation, *Obstet Gynecol* 82(2):270–275, 1993.

Research

Carter S: Themes of grief, *Nurs Res* 38(6):354–258, 1989.

Cleiren M: *Bereavement and adaptation,* Washington, DC, 1992, Hemisphere.

DeVries B, Dalla Lana R, and Falk V: Parental bereavement over the life course: a theoretical intersection and empirical review, *Omega* 29:47, 1994.

Discher T, Haggerty P: *The bereavement needs of family members in a hospital setting.* Poster session presented at RTS Bereavement Conference, Naperville, Ill, October 1995.

Gilbert K: Interactive grief and coping in the marital dyad, *Death Stud* 13:605, 1989.

Goldbach K and others: The effects of gestational age and gender on grief after pregnancy loss, *Am J Orthopsychiatry* 61(3):461–467, 1991.

Harper M, Wisian N: Care of bereaved parents: a study in patient satisfaction, *J Reprod Med* 39(2):80–86, 1994.

Janssen H and others: Controlled prospective study on the mental health of women following pregnancy loss, *Am J Psychiatry* 153(2):226–230, 1996.

Lasker J, Toedter L: Satisfaction with hospital care and interventions after pregnancy loss, *Death Stud* 18(1):41–64, 1994.

Lemmer C: Parental perceptions of caring following perinatal bereavement, *West J Nurs Res* 15:199, 1993.

Moos N: An integrative model of grief, *Death Stud* 19:337, 1995.

Ponzetti J: Bereaved families: a comparison of parents' and grandparents' reactions to the death of a child, *Omega* 25(1):63, 1992.

Schaefer C, Quesenberry C, and Wi S: Mortality following conjugal bereavement and the effects of a shared environment, *Am J Epidemiol* 141(12):1142–1152, 1995.

Solari-Twadell P and others: The pinwheel model of bereavement, *Image J Nurs Sch* 27(4):323–326, 1995.

Swanson K: Empirical development of a middle range theory of caring, *Nurs Res* 40(3): 161–166, 1991.

Theut S and others: Resolution of parental bereavement after a perinatal loss, *J Am Acad Child Adolesc Psychiatry* 29(4):521–525, 1990.

Standards/Guidelines

Association of Women's Health, Obstetric, and Neonatal Nurses: *AWHONN standards for the nursing care of women and newborns,* ed 4, Washington, DC, 1991, AWHONN.

Association of Women's Health, Obstetric, and Neonatal Nurses: *Competencies and program guidelines for nurse providers of perinatal education,* Washington, DC, 1993, AWHONN.

Association of Women's Health, Obstetric, and Neonatal Nurses: *Didactic content and clinical skills verification for professional nurse providers of perinatal home care,* Washington, DC, 1994, AWHONN.

Freeman R, Poland R, editors: *Guidelines for perinatal care,* ed 3, Washington, DC, 1992, AAP and ACOG with March of Dimes.

Gracey K and others: Certification: hospital versus national standards, *J Nurs Staff Dev* 12(2):93–97, 1996.

Joint Commission on Accreditation of Healthcare Organizations: Patient rights and organizational ethics. In *1995 Accreditation manual for hospitals,* vol 2, No. 1, Oakbrook Terrace, Ill, 1994, JCAHO.

Stillbirth

Dalla Grana W: Stillbirth: the silent birth cry, *Bereavement Magazine,* p 24, 1993.

DeFrain J: *Stillborn: the invisible death,* Lexington, Mass, 1986, Heath and Co.

Mitchell S: Stillbirth: a patient's perspective, *Practitioner* 232:1368, 1988.

Reid J: *Lifeline: a journal for parents grieving miscarriage, stillbirth or early infant death,* St John's, Mich, 1994, Pineapple Press.

Subsequent Pregnancy

Bourne S, Lewis E: Delayed psychological effects of perinatal deaths: the next pregnancy and the next generation, *Br Med J (Clin Res Ed)* 289(6438):147–148, 1984.

Bourne S, Lewis E: Pregnancy after stillbirth or neonatal death: psychological risks and management, *Lancet* 2(8393):31–33, 1984.

Brost L, Kenney J: Pregnancy after perinatal loss: parental reactions and nursing intervention, *J Obstet Gynecol Neonatal Nurs* 21(6):457–463, 1992.

Parker L, O'Leary J: Impact of prior prenatal loss upon subsequent pregnancy: the function of the childbirth class, *Int J Childbirth Educ* 7, August 1989.

Schwiebert P, Kirk P: *Still to be born,* Portland, Ore, 1986, Perinatal Loss.

Stumpf V: The promise of tomorrow: subsequent pregnancy after prenatal loss, *Int J Childbirth Educ* 9:29, 1994.

Theut S and others: Pregnancy subsequent to perinatal loss: parental anxiety and depression, *J Am Acad Child Adolesc Psychiatry* 27(3):289–292, 1988.

Wheeler S: A loss of innocence and a gain in vulnerability: subsequent pregnancy after a loss, *Illness, Crisis, Loss* 8(3):310, 2000.

Support Groups

Braun L, Coplon J, and Sonnenschein P: *Helping parents in groups: a leader's handbook,* Boston, 1984, Resource Communications.

Guillory B, Riggin O: Developing a nursing staff support group model, *Clin Nurse Spec* 5(3):170–173, 1991.

Holm M: Strategies for developing a family support group, *Focus Crit Care* 18(6):444, 1991.

Humm A: *How to organize a self-help group,* New York, 1979, National Self-Help Clearinghouse.

Kellett J: Facilitating support groups: a pilot study, *Nurs Stand* 6(23):34, 1992.

Limbo R, Wheeler S: *A parent support group guide,* La Crosse, Wisc, 1994, Bereavement Services/RTS.

Nugent K and others: A practice model for a parent support group, *Pediatr Nurs* 18(1): 11–16, 1992.

Overbeck B, Overbeck J: *Starting/running support groups,* Dallas, 1992, TLC Group.

Rootes L, Aanes D: A conceptual framework for understanding self-help groups, *Hosp Community Psychiatry* 43(4):379–381, 1992.

Ryan P, Cote-Arsenault D, and Sugarman L: Facilitating care after perinatal loss: a comprehensive checklist, *J Obstet Gynecol Neonatal Nurs* 20(5):385–389, 1991.

Wheeler S, Limbo R: Bereavement support: keep it going and keep it growing, *The Director,* p 34, Jan 1991.

III

Ethical Dilemmas and Legal Considerations in Perinatal Nursing

A s technologic advances have occurred, new methods of maternal and fetal diagnoses and medical therapies have emerged. Nurses are confronted daily with unexpected ethical dilemmas for which they may be unprepared.

The first chapter in this unit provides a basis for understanding the elements of ethical decision making and lists some possible clinical examples in perinatal nursing care. The rapid expansion of available technology in perinatal medical management and nursing care has also had an impact on the increase in litigation when unexpected outcomes occur. Legal considerations have become a common concern for the perinatal team. The second chapter in this unit discusses professional liability, related legal terminology, risks, and litigation processes and lists examples of common clinical concerns.

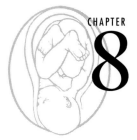

Ethical Decision Making

P erinatal nurses are confronted daily with ethical dilemmas. This chapter examines the nature of values clarification, introduces a framework for ethics, provides a model for ethical decision making, outlines the individual nurse's responsibility for participation and involvement, and lists the relevant clinical perinatal examples that commonly confront the perinatal nurse.

VALUES CLARIFICATION

Educators, psychologists, anthropologists, sociologists, and theologians have influenced the definition of values. They consider values to be attitudes, beliefs, and moral judgments that are chosen freely and thoughtfully and are prized and acted on (Beauchamp and Childress, 2001; Albert and others, 2002).

Process of Valuing

The process of valuing has three aspects: choosing, prizing, and acting.

Choosing

Choosing involves the cognitive component of valuing. Logical, critical, creative thinking and moral judgment development are included. Important elements of choosing include the following:
- Chosen freely
- Chosen from available alternatives
- Chosen after considering the consequences of each alternative
- Complements other values previously internalized

Prizing

Prizing involves the affective component. This feeling component of valuing includes the following aspects (Beauchamp and Childress, 2001):
- Being aware of one's position on the matter
- Expressing one's value

- Experiencing positive self-esteem as a result of the expression of the value
- Communicating and sending clear messages about the value
- Empathetic listening
- Feeling pride and happiness with the choice

Acting

Acting involves the behavioral component and results in the following (Beauchamp and Childress, 2001):

- Personal, professional, and academic competence
- Conflict resolution
- Willingness to affirm the choice publicly
- Assimilation of the choice as part of personal behavior
- Consistent repetition of the choice

MORAL JUDGMENT DEVELOPMENT

Moral judgment development theory complements valuing. Kohlberg (1981) contributed to the study of moral development by expanding on the work of Piaget and describing six stages of moral development.

Stages

Preconventional Level

The child at the preconventional level is responsive to cultural rules and labels of good and bad, right and wrong. These labels are considered by the child in the context of punishment, reward, or exchange of favors. This level is divided into two stages.

Stage 1. Stage 1 is the stage of punishment and obedience. Avoidance of punishment and deference to power are ends in themselves. The physical consequences of an action determine whether it is good or bad. For example, the reason for doing right is to avoid punishment from those with more power.

Stage 2. Stage 2 is the stage of instrumental purpose and exchange. Right action is that which pragmatically satisfies one's own needs and occasionally the needs of others. Right is following the rules because it is in the immediate interest. Right is also what is fair, equal, a deal, or an agreement. Reciprocity is given for the actual reward rather than out of loyalty or gratitude.

Conventional Level

At the conventional level of moral judgment development, the person considers the expectations of others and conformity as valuable in their own right, regardless of the immediate consequences. There is an attitude of not only conformity but also active maintenance, support, and justification of the order. Stages 3 and 4 are at this level.

Stage 3. Stage 3 is the stage of mutual interpersonal expectations, relationships, and conformity. Good behavior is that which pleases and helps others and is approved by them. Conformity to stereotypes is common.

Behavior is frequently judged by intention, as in meaning well. Right behavior is being nice and living up to what is expected.

Stage 4. Stage 4 is the stage of social system and conscience maintenance. Right action is doing one's duty in a group, showing respect for authority, and upholding the prescribed social order for its own sake. Orientation is toward authority, fixed rules, and maintenance of the social order.

Postconventional Level

The postconventional level is also called the autonomous or principled level. The individual attempts to define moral values and principles that have validity and application apart from the authority of society and the individual's identity with societal groups. There are two stages at this level.

Stage 5. Stage 5 is the stage of *a priori* rights and social contract or utility. This stage has utilitarian overtones. Right action is defined in terms of standards that have been agreed on by society in terms of individual rights. Right action is described as upholding basic rights, values, and legal contracts of society even when they conflict with concrete rules and laws of the group.

Awareness of relativism of personal values and opinions exists, with an emphasis on reaching consensus. Right action is also a matter of personal values aside from what is constitutionally agreed on. There is an emphasis on the legal point of view, with the possibility of changing law in terms of rational consideration of societal utility (Douglas, 2001).

Stage 6. Stage 6 is the stage of universal ethical principles. Right action is defined by a decision of conscience in accord with self-chosen ethical principles. Specific laws usually rest on these principles. When, however, laws violate these principles, acts must be in accord with principles rather than law. Principles are abstract, ethical, and universal, such as the principles of justice, reciprocity, equality, and respect for human dignity.

Qualities

In addition to the six stages of moral development, Kohlberg (1981) described six qualities of the stages of moral development:

- The development of morality proceeds in an invariant sequence as the individual matures and as the environment offers the necessary stimulation and opportunities to learn.
- Subjects cannot comprehend moral reasoning at a level more than one stage beyond their development.
- Subjects are cognitively attracted to reasoning one level above their own predominant level.
- Movement through stages is effected when cognitive disequilibrium is created by conflicting values.
- Although the time it takes to move through the stages varies, the sequence is always the same.
- Movement to higher stages of moral development is advantageous for the individual and society.

FRAMEWORK FOR ETHICS
Definitions
Ethics
Ethics is the study of values in human conduct or the study of right conduct. It is a branch of philosophy that attempts to state and evaluate principles by which ethical dilemmas may be resolved. It is not a science with right or wrong answers but rather a systematic, critical, rational, defensible, intellectual approach to determining what is best in a situation with conflicting values. The result will ultimately be unfavorable and pit one or more ethical principles against another (Albert and others, 2002).

Metaethics
Metaethics is the part of ethics that focuses on the extent to which ethical judgments are reasonable or justifiable.

Normative Ethics
Normative ethics is the part of ethics that raises questions about what is right or ought to be done in a situation that calls for an ethical decision.

Ethical Principles
Several basic principles help to identify values, morals, beliefs, and attitudes and to clarify ethical dilemmas (Table 8-1). Ethical principles comprise the sixth stage of Kohlberg's (1981) moral development. The characteristics of ethical principles follow:
- They suggest direction or propose certain behaviors.
- They serve as guides to organizing and understanding ethically relevant information in an ethical dilemma.
- They propose how to resolve competing claims.
- They are the reasons justifying moral actions.
- They are universal in nature. They are not absolute; they do have exceptions.
- They are neither rules (means) nor values (ends).
- They are unchangeable and discovered by human beings rather than invented.

MODEL FOR ETHICAL DECISION MAKING
Characteristics of Ethical Dilemmas
We live in an era in which technologies develop faster than we can consider consequences. Changes affect clinical practice before guidelines for use are developed and before the social and ethical impact can be considered. Recent technologic advances in endocrinology, genetics, reproductive therapy, neonatal and maternal-fetal medical care, and fetal therapy have created numerous ethical dilemmas for the recipient of care and the caregiver. These dilemmas and the resultant decisions have a considerable impact on society.

Table 8-1   Definitions of Ethical Principles

Ethical Principle	Definition
Autonomy	Being one's own person without constraints by another's action or psychologic and physical limitations
Beneficence	Duty to do good
Confidentiality	Holding information entrusted in context of special relationships as private
Fidelity	Duty to keep one's promise or word
Finality	May override demands of law and custom
Generality	Must not refer to specific people or situations
Informed consent	Contains four elements: Disclosure of sufficient information Comprehension Voluntary agreement Competency to make decision
Justice	Equitable distribution of risks and benefits
Nonmaleficence	Duty to do no harm
Ordering	Ethical principles must be prioritized even though they may be conflicting
Publicity	Principles must be known and recognized by all
Reparation	Duty to make up for a wrong
Universality	Same principle must hold for everyone, regardless of time, place, or people involved
Utility	Greatest good or least harm for the greatest number
Veracity	Duty to tell the truth

The characteristics of an ethical dilemma follow (Albert and others, 2002):
- The choice is between equally undesirable alternatives.
- Real choices exist between possible courses of action.
- The people involved place a significantly different value judgment on possible actions or the consequences.
- Data alone do not help to resolve the dilemma.
- "Answers" to the dilemma come from a number of different disciplines, such as psychology, sociology, and theology.
- Actions taken in an ethical dilemma result in unfavorable outcomes or constitute a breach of one's duty to another individual.
- The choices made in an ethical dilemma have far-reaching effects on our perception of human beings and our definition of personhood, our relationships, and people and society as a whole.
- Any ethical decision involves the allocation and expenditure of resources that are finite.
- Ethical dilemmas are not solvable but rather resolvable.
- There is no right or wrong when dealing with two equally unfavorable actions.

Theories in Ethics

Two classic schools of thought—teleology and deontology—dominate ethical theory (Follin, 2004).

Teleology

According to the theory of teleology, the rightness or wrongness of an action is determined by the consequences, not by whether it is inherently right or wrong. This approach to decision making is risk-to-benefit–based. It is also called utilitarianism or consequentialism.

Deontology

The theory of deontology holds that the inherent characteristics of the decision can be judged independent of its outcome or consequences. Duty-based or rights-based approaches are examples of deontologic thoughts.

Moral Relativism

A pure application of either teleology or deontology may not be useful. Aspects of both theories are usually combined when making ethical decisions blended with moral relativism. Moral relativism adds the notion of personal interpretation. The application of paradigm cases, anecdotal experiences, and ethical principles to clinical problems exemplifies relativism.

The root principles of ethical theory are beneficence, justice, and autonomy (see Table 8-1). Decision making is always colored by the individual's values, attitudes, knowledge, desires, cultural mores, experiences, and background (Beauchamp and Childress, 2001).

Steps in Decision Making

The steps in ethical decision making are described in Box 8-1.

Nursing Responsibility

The concepts central to nurses' responsibility in participation in ethical decision making are caring, coordination, and advocacy. These concepts are based on the unique relationship between the nurse and the patient. Clinical ethics, existing aside from medical ethics, incorporates the ethical problems the nurse encounters in the independent and collaborative domains of practice. Nursing is owned by society and as such is an essential part of society with a responsibility to the whole.

Caring

Caring, described by Swanson (1993), provides the first mandate for nurses' participation in and assumption of ethical practice. The second mandate is derived from the social contract and the American Nurses Association (ANA) code for nurses (Box 8-2). The third mandate for participation in ethical decision making is the pivotal position of nursing within the health care organization. Professional nursing practice is ethical nursing practice.

Box 8-1   Steps in Ethical Decision Making

Identify the Problem:
- Who are the people involved?
- How are they interrelated?
- What is involved?

Identify the Values, Issues, or Ethical Dilemmas, and Make a Concise Statement of the Problem and Conflicts in Values:
- State your values and ethical position related to the case.
- Generate alternatives for resolving the dilemma or dilemmas.

Examine and Categorize the Alternatives:
- List alternatives.
- Identify those consistent and those inconsistent with your own values and ethics.

Predict the Possible Consequences for those Acceptable Alternatives:
- Identify physical, psychologic, social, spiritual, and short- and long-range consequences.
- Identify those consequences consistent with your values and ethics.

Prioritize Acceptable Alternatives:
- Develop a plan of action.
- Implement the plan.
- Evaluate the action taken.

PATIENT SELF-DETERMINATION ACT

A federal law, the Patient Self-Determination Act, went into effect in December 1991 for all health care facilities receiving federal monies. This act requires that all patients be informed of their rights to make decisions concerning their health care.

ADVANCE DIRECTIVE

An advance directive, also known as a living will or a durable power of attorney, recognizes the patient's right to control decisions relating to acceptance or refusal of aspects of his or her own medical care. When the patient has decision-making capacity, that control can be exercised by formulating an advance directive.

If the patient loses decision-making capacity, a durable power of attorney can appoint another person to make those decisions. A living will can direct the physician to provide, withhold, or withdraw life-sustaining care.

In the case of a pregnant woman, however, the advance directive does not allow her to make decisions in advance that may affect fetal survival or quality of life. For example, if a pregnant woman is involved in a motor vehicle crash and sustains a head injury that permanently affects her cardiorespiratory center, she may be kept on life-sustaining care despite instructions in her living will to the contrary. If sustaining her on life support can successfully maintain the pregnancy, which shows no evidence of fetal compromise, her living will requesting no life support will be disregarded. In such situations it has been

> **Box 8-2** American Nurses Association Code of Ethics
>
> - The nurse, in all professional relationships, practices with compassion and respect for the inherent dignity, worth, and uniqueness of every individual unrestricted by consideration of social or economic status, personal attributes, or nature of the health problems.
> - The nurse's primary commitment is to the patient, whether an individual, family, group, or community.
> - The nurse promotes, advocates for, and strives to protect the health, safety, and rights of the patient.
> - The nurse is responsible and accountable for individual nursing practice and determines the appropriate delegation of tasks consistent with the nurse's obligation to provide optimum care.
> - The nurse owes the same duties to self as to others, including the responsibility to preserve integrity and safety, to maintain competence, and to continue personal and professional growth.
> - The nurse participates in establishing, maintaining health care environments and conditions of employment conducive to the provision of quality health care and consistent with the values of the profession through individual and collective action.
> - The nurse participates in the advancement of the profession through contributions to practice, education, administration, and knowledge development.
> - The nurse collaborates with other health professionals and the public in promoting community, national, and international efforts to meet health needs.
> - The profession of nursing, as represented by associations and their members, is responsible for articulating nursing values, for maintaining the integrity of the profession and its practice, and for shaping social policy.

From American Nurses Association: *Code of ethics for nurses with interpretive statements,* Silver Springs, MD, 2001, American Nurses Publishing. Retrieved from *http://www.nursingworld.org/ethics/chcode.htm*

determined that postponement of maternal death does less harm to her when balanced against the fetal right to survive.

ETHICS COMMITTEE

Most tertiary institutions have a review board or ethics committee in place for situations in which individuals/families need assistance in dealing with difficult decisions regarding what is right or fair care or when ethical decisions collide with legal and moral obligations of the institution. These committees are usually multidisciplinary and composed of physicians and nurses from the various settings where many of the dilemmas arise, along with allied health care professionals such as an administrator, a member of the clergy, a social services representative, an attorney or risk management representative, and an ethicist (who actually may be one of the professionals previously listed) (Beauchamp and Childress, 2001). A layperson may be asked to serve on the committee as well.

In the beginning of the formation of a board, there are usually some requirements for the prospective members to receive formalized education in the process of ethical decision making. There typically is also some time set aside to educate the members and for them to become accustomed as a group to the processes they will follow. The main functions of the committee are:

- To develop and revise ethical policies and procedures such as informed consent, confidentiality, and advance directives
- To assist with difficult ethical decisions related to health care

It is recommended that there be a process in place for handling emergency situations and specified people who must serve on the board to make decisions. The family should always be invited to provide input and to attend some part of the session when possible and when desired.

CLINICAL EXAMPLES OF ETHICAL DILEMMAS

Some clinical examples of ethical dilemmas that perinatal nurses face are listed in Box 8-3.

Box 8-3   Clinical Examples of Perinatal Ethical Dilemmas

- Voluntary pregnancy termination
- Second trimester abortions
- Selective reduction in multiple gestation
- Emergency contraception
- Previable termination of pregnancy for maternal reasons
- Harvesting of fetal organs or tissue
- In vitro fertilization and decisions for disposal of remaining fertilized ova
- Allocation of resources in pregnancies complicated by substance abuse and other antisocial behaviors
- Allocation of resources in pregnancy care during previable period
- Fetal surgery
- Treatment of genetic disorders or fetal abnormalities found on prenatal screening
- Routine use of electronic fetal monitoring (EFM) for cesarean delivery indication in cases of previous cesarean delivery
- Equal access to prenatal care
- Health care rights
- Maternal rights versus fetal rights
- Extraordinary medical treatment for pregnancy complications
- Court-ordered cesarean section
- Using organs from an anencephalic infant
- Genetic engineering
- Cloning
- Surrogate motherhood
- Mandatory drug testing
- Sanctity of life versus quality of life for extremely premature or severely disabled infants

CONCLUSION

The list of perinatal ethical decisions is much longer than that given in Box 8-3. Some dilemmas are everyday issues. Others are likely to be encountered infrequently and then only in select tertiary perinatal centers. However, it is impossible to work in perinatal nursing and not become involved in ethical dilemmas or participate in ethical decision making. The nurse must not only examine issues in light of the level of participation she or he is willing to have but also facilitate an environment in which colleagues and patients can participate in ethical decisions. The nurse functions as educator, support person, counselor, administrator, researcher, and care provider. Nurses spend more time with patients than any other health care team members do. As a result, nurses must take an active and assertive role in the development of ethical guidelines for areas of perinatal practice (Beauchamp and Childress, 2001; Follin, 2004).

BIBLIOGRAPHY

Albert R and others: *Clinical ethics: a practical approach to ethical decisions in clinical medicine,* ed 5, New York, 2002, McGraw-Hill.

American College of Obstetricians and Gynecologists: *Position statement: practice patterns of emergency contraception,* Washington, DC, 2001, ACOG.

American Nurses Association: *Code of ethics for nurses with interpretive statements,* Silver Springs, MD, 2001, American Nurses Publishing. Retrieved from *http://www.nursingworld.org/ethics/chcode.htm*

Association of Women's Health, Obstetric, and Neonatal Nurses: *Position statement: emergency contraception: the nurses' role in providing postcoital options,* Washington, DC, 1998, AWHONN.

Association of Women's Health, Obstetric, and Neonatal Nurses: *Position statement: pregnancy discrimination act,* Washington, DC, 2000a, AWHONN.

Association of Women's Health, Obstetric, and Neonatal Nurses: *Position statement: access to health care issues,* Washington, DC, 2000b, AWHONN.

Beauchamp T, Childress T: *Principles of biomedical ethics,* ed 5, New York, 2001, Oxford University Press.

Brent N, editor: *Nurses and the law: a guide to principles and applications,* ed 2, Philadelphia, 2001, Saunders.

Douglas M: Ethics in nursing practice. In Brent N, editor: *Nurses and the law: a guide to principles and applications,* ed 2, Philadelphia, 2001, Saunders.

Follin S, editor: *Nurse's legal handbook,* ed 5, Philadelphia, 2004, Lippincott Williams & Wilkins.

Kohlberg L: *Essays on moral development: Vol I, the philosophy of moral development; Vol II, the psychology of moral development: moral stages the life cycle; Vol III, education and moral development: moral stages and practice,* San Francisco, 1981, Harper & Row.

Pryde P and others: Determinants of parental decision making to abort or continue after non-aneuploid ultrasound detected fetal abnormalities, *Obstet Gynecol* 80(1):52–56, 1992.

Swanson K: Nursing as informed caring for the well-being of others, *Image J Nurs Sch* 25(4):352–357, 1993.

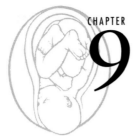

Legal Issues and Risk Management

*P*rofessional liability is a concept that explains a system of accountability. This system is expected to compensate for losses and deter negligent or substandard practices by the professional. Unfortunately, the professional liability system does a poor job of both compensation and deterrence.

The system does not focus so much on poor performance and incompetence as it does on unexpected outcomes. Litigation in health care fields has increased sharply in the past 15 years, both in the number of lawsuits and in the amount of awards.

Approximately 80% of all lawsuits in American history have occurred since 1970 (Shiffrin, 2001). More than 75% of obstetricians and gynecologists are sued over the course of their professional careers, and more than one third of them are sued more than three times. More than half the cost of insurance premiums and award amounts is derived from transaction costs to pay attorney fees and court costs (Shiffrin, 2001).

MALPRACTICE INSURANCE

Nurses are more frequently being included among the separately named parties in lawsuits (Brent, 2001). As a result, more nurses carry their own malpractice insurance. Insurance premiums are higher for specialty nursing practice, such as perinatal care, than for other less litigious nursing specialties. Nurses in the specialty of perinatal care find themselves in a difficult position because they are part of the team; therefore they do not often act independently to reduce personal risk (AWHONN, 1999).

Some issues a nurse needs to examine before deciding to carry a personal insurance policy (Brent, 2001) include the following:

- Is there a high frequency of exposure to lawsuits in the setting in which I practice? High exposure may occur where there are high risk patients more than 25% of the time.
- Do the policies and procedures represent a safe standard of care?
- Do I sometimes practice outside a hospital setting in independent practice or always as an employee where liability insurance includes nurse practice?

A physician's malpractice insurance does not cover the practice of office nurses. Examples of practice outside the hospital setting include teaching childbirth preparation classes, giving frequent telephone advice, doing outreach education, or providing contract care.

- Am I working in a setting where physician response is not timely or where physicians are overworked?
- Is the staff-to-patient ratio commonly lower than standard?
- Are continuing education programs encouraged, and are they supported?

REASONS PARENTS SUE

One reason for increased frequency and severity of perinatal litigation is that patients have unrealistic and inflated expectations of the health care system to correct all ills. Another cause is the health care professional's overconfidence.

Reasons parents sue vary. Some common reasons (Brent, 2001) include the following:

- Injured or dead infant
- Advice of family and friends, who believe that if fault can be found, parents will feel better or at least feel that justice has been done
- Monetary concerns related to the expense of continued care for an injured infant
- Anger, a need to blame, and belief that the provider is at fault
- Complicated grief
- Surprise that anything could go wrong, unrealistic expectations, or inadequate information before giving consent for care
- Belief that litigation will be profitable
- Poor communication with health care providers

When parents sue because their child is injured, the award sought is generally for the expenses involved in the continued and future care of that child. A small amount of the award may be for the emotional damages the parents have suffered; this must be proved separately from the child's damages. When parents sue because their child is dead, the award is almost solely for the emotional damages suffered from loss of the relationship and for any impairment in other relationships. The nurse must assess the family to discover whether any of the members are unable to deal with death constructively, to meet their basic needs, to accept and receive needed help, or to express and accept various family members' individualized expressions of feelings.

LITIGATION RISK

There are three common sources of litigation risk:

- Failure to keep current
- Inadequate supervision, management, or administration of services
- Communication inadequacies, errors, or inaccuracies

Failure to Keep Current

Ways to keep current include the following:

- Exercising professional responsibility by attending continuing education programs consistently
- Participating in a detailed orientation program when employed in a new setting
- Maintaining familiarity with relevant policies and procedures (AWHONN, 2000)
- Being aware of sources of and relevant guidelines for standards of care
- Keeping abreast of current relevant legal issues and decisions

Inadequate Supervision

The following aspects help to make sure that supervision is adequate:

- The immediate supervising nurse who is present (head nurse, charge nurse, team leader, designee, or nurse of other similar title) is required to respond to all questions the nurse at the bedside has regarding supervision. This includes responding to issues related to who was informed of any difficulties or immediate identification of problems.
- Nurses must know the chain of command to follow when a problem is identified; this is especially important when there is conflict regarding who should respond to patient care issues.
- Nurses should consult with other staff members who are more experienced or who are experts; in cases of litigation, this may help their defense.
- Nurses should report problematic staffing patterns or ratios to the supervisor. Areas that are potentially problematic include nurse-to-patient ratios that are too low, staff shifts on rotation or on call that are too long, inadequate staff orientation, too many inexperienced staff members, and staff members who are not qualified for their assignments. These problematic patterns must be considered and responded to by the supervisor.

Sinclair (2000) cited six reasons for the shortage of nurses in the health care system:

- Changes in the type and place of nursing care
- Inadequate staffing ratios
- Inadequate salary increases
- Inflexible hours
- Insufficient control over nursing activities
- Relatively poor communication within the organizational infrastructures

This nursing shortage and the reasons definitely affect the legal climate. The nursing shortage contributes to increased personal liability and to the liability of the institution in which the nurse is practicing. It affects the physician's practice and liability secondary to dependence on adequate patient supervision and collegiality in practice.

Inadequate Communication

Patient/Family and Nurse

Some areas of patient and nurse communication risks are described in the following sections.

Patient education and childbirth preparation. There may be risks associated with misinformation, incomplete information, or no information provided in patient education and childbirth preparation situations.

Telephone advice. Generally, it is best to view a patient's telephone call requesting advice as an opportunity to help the patient focus on the key elements of the complaint and to empower the patient in self-advocacy with the concerns. When much of the nurse's time is used to take calls and give telephone advice, clear guidelines should be established for what the nurse is allowed to discuss and what the patient is supposed to do with the advice. The advice and recommendations, any consultation with the physician, and the patient's statement of understanding should be documented on a specific form intended for this purpose, and this form should then be filed in the permanent record.

Amount of information. Exercise caution when giving information; providing too little or too much information, giving vague responses, giving misinformation or conflicting information, and withholding information are all practices to avoid.

Nurse to Physician

When there is disagreement between the nurse and the physician, the nurse should do the following:
- Settle it privately.
- Get agreement before documenting.
- Use "I" messages rather than "you" messages. For example, "I am concerned that this problem is not being evaluated" or "I need a physician to see this strip and evaluate the patient."
- Follow the chain of command when differences cannot be immediately resolved.
- Document the situation (just the facts), but not in the patient record.

Verbal Orders

There are increased risks involved with giving verbal orders because of issues related to translation and transmission. Also, some risk exists with telephone orders because the physician relies entirely on relayed information to diagnose the problem. This increases potential errors in treatment decisions. It is the nurse's responsibility to acknowledge that the physician's response seems to be in error.

Refusal or Inability to Comply

When the nurse clearly believes that to follow the physician's orders, to fail to obtain orders, or to fail to convince a physician of the necessity to see the patient will result in harm to the patient, the nurse has an obligation to follow through with a series of actions in a timely manner commensurate with the potential for harm. The nurse should always start by attempting to resolve the conflict and by firmly stating the expectation of a response from the physician involved. If that response is not quickly forthcoming, the nurse must follow the administrative chain of command with alternative notification of medical team members.

MID-LEVEL PROVIDERS

Mid-level providers (nurse practitioners, midwives, nurse anesthetists, clinical nurse specialists) have only one clear thing in common from state to state and from specialty to specialty: all mid-level providers are registered nurses who have completed an advanced level of education and therefore have an increased level of responsibility and accountability as advanced practice nurses (APNs). Different states regulate the level of educational degree required to practice as an APN. More than 30 states now require APNs to have a graduate (i.e., master's) degree in their specialty. Many of those states also require these individuals to take and pass a certification examination from a specified certifying agency and to hold a current registered nurse licensure.

If the APN is prepared in adult health areas, he or she may not practice in pediatrics and vice versa. An adult health nurse practitioner may practice in all areas of adult health but not in obstetrics. A family nurse practitioner may remain generalized or choose to primarily specialize in one or two areas. However, a family nurse practitioner may not certify by examination in any of the specialty areas if one of the usual certifying agencies is used and can only certify as a generalist. Scope of practice issues vary little from state to state for APNs.

Certified nurse midwives must be RNs, must obtain a master's degree, and must pass certification consisting of oral and written board examinations. There is a great deal of consistency in practice privileges for nurse anesthetists from state to state, but the educational degree granted varies. Physician assistants may or may not start out as nurses. They usually have a master's degree, which is required by most states, and they do not hold an independent license from their co-practice physician. Again, state laws vary as to privileges granted and withheld.

States vary in how and what they regulate for those APNs who have prescribing privileges. They usually also describe the degree of autonomy the APN may have, from requiring the APN to list a supervising physician to not requiring them to do so at all. In the latter case, the APN has even greater legal responsibility and accountability for understanding the law in the state in which he or she practices. An APN must take seriously the ethical and legal obligation to practice and provide optimal care within those laws, understand the scope of practice, and not overstep the boundaries of that practice as defined by the state and certifying agencies involved in the licensure (Brent, 2001).

EFFECT OF INCREASED LITIGATION ON HEALTH CARE

The following risks and the failure to reduce them affect cost and practice in health care:
- Increased cost of health care premiums
- Increased cost of health care
- Increased cost of malpractice/liability insurance

- Decreased access to prenatal care as physicians limit their practice
- Decreased quality of care as access is limited, especially for the medically indigent for whom risk is often the greatest

Rather than deterring incompetent or substandard care, increased litigation has led to defensive medical practices that include more costly and often questionably indicated testing. In addition, the personal, trusting relationship patients once shared with providers has become less trusting, with referrals to specialists who do not have a long-term care relationship with the patient. Fragmented care with increased referrals may actually result in less continuity and thus increased risk for negligence (Sinclair, 2000; Brent, 2001).

SYSTEMS OF LAW

The four systems of law in the United States are martial, military, criminal, and civil law.

Martial Law

Martial law is invoked only in times of social emergency. An example of a social emergency is a national disaster. Under martial law, civil rights can be selectively suspended.

Military Law

Military law operates in the military services and supersedes laws of states or other countries.

Criminal Law

Criminal law is the system by which the state prosecutes criminal behavior. It is subject to the court of appeals and is based on precedent. Intent is an important element of proof, as is proof of the criminal act itself. The defendant is considered innocent until proven guilty by the state as plaintiff.

Civil Law

Civil law serves for noncriminal behavior and seeks to recover compensation for proven damages. It is guided by torts, which put some of the burden of proof on the defendant. There are four elements to be proven and defended: duty, breach of duty, proximate cause, and damages (Brent, 2001).

Duty

Duty is that special relationship, recognized by law, that establishes the duty of the health care professional to render a degree of care that can be reasonably expected by a professional with the same or similar experience in the same or similar situation.

Breach of Duty

Breach of duty is a failure to meet the minimum standard of care as defined by the bodies that set the standards.

Proximate Cause

Proximate cause is an act or omission that, unbroken by any intervening cause, produces an injury. In a medical malpractice case, failure to adhere to the minimum standard of care must be the proximate cause of the injury.

Damages

Damages are the sum of money a court or jury awards as compensation. The law recognizes certain, often imprecise and inconsistent, categories of damages (Brent, 2001):

- *General damages.* Typically intangible damages such as pain and suffering, disfigurement, and interference with ordinary enjoyment of life.
- *Special damages.* Out-of-pocket expenses for medical expenses, lost wages, and rehabilitation.
- *Punitive exemplary damages.* Damages awarded to the plaintiff for intentional acts or gross negligence and used to punish the defendant or act as a deterrent to others.

Table 9-1 defines common terms used during the litigation process, terms with which nurses may be unfamiliar.

LITIGATION SEQUENCE

Once parents decide to sue, the following sequence of events occurs:

- Parents seek the services of a lawyer. They explain their view of the situation and events. During that conference, the parents name the physicians, one or more hospitals, and the nurses involved. They may bring medical records from current providers with documentation of existing problems.
- The attorney reviews the information, files the complaint, and requests records. The defense attorneys are notified.
- The attorney notifies the court of intent to bring suit and states the elements of the complaint.
- During this period, called *discovery* (Brent, 2001), a list of all possible parties to be deposed is reviewed.
- The defense attorneys for the listed parties also begin discovery.
- Potential experts for the physicians, the hospital, and the nurses are contacted to begin reviewing records.
- Some depositions are taken. The plaintiff's attorney takes the depositions of the physician(s) and the most closely involved nurses. The defense attorneys are present.
- The defense attorney or attorneys take depositions of the parents. The plaintiff's attorney is present.
- Experts are named with the court after their agreement is obtained. Some attorneys give the experts an affidavit, which is a legal document stating in general terms what the expert is prepared to stipulate as expert opinion. This statement usually involves his or her opinion of whether the standards of care were met.

Table 9-1   Definitions of Commonly Used Legal Terms

Terms	Definitions
Accreditation	The official authorization providing credentials for maintaining standards and ensuring quality of care
Case law	Legal principles derived from judicial decisions; differs from statutory law
Complaint	Legal document that is initial pleading on part of plaintiffs in a civil lawsuit; purpose is to give defendant notice of alleged facts constituting cause of action
Court trial	Trial without jury
Credentialing	System based on accepted standard criteria for determining competence and capabilities of a professional to provide consistent quality care and to minimize risks
Defendant	Individual who is named in a suit by plaintiff; medical malpractice or professional negligence cases usually include multiple defendants, such as hospital, physician or physicians, and potentially nurse or nurses if they are insured separately from the hospital
Deposition	A discovery procedure whereby each party may question the other party or any person who may be a possible witness
Evidence	Facts presented at trial through witnesses, records, documents, and concrete objects for purpose of proving or defending a case, such as standard of care testimony in medical malpractice case or opinion, which is testimony of an expert witness based on special training or background, rather than on personal knowledge of facts at issue
Expert opinion	Testimony of person who has specialized knowledge, training, skill, and experience in area relevant to resolution of the legal dispute
Foreseeability	Requirement that case be judged on facts as they were known at the time of the occurrence, not in retrospect, with hindsight, or with knowledge gained since that time
Incident report	Term for report of situation that is not consistent with entire operation of hospital or routine care of patient; more appropriately termed *occurrence* or *situation report*; usually privileged, protected from discovery unless described in patient record
Malpractice and negligence	Legal cause of action involving failure to exercise degree of diligence and care that a reasonable and ordinarily prudent person in same specialty would exercise acting under similar circumstances
Plaintiff	Individual initiating lawsuit; in case of injured minor, parents or state brings suit

Continued

Table 9-1   Definitions of Commonly Used Legal Terms—cont'd

Terms	Definitions
Professional negligence	In medical terms, malpractice is failure to exercise that degree of care, as it is used by reasonably careful health care professionals in same or similar situation or with like qualifications; failure to meet this acceptable standard of care must be direct cause of injury
Respondent superior	Legal principle that makes employer liable for civil wrongs committed by employees within course and scope of their employment
Risk management	Systems approach to prevention of malpractice claims; involves identification of system problems, analysis, and treatment of risks before a suit is brought, as well as identification of patients who may sue
Standards of care	Norms of behavior and action defined by a particular profession and described and applied by professional and accrediting organizations
Statutory law	Law enacted by legislature
Statute of limitations	Time period in which plaintiff may file lawsuit; varies from state to state and is extended in most states for birth injury for discovery to take place after school age has been reached; then time is specified for complaint to be filed after discovery

- Depositions are taken from experts and from other persons listed in the medical records.
- Some states have a system for screening cases before deciding to settle or go to court.
- The attorneys for both sides begin to make offers and counteroffers for settlement out of court.
- If no settlement is reached, the plaintiff's attorney files a court date.
- All filings of complaints, experts named, and court dates have deadlines that need to be met in order to be within the statute of limitations.
- The attorneys orchestrate the timetable for presentation of witnesses and experts. The plaintiff has the first and last word in presentation of the case.
- Subpoenas are issued to the witnesses. The attorneys who issue the subpoenas pay experts. The defense attorney recovers those costs from the insurance companies for the physicians, the hospital, or the nurse or nurses (Brent, 2001).

NURSE'S DEPOSITION

Players

People involved in the nurse's deposition are the hospital's attorney, plaintiff's attorney, physician's attorney, various paralegals and nursing consultants, a court recorder, and the witness.

Process

Swearing In

The court recorder swears in the witness by having the witness state name and current address and then swear or promise to tell the truth.

Introductory Questioning

The plaintiff's attorney begins by asking general questions such as name, marital status, current and past employment, and schooling. These questions are designed to put the nurse at ease, gain his or her trust, and evaluate body language when telling the truth for comparison against later answers about sensitive issues.

Questioning Regarding the Case

The rest of the questions are related to the care given by that nurse to the mother. These questions usually are designed to nail down the facts from the witness or the opinions of the expert. They vary in style and associated pitfalls.

Helpful Guidelines

- *Answering "yes or no" questions:* If the plaintiff's attorney asks for a "yes or no" response, and the question does not lend itself to either, the best answer is "I don't understand the question" or "I don't know." It is not wise to rephrase the question or answer "yes or no" and then try to explain the conditions. Sometimes the questions are fired in rapid succession, with the goal of eliciting a string of "yes" or "no" answers. The tendency in this situation is to answer "yes" or "no"; however, if the witness stops to think, the answer might vary. The best strategy is to stop, rephrase the question silently, and then answer thoughtfully.
- *Answering long, difficult, complex questions:* Do not answer the question in its long form. State that the question is confusing. If asked to explain the confusion, ask for the question to be separated into smaller parts; do not rephrase it.
- *Response when hospital's attorney objects to question:* If the hospital's attorney objects to a question, remember that there is no judge to arbitrate. You must have a response. Consider the objection to be a clue to think carefully about your response. Two common problems that may cause the attorney to object are (1) that the question is phrased to force you to contradict yourself or (2) that the question asks for an opinion that is not in your purview. In either of these cases, the two best answers are "I don't know (understand)" and "the question is confusing."
- *Always answer truthfully:* Even when the answer is perceived by you as less than helpful to the defense, a truthful answer is always best.
- Always look directly at the plaintiff's attorney.
- *Dress professionally and comfortably:* Position your body to occupy all of your allotted space with glasses, tissues, small purse, or a glass of water to mark

boundaries. Do not curl into a small space in the chair; *occupy* it. Avoid caffeinated beverages before or during the deposition.

- *Never argue:* Do not argue with the attorney if he or she mistakenly rephrases your responses; state that you did not understand your response to have been given as repeated.
- *Simply answer the question being asked:* Never explain unless specifically requested to do so.
- *Preparation before deposition:* Study the scientific principles underlying the situation. Study the applicable standards and policies and procedures in force at the time of the incident (Ramos, 2003).

TRIAL

Players

The same players exist for the trial as for the deposition; in addition, a judge and jury are present. There may be some onlookers, including the parents and hospital staff, if approved by both attorneys.

Process

- All attorneys read opening statements.
- The plaintiff presents his or her case first; then the defense presents. The plaintiff has some rebuttal time.
- The judge may sustain or overrule attorneys' objections. If the objection is overruled, you answer; if it is sustained, you do not.
- Look at the attorney when he or she questions you, and look at the jury when you answer.

The trial can be very threatening to self-esteem. A lawsuit may require giving information to the state board of nursing, and you may be required to take continuing education or assertiveness training and your practice scope may be limited. View the experience as an opportunity for professional growth. Support groups or individual therapy is available through many employee assistance programs. Be aware of vulnerability in the practice concurrent with the events of the lawsuit. Avoid discussing the case with any other involved staff members for your protection and theirs.

Prevention

Nurses have the following professional and personal responsibilities for preventing litigation and for assisting in the reduction of awards:

- Use practice that is evidence-based (Kardong-Edgren, 2001).
- Know the sources of standards of care and what the specific standards are. Table 9-2 describes relevant sources.
- Participate in formulating and writing nursing policies and procedures. Box 9-1 describes elements of policies and procedures to be considered.
- Know and apply components of risk management and quality assurance in clinical practice. Box 9-2 describes components of risk management and quality assurance.

Table 9-2   Sources of Standards

Organization	Description
Joint Commission on the Accreditation of Healthcare Organizations (JCAHO)	JCAHO accreditation is a voluntary and paid-for service. Among other things, it scrutinizes specialty services and requests proof of quality assurance, staff education, policies and procedures, staff ratios, and nursing procedures.
American Nurses Association (ANA)	The ANA provides statements of standards of maternal child nursing care and the Code for Nurses, 1976. It provides guidelines for minimum care standards in the specialty area of maternal child nursing.
Association of Women's Health, Obstetric, and Neonatal Nurses* (AWHONN, formerly NAACOG)	AWHONN promotes excellence in nursing practice to improve the health of women and newborns. It publishes standards of practice and education.
Community standards	Community standards are superseded by a national standard. However, a like-level designation is compared with similar-level designations. Where designation has not been requested by state accreditation such as through health department or perinatal association, the facility remains undesignated. It is compared to the level I (primary care) facilities in that state.

*For more information, contact AWHONN, 2000 L Street, NW, Suite 740, Washington, DC, 2003 6; (800) 673–8499.

- Document clinical practice that is complete, concise, and accurate and that reflects communication among health team members and with patients and family. There is some controversy regarding whether charting on monitor strips should be done at all beyond identifying the patient and medical record. This is particularly true when it pertains to recording time for certain events. Most experts agree that, in general, charting needs to be simplified so that events do not have to be charted in multiple places. Multiple charting increases the likelihood of inconsistencies in the time something was recorded on various charts. Times are recorded from a variety of sources such as a clock on a graph, a nurse's watch, and clocks on the walls of any room the patient occupies or to which she may be moved in an emergency. On the other hand, there are those who argue that the increased use of computerized charting and or the use of checklists with little or no space for narrative leave little or no room to document emergent events in sequential order and detail. Therefore the thinking processes that went into nursing decisions are easily overlooked and

---

Box 9-1   Policy and Procedure Writing

Practice Statements
- Write policies so that a wide range of acceptable practice is possible and flexibility is allowed.
- When restrictions or limitations for acceptable practice are necessary, they should be specified (ACOG, 1997).

Policy Statements
- Specific care to be rendered

Staff
- Patterns of staffing
- Educational preparation
- Special credentialing/certification/validation
- New orientation and continuing education

Equipment
- Care, repair, and testing
- Cleaning and storage
- Environment where care can or cannot be provided

Suggested Organization of Policy and Procedure
- Institution name
- Department
- Title
- Dates of origination, review, and revision
- Approval signature/committee
- Date of approval
- Purpose and patient's desired outcomes
- Practice and policy statements
- Equipment
- Procedure
- Additional information
- Cross index
- References

---

misinterpreted, and the timing of actions is often impossible to determine. It is my opinion that emergent events surrounding an electronically monitored patient should always be written on the monitor strip. If the times are missing on the computerized chart forms or the checklist forms, the timing can easily be explained from the monitor strip. It is this timing that often explains the thinking processes and the understanding of the nurse of the emergent nature of the event (Rostant and Cady, 1999). Box 9-3 describes guidelines for documentation.

- Be aware of potential risks in clinical practice. Box 9-4 lists some clinical examples of common issues.

Box 9-2   Components of Risk Management: Continuous Quality Assurance

Policy Revision

- Write new or review/revise existing policies and procedures based on national evidence-based guidelines, when available.
- Reflect achievable goals that can lead to reliable patient outcomes.
- Update the policy to reflect current practice and to meet current standards of care.
- Have a policy regarding staffing ratios and chain of command for conflict resolution.
- Educate and provide in-service education for staff about new or revised policies and procedures.
- Keep old policies until the statute of limitations expire.

Monitoring Quality Assurance

- Document a quality assurance program with provision for monitoring patient outcomes, process outcomes if patient outcomes do not meet established levels, and operational and administrative outcomes.
- Conduct patient satisfaction surveys.

Risk Management Plan for Problematic Perinatal Clinical Risks

- Fetal heart rate (FHR) monitoring as to method, frequency, and documentation data
- Oxytocin administration and safe use of labor stimulants
- Fundal versus suprapubic pressure
- Nursing response to obstetric emergencies such as
  - Fetal intolerance/nonreassuring response to labor or antepartum events
  - Maternal hemorrhage
  - Eclamptic seizures
  - Hypertensive emergencies
  - Precipitous delivery
  - Uterine rupture
  - Umbilical cord prolapse
  - Hypoglycemia
  - Maternal and fetal resuscitation
- Cardiac and respiratory emergencies
- HIV issues of reasonable accommodations and privacy
- Newborn safety (e.g., kidnapping)
- Perinatal grief support
- Advice during telephone triage
- Staffing

Sources of Liability

- Deficiency in monitoring patient status
- Failure to appropriately intervene
- Failure to accurately document (see section below)
- Failure to validate informed consent
- Failure to use appropriately current technology
- Neglect to follow advance directives
- Improper administration of medication

Continued

Box 9-2   Components of Risk Management: Continuous Quality
Assurance—cont'd

Documentation
- Patient status
- Care provided according to the nursing process and professional standards of care
- Quality assurance indicators
- Monitoring results
- Correction plan and implementation

Adapted from Rostant D, Cady R: *AWHONN: liability issues in perinatal nursing*, Philadelphia, 1999, Lippincott Williams & Wilkins; Sprague A, Trepanier M: Charting in record time, *AWHONN Lifelines* 3(5):25, 1999.

Box 9-3   Guidelines for Documentation

Documentation on Fetal Monitor Strip
- Identifying patient information
- Dates, times, and strip sequence information
- Monitoring mode, equipment used, adjustments, and calibrations
- Maternal status: vital signs, activity/position changes, vaginal examinations, status of membranes
- Medications: route, dosage, time of analgesics/anesthesia, oxytocin (Pitocin), tocolytics
- Cervical assessment
- Interventions and treatments: position changes, oxygen, oxytocin, hydration
- Delivery information: time and type of delivery
- Infant information: gender, Apgar scores, weight, newborn findings, cord pH

Documentation on Maternal Record
- Time electronic fetal monitor (EFM) was applied and mode of monitoring
- Patient status and activity
- Fetal heart rate (FHR)
- Baseline FHR to include range, stability, and variability
- Presence of accelerations, including amplitude and duration
- Presence of decelerations as to type, depth, duration, time to recovery, and completeness of recovery
- Uterine activity
- Presence, frequency, and duration
- Intensity and resting tone if intrauterine pressure catheter (IUPC)
- Assessment
- Vital signs
- Cervical assessments
- Interventions, including patient response and time of physician notification
- Communication between nurse and physician
- Antepartum and postpartum patient education, verbalization and demonstration of understanding
- Referrals

Box 9-3   Guidelines for Documentation—cont'd

Terms to Be Avoided*
- Uteroplacental insufficiency (UPI)
- Hypoxia
- Fetal distress or stress

Storage
- Safe and confidential storage of patient records must be provided by the hospital to last for at least the statute of limitations; fetal monitor strips are the fetal record and should be stored with the maternal record.

Purpose of Documentation
- Provides record of patient assessment and assists with planning care
- Evaluates patient condition and ongoing response to treatment
- Allows assessment of developing patterns in patient condition
- Provides a history for future admissions
- Provides communication among health care professionals contributing to patient care and documents that communication
- Explains diagnosis and course of illness management and treatment
- Assists in utilization review for appropriate use of hospital and resources
- Provides data in continuing education and research
- Provides information for Joint Commission on the Accreditation of Healthcare Organizations (JCAHO)
- Provides information for billing and reimbursement
- Possibly constitutes a legal document
- Identifies and provides necessary information for incident management
- "Decreased" variability

---

* These terms have not been given consistently accepted definitions.
From Brent N: *Nurses and the law: a guide to principles and applications*, Philadelphia, 2001, Saunders; Rostant D, Cady R: *AWHONN: liability issues in perinatal nursing*, Philadelphia, 1999, Lippincott Williams & Wilkins; Sprague A, Trepanier M: Charting in record time, *AWHONN Lifelines* 3(5):25, 1999.

CONCLUSION

Prospective risk management is currently our only protection in a litigious society. With high expectations for the outcome of any pregnancy being the norm for human nature, and with the forces promoting increased numbers of and amounts of awards in birth injury cases, it is little wonder that health care costs have soared.

Nurses are increasingly exposed to the risk for being named as a party to a birth injury case. It is important to realize that being found liable does not necessarily mean one is considered incompetent or likely to be punished by loss of employment or licensure. Becoming educated in terminology and the litigation process can help the nurse to maintain his or her self-esteem in this difficult and threatening experience.

Box 9-4	Clinical Examples of Common Issues

- Amniotomy and placement of internal fetal electrode through intact membrane
- Electronic fetal heart rate monitoring: continuous or intermittent
- Nurse's responsibilities and management of induction/augmentation
- Nurse's response to obstetric, cardiac, or respiratory emergencies
- Patient education for self-care antepartum and postpartum
- Birth plans
- Childbirth education and patient expectations
- Genetic or teratogenic advice
- Preterm labor response to need for treatment
- Precipitous delivery
- Role of the nurse in the care of the pregnant woman receiving analgesia and anesthesia
- Nursing care impact on cesarean birth rate
- Maternal stabilization and transport; regionalized care
- Standards for three levels of perinatal care

From Association of Women's Health, Obstetric, and Neonatal Nurses: *Clinical position statement: amniotomy and placement of internal fetal spiral electrode through intact membranes,* Washington, DC, 2002, AWHONN; Brent N: *Nurses and the law: a guide to principles and applications,* Philadelphia, 2001, Saunders; Sprague A, Trepanier M: Charting in record time, *AWHONN Lifelines* 3(5):25–30, 1999; Kardong-Edgren S: Using evidence-based practice to improve intrapartum care, *J Obstet Gynecol Neonatal Nurs* 30(4):371–375, 2001; Mahlmeister L: Legal implications of fetal heart assessment, *J Obstet Gynecol Neonatal Nurs* 29(5):517–526, 2000; Haggerty L, Nuttall R: Experienced obstetric nurses' decision-making in fetal risk situations, *J Obstet Gynecol Neonatal Nurs* 29(5):480–490, 2000; Maloni J: Preventing preterm birth: evidence-based interventions shift toward prevention, *AWHONN Lifelines* 4(4):26–33, 2000.

Nurses have an evolving role as expert witnesses as well. In the past, physicians most often gave expert testimony about the nurse's duty and standard of care. As nurses have become better educated about the process and their responsibilities as professionals and as citizens, it is appropriate for them to give expert testimony in malpractice cases involving specific nurses or the hospital's quality of nursing care.

BIBLIOGRAPHY

American Academy of Pediatrics (AAP) and Association of Obstetricians and Gynecologists (ACOG): *Guidelines for perinatal care,* ed 4, Elk Grove Village, Ill, 1997, AAP and Washington DC, 1997, ACOG.

Association of Obstetricians and Gynecologists: *Position statement: quality improvement in women's health care,* Washington, DC, 2000, ACOG.

Association of Women's Health, Obstetric, and Neonatal Nurses: *Access to health care issues,* Washington, DC, 2000, AWHONN.

Association of Women's Health, Obstetric, and Neonatal Nurses: *Fetal assessment, fetal monitoring, principles and practices,* Washington, DC, 1997, AWHONN.

Association of Women's Health, Obstetric, and Neonatal Nurses: *Position statement: insurance coverage, position statement,* Washington, DC, 1999, AWHONN.

Association of Women's Health, Obstetric, and Neonatal Nurses: *Position statement: translating standards and guidelines into practice,* Washington, DC, 2000, AWHONN.

Association of Women's Health, Obstetric, and Neonatal Nurses: *Standards for professional nursing practice in the care of women and newborns,* ed 6, Washington, DC, 2003, AWHONN.

Brent N: *Nurses and the law: a guide to principles and applications,* ed 2, Philadelphia, 2001, Saunders.

Haggerty L, Nuttall R: Experienced obstetric nurses' decision-making in fetal risk situations, *J Obstet Gynecol Neonatal Nurs* 29(5):480–490, 2000.

Kardong-Edgren S: Using evidenced-based practice to improve intrapartum care, *J Obstet Gynecol Neonatal Nurs* 30(4):371–375, 2001.

Mahlmeister L: Legal implications of fetal heart assessment, *J Obstet Gynecol Neonatal Nurs* 29(5):517–526, 2000.

Maloni J: Preventing preterm birth: evidenced-based interventions shift toward prevention, *AWHONN Lifelines* 4(4):26–33, 2000.

Ramos F: Preparing for a deposition, *Advance for nurse practitioners* 11(11):23, 2003.

Rostant D, Cady R: *AWHONN: liability issues in perinatal nursing,* Philadelphia, 1999, Lippincott Williams & Wilkins.

Shiffrin B: *Obstetrical malpractice: whose side are we on?* Presentation at the OB Challenges of the Millennium meeting, Phoenix, Ariz, April 2001.

Sinclair B: Where are the nurses? Perspectives, *AWHONN Lifelines* 4(4):7, 2000.

Sprague A, Trepanier M: Charting in record time, *AWHONN Lifelines* 3(5):25–30, 1999.

IV

Health Disorders Complicating Pregnancy

V arious health disorders can complicate pregnancy. In the past, major medical disorders precluded pregnancy either because maternal well-being could not be guaranteed or because the fetal effects were devastating. Now, with more sophisticated medical management of maternal conditions and with high technology for fetal surveillance, outcomes for both the mother and the neonate have improved. Common health disorders complicating pregnancy that are discussed in this unit are diabetes, cardiac disease, renal disease, and connective tissue disease.

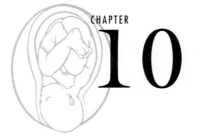

CHAPTER

10

Diabetes

D iabetes is a disease characterized by the inability to produce or use sufficient endogenous insulin to metabolize glucose properly. This inability to metabolize glucose leads to altered metabolism. Pregnancy is a diabetogenic state. Metabolism of glucose, fats, and proteins is altered, and antiinsulin forces are present. This may affect the already altered metabolism.

According to the National Diabetes Data Group Classification, there are three types of diabetes: type 1, type 2, and type 3, gestational diabetes mellitus (GDM) (ADA, 2005a). Types 1 and 2 diabetes are pregestational, that is, the woman has diabetes before becoming pregnant. In type 1 diabetes mellitus, there is absolute insulin deficiency related to a cellular-mediated autoimmune destruction of the islet cells. In type 2 diabetes mellitus, there is insulin resistance because receptor sites at the tissue level are not responsive to insulin. Therefore it takes more insulin to shut off the release of glucose from the liver. Furthermore, it takes higher levels of insulin to open the receptors and facilitate muscle glucose uptake. The pancreas is overworked to meet the increased demand of extra insulin, and hyperglycemia develops.

GDM is defined as carbohydrate intolerance that is first recognized during pregnancy (ADA, 2004b). *Impaired glucose tolerance (IGT)* and *impaired fasting glucose (IFG)* are levels of impaired glucose metabolism that are not severe enough to be diagnosed as type 1 or 2 or GDM. IGT and IFG are intermediate stages between normoglycemia and diabetes. *IGT* is defined as a 2-hour postprandial blood sugar level higher than 140 mg/dl but lower than 200 mg/dl. *IFG* is defined as a fasting blood sugar level that is 100 or higher but lower than 126 mg/dl.

During pregnancy, IFG and IGT are considered to be clinical entities of their own. Otherwise, they are considered risk factors for future diabetes and cardiovascular disease because they are associated with the insulin resistance syndrome also referred to as *syndrome X* or *metabolic syndrome*. This syndrome consists of insulin resistance and compensatory hyperinsulinemia. Inherent characteristics are obesity (especially abdominal), dyslipidemia that includes high triglycerides, low high-density lipoprotein (HDL) and high low-density lipoprotein (LDL), hypertension, prothrombotic state, and impaired glucose tolerance (National Guideline Clearinghouse, 2004).

In pregnancy, diabetes is also classified according to the age at which it was diagnosed, the length of time the disease has been present, and the degree of vascular changes that have occurred. This classification was helpful in the past to provide prognostic indicators for neonatal outcome (Table 10-1). Research indicates that the degree of metabolic control and the presence or absence of long-term complications better delineate maternal and fetal risk (ADA, 2005c).

Table 10-1   Guide to Classification of Perinatal Diabetes: Revised White's Classification

Class	Description	Vascular Disease	Treatment
A1	GDM characterized by abnormal GTT without other symptoms; fasting glucose normal	None	Diet control
A2	GDM characterized by abnormal GTT; fasting glucose elevated insulin required to control	None	Diet and insulin
B	Diabetes onset at age 20 years or older or diabetes of less than 10-year duration	None	Diet and insulin
C	Diabetes onset between ages 10 and 19 years or duration of 10–19 years	None	Diet and insulin
D	Diabetes onset before 10 years of age or duration of more than 20 years	Benign retinopathy	Diet and insulin
E	Diabetes onset at any age	Pelvic vascular disease	Diet and insulin
F	Diabetes onset at any age	Nephropathy	Diet and insulin
R	Diabetes onset at any age	Proliferative retinopathy	Diet and insulin
RF	Diabetes onset at any age	Nephropathy and retinopathy	Diet and insulin
H	Diabetes onset at any age	Atherosclerotic heart disease	Diet and insulin
T	Diabetes onset at any age	After renal transplant	Diet and insulin

Data from American College of Obstetricians and Gynecologists: Management of DM in pregnancy, *ACOG Technical Bulletin*, No. 92, Washington, DC, 1986, ACOG Resource Center.
GDM, Gestational diabetes mellitus; *GTT*, glucose tolerance test.

INCIDENCE

Diabetes in pregnancy has long been recognized as a serious problem for both the mother and fetus. Before the availability of insulin in the 1920s, women with diabetes rarely became pregnant. Those who did rarely carried a fetus to viability. According to the National Center for Health Statistics (2004), diabetes now occurs in approximately 4% to 14% of pregnant women. GDM represents almost 90% of this group (ACOG, 2005).

CAUSES

The causes of diabetes are inherent in pancreatic inability to produce sufficient insulin to transport glucose into the cells. Insulin deficiency may result from pancreatic beta-cell damage, inactivation of insulin by antibodies, or increased insulin requirements. Type 1 diabetes is a chronic autoimmune disorder of the pancreatic islet cells that develops in individuals who carry a genetic marker that has been identified on chromosomes 6 and 11 and possibly 10 other genes (EPGO, 2004; ADA, 2005a). Viral-induced, immune-stimulated antibodies against the beta cells form. This autoimmune response causes gradual destruction of the pancreatic beta cells.

People with type 2 diabetes do not carry a genetic marker but, rather, have a genetic susceptibility. Insulin resistance and pancreatic islet cell dysfunction characterize type 2 diabetes. When insulin resistance occurs, there is increased insulin secretion but ineffective insulin postreceptor binding (ADA, 2005a). Thus glucose uptake by cells is decreased and hyperglycemia results. In 80% to 85% of patients with type 2 diabetes, obesity, especially in the abdominal region, causes their insulin resistance.

NORMAL PHYSIOLOGY

Pregnancy is a diabetogenic state characterized by mild fasting hypoglycemia, postprandial hyperglycemia, and hyperinsulinemia. These changes occur to ensure a continuous supply of glucose to the fetus. There is marked individual variation in the renal threshold for glucose.

Hyperinsulinemia: Increased Insulin Production

Estrogen and progesterone stimulate pancreatic beta-cell hyperplasia. As insulin secretion is increased, peripheral glucose utilization is enhanced, leading to a decreased fasting blood glucose level in the first trimester. During the second and third trimesters, rising placental hormones increase insulin resistance; decreased hepatic glycogen stores and an increased hepatic production of glucose cause elevated postprandial blood sugar levels. This increased glucose presence further stimulates pancreatic islet cell hypertrophy, increasing insulin levels.

Increased Tissue Resistance to Insulin

During the second and third trimesters, pregnancy hormones (estrogen, progesterone, human placental lactogen hormone, and cortisol) antagonize insulin's effectiveness because of postreceptor cellular changes and stimulate hepatic glucose production. In addition, the placental enzyme *insulinase* accelerates degradation of insulin. The net effect is decreased insulin effectiveness, causing reduced peripheral uptake of glucose, which facilitates glucose availability to the fetus for accelerated fetal growth (Moore, 2004).

PATHOPHYSIOLOGY
Pregestational Diabetes
In theory, the cause of faulty metabolism in the person with diabetes is one or more of the following:
- Production of defective insulin
- Overproduction of insulin antagonist
- Increased tissue resistance to insulin
- Underproduction of insulin
- Inappropriate timing of insulin release

When insulin is not available or effective in transporting glucose into the cell, glucose remains in the bloodstream in abnormal quantities. Because of cellular starvation, the body begins breakdown of fats (*ketogenesis*) and proteins (*gluconeogenesis*) for energy.

If hyperglycemia is allowed to become severe, ketoacidosis can develop. The resultant diuresis causes loss of water and electrolytes, hyperosmolarity, and volume depletion. This in turn causes a release of stress hormones such as glucagon, catecholamines, cortisol, and growth hormones; impairs insulin action; and contributes to insulin deficiency.

When hyperglycemia becomes a long-term or recurrent event, long-standing vascular effects (Table 10-2) can occur.

Table 10-2 Long-Standing Vascular Effects

Consequences	Manifestations
Microvascular	
Autonomic neuropathy	Gastrointestinal, genitourinary, CV, sexual dysfunction
Peripheral neuropathy	Decreased perception of pain; foot ulcers
Nephropathy	Proteinuria, oliguria, renal failure
Retinopathy	Visual changes that can lead to blindness
Macrovascular	
Atherosclerotic heart changes	Cardiovascular disease, coronary artery disease
Atherosclerotic peripheral vascular changes	Hypertension, hyperlipidemia; poor healing and gangrene

When glucose is low in relation to the amount of insulin, a person with diabetes experiences different physiologic responses, manifested by hypoglycemia. During pregnancy, hypoglycemia is characterized by rapid onset. Hypoglycemia can also be exaggerated in early control of hyperglycemia. A high blood sugar level rapidly brought down to normal ranges can cause an excessive blood sugar response, and wide variations from low to high blood sugar levels can result. It is extremely important that hypoglycemia be treated with a measured amount of complex carbohydrate and protein. Thus the body does not rapidly use the glucose and then drop blood sugars even lower than the previous levels because no other source of glucose is being gradually formed and released from fats and proteins.

Women with Gestational Diabetes

GDM is defined as carbohydrate intolerance of variable severity with onset or first recognition during pregnancy (ADA, 2005a). The pancreatic beta-cell functions are impaired in response to the increased stimulation and induced insulin resistance. It is a disorder typically of late gestation. Hyperglycemia during the first trimester usually means type 2 diabetes mellitus (ADA, 2001b).

SIGNS AND SYMPTOMS

Gestational Diabetes

Signs of GDM in a previous pregnancy are as follows:
- Prior delivery of an infant weighing more than 9 pounds
- Previous stillbirth or an infant with congenital defects
- History of polyhydramnios
- History of recurrent monilial vaginitis
  Signs of GDM in the current pregnancy are as follows:
- Glycosuria on two successive office visits
- Recurrent monilial vaginitis
- Macrosomia of the fetus on ultrasound
- Polyhydramnios

Pregestational Diabetes

In the woman with pregestational diabetes, diabetic symptoms vary by trimester. Acanthosis nigrican, a hyperpigmentation and thickening of the skin of the neck or axilla area, is a common sign of insulin resistance (Ramchandani, 2004). Table 10-3 outlines the trimester manifestations and consequences.

Ketoacidosis

Signs and symptoms of ketoacidosis in the pregnant woman include the following:
- Hyperventilation or Kussmaul respirations
- Mental lethargy
- Dehydration
- Hypotension unless complicated by pregnancy-induced hypertension

Table 10-3 Trimester Manifestations and Consequences of Diabetes

	Insulin Requirements	Blood Glucose Alterations	Complicating Factors
First trimester	Reduced, related to inhibition of anterior pituitary hormones Developing embryo is glucose drain Decreased maternal caloric intake Increased insulin production	Frequent low blood glucose levels leading to increased numbers of hypoglycemia episodes, increased incidence of starvation, ketosis, and ketonemia	Loss of appetite, nausea, or vomiting common in any early pregnancy Recovery from an acidemic state is more difficult because of insulin antagonists
Second trimester	Increase related to placental hormones (cortisol, insulinase) and their antiinsulin properties	Hyperglycemia leading to ketonemia, aminoacidemia	Exaggerated ketone response to caloric restriction Decreased renal threshold from increased blood flow makes urine sugar levels meaningless Body produces lactose or milk sugar, which further increases urinary sugar
Third trimester	Marked increase related to increased placental hormones but level off after 36 weeks of gestation	Hyperglycemia leading to ketonemia, acidemia	Same as second trimester
Labor	Decrease related to workload of labor and increased metabolism	Hypoglycemia, acidemia from starvation ketosis	Usually nothing by mouth pending cesarean delivery
Postpartum	Decrease markedly related to loss of placental hormones	Hypoglycemia	Lactation lowers insulin; can initially complicate because supply is established and scheduled

- Abdominal pain; nausea and vomiting
- Fruity odor to the breath
- Ketonuria

MATERNAL EFFECTS

In general, the diabetic state in the mother does not deteriorate because of the pregnancy itself. In fact, most women, regardless of their classification during pregnancy, are in better control of their diabetes than when they are not pregnant. Despite the antagonistic forces of hormones, control is often better because of the close observation of blood sugar levels by the patient and health care team.

However, a diabetic pregnancy is more vulnerable to certain complications. The woman with diabetes who develops hyperemesis gravidarum is at risk for severe metabolic disturbances. In addition to the obvious risks of dehydration and electrolyte imbalance that are always encountered with hyperemesis, starvation ketosis becomes a very real threat to the mother and the developing fetus. Hospitalization with appropriate intravenous (IV) therapy for fluids and calories is essential to prevent complications.

A pregnancy complicated by diabetes is at significant risk for the complications outlined below. However, the risk is directly related to glucose control initiated before conception and continued throughout the pregnancy (ADA, 2004d).

Spontaneous Abortion

Diabetes mellitus increases the risk for miscarriage related to inadequate glycemic control during the embryonic phase (first 7 weeks of gestation) indicated by an elevated Hb A1c (Unger, 2001). A pregnant woman with poorly controlled diabetes has a 30% to 60% risk for spontaneous abortion (Unger, 2001).

Preeclampsia

The pregnant woman with diabetes has two times the normal risk for preeclampsia (Sibai and others, 2000). This is particularly true when there is already evidence of renal and vascular compromise. Hypertension and the resultant vasospasm can be the final blows to an already marginally effective placenta.

Preterm Labor

The woman with diabetes has a 25% risk for developing preterm labor if she has increased uterine volume, has a hypertensive disorder, develops a kidney or urinary tract infection (UTI), or has vascular compromise (Walkinshaw, 2004).

Polyhydramnios

Polyhydramnios is also more frequently encountered in the pregnant woman with diabetes than in the general population. Approximately 18% of all women with diabetes develop polyhydramnios during pregnancy. Although the mechanism for this is not fully understood, fetal hyperglycemia is thought to result in increased fetal diuresis. The significance of polyhydramnios varies depending on its source. Polyhydramnios may threaten premature rupture of the membranes because of uterine overdistention, and polyhydramnios is known to be associated with an increased incidence of fetal anomalies. In women with severe polyhydramnios, repeated therapeutic amniocenteses can be performed to relieve the pressure. Amniocentesis, when repeated, places the mother at increased risk for rupture of the membranes and infection.

Infection

The pregnant woman with diabetes is at significant risk for development of an infection involving almost any organ system. Approximately 80% of all pregnant women with diabetes develop at least one infection as compared with 26% of women who do not have diabetes (Stamler and others, 1990). These infections can occur during the antepartum or postpartum period. Vaginitis, especially monilial, occurs frequently. This is related primarily to the altered pH of the vaginal canal common in all pregnancies. Because of the increased incidence of vaginitis, which makes a prime medium for bacterial growth, the pregnant woman with diabetes has an increased risk for pyelonephritis and UTIs. These infections can be dangerous to health and increase the likelihood of preterm labor. Insulin-dependent women with diabetes are 2.5 times more likely to develop postpartum endometritis or a wound infection (Takoudes and others, 2004).

Related to the increased susceptibility and the increased risk for morbidity related to influenza, the American Diabetes Association (ADA) (2004e) recommends that persons with diabetes be immunized yearly against influenza. Pregnant women can be vaccinated after 12 weeks gestation (Weiner and Buhimschi, 2004).

Diabetic Ketoacidosis

Because of the increased risk for infection, added stress, and antiinsulin placental hormones of pregnancy, diabetic ketoacidosis (DKA) is a real risk, especially in patients with type 1 diabetes. Maternal mortality is about 1% (Trout, 1998). In DKA, glucose cannot enter the cell because of insufficient active insulin; therefore the cell starves. The result is increased lipolysis (breakdown of fat in adipose tissue). Free fatty acids are then produced in the liver and ultimately more ketone bodies are produced and build up in the bloodstream. A vicious cycle is created: the increase in ketone bodies leads to dehydration, acidosis, further breakdown of fats, and increased ketones; thus the cycle begins again. This cycle ultimately ends with decreased cardiac preload, hypertension, and shock followed by death (Foley, 1997).

Cesarean or Instrumental Birth and Induction

The pregnant woman with diabetes is more likely to deliver by the cesarean route because of concurrent complications, fetal distress, fetal macrosomia, and induction failures before term.

Retinopathy

Diabetic retinopathy may accelerate during pregnancy, especially if hypoglycemia develops with rapid institution of strict glucose control (ACOG, 2005; ADA, 2005c). This risk can be controlled by gradual attainment of normal glycemic levels and preconceptual laser photocoagulation therapy if indicated.

Hypoglycemia

The Diabetes Control and Complications Trial Research Group (1996) demonstrated that there is a greater risk for hypoglycemia when tight control is attempted (ADA, 2004d).

FETAL AND NEONATAL EFFECTS

The effects of maternal diabetes on the fetus depend somewhat on the presence of maternal vascular complications. If the mother has class D or more advanced disease, vascular deficits can affect the sufficiency of the placenta. Placental insufficiency can also cause varying degrees of nutritional or hypoxic damage to the fetus. It is manifested by intrauterine growth restriction (IUGR) and oligohydramnios.

Hypoglycemia

Hypoglycemia normally has a minimal effect on the fetus if the mother is treated appropriately. The embryo draws its glucose from stores in the lining of the uterus, and the fetus draws from stores in the placenta. In selective transfer, glucose is transferred across the placental membrane. The immediate effects of maternal hypoglycemia on the fetus are therefore minimized over time. However, severe episodes of maternal hypoglycemia that result in ketosis have been shown to cause abnormal postnatal neurologic development (Moore, 2004).

Hyperglycemia

Hyperglycemia can have numerous deleterious and sometimes fatal effects. Maternal ketonemia is transferred into the circulating amniotic fluid and therefore can induce a ketotic state in the fetus. Maternal dehydration can lead to markedly diminished amniotic fluid production and thus the loss of amniotic fluid function. Maternal hypotension can cause major shunting of blood flow away from the uterus and therefore considerably decreased oxygenation for the fetus (Moore, 2004).

Congenital Defects

The risk for congenital defects occurring in the infant of a mother with diabetes is 6% to 12%, which is four times more often than in the general population (Unger, 2001; ACOG, 2005). Hyperglycemia can be teratogenic by directly effecting the yolk sac development and interfering with free radical functioning (Walkinshaw, 2004; Kendrick and others, 2005). Faulty carbohydrate, protein, and fat metabolism also occur in the embryo and adversely affect organ development. Common fetal anomalies found in infants of mothers with diabetes include skeletal and central nervous system defects such as neural tube defects, congenital cardiac anomalies, gastrointestinal malformations, and congenital renal anomalies. Congenital anomalies are directly related to diabetic control in the 3 months before conception and during the first 2 months of pregnancy as indicated by glycosylated hemoglobin levels (ACOG, 2005).

Macrosomia

Elevated maternal glucose results in elevated fetal glucose. This stimulates fetal pancreatic production of insulin, which causes fetal hyperinsulinemia. Hyperinsulinemia increases growth and fat deposition, which are referred to as *macrosomia*. This is seen especially in classes A to C diabetes. These large-for-gestational-age (LGA) infants are at greater risk for birth trauma, particularly shoulder dystocia, brachial plexus injuries, facial nerve injuries, and asphyxia.

Intrauterine Growth Restriction

Intrauterine growth restriction (IUGR) is less frequent than macrosomia, occurring in conjunction with placental insufficiency resulting from maternal diabetic vascular disease. This is seen especially in women with class D or higher diabetes and in those with existing vascular disease before their pregnancy.

Intrauterine Fetal Death

There is an increased risk for unexplained and explainable stillbirths in women with diabetes. When placental insufficiency occurs as the result of vascular complications or an abruption, there is a clear reason for stillbirth. However, stillbirth occurs at times without obvious placental insufficiency as would be indicated by decreased fetal growth and oligohydramnios. These infants are usually LGA with polyhydramnios. It appears that severe prolonged hyperinsulinemia interferes with the transport of oxygen and carbon dioxide, leading to decreased fetal pH and increased P_{CO_2}, lactate, and erythropoietin incompatible with life (Walkinshaw, 2004).

Ketoacidosis

DKA can be life-threatening to the mother and the fetus. Fetal mortality is approximately 10% to 35% if ketoacidosis develops (ACOG, 2005). The acidotic state of DKA leads to decreased uterine blood flow, which thereby reduces fetal oxygenation.

Delayed Lung Maturity

Various studies have suggested that hyperglycemia and hyperinsulinemia cause a delay in fetal lung maturity (Walkinshaw, 2004). Elevated blood glucose appears to interfere with the production of phosphatidyl glycerol. This indicates that a mature fetal surfactant may not be present until 38 to 39 weeks of gestation (Piper and Langer, 1993).

Neonatal Hypoglycemia

The fetus is programmed to produce high quantities of insulin, and the neonate does not turn this off immediately. At birth, the supply of increased glucose is suddenly cut off, but increased production of insulin continues, resulting in neonatal hypoglycemic episodes.

Neonatal Hyperbilirubinemia

Because of possible long-term stress, the compensatory mechanism of increased production of red blood cells is stimulated. After delivery the increased red blood cell breakdown frequently overworks the young hepatic system, resulting in hyperbilirubinemia.

Neonatal Polycythemia

Polycythemia is the result of decreased oxygenation, stimulating the fetal kidneys to release glycoprotein hormone. This hormone stimulates the production of erythrocytes as a compensatory mechanism to increase the oxygen-carrying capacity of the blood. Therefore in the presence of uteroplacental insufficiency, the newborn may have polycythemia.

Learning Disabilities

Fetal brain cell damage and decreased brain growth result from prolonged exposure to hyperglycemia. This will increase the incidence of learning disabilities, lower intelligence quotient (IQ), and motor impairment (Cousins and others, 1991).

Childhood Obesity and Type 2 Diabetes Later in Life

The risk for a child of a mother with type 2 diabetes to develop type 2 diabetes later in life is 70% (Dabelea, Knowler, and Pettitt, 2000). Children who were exposed to hyperglycemia in utero have a greater risk for developing childhood obesity and childhood type 2 diabetes because they may have suffered islet cell injury (Dabelea, Knowler, and Pettitt, 2000; Vohr, McGarvey, and Tucker, 1999; Lindsay and others, 2000). Breastfeeding, diet, exercise, and prevention of obesity decrease the child's risk significantly (ADA, 2005c; Kendrick and others, 2005).

DIAGNOSTIC TESTING

Diabetes Mellitus, Type 1 and Type 2

Criteria for the diagnosis of diabetes mellitus (Expert Committee, 2001) follow:

- Fasting plasma glucose (FPG) 126 mg/dl or greater after at least an 8-hour fast
- Two-hour postprandial glucose (PG) greater than 200 mg/dl after a 75-g glucose load

- Symptoms of diabetes such as polyuria, polydipsia, and unexplained weight loss plus casual plasma glucose concentration greater than 200 mg/dl

The diagnosis is made after these criteria are confirmed by a repeat positive test on a different day.

Gestational Diabetes

According to a position statement of the American Diabetes Association, all patients except women at low risk should be screened for GDM between 24 and 28 weeks of gestation. The low risk group (ADA, 2004b) includes women who meet the following criteria:

- Younger than 25 years
- Normal body weight prior to pregnancy
- Negative family history of diabetes (no first-degree relative with the disease)
- No history of IGT or IFG
- No history of poor obstetric outcome
- Not a member of a high risk ethnic or racial group, such as African American, Asian, Hispanic, or Native American

Any pregnant woman whose history indicates that she is at high risk for developing GDM should be screened at her first prenatal visit, as well as the prenatal visit between 24 and 28 weeks of gestation (ADA, 2004b). High risk factors include the following:

- Positive family history for diabetes in parents or siblings
- Positive history of poor obstetric outcome such as unexplained stillbirth, prior fetal anomaly, or recurrent spontaneous abortion
- Prior infant with a birth weight of 9 pounds or more
- Obesity
- Multiple gestation
- Polycystic ovary syndrome (PCOS)
- Hypertensive disorder
- Recurrent monilial vaginitis
- Polyhydramnios without demonstrated fetal anomalies
- Glycosuria on two consecutive office visits
- Native American, Hispanic American, Asian American, African American, or Pacific Islander ethnic descent

Screening for GDM takes one of two forms.

Two-Step Approach: Glucose Challenge Test

A glucose challenge test is performed by initially giving 50 g of oral glucose and 1 hour later testing the blood sugar. Boyd and others (1995) found 18 jelly beans to be an acceptable alternative to 50 g of glucose. A blood sugar level of 130 mg/dl or greater should be followed up with an oral glucose tolerance test (OGTT) to confirm GDM.

One-Step Approach: Oral Glucose Tolerance Test

An OGTT is performed without prior glucose challenge test to screen for GDM.

Table 10-4   Normal Serum Values of Oral Glucose Tolerance Test in Pregnancy

Time of Measurement	100 g Blood Glucose (mg/dl)	75 g Blood Glucose (mg/dl)
Fasting	Less than 95	less than 95
1 hr	Less than 180	less than 180
2 hr	Less than 155	less than 155
3 hr	Less than 140	

Data from American Diabetes Association: Position statement: Gestational diabetes mellitus, *Diabetes Care* 27(Suppl 1):S88–S90, 2004b.

Two- or Three-Hour Glucose Tolerance Test

In either approach, GDM is diagnosed with an OGTT of either a 3-hour, 100-g glucose load or a 2-hour, 75-g glucose load. The 100-g OGTT is preferred because the 75-g glucose load is not as well validated. Before either OGTT, 150 g of complex carbohydrate should be eaten for 3 days. Instruct the woman to abstain from eating, drinking, and smoking for 8 hours before the test. Have her rest for approximately 30 minutes before the test. Begin the test by drawing a fasting blood sugar sample. Start the timer and have the patient drink 100 g of glucose solution within 5 minutes. Subsequent blood samples are drawn at 1, 2, and 3 hours. During the test, the patient should rest and abstain from smoking. GDM is diagnosed if two or more plasma glucose blood values exceed the values listed in Table 10-4 (ADA, 2004b; ADA, 2005c). A single abnormal value indicates IGT.

Detection of Maternal Complications

Women who have already been diagnosed with diabetes, either during a previous pregnancy or in the absence of pregnancy, are usually classified as previously described (see Table 10-1). If the woman is insulin-dependent, she should be screened for hypertension; dyslipidemia; peripheral and autonomic neuropathy; and renal, retinal, peripheral vascular, and cardiac involvement. Some commonly ordered tests are blood urea nitrogen (BUN) and serum creatinine, fasting lipid profile, microalbuminuria with a 24-hour albumin excretion with creatinine clearance or collection for albumin-to-creatinine ratio, electrocardiogram (ECG), ophthalmic examination for retinopathy, and treadmill test. Women with type 1 diabetes should have thyroid function studies.

Glycosylated Hemoglobin

Hemoglobin A is a normal minor hemoglobin that has a glucose link. Glucose attaches to this hemoglobin during its normal 120-day life span. The amount depends on the glucose in the bloodstream. Glycosylated hemoglobin (Hb A1c) is a blood test to determine the level of hemoglobin A that has become "sugar coated." Therefore the test reflects adequacy of glucose control for the previous 4 to 6 weeks. Hb A1c levels above 7 indicate elevated glucose during the past 4 to 6 weeks and are associated with an increased incidence of congenital anomalies. Therefore this test is used to screen women with diabetes before conception or at the initial prenatal visit. Some endocrinologists continue to screen for adequacy of control every 2 to 3 months throughout the pregnancy.

USUAL MEDICAL MANAGEMENT AND PROTOCOLS FOR NURSE PRACTITIONERS

Preconception Management

Preconception planning is the key to a successful pregnancy; planning decreases risks for the woman and her fetus with pregestational diabetes. This involves evaluating the treatment of any existing complications of DM, as outlined below.

Hypertension

Ideally, blood pressure should be stabilized prior to pregnancy. In the nonpregnant person with diabetes, angiotensin-converting enzyme inhibitors (ACE inhibitors), diuretics, or angiotension II receptor blockers (ARBs) are the drugs of choice. However, none of these drugs should be used during pregnancy. ACE inhibitors and ARBs increase the risk for congenital malformations. Diuretics may decrease maternal plasma volume decreasing uteroplacental perfusion. Beta-blockers are not recommended since they can interfere with glucose control. Approximately 5% to 10% of pregnant patients with diabetes have chronic hypertension (Hinton and Sibai, 2004). The antihypertensive medications of choice during pregnancy are methyldopa, calcium channel blockers such as nifedipine, or alpha-adrenergic blockers. Ideally, the blood pressure should be kept between 110–129 mm Hg systolic and 65–79 mm Hg diastolic (ADA, 2005c). Pregnant patients with diabetes and hypertension are at increased risk for preeclampsia, UPI, and stillbirth if the blood pressure is elevated. In contrast, a blood pressure that is too low may interfere with uteroplacental perfusion, thus interfering with fetal growth as well.

Preeclampsia is a common complication in the pregnant patient who has diabetes, with or without chronic hypertension, especially if glucose control is poor. Therefore close monitoring of the blood pressure throughout pregnancy is important.

Dyslipidemia

Many patients with diabetes are on a lipid-lowering agent such as a HMG-CoA reductase inhibitor (statin) to decrease coronary and cerebrovascular events. However, statins are a pregnancy category X drug, and their use should be stopped prior to pregnancy. Dyslipidemia is a chronic disorder. Cessation of therapy during pregnancy does not significantly affect the long-term sequela (Weiner and Buhimschi, 2004).

Platelet Aggregation

Many patients with diabetes have increased production of thromboxane, a potent vasoconstrictor and platelet aggregate. Low-dose aspirin (75 mg) is being used as primary and secondary prevention strategy for patients with diabetes who have CV risk without contraindications such as aspirin allergy, bleeding disorder, hepatic disease, or on anticoagulant therapy (ADA, 2004a). Low-dose aspirin use in the second and third trimester may decrease the risk for preeclampsia and IUGR (see Chapter 21). Aspirin therapy should be avoided during the first trimester related to the risk for fetal abnormalities (Weiner and Buhimschi, 2004).

Autonomic Neuropathy

Autonomic neuropathy can cause cardiovascular, gastrointestinal track, or bladder dysfunction and increase the risk for pregnancy complications. Orthostatic blood pressure changes, a flat pulse rate during position change, dizziness, lightheadedness, and weakness on standing are signs of possible cardiovascular neuropathy indicating a referral. Bloating, epigastric pain, nausea, vomiting, diarrhea, and postprandial hypoglycemia are signs of gastroparesis indicating a referral to the gastroenterologist.

Peripheral Sensory Neuropathy

Because diabetes can cause peripheral sensory neuropathy leading to nerve damage to the feet, conduct a comprehensive foot screen using the LEAP assessment. The assessment includes sensory testing of the feet for position sense, vibratory sensation, and monofilament tactile perception (Birke and Rolfsen, 1998). Details about the LEAP assessment can be found online *(http://www.bphc.hrsa.gov/leap/LEAPFilament.htm)*. Assess also the dorsalis pedis pulse, posterior tibialis pulse, capillary refill, and ankle reflexes. Any negative finding indicates a referral.

Nephropathy

Renal insufficiency can increase the risk to mother and fetus during pregnancy. Therefore all patients with diabetes should be screened before conception or at the first prenatal visit. Serum creatinine, creatinine clearance, or microalbuminuria are tests that evaluate renal function.

Retinopathy

A preconception dilated retinal examination by an ophthalmologist is recommended to assess for microaneurysms, small retinal hemorrhages, cotton wool spots, and exudates. Pregnancy can cause retinopathy to worsen.

Antepartum Glycemic Management

According to the American Diabetes Association (2000), the goals of management of the pregnant woman with diabetes using whole blood values are as follows (add 15% if plasma values are used):
- Maintain fasting glucose levels between 60 and 90 mg/dl
- Maintain glucose levels before lunch and dinner between 60 and 105 mg/dl
- Bedtime glucose between 90 and 120 mg/dl
- Keep 1-hour postprandial glucose levels between 100 and 120 mg/dl
- Keep 2-hour postprandial glucose levels between 90 and 120 mg/dl

- Keep the 2 AM to 4 AM blood glucose between 60 and 120 mg/dl
- Achieve a treatment Hb A1c concentration (6.1%)
- Prevent episodes of hypoglycemia
- Prevent DKA

Home monitoring and control consist of the following six facets in the patient with diabetes: blood glucose monitoring, urine testing, insulin management, diet management, exercise recommendations, and antepartum fetal surveillance. Hospitalization may become necessary if euglycemia cannot be maintained with home monitoring and outpatient surveillance. Care is provided in collaboration with an endocrinologist and obstetrician or perinatologist.

Blood Glucose Monitoring

Monitoring blood glucose during pregnancy is a cornerstone to glycemic control (ADA, 2005c). It is primarily accomplished by daily self-monitoring of blood glucose (SMBG) by the patient and Hb A1c tests every 4 to 6 weeks to confirm glycemic control of the previous 120 days. Periodic laboratory measurements of plasma glucose are used only to supplement or test the accuracy of SMBG (ADA, 2001e).

SMBG should be done 2 to 10 times a day, depending on difficulty of control, but postprandial must be assessed. The capillary blood glucose samples are taken before meals and snacks, 1 to 2 hours after meals, at bedtime, and between 2 AM and 4 AM. The typical management plan consists of blood glucose monitoring at four separate times throughout the day and evening:

- Morning fasting
- Two hours after breakfast
- Two hours after lunch
- Two hours after dinner (may count as the bedtime glucose monitoring)
- Bedtime checks (optional, unless there are problems with morning hyperglycemia)

Glucose monitoring should begin before conception. If this is not possible, it should begin as soon as pregnancy is suspected or determined. A portable blood glucose reflectance meter is readily available to rent or buy. The meter is used to read chemical test strips. The results should be recorded in a logbook and brought to each prenatal visit. For correct interpretation of blood glucose, it is critical to know whether the home monitor and strips provide whole blood or plasma results. The laboratory blood glucose test uses plasma, and many home capillary monitors measure whole blood glucose. Whole blood glucose values are about 15% lower than plasma; this is related to dilution (Chernecky and Berger, 2001). (See Self-Monitoring of Blood Glucose, p. 259.)

Two new continuous glucose monitoring systems are currently available: Glucowatch G2 Biographer (GW2B) and the Continuous Glucose Monitor system by Medtronic Minimed. The GW2B is a noninvasive device worn as a wristwatch with a disposable autosensor that pulls glucose through the skin. (For additional information, go to *http://www.glucowatch.com*) The Continuous Glucose Monitor system uses a subcutaneous sensor to perform ongoing glucose measurements throughout the day. The device is worn for 3 days and the information obtained is then downloaded into a computer, which graphically prints out the blood glucose levels. Both devices can be helpful in determining at what time during the day the blood sugars are abnormal (Loon, 2004).

Urine Testing

Ketones. Urine testing for ketones should be done three times a week during pregnancy on the first void of the day. A slight ketonuria may indicate nocturnal hypoglycemia. If the patient becomes ill or if blood glucose levels are greater than 200 mg/dl, it should be done daily. In pregnancy, ketonuria may be caused by dietary insufficiencies such as low carbohydrate intake, low calorie intake, or skipped meals or snacks; it can also occur when ketoacidosis is present.

Sugar. Because of the lowered renal threshold for glucose, glucosuria is not used as a means of determining management.

Insulin Management

Normal insulin needs change during pregnancy related to insulin-antagonistic placental hormones. Table 10-5 outlines the normal changes in insulin need during pregnancy. Early in pregnancy, insulin requirements may decrease slightly. At about 18 to 24 weeks of gestation, the insulin requirements begin to gradually increase until approximately 36 weeks of gestation, when insulin requirements usually level off. Around 38 weeks of gestation, requirements may

Table 10-5   Changes in Insulin Need During Pregnancy

Trimester	Insulin Need	Common Problems
First	Decrease 10%–25% to avoid hypoglycemia	Blood sugar very unstable Nocturnal hypoglycemia common
Second 18–24 wk	Daily insulin requirement increases gradually Typically, over pregnancy baseline: • Type 1 increase 10%–20% • Type 2 increase 30%–90%	Mother switches from a glucose-based to a lipid-based energy to spare glucose for fetal growth
Third	0.9–1.2 units/kg/day	Related to diminished responsiveness to insulin
36 weeks of gestation	Insulin levels plateau and may slightly decrease	
Labor and delivery	In active labor may decrease to 0	
Postpartum	Decrease markedly related to loss of placental hormones	Hypoglycemia

slightly decrease. A rapid decrease may indicate placental compromise. See Insulin Administration, under Nursing Management.

Types of insulin. The usual type of insulin used for the pregnant woman with diabetes is a biosynthetic human insulin (Humulin), made by genetically programming *Escherichia coli* bacteria to produce insulin. Adverse reactions to insulin, which include hypersensitivity or allergic skin reactions, lipodystrophy, and tissue resistance, rarely occur with biosynthetic human insulin as compared with the animal-based insulins (ACOG, 2005).

Insulin classifications. The current classifications of insulin today are rapid-acting lispro (Humalog), short-acting regular (Humulin R), intermediate-acting neutral protamine Hagedorn (NPH; Humulin N), and Lente (Humulin L) or long-acting Ultralente (Humulin U).

Lispro can be substituted for regular insulin at a 1:1 rate and is preferred during pregnancy and lactation (Weiner and Buhimschi, 2004). The advantages of lispro are that it works faster (within 15 minutes) and has a shorter duration (lasting only 3 hours) than regular insulin. Therefore lispro matches the body's insulin needs at mealtime.

In contrast, the onset of regular insulin is slower, taking 30 minutes or longer, and it has a longer duration time of 6 to 8 hours, which lasts past the mealtime. Therefore lispro causes less postprandial hyperglycemia and decreases the rate of hypoglycemia. However, the patient must eat as soon as she takes her injection unless she is lowering a high blood glucose. High glycemic index foods such as bread, rice, potatoes, and sucrose products are covered much better with lispro than with regular insulin, but with slow glycemic foods lispro may cause hypoglycemia. When regular insulin is used, snacks are essential in the morning, in the afternoon, and at bedtime to prevent premeal hypoglycemia because it peaks at 4 hours. See Table 10-6 for onset, peak, and duration of insulins.

Newer insulins are available, such as the delayed-absorption peakless basal insulin glargine (Lantus) and a new rapid-acting insulin aspart (Novolog). Research needs to be done to direct the use of these newer insulins for the

Table 10-6   Comparison Chart for Human Insulins

Type	Preparation	Appearance	Onset	Peak (hr)	Duration (hr)
Rapid-acting Humalog	Lispro	Clear solution	15.0 min	1½	3–4
Short-acting Humulin	Regular insulin	Clear solution	0.5 hr	3–4	6–8
Intermediate-acting	NPH	Cloudy suspension	2–4 hr	4–12	12–24
Humulin	Lente	Cloudy suspension	2–6 hr	6–15	14–24

NPH, Neutral protamine Hagedorn (insulin).

pregnant or lactating woman with diabetes. When Lantus is used, it is administered at bedtime and cannot be mixed with any other insulin in the same syringe or at the same site.

Insulin dosage. Insulin doses must be constantly adjusted as the pregnancy progresses. The patient's 24-hour insulin dosage is usually calculated according to trimester. Table 10-7 provides calculation guidelines for insulin dosage during the three trimesters. Table 10-8 presents common causes and treatment for early morning hyperglycemia. Individualized modifications of insulin need depend on various factors. For women with GDM or class B

Table 10-7 Calculation Guidelines for Insulin During Pregnancy

Trimester	Insulin Dosage (Units/kg Body Weight)
Prepregnant	0.5–0.6
First trimester	0.7–0.8
Second trimester	0.8–1.0
Third trimester until 36 weeks	0.9–1.2
Postpartum	0.6

Data from American College of Obstetricians and Gynecologists: *Pregestational diabetes mellitus, clinical management guidelines for obstetrician-gynecologists,* No. 60, 2005, ACOG.

Table 10-8 Early Morning Hyperglycemia

Cause	Definition	2–4 AM Blood Sugar	Treatment
Somogyi effect	Nocturnal hypoglycemia causes a surge of counterregulatory hormones that increase the morning blood glucose	Low	Decrease evening NPH or increase kilocalories of bedtime snack OR Change the evening NPH from predinner to prebedtime snack
Dawn phenomenon	Exaggerated growth hormone effect between 5 AM and 8 AM in conjunction with the waking process	Normal	Change the evening NPH from predinner to prebedtime snack Cautious use of early morning regular insulin (3–6 AM)
Waning insulin	Inadequate insulin coverage relative to evening caloric intake	Elevated	Increase evening NPH dose Change evening NPH dose from predinner to prebedtime snack

NPH, Neutral protamine Hagedorn (insulin).

diabetes that had been controlled with oral agents, the 24-hour insulin dosage is usually calculated according to the patient's present weight and weeks of gestation. If the patient is thin, her need is lower than normal. However, if she is extremely overweight, her need is increased from the norm. For pregestational women with diabetes already on insulin, the insulin dosage is evaluated and adjusted based on current control and weeks of gestation.

Dosage distribution. The 24-hour insulin requirement is divided into two components: basal (long-acting) and bolus (rapid- or short-acting) insulin. Of the total 24-hour insulin dose, 50% should be provided as basal insulin and 50% as bolus insulin.

The 24-hour insulin requirement is further divided into two to four injections each day, to be given 20 to 30 minutes before a meal if regular insulin is used or just before the meal if lispro is used. Patients with type 1 diabetes most likely need three or more injections per day.

For a *two-dose regimen*, the morning dose is usually two thirds of the woman's 24-hour dose, of which one third is regular insulin and two thirds is NPH. Her predinner dose is the remaining one third of her 24-hour dose, of which one half is rapid- or short-acting insulin and one half is NPH. The greatest risk with this type of dosing is the evening intermediate-acting insulin peaking during the middle of the night.

A *three-dose regimen* is similar to the two-dose regimen, but the evening intermediate-acting insulin (NPH) is held to bedtime to decrease nocturnal hypoglycemia.

For a *four-dose regimen*, rapid- or short-acting insulin is to be given before each meal and NPH before the bedtime snack.

A *multiple-injection method* is an insulin dosage based on premeal blood glucose levels and grams of carbohydrate in the meal to be eaten. A basal dose of insulin of approximately 50% of the day's total insulin requirement is given as a long-acting insulin, such as Ultralente insulin in the morning and evening. The morning dose is one third of the long-acting dose, and the predinner dose is two thirds of the long-acting dose. The patient then gives herself a rapid- or short-acting insulin before each meal, based on the number of carbohydrate grams in the planned meal and her premeal blood glucose level. The equation used is 1.5 units of regular insulin per 10 carbohydrate grams at breakfast and one unit of regular insulin per 10 carbohydrate grams at lunch and dinner. No additional insulin is given if the blood glucose is in the normal range (70 to 100 mg/dl). If the blood glucose is lower than 70 mg/dl, the dose is decreased by two units of regular insulin. If the blood sugar is between 100 and 140 mg/dl, two extra units of regular insulin are given, and if the blood sugar is greater than 140 mg/dl, four extra units of regular insulin are given (ADA, 2000).

Dosage adjustments. Adjustments in insulin may need to be made every 5 to 10 days during pregnancy to achieve target glucose control, based on SMBG. Always start by fixing the fasting blood sugar first. Usually, adjust by one to two units or 10% of dosage, not to exceed four units, in response to a pattern of blood glucose levels. Usual insulin changes recommended on an outpatient basis are described in Table 10-9. However, if early morning hyperglycemia occurs, refer

Table 10-9   Changes with Split-Dose Insulin

Time	Blood Sugar Level (mg/dl)	Action
Fasting blood sugar	Less than 60	Call physician for adjustment
	60–120	No change in 4 PM dose
	120–150	Increase evening NPH insulin by 2 units; check fasting blood sugar next day
	150–210	Increase evening NPH insulin by 4 units; check fasting blood sugar next day
	Greater than 210	Call physician for adjustment
Lunch blood sugar	Less than 60	Call physician for adjustment
	60–120	No change in morning regular insulin
	120–150	Increase morning regular insulin by 2 units
	200–240	Increase morning regular insulin by 6 units
	Greater than 240	Call physician for adjustment
Dinner (PM) blood sugar	Less than 60	Call physician for adjustment
	60–120	No change in morning dose
	120–150	Increase morning NPH insulin by 2 units; check 4 PM blood sugar next day
	200–240	Increase morning NPH insulin by 6 units; check 4 PM blood sugar next day
	Greater than 240	Call physician for adjustment
Bedtime snack blood sugar	Less than 60	Call physician for adjustment
	60–120	No change in evening regular insulin
	120–150	Increase evening regular insulin by 2 units
	200–240	Increase evening regular insulin by 6 units
	Greater than 240	Call physician for adjustment

Private practice protocols of Drs. D. O'Keeffe and J. Elliott, perinatologists, Phoenix, 1991.
NPH, Neutral protamine Hagedorn (insulin).

to Table 10-8 for common causes and treatment. Nocturnal hypoglycemia is more common during pregnancy. Symptoms such as night sweating, nightmares, difficulty sleeping, or morning headaches may indicate nocturnal hypoglycemia.

To treat a temporary loss of control, the current insulin dose of rapid- or short-acting insulin is adjusted using an insulin sensitivity factor formula to determine the amount the blood sugar will be lowered by one unit of insulin. This is determined by using the rule of 1500 if regular insulin is used and rule of 1800 if Humalog (Lispro) is used. According to these rules, either 1500 or 1800 divided by the daily insulin dosage the patient is taking. This equals the amount the glucose level will drop with one unit of regular insulin.

Insulin Therapy for Gestational Diabetes Mellitus

When medical nutritional therapy (MNT) with exercise does not keep the fasting plasma glucose lower than 95 mg/dl or the 2-hour postprandial lower than 120 mg/dl, insulin should be initiated (ADA, 2000; EPGO, 2004). An average starting insulin dose is between 20 and 30 units, divided into two thirds intermediate-acting insulin and one third regular insulin. Adjustments are necessary based on such variables as follows:

- Dosage is less if started before third trimester related to less insulin resistance
- Dosage is increased in obese women because of increased insulin resistance

Insulin pump. The usual means of administering insulin at home is through multiple subcutaneous injections. However, a device for continuous infusion is used in some circumstances. It is recommended only if the woman cannot achieve adequate control with multiple-dose injections because of the risk for nocturnal hypoglycemia with the use of the pump during pregnancy. The open-loop system infuses insulin at a basal rate and, before meals, delivers a bolus of insulin. The basal rate is generally 2.5 to 5 mU/kg/hr. Some open-loop systems require resetting after each bolus dose; others do this automatically. These systems are small and portable, usually worn around the waist with a belt. Indications for its use includes erratic blood glucose levels, need for flexibility in meal and sleep schedules, or difficulty controlling postprandial blood glucose levels (Doyle and others, 2004).

Glyburide. Oral glucose-lowering agents have not been recommended during pregnancy because of the risk for fetal anomalies and reactive hypoglycemia. However, one randomized control trial compared glyburide, a type of sulfonylurea drug, with insulin in women with GDM who were unable to meet glycemic control on MNT. Both treatments resulted in similar perinatal results (Kremer and Duff, 2004). This particular sulfonylurea does not cross the placenta to the fetus. Glyburide has not been FDA-approved for use during pregnancy; therefore its use is restricted to investigational research. It should not be concluded that other sulfonylurea drugs are safe to be used during pregnancy.

Diet Management

Diet is another cornerstone of therapy in the management of diabetes. The current diabetic diet is less restrictive and encourages individualization (ADA, 2001d). Consideration must be given to prepregnancy weight, general health status, dietary habits, activity level, and insulin therapy. Folic acid supplements of 400 mcg/day are recommended before conception and throughout the first trimester to decrease the risk for neural tube defects. (See Medical Nutrition Therapy, under Nursing Management, for in-depth diabetic dietary guidelines.)

Caloric Needs

During pregnancy, caloric intake should be increased by approximately 300 calories daily and modified to provide at least a 25-pound weight gain plus additional nutrients for mother and fetus. Daily caloric intake for a pregnant woman whose preconception body weight was ideal for her height and body frame is calculated as 30 to 35 cal/kg of body weight per day. If the woman was underweight before conception, her daily caloric intake is calculated as 36 to 40 cal/kg of body weight. When the pregnant woman was heavier than her ideal weight starting pregnancy, her daily caloric intake is calculated as 24 cal/kg or as low as 12 to 18 cal/kg if she is extremely obese (greater than 150% of ideal body weight) (ACOG, 2005).

Exercise Recommendations

Exercise is an important component in establishing and maintaining glucose control; improved insulin sensitivity is evident after 4 weeks of exercise (ADA, 2001a; Cunningham and others, 2005). See Activity and Exercise Functional Health Pattern, under Nursing Management, for specifics on exercise during pregnancy complicated with diabetes. However, if the pregnancy is also complicated with hypertension or vascular disease, a regular exercise program may be contraindicated (ADA, 2000).

Maternal Surveillance with Preexisting Diabetes

Frequent laboratory tests to be done during pregnancy to monitor the patient's diabetes status follow:
- Hb A1c test every 4 to 6 weeks
- Blood glucose fingerstick each prenatal visit to evaluated accuracy of SMBG
- Urine for protein, sugar, ketones, nitrate, and leukocyte esterase at each prenatal visit (Positive for nitrates and leukocyte esterase indicates possible UTI and should be followed up with a urine culture and sensitivity. Positive for protein indicates further evaluation for preeclampsia. Positive for ketone indicates further dietary workup to evaluate eating habits.)
- Kidney function with a 24-hour creatinine clearance and total protein to be done each trimester
- Retinal examination in the first trimester and then as indicated
- Thyroid panel for women with type 1 diabetes in the first trimester to include free thyroxine (T_4), thyroid-stimulating hormone, and antimicrosomal antibodies and then as indicated

In the presence of cardiovascular disease, a cardiologist should be a part of the health care team.

Antepartum Fetal Surveillance

Antepartum monitoring is essential to evaluate early and periodic fetal condition and to help time the delivery to coincide with optimal outcome.

Ultrasound. Ultrasound examinations are usually done at intervals throughout the pregnancy. They are done to help accurately predict gestational age and to provide reassurance about fetal organ development. They also give information about fetal growth rate, activity quality, amniotic fluid volume, and biophysical profile evaluation.

Alpha-fetoprotein. Alpha-fetoprotein helps detect open fetal defects such as open neural tube or ventral wall defects of omphalocele or gastroschisis. The fetus of a woman with type 1 diabetes is at increased risk for these defects.

Fetal movement. Fetal movement counts are a valuable component of fetal surveillance. They should be used for daily surveillance of fetal well-being from 28 weeks of gestation until delivery. Several methods can be used (see Chapter 3).

Fetal echocardiogram. If the initial Hb A1c test was elevated, a fetal echocardiogram may be considered between 20 and 22 weeks of gestation to rule out a cardiac anomaly (Moore, 2004).

Biophysical profile. Biophysical profiles are the primary means of surveillance of fetal well-being and uteroplacental adequacy. For classes A_2, B, C, and D diabetes, the biophysical profile is started at or near week 32 and is done weekly until delivery. For more advanced disease indicated by proteinuria, IUGR, or hypertension, it is started by week 26 to 28. For class A diabetes, biophysical profiles should be started by week 40 (Moore, 2004).

Contraction stress test. The contraction stress test (CST) may be the primary means of fetal surveillance when biophysical profiles are not readily available.

Nonstress test. Because the nonstress test (NST) is not as sensitive as the CST, the NST may be done between weekly CSTs so that testing is performed every 3 to 4 days (Moore, 2004). In some centers, NSTs are used in place of CSTs. If so, NSTs should be done twice each week instead of weekly.

Doppler umbilical artery velocimetry. Doppler umbilical artery velocimetry may be used early to detect IUGR. If the mother has vascular insufficiency, risk is increased for placental vascular disease. In these cases, Doppler studies may be done.

Amniocentesis. Amniocentesis is usually used to ascertain the lecithin/sphingomyelin (L/S) ratio and the presence of phosphatidyl glycerol (PG). An L/S ratio of 2.0 or greater when PG is present is sufficient to expect that surfactant levels are high enough in the fetus to prevent the development of respiratory distress syndrome (RDS). Amniocentesis is generally done if elective delivery is planned in a patient with poor glycemic control. It is not necessary in patients who have had consistent glycemic control (Moore, 2004).

Management of Ketoacidosis

DKA is caused by ineffective insulin combined with an elevation of counter-regulatory hormones such as glucagon, catecholamines, cortisol, and growth hormone to move glucose into cells, leading to hyperglycemia (diabetes). The liver tries to compensate by increasing its production of glucose, only to further raise blood glucose levels. The lack of glucose for cell use causes the body to break down fat for energy, which results in ketone (acetone) release, ketosis (serum acetone at a 1:2 dilution or greater). The respiratory system attempts to compensate by increasing the respiratory rate and depth (Kussmaul respirations), blowing off carbon dioxide. A decline in pH (less than 7.3), a drop in serum bicarbonate (less than 15 mg/dl), and an abnormal elevated anion gap (greater than 12) results.

When the woman's buffering system is unable to compensate, metabolic acidosis develops. The excessive glucose and ketone bodies result in osmotic diuresis and ketonuria with subsequent fluid and electrolyte loss, volume depletion, and cellular dehydration. Infections of urine, skin, lungs, or amniotic fluid; noncompliance with insulin administration; or dietary indiscretion are precipitating factors.

Nonreassuring fetal heart rate tracings are very common. In deciding the plan of care, keep in mind that the fetal heart rate usually improves as the maternal DKA is corrected (ADA, 2000).

The critical care management protocols for ketoacidosis are summarized in Critical Care Intervention for Perinatal Ketoacidosis, under Nursing Management.

Preterm Labor Management

Nifedipine is the preferred tocolytic drug as to effectiveness and safety (Weiner and Buhimschi, 2004). Magnesium sulfate or indomethacin may also be used to allow for the administration of corticosteroids. If corticosteroids are needed to enhance fetal lung maturity, close assessment of maternal glucose levels and IV insulin may be necessary. The daily dose of insulin may need to be doubled (ADA, 2000). Because beta-sympathomimetics can stimulate hyperglycemia and even cause ketoacidosis, their use is not recommended for the patient with diabetes.

Intrapartum Management

The woman with well-controlled diabetes who has no complications does not need to deliver before term if the fetus is not macrosomic and the biophysical profile is reassuring. Early delivery may be necessary if the woman has not had good glucose control, has a history of a stillbirth, or has developed complications such as a hypertensive disorder of pregnancy or vasculopathy or if the fetal estimated weight is LGA or there is an indication of fetal compromise (Moore, 2004). In any of these cases, an induction or cesarean birth may be scheduled.

Otherwise, according to the Cochrane review, there is little evidence to support either active induction of labor at the end of 38 weeks of gestation or expectant management until week 42 (Boulvain, Stan, and Irion, 2001). During an induction or spontaneous labor, intermittent subcutaneous insulin or a continuous insulin infusion is required. Most women with GDM do not require insulin during labor. See Intrapartum Management, under Nursing Management.

Insulin Infusion

If a continuous insulin infusion is needed, 25 units of regular insulin are added to 250 mg of normal saline (NS) (ACOG, 2005). Piggyback insulin is infused to the main IV line of D_5LR. The IV rate and supplemental regular insulin vary based on every 1- to 2-hour capillary blood glucose value. See Potential Complication: Hypoglycemia, Intrapartum.

Intermittent Subcutaneous Insulin

If intermittent subcutaneous injections are used, one third to one half of the patient's prepregnancy dosage of insulin may be given the morning of the induction. A long-acting insulin most likely is not used because of the drop in insulin requirement after delivery (Moore, 2004). A continuous 5% glucose infusion is started at approximately 100 ml/hr. Supplemental regular insulin is given based on glucose values obtained every 1 to 2 hours to maintain plasma glucose between 80 and 120 mg/dl or capillary whole blood glucose between 70 and 110 mg/dl.

Cesarean Birth

In the event a cesarean birth is planned, fetal lung maturity is usually predetermined. The cesarean is scheduled for early morning. The woman should drink nothing after midnight and hold her evening and morning dosages of insulin. Her capillary glucose level should be checked before and immediately following the delivery. Glucose is administered IV.

Postpartum Management

At delivery there is an abrupt loss of the antagonistic placental hormones and suppression of the anterior pituitary growth hormone. Therefore there is a significant decrease in insulin need during the immediate postpartum period. Insulin requirements for the patient with GDM disappear in 90% of the women (ADA, 2000). For the woman with type 2 diabetes, the insulin dose is typically minimal for 1 to 3 days. The woman with type 1 diabetes may require small doses, which are determined by the blood glucose levels. By the third or fourth postpartum day, insulin requirements usually increase to about two thirds of the prepregnancy dosage.

Frequent blood glucose monitoring may be necessary for the first 48 hours postpartum to determine the individual patient's insulin need. Women who were not insulin-dependent before pregnancy most likely do not need insulin. During the early postpartum period, the importance of ongoing glycemic control should be stressed. The Diabetes Control and Complications Trial Research Group (1996) showed that keeping blood glucose levels within normal limits reduced the risk for diabetic complications such as retinopathy by 76%, nephropathy by 50%, neuropathy by 60%, and cardiac problems by 35%.

To maintain normal blood glucose levels after delivery, ongoing SMBG, comprehensive meal planning as outlined for pregnancy, and regular exercise along with possible oral hypoglycemic agents or insulin regimen are required. (See Table 10-10 for a summary of newer oral hypoglycemic agents.)

All women, following a pregnancy complicated with GDM, must understand the need for ongoing, long-term follow-up. Women who have had GDM have a 40% to 60% risk for developing type 2 diabetes mellitus within the next 20 years (O'Sullivan, 1991; ADA, 2000). Maintaining a normal weight and exercising regularly have been shown to decrease the risk to 25% (ADA, 2000;

Table 10-10   Oral Antidiabetic Agents

Drug	Method of Action	Dosages	Side Effects	Use During Pregnancy and Lactation	Contraindications
Second-Generation Sulfonylureas • Glyburide • Micronase • DiaBeta	Sensitizes pancreas to secrete first-phase insulin appropriately; therefore normalizes postprandial blood glucose Increases number of insulin receptors Improves the postreceptor defect production; therefore decreases fasting hyperglycemia	1.25–20 mg in 1–2 doses Max dose: 20 mg/day With first meal	Hypoglycemia Weight gain Skin rash Headache Dizziness Occasional nausea Thrombocyopenia Aplastic/hemolytic anemia Hyponatremia Photosensitivity	Glyburide has been used to effectively treat GDM (Gutzin and others, 2003; Langer and others, 2000) Ongoing research to determine use during pregnancy as an alternative or supplement to insulin	Allergic to sulfa drugs History of alcohol abuse Liver disease Renal dysfunction Thyroid disease Adrenal insufficiency
Meglitinides • Repaglinide (Prandin)	New class of beta-cell stimulators; depends on glucose presence to exert action Reduces blood glucose by simulating insulin release from pancreas	0.5–4.0 mg/meal Max dose: 16 mg/day Take 5 to 30 min before each meal	Hypoglycemia Nausea/vomiting Constipation/diarrhea Dyspepsia Myalgias Hemolytic anemia Elevated hepatic	Avoid during pregnancy and lactation until further research	Hypersensitivity Ketoacidosis Renal disease

| Biguanides Metformin (Glucophage) | only if elevated; therefore does not cause hypoglycemia Decreases hepatic glucose production; therefore decreases fasting hyperglycemia Increases glucose utilization by muscle cells Does not stimulate insulin secretion; therefore provides rest for the pancreas Improves lipid profile by decreased total cholesterol; decreased LDLs; decreased triglycerides Decreases appetite | mg daily or 500 mg bid; Titrate up: 500 mg q week or 850 mg q 2 weeks Usual dose: 850 mg bid Max dose: 2550 mg/day | Nausea/abdominal discomfort Indigestion Diarrhea Metallic taste Headache Megaloblastic anemia Lactic acidosis (rare) Rash Temporarily withhold if undergoing: Radiologic studies with iodinated material (stop 6 hr before) Surgical procedure (stop 48 hr before) Wait 48 hr postprocedure to ensure adequate renal function Restart only after checking renal function | throughout pregnancy in presence of PCOS; reduces first-trimester spontaneous abortion and GDM (Heard and others, 2002; Glueck and others, 2004) Under research for treatment of GDM during pregnancy | Kidney disease Cardiopulmonary insufficiency Lactic acidosis History of alcoholism Binge drinking Test renal function before starting the medication |

Continued

Table 10-10   Oral Antidiabetic Agents—cont'd

Drug	Method of Action	Dosages	Side Effects	Use During Pregnancy and Lactation	Contraindications
Insulin Sensitizers • Thiazolidinediones • Pioglitazone (Actos) • Rosiglitazone (Avandia)	Binds to receptors that activate genes involved in fat synthesis and carbohydrate metabolism Enhances glucose transport into the cell Reduces hepatic glucose production	15 to 30 mg in 1 dose per day May increase after 12 weeks if inadequate response Max dose: 45 mg/day *Monitor:* Liver enzymes (AST/ALT) Before starting Every 2 mo for 1 year	Hypoglycemia Headache Edema URI/sinusitis/pharyngitis Myalgia Dyspepsia	Use only if the benefit justifies the potential perinatal risk	Hypersensitivity to the drug Ketoacidosis CHF class III or IV Liver disease

				for research to determine use during pregnancy and lactation	the drug Intestinal malabsorption syndrome Inflammatory bowel disease Intestinal obstruction
• Acarbose (Precose) • Miglitol (Glyset)	carbohydrates; therefore smaller rise in blood sugar Does not increase insulin production Does not cause hypoglycemia alone, but can occur in combination therapy May decrease FPG 10–15 mg/dl Decreases postprandial 25–45 mg/dl Decreases Hb A1c 0.4%–0.8%	every day to TID AC Increase every 4–8 wk 50–100 mg TID AC Max dose: 300 mg/day	symptoms Flatulence (50%–75%) Diarrhea (20%–30%) Abdominal pain (20%) Elevated AST/ALT Hypoglycemia if in combination therapy Hypoglycemia cannot be treated with food; use glucose tablets or gel Measure serum ALT every 3 mo/first year		

Data from Weiner C, Buhimschi C: *Drugs for pregnant and lactating women*, Philadelphia, 2004, Churchill Livingstone.
ALT, alanine aminotransferase; *AST*, aspartate aminotransferase; *CHF*, congestive heart failure; *FPG*, fasting plasma glucose; *GDM*, gestational diabetes mellitus; *LDLs*, low-density lipoproteins; *PCOS*, polycystic ovary syndrome; *TID*, three times daily; *URI*, upper respiratory infection.

Care Management Institute, 2004). See Postpartum Nursing Interventions for appropriate postpartum teaching.

NURSING MANAGEMENT
Prevention

The two major goals of care for pregnant women with diabetes are to promote a healthy, normally developed newborn and to prevent complications of diabetes from adversely affecting the pregnant woman. Counseling before conception is aimed at planning a pregnancy rather than simply allowing it to occur. Euglycemia should be attained and maintained for a minimum of 1 to 2 months before conception to reduce the risks of birth defects and congenital abnormalities to no more than the general population.

Education about diet, glucose monitoring, exercise, and insulin adjustments is necessary for the woman to self-manage diabetes during pregnancy. Education and referrals should be aimed at promoting as much independence as the woman is willing and cognitively able to assume.

Preconception Nursing Interventions for Diabetes*
Goals

- Achieve euglycemia for 1 to 2 months before conception to prevent fetal anomalies. Determine glucose control by reviewing the patient's home SMBG record and Hb A1c. Achieve Hb A1c test of less than 6.1%. Obtain health history of the following:
- Determine the type and duration of diabetes.
- Assess the current diabetes management, including insulin usage, prior or current use of oral glucose-lowering agents, SMBG pattern and results, medical nutrition therapy (MNT), and physical exercise pattern. Medication change may be needed if the patient is using oral agents.
- Review the known chronic complications of diabetes such as retinopathy, autonomic neuropathy (gastroparesis, urinary retention, hypoglycemic unawareness, or orthostatic hypotension), peripheral neuropathy, and nephropathy and macrovascular changes such as hypertension or atherosclerotic vascular disease. Note: Angiotensin-converting enzyme inhibitor hypertensive agent is contraindicated during pregnancy. Avoid beta blockers and diuretics as well.
- Determine whether the patient has a recent history of severe ketoacidosis or hypoglycemic episodes.
- Determine any history of recent infections.
- Ask about other medications being taken, such as antihypertensive agents, lipid-lowering agents, or aspirin therapy. Also ask whether alternative therapy practices are being used.

---

*ADA, 2004d.

- Inquire about the patient's patterns of using health screenings such as physical, dental, and eye checkups, Pap smears, and immunizations (especially rubella).
- Assess for negative health behaviors such as substance abuse, smoking, subclinical food issues, and alcohol intake. Encourage lifestyle changes as indicated.

Physical Examination

- *General.* Determine age, weight, body mass index, and height to attain or maintain reasonable body weight to enhance glycemic control.
- *Vital signs.* Determine temperature, pulse, respiration, and blood pressure (BP) (hypertension), including orthostatic BP changes (autonomic neuropathy). The BP goal for the patient with diabetes is lower than 130/80 mm Hg.
- *Skin.* Observe visible rashes or lesions, and select injection sites.
- *Eyes.* Refer to ophthalmologist for a dilated eye examination to rule out retinopathy.
- *Oral examination.* Evaluate oral and dental health, and emphasize importance of biannual dental checkup with cleaning.
- *Thyroid palpation.* Rule out hypothyroidism or hyperthyroidism.
- *Cardiovascular disease.* Evaluate for angina, claudication, decreased pulses, vascular bruits, and ECG abnormalities to rule out coronary heart disease. If found, refer for screening tests for coronary artery disease such as exercise stress testing, stress perfusion imaging, stress echocardiography, or catheterization.
- *Abdomen.* Rule out abnormal pulsations and organomegaly, especially of the liver.
- *Genital.* Perform a pelvic examination and Pap smear to rule out vaginal infection.
- *Neurologic.* Assess for signs of peripheral neuropathy; include ankle and knee reflexes, vibratory sensation below knee with tuning fork, light touch and pinprick sensation, and foot screening. Foot screening includes history of foot problems, deformity, muscle atrophy, calluses, swelling, blisters, ingrown or thick toenails, and use of appropriate footwear. Check protective foot sensation with monofilament testing instrument. Refer to podiatrist as indicated (LEAP, 2000).
- *Autonomic neuropathy.* Evaluate gastrointestinal and genitourinary functions.
- *Peripheral vascular disease.* Screen for intermittent claudication (intermittent pain or cramps in legs), loss of heat sensitivity in feet, dorsalis pedis and posterior tibial pulses by palpation and auscultation, hair growth on legs and big toes, and tingling or numbness in feet.

Psychosocial Assessment

- Determine any psychosocial stressors and compliance issues.

Laboratory Evaluation

- Fasting plasma glucose level
- Hb A1c
- Serum creatinine
- Fasting lipid profile: total cholesterol, LDL, HDL, triglycerides to rule out dyslipidemia; goals: LDL lower than 100 mg/dl; triglycerides lower than 200 mg/dl; HDL higher than 55
- Thyroid panel: T_4 thyroid-stimulating hormone, antimicrosomal antibodies (antithyroid) because of a 5% to 10% chance of concurrent hyperthyroidism or hypothyroidism with type 1 diabetes
- Rubella titer to check for immune status
- Microalbuminuria with a 24-hour albumin excretion with creatinine clearance or a random spot collection for albumin/creatinine ratio to evaluate for nephropathy
- Urinalysis for glucose, ketones, protein, sediment, and culture if sediment is abnormal or if symptoms are present
- Electrocardiogram (ECG)
- Treadmill test if diabetes mellitus has persisted for more than 10 years or signs and symptoms of cardiac disease are present

Education Regarding Interaction of Family Planning, Diabetes, and Pregnancy

- Importance of effective contraception until tight glycemic control is achieved
- Risk and prevention of congenital anomalies and spontaneous abortion by tight glycemic control and avoidance of substance use
- Tight glycemic control increases risk for hypoglycemia especially in type 1 diabetes
- Effects of pregnancy on maternal diabetic complications: pregnancy may accelerate retinopathy; in the presence of incipient renal failure, pregnancy may worsen the disease process; untreated coronary artery disease may cause maternal death during pregnancy
- Increased risks of obstetrical complications such as pregnancy-induced hypertension
- Risks to fetus and neonate
- Referral to diabetes educator, counselor, and social worker as indicated

Education in Self-Management

- Significance of tight glycemic control
- Five keys to tight control: diet, exercise, SMBG, stress control, and insulin administration and regulation to be adjusted based on SMBG
- SMBG before meals, 1 to 2 hours after meals, and at bedtime
- Use the Hb A1c test every 4 to 6 weeks to determine stable glycemic control
- Effect of stress and illness on glycemic control
- Use of record-keeping system to include blood glucose values with times, insulin dosages with times, foods eaten, activity with time and duration, and urine testing when needed

Nursing Interventions for Diabetes During Pregnancy

Health Perception Functional Health Pattern

- **Confirmation.** Confirm pregnancy as early as possible.
- **Interventions.** Reevaluate or initiate preconceptual interventions as stated earlier.
- **Testing.** Do Hb A1c test routinely every 2 to 3 months to determine ongoing glycemic control. Use a laboratory that uses glycosylated hemoglobin assay methods that have passed certification testing by the National Glycohemoglobin Standardization program so that the results are traceable to the Diabetes Control and Complications Trial reference method. The glycated hemoglobin assay method uses whole blood specimens in addition to lyophilized specimens *(http://web.missouri.edu/~diabetes/ngsp.html)*.

Nutrition Functional Health Pattern-Medical Nutritional Therapy (Franz and others, 2002; ADA, 2003)

- **Goal.** Maintain normal glycemic control, reach a reasonable body weight, and achieve optimal serum lipid levels while obtaining adequate calories and nutrients for increased metabolic needs during pregnancy.
- **Key dietary points**
    - There is not a diabetic diet; there is just good nutrition.
    - Total carbohydrates are more important than type of carbohydrates.
    - Consistent carbohydrate intake from day to day and at each meal and snack is essential.
    - Saturated fat and sugary foods must be limited.
    - Reasonable body weight should be achieved and maintained; moderate weight loss (10 to 20 pounds), regardless of starting weight, has been shown to reduce hyperglycemia, dyslipidemia and hypertension.
    - Eat at about the same time each day.
    - Eat foods from all food groups.
    - Use portion control.
    - Eat healthy snacks to prevent low blood sugar.
- **Ideal body weight (IBW).** The following formula determines the IBW: 100 pounds for first 5 feet of height + 5 pounds per inch for each 1 inch over 5 feet (+10% for large frame) (−10% for small frame).
- **Percentage of body fat.** Calculating the body mass index, waist-to-hip ratio, and the percentage of body fat by underwater weighing, skinfold measurements, or bioelectric impedance determines the percentage of body fat.
- **Detailed dietary history.** The following formula calculates caloric needs:
    - Baseline calories = IBW × 10
    - Activity calories
        Sedentary = IBW × 3
        Moderate = IBW × 5
        Strenuous = (IBW × 7) − 10

- Obesity −500 calories
- Pregnant +300 calories

Kcal = baseline calories + activity calories − obesity + pregnancy

- Calorie distribution (ACOG, 2005)
  - 10% to 20% at breakfast
  - 5% to 10% at midmorning snack
  - 20% to 30% at lunch
  - 5% to 10% at midafternoon snack
  - 30% to 40% at dinner
  - 5% to 10% at bedtime snack
- **Division of calories from protein.** Protein should be 12% to 20% of total calories unless kidney disease exists; if this is the case, then restrict to 0.8 g/kg/day normal recommended dietary allowance (RDA).
- **Division of calories from lipids.** Lipids should be 30% to 40% of total calories; individualized on the basis of weight, blood sugar level, and blood lipid level. Emphasize lipids from monounsaturated fats, such as avocados, olive, peanut, and canola oils. Saturated fats are to be less than 7%, and polyunsaturated fats are to be approximately 10% of total calories.
- **Division of calories from carbohydrates.** The percentage of carbohydrates to lipid ranges from 40% to 50%, depending on weight, lipid profile, and type of diabetes. For example, if triglyceride level and very low density lipoprotein (VDLD) level are high, decrease carbohydrate and increase monounsaturated fat intake, unless triglyceride levels are greater than or equal to 1000. If this is the case, reduce dietary fat to less than 10% to reduce the risk for pancreatitis. Emphasize low glycemic index carbohydrates and soluble fiber foods such as whole grains, fruits, vegetables, and legumes. Limit simple sugars to less than 10% of the total calories. Consistent carbohydrate intake from day to day and at each meal and snack is important for glucose control. Postprandial blood glucose level is dependent on the carbohydrate content of the meal and contributes most to neonatal macrosomia.
- **GDM dietary guidelines.** Women with gestational diabetes are sensitive to carbohydrates, especially at breakfast, and should limit sugary and concentrated sweets, as well as processed convenience foods. Better control is achieved if total carbohydrates are around 40%, protein around 20%, and fat around 40%, and monounsaturated and polyunsaturated fat intake is increased (Wang and others, 2000; ADA, 2003). Eating a small breakfast (less than 10% of the daily total calories) made up of whole grains and protein rich foods might help control blood sugar because the morning blood glucose level is likely to be high. "Free foods" such as cabbage, cucumbers, green onions, mushrooms, zucchini, spinach, celery, green beans, radishes, and lettuce may be eaten as desired.
- **Water.** One glass of water is to be consumed every waking hour until 2 hours before bedtime. This is important because it keeps the kidneys healthy and decreases preterm labor contractions.

- **Vitamin and minerals.**
  - Magnesium decreases insulin resistance and carbohydrate intolerance and decreases BP. The woman may benefit from magnesium supplementation.
  - Chromium has a slight effect on blood sugar level if deficient; however, most people do not have a chromium deficiency.
  - Folate in dosages of 400 mcg/day is needed to decrease the incidence of small-for-gestational-age babies and neural tube defects.
- **Fiber.** Soluble fiber such as legumes, fruit, and oat bran form gels that delay the absorption of nutrients from the intestine. This helps control diabetes by preventing dramatic swings in blood glucose levels. Insoluble fiber, such as wheat bran, cannot be digested and speeds the movement of food through the intestines, decreasing the risk for constipation. If carbohydrate counting is being used for meal planning, subtract fiber from total carbohydrate grams if a food contains 5 g or more of dietary fiber.
- **Sodium.** A normal intake of sodium is 2400 to 3000 mg each day unless the woman with diabetes has chronic hypertension. In this situation, the sodium should be limited to less than 2400 mg.
- **Meal plan**. Translate all of this information into a meal plan using the exchange list, carbohydrate counting, food pyramid, or plate method.
- **Exchange system.** The exchange system divides foods into seven categories: starch and bread, fruit, vegetables, meat, fat, and other carbohydrates that are the simple sugary foods. Each food within a category provides similar amounts of carbohydrate, protein, fat, and calories; therefore any food within a group can be exchanged for any other food in the same group. See Table 10-11 for meal planning guidelines and Table 10-12 for a sample exchange plan summary.

  By noting the proper serving size within a group, the patient can choose different foods within a group and still consume the same division of foods and similar calories each day. A dietitian usually initiates the number of servings in each group. The other carbohydrate group was added in 1995. When a patient decides to have a dessert, she notes the number of grams of carbohydrate and then decreases other carbohydrate servings by that amount. In this way, carbohydrate consistency is maintained from day to day.
- **Carbohydrate counting.** There are three levels of carbohydrate counting. Level 1 focuses on carbohydrate consistency only. Level 2 focuses on the relationships among food, diabetes medications, physical activity, and blood glucose levels and takes appropriate action by adjusting the appropriate diabetes management. Level 3 adds the component of matching short-acting bolus insulin dosing to the carbohydrate amount of that meal. There is a consistent basal dose of long-acting insulin given daily, usually 50% of the total daily insulin requirement given in divided doses: one third in the morning and two thirds before dinner. Then the short-acting insulin is given before each meal based on the number of carbohydrates in the meal: usually, 1.5 units per 10 grams of carbohydrate

Table 10-11   American Diabetes Association and American Dietetic Association: New Exchange List* for Meal Planning

Group	Carbohydrates	Protein	Fat	Calories/ Serving
Carbohydrates				
Starch	15	3	1 or less	80
Fruit	15	0	0	60
Vegetables	5	2	0	25
Other carbohydrates	15	Varies	Varies	Varies
Milk				
Skim	12	8	0–3	90
Low fat	12	8	5	120
Whole	12	8	8	150
Meat and Meat Substitutes				
Very lean	0	7	0–1	35
Lean	0	7	3	55
Medium fat	0	7	5	75
High fat	0	7	8	100
Fat group	0	0	5	4

*In grams.

eaten at breakfast and 1 unit per 10 grams eaten at lunch and dinner. The reason more insulin is required in the morning is that the body is more insulin-resistant at that time. If carbohydrates are being counted, subtract fiber from total carbohydrate grams if a food contains 5 g or more dietary fiber. If the premeal blood sugar is above or below normal, add or subtract insulin as outlined under insulin dosage distribution earlier in this chapter. It might be necessary to check blood sugar in 2 hours to evaluate the plan.

- **Food pyramid.** Individuals with diabetes use the new food pyramid as a meal plan (*http://MyPyramid.gov*). Whole grains, fresh fruit and vegetables, and low-fat dairy products and meat are emphasized. Starchy vegetables such as corn, potatoes, and peas are treated as bread, and grains and cheese are considered protein. Special attention is needed to keep the number of servings of carbohydrates consistent from day to day, limiting fat and simple sugar.

- **Plate method.** To use this method, imagine that the plate is divided into three sections to determine similar serving sizes of protein, a starch food, and a vegetable. Then add a fruit or a beverage to the meal. If the diet allows more carbohydrates for the meal, add a bread or starch serving.

- **Referral.** Refer the patient to a registered dietitian or nutritionist for development of an individualized dietary plan. Discuss problems associated with strict adherence to the prescribed diet.

Table 10-12   Exchange Plan Summary

Food Exchange Groups	Nutrients Provided	Calories per Serving	Serving Sizes
Starch (bread, cereals, grains, starchy vegetables)	15 g carbohydrate 3 g protein 3 g fiber	80	½ cup cereal, grain, or pasta 1 slice bread
Fruits	15 g carbohydrate 3 g fiber	60	½ cup fresh fruit ½ cup fruit juice ½ cup dried fruit
Vegetables	5 g carbohydrate 2 g protein 2–3 g fiber	25	½ cup cooked vegetables ½ cup vegetable juice 1 cup raw vegetables
Other carbohydrates: snack foods and sweet desserts	15 g carbohydrates Protein varies Fat varies	Varies	2 small cookies ½ cup ice cream
Milk			
Skim; very low fat	12 g carbohydrate 8 g protein Trace grams of fat	90	1 cup skim milk 8 oz plain nonfat yogurt
Low fat	12 g carbohydrate 8 g protein 5 g fat	120	1 cup 2% milk 8 oz plain low-fat yogurt
Whole	12 g carbohydrates 8 g protein 8 g fat	150	1 cup whole milk 8 oz whole plain yogurt
Meat and substitutes			
Very lean	7 g protein 0–1 g fat	35	1 oz chicken: white meat, no skin ¼ cup nonfat cottage cheese 2 egg whites
Lean	7 g protein 3 g fat	55	¼ cup 4.5% fat cottage cheese 1 oz lean pork or beef 1 oz chicken: white meat with skin
Medium fat	7 g protein 5 g fat	75	1 egg 4 oz tofu

Continued

Table 10-12   Exchange Plan Summary—cont'd

Food Exchange Groups	Nutrients Provided	Calories per Serving	Serving Sizes
High fat	7 g protein 8 g fat	100	1 oz roast beef, pork, or lamb 1 oz processed sandwich meats 1 oz American, cheddar, or Swiss cheese 2 Tbsp peanut butter
Fat	5 g fat	45	Varies

Developed from American Dietetic Association: *Exchange lists to meal planning,* Chicago, 1995, ADA.

Elimination Functional Health Pattern

- **Urine testing.** Urine is tested for protein and ketone levels.
- **UTI.** Prevent infection by drinking 8 to 10 glasses of water a day and emptying the bladder every 2 hours.

Sleep and Rest Functional Health Pattern

- **Fatigue.** Obtain enough rest and sleep to prevent fatigue.

Activity and Exercise Functional Health Pattern*

- **Amount and type of exercise.** If patient is older than 35 years of age or shows signs of cardiovascular disease, a stress ECG can be used to evaluate cardiovascular status to prevent silent myocardial infarction.
- **Regular exercise program.** Increasing the uptake of glucose into the cells and decreasing central obesity, hypertension, and dyslipidemia decrease insulin requirements.
- **Water consumption.** Ingesting water before, during, and after exercising prevents dehydration.
- **Abdominal injection site.** Exercising the area of insulin injection increases absorption of insulin from that area.
- **Postexercise hypoglycemia.** Check blood sugar before and after exercise; then add 15 g carbohydrate to the diet for every 30 to 60 minutes of strenuous exercise or adjust the insulin at the time of exercise by 10% of total daily dose. For example, exercise in the morning, decrease morning regular insulin; exercise in the afternoon, decrease the morning NPH. If the pre-event blood sugar level is lower than 100 mg/dl and the exercise period lasts more than 1 hour, add 1 to 2 ounces of protein to the increased carbohydrate snack.

*ADA, 2001a.

- **Low blood sugar level.** The patient should be encouraged to carry a snack designed to treat low blood sugar.
- **Aerobic exercise.** Aerobic exercise with resistance training at 60% to 80% of maximum heart rate for a minimum of 30 minutes two times a week is the best type of exercise (220 − age = maximum heart rate).
- **Exercise.** Exercise must not cause fetal stress, low infant birth weight, or uterine contractions. The patient should be taught to palpate the uterus for contractions during exercise and stop if any occur.
- **Protecting the feet.** Wearing properly fitted shoes with silica gel or air midsoles and wearing cotton and polyester socks to prevent blisters and keep the feet dry helps to protect the feet from injury.
- **Diabetic identification bracelet.** Encourage the patient to wear a diabetic identification bracelet.
- **Limited activity.** If hypertension, ketonuria, or vascular disease is present, limit activity to decrease metabolic needs.

Self-Perception Functional Health Pattern
- **GDM.** Assess feelings about diagnosis of GDM.
- **DM.** Assess feelings about managing a pregnancy complicated with DM.
- **Family response.** Assess family and partner responses.

Role Relationship Functional Health Pattern
- **Relationship responsibilities.** Assess how pregnancy and the management of DM will affect relationship responsibilities.
- **Work absences.** Assess ability to interrupt occupation, such as accommodations for job absences.
- **Economic considerations.** Assess economic considerations, such as insurance coverage.

Sexuality Functional Health Pattern
- **Assessment.** Assess for sexuality problems.
- **Obstetric history.** Assess for preeclampsia, preterm labor, cesarean birth, congenital anomalies, macrosomia, birth injury, and neonatal metabolic abnormalities.

Coping Functional Health Pattern
- **Life stresses.** Ask patient about perceived life stresses, such as adjusting to GDM; managing DM; and juggling family, job, and financial concerns. Good questions include, "Is there anything in particular that is worrying you about yourself, your significant other, or your baby?" and "How do you feel about being pregnant and having DM?"
- **Patient concerns.** Discuss issues that cause worry, such as the baby's health, need for ongoing insulin, and emotional peer support.
- **Patient support.** Provide emotional support.
- **Physical stresses.** Assess for domestic violence, inflammation, infection, and psychologic stress.

- **Patient understanding.** Assess understanding of the effects of stress on blood glucose levels. Stress increases blood glucose level via contrainsular hormones.
- **Patient fears.** Allay the fear that increased insulin needs equals worsening diabetes and educate that increased insulin needs really means a healthy, growing placenta.
- **Support referrals.** Make needed referrals to diabetes support groups, Sidelines National Network (a high risk pregnancy support group), social services, and American Diabetes Association. Advise of the importance of carrying a diabetic identification card and wearing a Medic-Alert bracelet or necklace.
- **Resource referrals.** Provide referrals to Lifescan telelibrary for information regarding diabetes (800-847-7226); American Diabetic Association (800-342-2382); National Institutes of Health for patient with diabetes information (*http://diabetes.niddk.nih.gov*).

Cognitive Functional Health Pattern

- **Visits.** Suggest more frequent prenatal visits.
- **Disease process.** Assess patient and family knowledge of the disease process and treatment, including the relationships among diet, exercise, insulin, illness, and stress. Determine patient and family understanding of the effects of diabetes on pregnancy and the effects of pregnancy on diabetes.
- **Complications.** Prevent complications with tight glycemic control using MNT, insulin administration, exercise plan, SMBG, urine test for ketones, early recognition and treatment for signs of hypoglycemia, and sick-day management.
- **Fetal evaluation.** Evaluate the fetus with periodic ultrasound scans to monitor for gestational age, structural growth, and fetal growth; take serum alpha-fetoprotein (AFP) measurements, take daily fetal movement count after 24 weeks of gestation, take fetal echocardiogram between 20 and 23 weeks of gestation to rule out congenital heart disease; make a biophysical profile with NST or CST and amniotic fluid volume (AFV) for fetal surveillance; and possibly perform amniocentesis to determine fetal lung maturity.

Insulin Administration

- **Types.** Two types of insulin are available: Humulin and pork insulins. Humulin is preferred for use in pregnancy because of less insulin antibody stimulation.
- **Insulin forms**
  - *Rapid-acting.* Humalog (Lispro) See Table 10-6.
  - *Short-acting.* Humulin R (Regular) See Table 10-6.
  - *Intermediate-acting.* Humulin N (NPH) and Humulin L (Lente) Refer to Table 10-6 for onset, peak, and duration.
  - *Long-acting.* Humulin U (Ultralente) Refer to Table 10-6 for onset, peak, and duration.

- **Storage**
  - Current vial can be stored at room temperature (36° to 86° F) for up to 1 month.
  - Insulin should not be stored in direct sunlight.
  - Unused vials should be stored in refrigerator until expiration date.
  - Insulin should not be frozen.
  - Prepared syringes are stable for 2 weeks in the refrigerator.
- **Strength.** Insulin is provided in different strengths: 100 to 500 units (very rare).
- **Mixing insulins.** Regular insulin with NPH insulins and Lispro with NPH or Ultralente can be mixed. After mixing, mixture can be used immediately or stored for future use. If stored, syringe is rotated 20 times before injection. It is not recommended to mix regular with Lente because it delays regular insulin's onset of action. Additionally, NPH (phosphate buffered) should not be mixed with Lente (zinc-buffered) because it causes precipitation and conversion to a short acting insulin.
- **Syringes.** The four capacities of insulin syringes are ¼ ml, ³/₁₀ ml, ½ ml, and 1 ml. There are two different lengths of needles, ½ inch and ⁵/₁₆ inch. The ⁵/₁₆-inch syringe is 8% thinner and 37% shorter and is designed to be used for very slender adults and children.
- **Syringe reuse.** The manufacturer recommends syringes be used once; however, some individuals reuse syringes until the needle is dull to save money. This practice does not cause increased infection if the syringe is effectively cleaned because insulin is prepared with bacteriostatic additives.
- **Syringe alternatives.** Alternatives to syringes are the pen injector, jet injector, and insulin pump.
- **Injection technique.** Injection technique should be demonstrated and a return demonstration of the correct technique using a systematic rotation pattern should be requested. A line drawing of the human body with an illustrated method of recording each injection is shown in Figs. 10-1 and 10-2. Each injection should be given 1 inch from the previous injection. The needle should be at a 90-degree angle to ensure deep subcutaneous administration unless the patient is very thin, in which case a 45-degree angle may be used to prevent an intramuscular injection.
- **Dose preparation.** Intermediate- and long-acting insulins are in a suspension and require mixing by gently rolling the vial between the palms of the hands.
- **Injection site.** Rotation of the injection site is important to prevent lipohypertrophy (fat bulges) and lipoatrophy. Absorption varies from site to site. The abdomen has the best absorption and is the preferred site. The next best site is the upper outer arm (no deltoid area), then the thigh, and last, the buttocks. It is best to rotate within one area to maintain a consistent absorption rate (ADA, 2001c). There should be 30 days between the uses of individual sites. It is important to remember that exercise accelerates absorption from extremity sites. Rate of insulin absorption is influenced by the injection site and smoking. Massage increases insulin

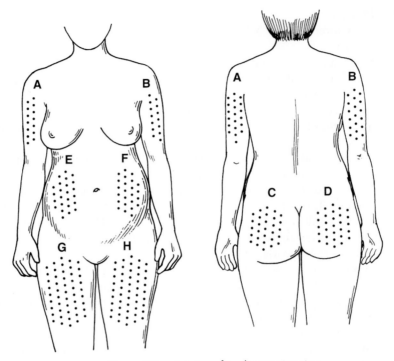

Figure 10-1 Rotation of insulin injection sites.

Area _____

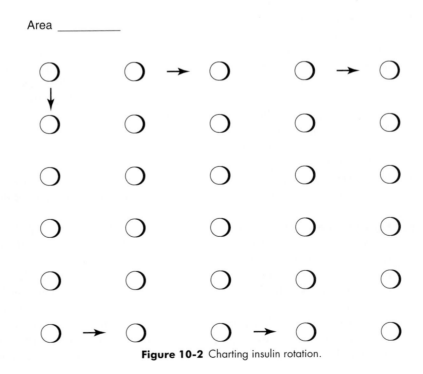

Figure 10-2 Charting insulin rotation.

absorption by increasing blood flow to the area. Smoking decreases insulin absorption (ADA, 2001c).

- **Injection procedure.** The injection should be given in the subcutaneous tissue at a 90-degree angle; there is no need to aspirate.
- **Dosing guidelines**
  - First trimester, reduce insulin dose by 10% to 25%.
  - Typical insulin dose first trimester is 0.7 units/kg body weight.
  - Type 1 DM insulin dosage usually increases 10% to 20% by 36 weeks of gestation.
  - Type 2 DM insulin dosage usually increases 30% to 90% by 36 weeks of gestation.
- **Distribution of rapid- or short-acting insulin to intermediate-acting insulin**
  - Two thirds total dose in morning, one third in evening.
  - NPH/R morning 2:1, NPH/R evening 1:1; NPH or Ultralente can be given at bedtime.
- **Distribution of basal.** Bolus injections are 50:50 in women who are not pregnant but 40:60 during pregnancy, related to the physiologic changes of pregnancy.
- **Injections.** During pregnancy, three or more injections per day are usually required.
- **Adjustments.** Adjustments are made to achieve target glucose control. During pregnancy, adjustments may be needed every 5 to 10 days. It is important to remember to fix the fasting blood sugar first.
- **Breastfeeding effects on insulin**
  - Hypoglycemia is common.
  - Nocturnal hypoglycemia is particularly common.
  - Caloric intake is increased from 500 to 800 kcal.
  - Insulin requirements are adjusted on the basis of SMBG.

Self-Monitoring of Blood Glucose

- **Self-monitoring.** Teach importance of self-monitoring. Explain or review the importance of SMBG using a reflectance meter and enzyme strips.
- **Technique.** Demonstrate proper technique, and observe a return demonstration. According to the American Diabetes Association (2000), proper technique includes the following:
  - Drop of blood should be large enough to cover the reaction area of the strip.
  - The strip should not be touched with the finger.
  - Proper timing of the test should be followed.
  - All the blood completely should be wiped off the strip when applicable.
  - The device should be calibrated and cleaned as outlined in the manual.
- **Pregnancy.** Ideally, pregnant women with diabetes, to obtain glycemic control, should test immediately after each meal (AC), 1 to 2 hours after meals, at bedtime, and between 2 AM and 3 AM.

- **Pregnancy**
  - Practicality means individualized frequency and time, but postprandial values must be assessed during pregnancy because they are better predictors of fetal macrosomia, decreased A1c, and decreased risk for neonatal hypoglycemia (de Veciana and others, 1995; Homko, Sivan, and Reece, 1998; Metzger and Coustan, 1998; Kjos and Buchanan, 1999).
  - Generally, pregnant women with diabetes test four to six times a day. A typical testing schedule involves a fasting measurement, 1 hour before breakfast, before and 1 hour after lunch, before dinner, and at bedtime.
- **Goals**
  - If fasting blood sugar is high, test blood sugar between 2 AM and 3 AM. (See Table 10-8 for common causes and treatment of this phenomenon.)
  - Women with GDM should test FPG and 1 to 2 hours after meal.
  - During illness, test every 4 to 6 hours.
  - When starting a new exercise program, test before and after activity to determine effect of exercise on insulin levels.
  - Adjust insulin dosages as indicated.
  - Have patient keep results in a logbook and bring it to each prenatal visit.
  - Measure A1C to confirm SMBG results every 4 to 6 weeks for type 1 DM. For GDM, a baseline Hb A1c may be reassuring; if elevated, it may indicate type 2 DM.
- **Urine ketone testing**
  - Individual urine ketone testing is performed to evaluate adequacy of calories and carbohydrates in the diet.
  - Voided AC morning specimen should be checked three times a week or daily if patient becomes sick or glucose levels exceed 200 mg/dL.
  - At each prenatal visit, clean-catch dipstick urine is checked for protein, ketone, leukocyte, and nitrite measurements.

Hypoglycemia Management

- **Significance.** The significance of hypoglycemia on the patient and fetus should be taught.
  - Teach symptoms such as sweating, irritability, tremulousness, headache, fatigue, tachycardia, hunger, bad dreams, and circumoral numbness.
  - Teach rule of 15:15 management: if blood sugar is low, take 15 g of fast sugar (carbohydrate), wait 15 minutes, then check blood sugar. If greater than 60%, eat a meal to stabilize sugar. If less than 60%, repeat the 15:15 rule. Choices of 15 g of carbohydrate are commercial glucose tablets, ½ cup of orange juice, 1 cup skim milk, ½ cup regular soda, or five to six hard candies.

- In the presence of hypoglycemia-induced nausea, 0.15 mg subcutaneous glucagon may elevate the blood sugar sufficiently to allow the patient to eat.
- Teach a family member or friend how to inject glucagon in case the patient losses consciousness due to hypoglycemia. The usual dose is 1 mg injected subcutaneously. If there are no signs of improvement in 15 to 20 minutes, contact emergency medical services.

Sick-Day Rule

- **Teaching points**
    - If she is unable to eat, she should continue to take insulin, check blood sugar levels, and check urine for ketones. Notify health care provider.
    - The stress of illness can cause blood glucose to rise related to counter hormones.
    - A plan that outlines when to call a health care provider should be provided.
    - Patient should continue to take insulin even which she is unable to eat, because the liver continues to make glucose.
    - Blood glucose should be checked.
    - A supplemental short-acting insulin plan based on blood glucose levels is normally used during illness.
    - The urine is tested for ketones.
    - The insulin dose is normally doubled if urine ketones are present.
    - An easily digestible liquid diet containing fluids, carbohydrates, and salt is initiated. Carbohydrate food choices are cola, lemon-lime soda, or orange juice. Replace sodium and potassium with foods such as broth, tea, or saltine crackers. Take fluids in small amounts every hour.
    - Vomiting episodes are immediately reported to the health care provider.

Critical Care Intervention for Perinatal Ketoacidosis*

- **Hydration.** A dose of 1 L of NS is administered over the first hour. Then 200 to 500 ml/hr is given until 80% fluid deficit is corrected in approximately 24 hours. If hypernatremia develops, 0.45% saline is used to hydrate. Note: NS is the preferred fluid initially because the hypotonic solutions such as Ringer's lactate or 0.45% NS can cause a rapid decline in plasma osmolarity, which may lead to cellular swelling and resultant cerebral edema (Foley, 1997).
- **Reduce blood glucose levels with insulin.** An IV bolus is administered with 10 to 20 units of regular insulin. Then a continuous infusion of insulin is started to give 5 to 10 units of regular insulin per hour (50 units regular Humulin insulin in 500 ml of NS to run at 100–150 ml/hr). If serum glucose is not dropping by 20% in 2 hours, the insulin rate should be

---

*ADA, 2004b; ACOG, 2005.

doubled. The IV insulin should be continued until anion gap is normal (less than 12) and HCO_3^- is 18 to 31 mEq/L. To decrease risk for hyperglycemia, subcutaneous insulin is given before discontinuing IV drip.

- **Blood glucose levels.** Serum blood glucose testing is performed every 1 to 2 hours. The goal is to decrease blood glucose by 50 to 70 mg/dl/hr.
- **Ketones with glucose.** When serum glucose level is 250 mg/dl or less, insulin infusion is decreased by 50% and the IV line is changed to 5% dextrose. To give 5 to 10 g of glucose per hour, piggyback administration at approximately 100 ml/hr is provided. Once serum glucose is less than 150 mg/dl, patient is fed appropriate food.
- **Potassium (K^+) balance.** After the initial liter of fluid and urine output of at least 30 ml/hr, K^+ is added to each liter of fluid to prevent hypokalemia with the correction of the metabolic acidosis. When K^+ level is 4 to 5.5 mEq, 10 to 20 mEq/hr is given. If K^+ is less than 4 mEq, 30 to 40 mEq/hr is given. When K^+ level is low on admission, K^+ is immediately added to IV infusion to avoid arrhythmias or cardiac arrest and respiratory muscle weakness.
- **Bicarbonate (HCO_3^-).** If arterial pH is less than 7.1, 44 mEq is given every 2 hours until pH is greater than 7.1. If arterial pH is greater than 7.1 mEq, sodium bicarbonate is not given.
- **Monitoring.** Ongoing monitoring is provided every 2 to 4 hours until stable.
  - Arterial blood gases (pH, Po_2, $Paco_2$, O_2 saturation)
  - Serum electrolytes and anion gap (electrolytes panel). Goal: HCO_3^- 18 to 31 mEq/L, Na^+ above 150 mEq/L; K^+ 3.5 to 5.5 mEq/L; anion gap less than 12 mEq/L
  - Serum ketones (acetone)
- **General supportive measures**
  - Establish two IV access lines immediately.
  - Give oxygen by mask at 10 to 12 L/min.
  - Anticipate insertion of an arterial line for arterial blood gases.
  - Perform continuous peripheral pulse oximetry for noninvasive arterial blood oxygen saturation.
  - Insert Foley catheter for strict hourly output.
  - Evaluate kidney function with a serum BUN and creatinine to decrease risk for fluid overload.
  - Use invasive hemodynamic monitoring in the presence of renal compromise.
  - Initiate continuous ECG and monitor for ST segment depression, for inverted T waves, or for the appearance of U waves following the T wave.
  - Continuously monitor fetal heart rate and prepare for delivery if nonreassuring tracing persists after initial stabilization.
  - Keep mother positioned to avoid vena cava syndrome.
- **Treatment.** UTIs and infections of the skin, lungs, or amniotic fluid; noncompliance with insulin administration; or dietary indiscretion are

treated. Urinalysis is performed for culture and sensitivity to rule out URI; CBC with differential, chest radiograph, and amniocentesis may be considered.

- **Evaluation.** Condition is evaluated with ongoing physical assessment.
  - Provide neurologic checks every hour for signs of cerebral edema that include deteriorating mental status, sluggish pupillary light reflex, or headache.
  - Evaluate vital signs.
  - Assess for signs of pulmonary edema, including dyspnea, tachypnea, tachycardia, wheezing, or crackles on auscultation.
  - Assess for hypovolemia, including urine output less than 30 ml/hr, hypotension, or tachycardia.

Intrapartum Nursing Interventions for Diabetes

- **Preterm labor.** Preterm labor is treated with magnesium sulfate or indomethacin because beta-sympathomimetic agents can interfere with glucose control.
- **Corticosteroids.** If corticosteroids are used to enhance fetal lung maturity, two doses of 12 mg dexamethasone are administered orally 24 hours apart. Double the total insulin dosage on those 2 days and monitor blood glucose every 4 hours. Supplement with a short-acting insulin as blood sugar levels indicate (ADA, 2000).
- **Goal of insulin management during labor.** Maintain plasma glucose between 70 and 90 mg/dl or capillary whole blood concentrations 60 to 80 mg/dl to decrease neonatal hypoglycemia (ADA, 2000).
- **Insulin and glucose requirements**
  - Insulin requirements typically decrease with onset of labor; at onset of active labor, insulin is decreased to zero.
  - Glucose requirements in active labor are 2.5 mg/kg/min.
  - Determine last insulin dose to ascertain insulin peak.
  - Withhold usual morning insulin dosage and breakfast.
  - Give nothing by mouth except ice chips.
  - Obtain baseline blood glucose every 1 to 2 hours.
  - Start continuous IV infusion of D_5LR at 100 ml/hr unless urine ketone is present or blood glucose is less than 70 mg/dl. If so, then use D_5 at a rate of 2.5 mg/kg/min (ADA, 2000).
- Set up insulin solution by diluting 25 units of regular or lispro insulin in 250 ml of NS and flush line with 25 ml to decrease insulin-binding capacity of insulin to plastic surfaces.
- Piggyback insulin infusion to mainline IV at connection closest to insertion site. Use an infusion pump and adjust rate based on blood glucose levels as outlined in Table 10-13.
- Adjust the IV rate and supplemental regular insulin according to the every 1 to 2 hour blood glucose values.
- Keep 50% dextrose at the bedside to treat profound hypoglycemia.
- **Intermittent subcutaneous insulin method**. If used instead of the insulin infusion method, perform the following:

Table 10-13   Use an Infusion Pump and Adjust Rate Based on Blood Glucose Levels

Plasma/Capillary Blood Glucose (mg/dl)	Insulin Dosage (units/hr)
Less than 80	0.0
80–100	0.5
101–140	1.0
141–180	1.5
181–220	2.0
Greater than 220	2.5

Reference: Moore T: Diabetes in pregnancy. In Creasy R, Resnik R, Iams J, editors: *Maternal-fetal medicine: principles and practice*, ed 5, Philadelphia, 2004, Saunders.

- Be prepared to give one third to one half of the patient's pregnancy insulin dosage in the morning.
- Start a continuous infusion based on glucose levels.
- Administer regular insulin in 2 to 5 units per dose to maintain the blood sugar.
- **Continuous fetal monitoring.** Observe continuous fetal monitoring for reassuring or nonreassuring baseline fetal heart rate, variability, and patterns that develop in response to labor.
- **Labor progress**
  - Evaluate labor progress and ultrasound results for potential problems with dystocia, arrest of descent, or failure to progress (see Chapters 27 and 28).
  - Monitor and record vital signs every 15 minutes to every 1 hours; take temperature every 1 to 4 hours.
  - Maintain hourly input-output measurements.
  - Assess urine for ketones at every void or every 4 hours with indwelling catheter.
  - Assess for complications such as hypoglycemia, ketoacidosis, UTI, upper respiratory infection, polyhydramnios, which increases risk for fetal cord prolapse with rupture of membranes, and fetal macrosomia, which increases risk for shoulder dystocia.
- **Cesarean delivery**
  - Schedule for early morning.
  - Give nothing by mouth and hold morning insulin dose.
  - Monitor blood glucose levels every hour and administer short-acting insulin and glucose based on blood sugar levels.
  - After delivery; administer IV D_5W at a rate of 100 to 125 ml/hr.
  - Check blood glucose every 2 to 4 hours.
  - No insulin may be needed related to the sudden drop of the placental hormone, human placenta lactogen (HPL), after delivery of the placenta.

Postpartum Nursing Interventions for Types 1 and 2 Diabetes

- **Insulin.** Insulin is administered based on blood glucose level. The initial goal is to prevent hypoglycemia and severe hyperglycemia rather than achieve euglycemia (80 to 150 mg/dl). If the fasting or postprandial blood sugar is greater than 150 mg/dl, the dosage of insulin is recalculated at 0.6 units/kg/24 hr based on postpartum weight. When repeated rapid- or short-acting insulin is needed, the routine schedule of insulin or oral agents is resumed. New insulin dose is usually 50% to 60% of end-pregnancy dose. Tighter control is gradually resumed. Final goal is preprandial blood sugar 70 to 120 mg/dl.
- **Education**
  - Teach the importance of ongoing tight glycemic control with MNT, exercise plan, SMBG, glucose-lowering medications, and early detection of diabetic complications. (See Table 10-10 for a summary of the new oral hypoglycemic agents.)
  - Teach the need for family planning to ensure optimal glycemic control before the start of any subsequent pregnancy. According to the American Diabetes Association (2004d), when selecting a contraceptive method for the patient with diabetes, the same criteria are to be used as with any other patient. Low-dose estrogen-progestin oral contraceptives and IUDs are not contraindicated unless other co-morbidity factors exist (ACOG, 2005).
  - **Breastfeeding.** Breastfeeding should be encouraged. Breastfeeding decreases fasting and postprandial blood glucose levels and increases HDL cholesterol levels (ADA, 2000). Therefore during breastfeeding, the insulin requirement is usually considerably less, and protein and carbohydrate snacks are necessary. The woman's dietary needs will increase usually 500 to 800 calories. Teach the patient to expect fluctuations in her glucose levels during weaning and to continue close glucose monitoring. Reassure the mother that insulin does not cross into breast milk. However, elevated glucose levels are present in the breast milk if her blood glucose is high. Monitor for mastitis and nipple infections because of the increased risk they present. Sore nipples that do not respond to the usual nonspecific treatment are treated with nystatin ointment to the nipples and nystatin suspension for the infant as well.

Postpartum Nursing Interventions for Gestational Diabetes Mellitus

- **Monitoring.** For the patient with GDM, monitor blood sugar after delivery.
- **Education.** The woman with GDM has 40% to 60% increased risk for developing type 2 DM (O'Sullivan, 1991; ADA, 2000). The importance of the screening program for early detection of development of diabetes is advised. This includes a 75-g, 2-hour oral glucose tolerance test at the

Box 10-1	Nurse Practitioner Protocol for Postpartum Testing After Gestational Diabetes Mellitus

Glucose Tolerance Test
- Perform a 75-g glucose tolerance test at the first postpartum checkup between 6 and 8 weeks after delivery or shortly after the woman stops breastfeeding.

Test Preparation
- Instruct the patient to eat an additional 150 g of complex carbohydrates (e.g., 10 additional slices of bread each day) for 3 days before the test.
- Instruct the patient to abstain from eating, drinking (except water), and smoking for 8 hours before the test.
- Have the patient rest in the office for 30 minutes just before the test.
- Draw a fasting plasma glucose level.
- Administer 75 g of oral glucose drink.
- Draw plasma glucose at 2 hours.
- Interpret and reclassify gestational diabetes mellitus after pregnancy according to new criteria for the diagnosis of diabetes mellitus (Expert Committee, 2001).

Normal Results
- Medical diagnosis: previous abnormality of glucose tolerance
- Fasting plasma glucose, less than 110 mg/dl
- 2-hour postprandial, less than 140 mg/dl

Impaired Glucose Tolerance Results
- Fasting plasma glucose, 110–125 mg/dl
- 2-hour postprandial, 140–199 mg/dl

Type 2 Diabetes Mellitus Results
- Fasting plasma glucose, equal to or greater than 126 mg/dl
- 2-hour postprandial, greater than 200 mg/dl
- Random plasma glucose, equal to or greater than 200 mg/dl with symptoms (polyuria, polydipsia, and unexplained weight loss)

Follow-Up
- If results indicate impaired glucose tolerance, the annual well-woman examination should include a fasting blood glucose following a 3-hour fast. If the results of this test are 110 mg/dl or greater, further testing is needed.
- If the glucose levels are normal, glycemia should be reassessed annually.

6-week postpartum checkup and a random or fasting blood glucose annually (Box 10-1).
- **Lifestyle modifications.** There is a relationship between maintaining optimal weight and the decreased risk for later development of type 2 diabetes. If the woman stays lean and fit, her risk decreases to 25%. If the woman is or becomes obese, the risk for diabetes increases to 75% (ADA, 2004b). If the woman is obese, especially with increased abdominal fat, a weight loss of 5 to 10 pounds will make a difference in the amount of insulin the pancreas must produce. For example, an active thin person's

pancreas may produce only 35 to 40 units/day as compared with a person who is overweight, whose pancreas may be required to produce 150 units/day to clear the same amount of glucose. Encourage the woman to follow a nutritional diet and exercise regularly to decrease risk. A gradual weight loss of 0.5 to 1 pound per week is recommended.

- **Family Planning.** Progesterone-only oral contraceptive (Minipill) is contraindicated in breastfeeding mothers with a history of GDM because it increases the risk for later developing type 2 DM. Low-dose estrogen-progestin oral contraceptives and IUD may to considered (ADA, 2004b).

CONCLUSION

The ultimate goal of nursing care for a pregnant woman with diabetes is to minimize the effects of risks and complications. This is accomplished by educating the woman and her family to recognize early signs and symptoms of management failures and identify and solve management issues that they are capable of solving. It is also accomplished by promoting a relationship that encourages mutual work among the patient, her family, and members of the health care team.

The outcome of the pregnancy should be a mother without additional diabetic complications, a healthy newborn, and a family who is ready and able to integrate the new baby into their world. An added side benefit of educating the pregnant woman who is already insulin-dependent is that she commonly learns useful skills that aid in her self-management of diabetes for the remainder of her life.

BIBLIOGRAPHY

American College of Obstetricians and Gynecologists: *Pregestational diabetes mellitus: clinical management guidelines for obstetrician-gynecologists,* No. 60, 2005, ACOG.

American Diabetes Association: *Medical management of pregnancy complicated by diabetes,* ed 3, Alexandria, Va, 2000, ADA.

American Diabetes Association: Position statement: diabetes mellitus and exercise, *Diabetes Care* 24(Suppl 1):S51, 2001a.

American Diabetes Association: Position statement: gestational diabetes mellitus, *Diabetes Care* 24(Suppl 1):S77, 2001b.

American Diabetes Association: Position statement: insulin administration, *Diabetes Care* 24(Suppl 1):S94, 2001c.

American Diabetes Association: Position statement: nutrition recommendations and principles for people with diabetes mellitus, *Diabetes Care* 24(Suppl 1):S44, 2001d.

American Diabetes Association: Position statement: tests of glycemia of diabetes, *Diabetes Care* 24(Suppl 1):S80, 2001e.

American Diabetes Association: Position statement: evidence-based nutrition principles and recommendations for the treatment and prevention of diabetes and related complications, *Diabetes Care* 26(Suppl 1):S51–S61, 2003.

American Diabetes Association: Position statement: aspirin therapy in diabetes, *Diabetes Care* 27(Suppl 1):S72–S73, 2004a.

American Diabetes Association: Position statement: gestational diabetes mellitus, *Diabetes Care* 27(Suppl 1):S88–S90, 2004b.

American Diabetes Association: Position statement: hyperglycemic crises in diabetes, *Diabetes Care* 27(Suppl 1):S94–S102, 2004c.

American Diabetes Association: Position statement: preconception care of women with diabetes, *Diabetes Care* 27(Suppl 1):S76–S78, 2004d.

American Diabetes Association: Position statement: influenza and pneumococcal immunization in diabetes, *Diabetes Care* 27(Suppl 1):S111–S113, 2004e.

American Diabetes Association: Position statement: diagnosis and classification of diabetes mellitus, *Diabetes Care* 28(Suppl 1):S37–S42, 2005a.

American Diabetes Association: Position statement: standards of medical care in diabetes, *Diabetes Care* 28(Suppl 1):S72–S79, 2005b.

American Diabetes Association: National standards for diabetes self-management education, *Diabetes Care* 28(Suppl 1):S4–S36, 2005c.

Birke J, Rolfsen R: Evaluation of a self-administered sensory testing tool to identify patients at risk of diabetes-related foot problems, *Diabetes Care* 21(1):23–25, 1998.

Boulvain M, Stan C, and Irion O: Elective delivery in diabetic pregnant women, *Cochrane Database Syst Rev*, Issue 2: 2001.

Boyd K, Ross E, and Sherman S: Jelly beans as an alternative to a cola beverage containing 50 grams of glucose, *Am J Obstet Gynecol* 173(6):1889–1892, 1995.

Care Management Institute, Kaiser Permanente: *Adult diabetes clinical practice guidelines*, Oakland, Calif, Kaiser Permanente, Care Management Institute, p. 167, 2004.

Chernecky C, Berger B: *Laboratory tests and diagnostic procedures*, ed 3, Philadelphia, 2001, Saunders.

Cousins L and others: Screening recommendations for gestational diabetes mellitus, *Am J Obstet Gynecol* 165(3):493–496, 1991.

Cunningham G and others: *Williams' obstetrics*, ed 21, New York, 2005, McGraw-Hill Professional.

Dabelea D, Knowler W, and Pettitt D: Effect of diabetes in pregnancy on offspring: follow-up research in Pima Indians, *J Matern Fetal Med* 9(1):83–88, 2000.

de Veciana M and others: Postprandial versus preprandial blood glucose monitoring in women with gestational diabetes mellitus requiring insulin therapy, *N Engl J Med* 333(19):1237–1241, 1995.

Diabetes Control and Complications Trial Research Group: The effect of intensive treatment of diabetes on the development and progression of long-term complications in insulin-dependent diabetes mellitus, *N Engl J Med* 329(14):977–986, 1993.

Diabetes Control and Complications Trial Research Group: Effect of pregnancy on microvascular complications in the diabetes control and complications trial, *Diabetes Care* 23(8):1084–1091, 2000.

Diabetes Control and Complications Trial Research Group: Pregnancy outcomes in the Diabetes Control and Complications Trial, *Am J Obstet Gynecol* 174(4):1343–1353, 1996.

Diabetes Education Society: *Lifeskills teaching guides,* Denver, 1995, Diabetes Education Society.

Doyle E and others: A randomized, prospective trial comparing the efficacy of continuous subcutaneous insulin infusion with multiple daily injections using insulin glargine, *Diabetes Care* 27(7):1554–1558, 2004.

European Practice in Gynaecology and Obstetrics (EPGO): *Diabetes and pregnancy,* Amsterdam, The Netherlands, 2004, Elsevier.

Expert Committee on the Diagnosis and Classification of Diabetes Mellitus: Report of the Expert Committee on the Diagnosis and Classification of Diabetes Mellitus, *Diabetes Care* 24(Suppl 1): S5, 2001.

Foley M: Diabetic ketoacidosis in pregnancy. In Foley M, Strong T, editors: *Obstetric intensive care: a practical manual,* Philadelphia, 1997, Saunders.

Franz M and others: Evidence-based nutrition: principles and recommendations for the treatment and prevention of diabetes and related complications, *Diabetes Care* 25(1):148–198, 2002.

Glueck C and others: Height, weight, and motor-social development during the first 18 months of life in 126 infants born to 109 mothers with polycystic ovary syndrome who conceived on and continued metformin through pregnancy, *Hum Reprod* 19(6):1323–1330, 2004.

Gutzin S and others: The safety of oral hypoglycemic agents in the first trimester of pregnancy: a meta-analysis, *Can J Clin Pharmacol* 10(4):179–183, 2003.

Heard M and others: Pregnancies following use of metformin for ovulation induction in patients with polycystic ovary syndrome, *Fertil Steril* 77(4):669–673, 2002.

Hinton A, Sibai B: Hypertensive disorders in pregnancy. In Reece E, Coustan D, Gabbe S, editors: *Diabetes in women: adolescence, pregnancy, menopause,* ed 3, Philadelphia, 2004, Lippincott Williams & Wilkins.

Homko C, Sivan E, and Reece E: Is self-monitoring of blood glucose necessary in the management of gestational diabetes mellitus? *Diabetes Care* 21(Suppl 2):B118–B122, 1998.

Kahn R and others: The metabolic syndrome: time for a critical appraisal, *Diabetes Care* 28(9):2289–2304, 2005.

Kendrick J: Preconception care of women with diabetes, *J Perinal Neonat Nurs* 18(1): 14–25, 2004.

Kendrick J and others: Reliability of reporting of self-monitoring of blood glucose in pregnant women, *J Obstet Gynecol Neonatal Nurs* 34(3):329–334, 2005.

Kjos S, Buchanan T: Gestational diabetes mellitus, *N Engl J Med* 341(23):1749–1756, 1999.

Kremer C, Duff P: Glyburide for the treatment of gestational diabetes, *Am J Obstet Gynecol* 190(5):1438–1439, 2004.

Langer L and others: A comparison of glyburide and insulin in women with gestational diabetes mellitus, *N Engl J Med* 343(16):1134–1138, 2000.

Lindsay R and others: Secular trends in birth weight, BMI, and diabetes in the offspring of diabetic mothers, *Diabetes Care* 23(9):1249–1254, 2000.

Loon J: Technologic advances in glucose monitoring, *Adv Nurse Pract,* August, 49, 2004. Retrieved from *http://www.advanceweb.com*

Lower Extremity Amputation Preventive (LEAP): *Program for diabetic foot screening and free monofilament,* 2001. Retrieved from *http://bphc.hrsa.gov/leap/WhatIsLeap.htm*

Metzger B, Coustan D: Summary and recommendations of the Fourth International Workshop-Conference on Gestational Diabetes Mellitus, *Diabetes Care* 21(Suppl 2):B161–B167, 1998.

Miller E: Metabolic management of diabetes in pregnancy, *Semin Perinatol* 18(5):414–431, 1994.

Moore T: Diabetes in pregnancy. In Creasy R, Resnik R, Iams J, editors: *Maternal-fetal medicine: principles and practice,* ed 5, Philadelphia, 2004, Saunders.

National Center for Health Statistics: Summary health statistics for U.S. adults: National Health Interview Survey 2002, *Vital Health Stat* 10(222):1–160, 2004.

National Guideline Clearinghouse: *Screening for metabolic syndrome in adults,* Austin, Tex, University of Texas at Austin, School of Nursing, 2004, May. Retrieved from *http://www.guideline.gov*

Neiger R, Kendrick J: Obstetric management of diabetes in pregnancy, *Semin Perinatol* 18(5):432–450, 1994.

O'Sullivan J: Diabetes mellitus after GDM, *Diabetes* 40(Suppl 2):131–135, 1991.

Piper J, Langer O: Does maternal diabetes delay fetal pulmonary maturity?, *Am J Obstet Gynecol* 168(3 Pt 1):783–786, 1993.

Ramchandani N: Type 2 diabetes in children: a burgeoning health problem among overweight young Americans, *Am J Nurs* 104(3):65–68, 2004.

Sibai B and others: Risks of preeclampsia and adverse neonatal outcomes among women with pregestational diabetes mellitus, *Am J Obstet Gynecol* 182(2):364–369, 2000.

Stamler E and others: High infectious morbidity in pregnant women with insulin-dependent diabetes: an understated complication, *Am J Obstet Gynecol* 163:1217, 1990.

Takoudes T and others: Risk of cesarean wound complications in diabetic gestations, *Am J Obstet Gynecol* 191(3):958–963, 2004.

Trout W: Medical emergencies in obstetrics. In Zuspan F, Quilligna E, editors: *Handbook of obstetrics, gynecology and primary care,* St Louis, 1998, Mosby.

Unger J: Diabetes management in the new millennium, *Female Patient* 26(5):7, 2001.

Vohr B, McGarvey S, and Tucker R: Effects of maternal gestational diabetes on offspring adiposity at 4–7 years of age, *Diabetes Care* 22(8):1284–1291, 1999.

Walkinshaw S: Type 1 and type 2 diabetes and pregnancy, *Curr Obstet Gynaecol* 14:375, 2004.

Wang Y and others: Dietary variables and glucose tolerance in pregnancy, *Diabetes Care* 23(4):460–464, 2000.

Weiner C, Buhimschi C: *Drugs for pregnant and lactating women,* Philadelphia, 2004, Churchill Livingstone.

World Health Organization: *Medical eligibility criteria for contraceptive use,* ed 3, Geneva, 2004, WHO.

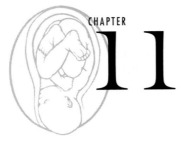

11

Cardiac Disease

P regnancy complicated with cardiac disease is potentially dangerous to maternal well-being. The understanding of normal and abnormal cardiovascular physiology in pregnancy can help enormously in anticipating problems and preventing complications.

INCIDENCE

The incidence of cardiac disease in the pregnant population ranges between 0.5% and 2%. Rheumatic fever, once responsible for 88% of cardiac disease cases in pregnancy, is now on the decline. Congenital disease now plays a more prominent role. Mitral stenosis is still the most frequently seen cardiac condition in pregnant women (Klein and Galan, 2004; Tan, 2004). However, because of better childhood management of congenital heart disease, pregnancy outcomes are generally positive. Nonetheless, cardiac disease accounts for 15% of maternal mortality during pregnancy (Chang and others, 2003). Pregnancy is contraindicated in the presence of the following cardiac conditions (Blanchard and Shabetai, 2004; Tan, 2004) related to the CV danger:
- Severe left ventricular dysfunction
- Complex cyanotic congenital heart disease
- Pulmonary hypertension
- Dilated cardiomyopathy
- Marfan syndrome with aortic involvement
- Eisenmenger's syndrome

ETIOLOGY

Cardiac disease in pregnancy takes a variety of forms and varies in functional severity. Some of the specific forms follow (Klein and Galan, 2004; Tan, 2004):
- Rheumatic heart disease
- Congenital heart disease
- Congestive cardiomyopathies
- Cardiac dysrhythmias
- Infective endocarditis

- Ischemic heart disease
- Valve deformities

NORMAL PHYSIOLOGY

Antepartum

Cardiac Output

In the antepartum period, *cardiac output* (the amount of blood pumped by the left ventricle into the aorta) rises significantly as early as the first trimester of pregnancy. It continues to rise and reaches a plateau between 28 and 34 weeks of gestation. It rises in response to the plasma volume increase, hormonal influences, and autonomic nervous system (ANS) influences. This increase in cardiac output can cause patients to report signs and symptoms that mimic, to some degree, those of cardiac disease (Klein and Galan, 2004; Tan, 2004), including the following:

- Dyspnea
- Orthopnea
- Dyspnea with exertion
- Edema
- Syncope
- Palpitations

Blood Volume

Blood volume increases by plasma volume expansion and red blood cell multiplication. The mean plasma volume increase is 45% over the prepregnant volume, and red cell multiplication is in proportion to volume expansion if nutritional requirements are met. In early pregnancy, the increased volume with each heart stroke increases cardiac output. As pregnancy continues, the heart rate increases to offset increased stroke volume. Increased volume maintains a dilated systemic vasculature.

Hormonal Influences

Hormonal influences affect resistance to blood flow and contractility of the myocardium. Increased estrogen leads to systemic vasodilation. Vasodilation increases cardiac output because of lowered peripheral resistance. Prolactin increases myocardial contractility (Blanchard and Shabetai, 2004; Tomlinson, 2005).

Autonomic Nervous System

During pregnancy, ANS influences on blood flow become more prominent. In the nonpregnant state, when the ANS is blocked, there is little effect on blood pressure. However, in pregnancy, when the ANS is activated or blocked, dramatic changes in the maternal blood pressure can result. The cardiovascular system is hyperfilled from increased blood volume and hyperdynamic because of the predominance of the ANS (see Chapter 1).

Venous Pressure

Increased venous pressure, especially in the lower extremities, occurs in pregnancy. This can lead to a normal finding of an accentuated jugular pulse.

Heart

A slightly enlarged heart sometimes occurs in pregnancy because of the upward and leftward anatomic displacement of the heart. Benign dysrhythmias can occur, presumably because of the normal influences on myocardial contractility.

Inferior Vena Cava

When the weight of the gravid uterus lies against the inferior vena cava, partial or total occlusion reduces return volume to the heart and subsequent output.

Intrapartum

Hemodynamic responses to labor are also important; labor can be a critical period in the care of a pregnant woman with cardiac disease. Uterine contractions normally increase cardiac output and stroke volume because of increased intravascular volume, which leads to an increase in the workload of the heart. The workload can be relieved by positioning the patient laterally and by administering pain relief, especially with epidural anesthesia (Klein and Galan, 2004).

Postpartum

In the immediate postpartum period, there is a high risk for fluid volume overload caused by remobilization of fluid into vascular compartments. It is important to be cautious with administration of intravenous fluids and oxytocin after birth, both of which may further complicate the risk.

Pathophysiology

To understand the pathophysiology of cardiac disease in pregnancy, one must understand what functional lesion is present. It is also necessary to understand various terms describing cardiac function.

Stroke Volume

Stroke volume is the amount of blood ejected with each contraction of the left ventricle. It is affected by four interrelated factors:
- Diastolic filling pressure (preload)
- Distensibility of the ventricle
- Myocardial contractility
- Aortic pressure, which is the amount of pressure the ventricle must overcome to push blood into the aorta (afterload)

Contractility

There is a direct relationship between diastolic volume and the amount of blood pumped during systole. The greater the diastolic filling pressure, the more the fibers of the left ventricle stretch during diastole and the harder they contract during systole, increasing stroke volume and cardiac output. However, if the muscle fibers are stretched beyond a certain point, there is a loss of distensibility. This loss decreases the force of contractions and therefore decreases cardiac output.

Preload

Preload is the force responsible for stretching the ventricular muscles. It is also called *diastolic filling pressure*. If the preload is low, the ventricular muscle will not stretch enough for effective contractility. This leads to decreased stroke volume. If preload is too high, the muscle fibers will be overstretched. This also results in decreased contractility, leading in turn to decreased stroke volume.

Afterload

Afterload is the amount of pressure resistance in the aorta to the emptying of the left ventricle. It is the volume in the ventricles at the end of diastole and is also called *systemic vascular resistance*. Systemic vascular resistance (or afterload) is measured by taking blood pressure readings. The higher the afterload, the greater the force required by the left ventricle to overcome aortic pressure with systolic pressure to force the aortic valve to open. A high afterload decreases stroke volume and cardiac output if the pressure cannot be effectively overcome. Right heart failure may result from persisting high afterload.

Signs and Symptoms

With cardiac disease in pregnancy, the actual lesion is responsible for the specific symptoms. Basically, cardiac disease causes problems with preload or afterload. The usual signs that the cardiac condition is deteriorating in a patient with preexisting cardiac disease are as follows:
- Dyspnea severe enough to limit usual activity
- Progressive orthopnea
- Paroxysmal nocturnal dyspnea
- Syncope during or immediately following exertion
- Chest pain associated with activity

In addition, a pregnancy with preexisting cardiac disease can increase predisposition to thromboembolic changes, palpitations, and fluid retention. These complications sometimes require prophylactic treatment or increases in dosage of current drug therapy. Other conditions of the cardiovascular system, such as chronic hypertension, can also rapidly deteriorate. Patients with chronic hypertension may develop cardiac functional compromise during pregnancy because of the increased volume expansion (see Chapter 21).

Symptoms of cardiac disease in general are classified by the functional incapacity. The classification does not change in pregnancy, although symptoms may worsen. The classifications of cardiac disease (Klein and Galan, 2004) follow:
- *Class I*: asymptomatic at all degrees of activity; uncompromised
- *Class II*: symptomatic with increased activity; slightly compromised

Box 11-1 Maternal Risk Subgroups

Group 1: Mortality Less than 1%
- Atrial septal defect
- Patent ductus arteriosis
- Mitral valve prolapse with regurgitation
- Tetralogy of Fallot (corrected with good repair)
- Mitral stenosis or aortic regurgitation NYHA class I and II

Group 2: Mortality 5% to 20%
- Mitral stenosis NYHA class III and IV or with atrial fibrillation
- Aortic stenosis
- Coarctation of aorta without valve involvement
- Uncorrected tetralogy of Fallot
- Previous myocardial infarction
- Marfan syndrome with normal aorta
- Artificial heart valve

Group 3: Mortality Approximately 50%
- Pulmonary hypertension
- Endocarditis
- Marfan syndrome with aortic involvement
- Eisenmenger's syndrome

NYHA, New York Heart Association.

- *Class III*: symptomatic with ordinary activity; markedly compromised
- *Class IV*: symptomatic at rest; incapacitated

These are prognostic indicators of maternal and fetal complications (Blanchard and Shabetai, 2004; Klein and Galan, 2004). Box 11-1 outlines the three maternal risk subgroups.

MATERNAL EFFECTS

Sudden, severe pulmonary edema occurs if afterload is high. If pulmonary hypertension is present in cardiac lesions such as mitral stenosis or tetralogy of Fallot, right cardiac failure occurs with a resultant increase in preload and decreased stroke volume.

Quite independent of hemodynamic changes, systemic emboli can occur. Patients with atrial fibrillation or mitral valve problems causing atrial fibrillation are particularly susceptible to embolic episodes if not treated adequately with anticoagulants.

Cyanotic heart disease generally does not decrease the pregnant woman's ability to oxygenate her blood unless there is pulmonary hypertension. In atrial or ventricular septal defects, pulmonary hypertension may progress and reverse existing shunts. The rate of maternal mortality is 50% if this occurs (Klein and Galan, 2004).

A dissecting aneurysm, either with coarctation of the aorta or in Marfan syndrome, is associated with a 50% maternal mortality. A dissecting aneurysm can develop suddenly as the pregnancy advances and fluid volume increases.

Pregnant patients with a mechanical heart valve need close monitoring related to the risk for thrombosis, despite anticoagulation (Chan, Anand, and Ginsberg, 2000; Ginsberg and others, 2003; Nassar and others, 2004). Warfarin is most effective in preventing valve thrombosis; however, it is teratogenic especially between 6 and 12 weeks of gestation, may cause CNS defects during the second and third trimester related to subtle bleeding episodes, and can cause cerebral hemorrhage if given too close to delivery. Unfractionated heparin (UH) or low-molecular-weight heparin (LMWH) does not cross the placenta and is very safe for the fetus but not as effective in preventing valve thrombosis. Therefore the safest medication for the fetus is not the best for the pregnant woman. Thus the treatment plan should always be decided in collaboration with the pregnant woman (Emery, 2004; Klein and Galan, 2004; Tan, 2004).

FETAL AND NEONATAL EFFECTS

Fetal effects are the result of decreased systemic circulation or decreased oxygenation. If maternal circulation is compromised because of cardiac functional incapacities, uterine blood flow may be reduced severely. In early pregnancy, this can result in spontaneous abortion. If the uterine blood flow reduction occurs with advancing pregnancy, the fetus can experience effects of deprivation ranging from growth retardation to central nervous system hypoxia. Preterm delivery may be necessary if maternal life is threatened, and the resultant neonatal morbidity associated with prematurity is high.

If maternal oxygenation is impaired, as in cyanotic heart disease or acute pulmonary edema, fetal oxygenation is also impaired. Depending on the severity and length of time of decreased oxygenation, fetal central nervous system hypoxia can result in degrees of mental retardation, fetal distress, or even fetal death (Klein and Galan, 2004).

If either parent has a congenital cardiac defect, the fetus has an increased risk for having a congenital cardiac defect. This could be devastating to the neonate already compromised by hypoxia or prematurity.

DIAGNOSTIC TESTING

Diagnosis of cardiac disease is made by the presentation of symptoms. If type of cardiac disease is unknown, the definition of the cardiac lesion is usually made by a cardiologist. An electrocardiogram (ECG), an echocardiogram, a series of laboratory tests including cardiac enzymes and electrolytes, and a chest radiograph are the usual means, during pregnancy, to define the lesion or assess current status. When the pregnant woman is given anticoagulant therapy, coagulation studies are done. If the woman is taking digitalis, therapeutic blood levels are measured.

USUAL MEDICAL MANAGEMENT AND PROTOCOLS FOR NURSE PRACTITIONERS
General Management

Usual medical management is accomplished with the obstetrician and cardiologist working as a team involving the pregnant cardiac patient in the management of her care. Cardiac medications are usually adjusted to be compatible with pregnancy, and dosages are adjusted when symptoms first present or worsen.

Early ultrasound of the fetus helps in accurate dating. Later, near 28 weeks of gestation, ultrasound can be used serially to document continued fetal growth and well-being. Fetal heart rate monitoring or biophysical profiles may be started by 24 weeks of gestation.

Bedrest, or at least restricted activity, is necessary throughout the last trimester for women with class III heart disease. If symptoms present in women with class I or II heart disease, limitations may be necessary for maternal comfort and well-being and also for adequate fetal oxygenation. The time of presentation of symptoms of cardiac decompensation is usually when maternal fluid volume expansion is greatest. This occurs during the pregnancy near 28 weeks of gestation or in the postpartum period as the then unneeded volume is remobilized.

When cardiac disease is caused by rheumatic fever, the patient has a prosthetic valve, or a history of previous endocarditis, prophylactic antibiotic therapy should be instituted during labor and continued into the postpartum period. Ampicillin or ampicillin plus gentamicin is the antibiotic usually used.

Throughout pregnancy and labor, care is aimed at reducing cardiac workload, especially the effects of tachycardia. During labor, pain relief is provided by regional anesthesia. Assistance with the delivery through the use of forceps in the second stage is often necessary. Vaginal delivery is preferred, if possible, because there are fewer hemodynamic disturbances. Sometime after 36 weeks of gestation a plan for labor induction is made after amniocentesis shows lung maturity.

In addition to other monitoring, an invasive line for hemodynamic monitoring of the mother is necessary during labor and during the unstable postpartum period. Central venous pressure and pulmonary wedge pressure readings aid in management of preload and afterload pressures. Careful titration of fluid volume can aid in preventing pulmonary edema and cardiac overload. Oxygen at 5 to 6 L/min may be needed if cyanotic cardiac disease is present. When decompensation of the cardiac disease occurs, placing the mother's life in jeopardy, termination of the pregnancy might be necessary. This procedure can occur before fetal viability or can result in extreme prematurity of the neonate. Consideration is first given to the safety of the mother.

Issues in the intrapartum period include advance planning of the route of delivery, thromboprophylaxis, hemodynamic monitoring, analgesia-anesthesia options, and antibiotic prophylaxis. Those issues are best addressed with the team, including representatives from perinatology, neonatology, cardiology, and anesthesiology (Tan, 2004).

Drug Therapy

The drug therapy chosen depends on the cardiac lesion. Consideration should be given to maternal benefits and fetal risks. Common anticoagulant drugs used in cardiac disease and pregnancy are low-molecular-weight heparin (LMWH) and unfractionated heparin (UFH). For some, warfarin sodium (Coumadin),

low-dose aspirin, furosemide (Lasix), digitalis, beta-blockers such as propranolol (Inderal), antidysrhythmics such as quinidine, or disopyramide phosphate
(Norpace) may be used. Drugs from newer classifications may be continued from
the prepregnant state if it is difficult to stabilize the mother when she is taking
the drugs just mentioned.

Heparin

Heparin is the most common anticoagulant recommended during pregnancy.
Warfarin crosses the placenta and may have teratogenic effects during the first
trimester and cause bleeding in the fetus, but it is used in the second trimester
and postpartum. Heparin does not cross the placenta and has no such problems
associated with its use.

Two types of heparin are used: low-molecular-weight heparin (LMWH)
and unfractionated heparin (UFH). According to the American College of
Obstetricians and Gynecologists (ACOG) and the Society for Maternal-Fetal
Medicine, low-molecular-weight heparin and unfractionated heparin are safe
for both mother and fetus and can be used for prophylactic or therapeutic
anticoagulation in pregnancy. Because of the longer half-life and increased
bioavailability of LMWH, it is a more efficient anticoagulant except for acute
management of pulmonary embolism and in women with mechanical heart
valves. It also has fewer side effects and a more favorable dosing schedule (daily
versus twice daily). LMWH requires less monitoring, and control can be
achieved rather quickly as an outpatient in comparison with unfractionated
heparin. However, LMWH costs more, and because its half-life is longer than
UFH, it must be stopped more than 24 hours before delivery and intravenous
heparin instituted to lessen the risk for hemorrhage, hematoma, or wound
dehiscence at the time of delivery (Emery, 2004). See Chapter 13 for more
complete information on use of anticoagulants in pregnancy.

Furosemide

Furosemide (Lasix) is a commonly used diuretic in pregnancy. Dosage can vary
from 40 to 80 mg one or two times daily subcutaneously. Intravenous dosage is
usually ordered by the single dose and is also 40 to 80 mg, depending on the
severity of fluid overload. Thiazides are rarely used because severe potassium
deficiency can result. Diuretics reduce amniotic fluid volume and cross the
placenta to the fetus.

Digitalis

Digitalis is a glycoside commonly used in cardiac disease because it increases
contractility and decreases heart rate. Although it does cross the placental
barrier, it does not affect fetal cardiac function. However, this crossing can
decrease maternal concentrations and require the dosage to be adjusted.

Tocolytics

The drug terbutaline is contraindicated for treatment of preterm labor in
women with cardiac disease. Beta-sympathomimetics increase cardiac rate and

workload, as well as the potential for pulmonary edema. Magnesium sulfate decreases calcium levels and has a direct effect on myocardial contractility. If magnesium sulfate is used to treat preterm labor, magnesium and calcium levels must be monitored frequently because magnesium may upset the delicate balance of cardiac electrolytes, cause vasodilation, and lead to decreased blood pressure and thus decreased cardiac output.

Beta-Blockers

Propranolol, labetalol, and other beta-blockers may be used to treat hypertension because they have a decreased pulsating effect on the aorta, or they may be used as antidysrhythmics. Beta-blockers can increase uterine tone and lead to preterm labor. They may also decrease cardiac output and therefore reduce uterine blood flow. Other antidysrhythmics used during pregnancy include quinidine and disopyramide phosphate. Most antidysrhythmics have not been well studied for their fetal effects. However, quinidine, verapamine, and beta-blockers have been used without evidence of teratogenic effects (Expert Consensus Document, 2004).

Quinidine

Quinidine is used as an antidysrhythmic because it depresses myocardial excitability, conductive velocity, and contractility. It has never been studied in animals for effects on the fetus. Therefore as with most antidysrhythmics, it is given when the benefits outweigh the risks. Because quinidine has been used for many years, there is clinical experience with it in pregnancy.

Disopyramide Phosphate

Disopyramide phosphate is an antidysrhythmic drug with effects similar to those of quinidine. However, it is chemically unrelated to any other antidysrhythmics. It decreases the sinus node recovery period and lengthens the response time in the atrium. It has no effect on alpha- or beta-adrenergic receptors, but it has been reported to cause increased uterine contractility. Its use in pregnancy has been studied in animals, and no fetal anomalies have been found.

NURSING MANAGEMENT
Tertiary Prevention

Nursing measures must be directed toward prevention of complications. Nutrition must be adequate in iron and folic acid to prevent anemia, which would increase cardiac workload. Sodium restriction may be necessary, but intake should not fall below 2.5 g/day during pregnancy. Increased dietary fiber can decrease the risk for constipation and thereby reduce heart workload. If the patient is taking a diuretic, she should be instructed in the dietary restriction of sodium and the increase of dietary sources of potassium to decrease the risk for potassium deficiency. This is particularly important when digitalis and diuretics are used together as part of the pharmacologic regimen.

A referral should be made to a registered dietitian for management of the dietary modifications with complex pharmacologic treatment. It is difficult to totally replace lost potassium dietarily or to take in high-fiber foods when bedrest complicates the management. Foods high in potassium (such as bananas, whole grains, and citrus fruits) should be included, but they may not provide the total therapeutic replacement. Supplementary iron and foods high in iron may be restrictively expensive for some patients, necessitating referral to the governmental supplementation program WIC (Women, Infants, and Children).

It is important to differentiate symptoms associated with blood volume increases in normal pregnancies from early signs of volume overload in the pregnant cardiac patient. The patient should be instructed to report any signs of infection and the potential need for antibiotics to prevent bacterial endocarditis. This is particularly important for patients with valve replacements.

Plans should be made early in the pregnancy for restriction of activities and possible prolonged bedrest. Relief from emotional stress can be facilitated if family care can be prearranged. During the pregnancy, attention must be directed at reducing and eliminating anxiety. The patient's anxieties regarding her own well-being, fetal well-being, and her family's care in her absence are likely to increase cardiac workload. Sedation provides only a partial solution. Realistic information about risks and benefits for mother and fetus facilitate adequate coping and reduce anxiety over uncertainties.

When pregnancy termination must occur for the mother's safety and well-being, consideration of potential future pregnancy is very important. Contraceptive means may be limited. Permanent surgical intervention is often not a safe procedure for a woman with class III or IV cardiac disease. Birth control pills also are often contraindicated because they have thromboembolic potential. For the sexually active couple, consistent use of a diaphragm, condoms, or foam might be a problem. Careful counseling in the area of contraception must include a realistic examination of the hazards of subsequent pregnancy to the health of the woman. Her sexual partner should be included in the counseling.

Nursing Interventions for Prevention of Cardiac Decompensation

- When taking the initial history, determine which drugs the patient is taking. (The nurse should be aware of specific drugs commonly used in cardiac disease that are contraindicated in pregnancy and note the dosage, which may need to be changed. Women are usually very aware of potential fetal harm from any drug therapy and often have numerous questions that the nurse should be prepared to answer.)
- At each prenatal visit, assess blood pressure, apical/radial pulses, lung sounds, weight gain, edema, Homans' sign, and chest pain.
- Diagnose and treat such contributing factors of cardiac decompensation as dysrhythmias, hypertension, anemia, or infection.
- Determine the patient's and her family's understanding of the effects of her heart disease on pregnancy and the effects of pregnancy on her heart disease.

- Assess for factors that increase stress.
- Report any signs of arrhythmia such as palpitations, irregular heart rate, apical and radial differences, and progressive edema.
- Report any signs of pulmonary edema such as crackles, abnormal heart sounds, a cough, and dyspnea.
- Report signs of thromboembolism such as pain, redness, tenderness, or swelling in the extremities or chest pain.
- Emphasize the importance of more frequent prenatal visits. During the first half of pregnancy, the patient is usually seen every 2 weeks. During the last half of pregnancy, she is usually seen weekly.
- Emphasize the importance of monitoring and immediate reporting of any signs of cardiac decompensation or congestive heart failure. Such signs are generalized edema, distention of neck veins, dyspnea, pulmonary crackles, frequent moist cough, or heart palpitations.
- Instruct the patient about the importance of daily weighing. A sudden weight gain indicates fluid retention.
- Provide the patient with information on the importance of avoiding constipation and straining during a bowel movement.
- Teach the importance of limiting activity (depending on the classification of heart disease). Patients with class I or II need 10 hours of sleep every night and 30 minutes of rest after meals in a semi-Fowler position. Patients with class III or IV usually need bedrest for most of each day.
- Refer to home health care or nurse specialists as indicated.
- Refer to a high risk pregnancy support group.

Nursing Interventions for Anticoagulation Therapy

In the event that anticoagulants become necessary, if injections are subcutaneous, be prepared to teach or reinforce heparin administration as follows (Johnson, 1997):

- The sites should be rotated in the fatty tissue of the thighs, hips, and abdomen.
- The area should be cleansed with alcohol in a circular motion and then iced for 1 minute with an ice cube to reduce bruising.
- The injection should be given in one motion without aspiration. A syringe with a short, 25-gauge needle should be used.
- The area should not be rubbed after the injection. Ice may be used following the injection.
- A return demonstration of the technique can be provided with normal saline.
- At least three correctly executed injections should be demonstrated by the woman and also by one family member.
- Instruct the woman to report side effects, such as bleeding gums, nose-bleeds, and easy bruising or excessive tissue trauma at injection sites.
- A pump designed for home use can also infuse heparin continuously subcutaneously. Home nursing care personnel should be involved in the setup and administration of heparin with this unit.

Nursing Interventions for Fetal Surveillance

- Monitor fetal heart rate (FHR) as indicated, depending on mother's condition and fetal gestational age.
- Use a combination of biophysical profile, nonstress tests (NSTs) and amniotic fluid volumes (AFVs) beginning between 28 and 32 weeks of gestation to assess fetal health.
- Teach mother to keep a daily fetal movement chart after 24 weeks of gestation.
- Explain rationale and procedure for fetal surveillance studies as ordered, such as biophysical profiles or NST.
- Use growth ultrasounds every 4 to 6 weeks to assess fetal growth.
- Evaluate and report any signs in the FHR of tachycardia, bradycardia, late or variable decelerations, and loss of long- or short-term variability during prenatal testing and during labor.
- During labor, encourage the mother to lie on her side with oxygen provided by face mask.

Nursing Interventions for Early Detection of Preterm Labor

- Assess the home situation for adequate help and support for modified bedrest.
- Evaluate for signs and symptoms of preterm labor through questioning on a routine basis.
- Educate the patient regarding recognition of signs and symptoms of preterm labor because most of the cardiac medications used in pregnancy are reported to increase uterine contractility.
- Teach the benefits of bedrest in reducing uterine irritability and improving uterine blood flow.
- Provide instructions as to what a contraction feels like, warning signs of preterm labor, and the importance of immediately reporting any of these signs.
- Assess the patient's risk for fear.

Nursing Interventions for Anticipatory Grieving

- Discuss loss- and grief-related issues in the antepartum period as appropriate.
- Include family members in the decisions made for medical management.
- Provide support and follow-up as indicated in Chapter 7.
- Take family and mother, if able, for a tour of the level III nursery.
- Discuss the couple's desires in the birth plan and explain any alterations such as epidural, episiotomy, and outlet forceps to decrease the workload on the heart.

Critical Care Nursing Interventions

- Potential complications that require critical care nursing interventions are dysrhythmias, congestive heart failure, thromboembolism, pulmonary edema, electrolyte and fluid imbalance, hypertension, disseminated intravascular coagulation, and superimposed pregnancy complications. These problems are related to increased circulating volume, increased workload during labor, and postpartum remobilization of fluid superimposed on an already compromised cardiac state (Koszalka, 1997; Blanchard and Shabetai, 2004; Anthony, 2005; Tomlinson, 2005).

- The complications are minimized or managed as indicated by a normal sinus rhythm without S_3 or S_4 heart sounds; no signs of congestive heart failure; normal pulmonary artery pressure, pulmonary arterial wedge pressure, and central venous pressure; absence of chest pain, frothy or bloody sputum, and pain or redness in lower extremity vascular beds; clear lung fields; and normal fluid balance and serum electrolytes.
- Continuous ECG monitoring of the mother is essential during any evaluation phase and during labor.
- Monitor vital signs every 15 minutes to 1 hour as indicated by the stability of the mother's condition.
- During labor, assess maternal temperature every 2 to 4 hours.
- Auscultate lung fields every 1 to 4 hours as indicated by the severity and stability of her condition. Report any signs of lung fluid immediately.
- Continuously monitor the FHR, after 24 weeks of gestation, during an acute phase of evaluation. In addition, monitor FHR during labor.
- Weigh the patient daily and assess her for peripheral edema.
- Assess the patient for fear and anxiety.
- At the first signs of fluid overload, be prepared to insert invasive monitoring lines to evaluate the degree of fluid overload and determine treatment.
- During insertion of monitoring lines, observe for dysrhythmias (especially premature ventricular contractions), for wave form changes indicating specific passage through the right atrium (low amplitude waves), for right ventricular wall (tall amplitude) waves, and for pulmonary wedge (smaller, lower pressures with diastolic and systolic) waves. Report abnormalities immediately to the provider (usually anesthesiologist) inserting the catheter.
- Following catheter insertion, continuous ECG monitoring for the cardiac rate is usual.
- Report S_3 and S_4 heart sounds, increased central venous pressure, pulmonary artery pressure, and pulmonary arterial wedge pressure or dysrhythmias, especially premature ventricular contractions. Evaluate every 15 minutes in the initial acute phase, then every 1 to 4 hours as appropriate to measure the degree of stabilization. (Table 11-1 outlines normal readings for each and the significance of low or high readings.)
- Inspect the site of arterial catheter insertion at least once each shift for signs of infection such as redness or drainage.
- Insert a Foley catheter and monitor intake and output hourly. (Urinary output of at least 30 ml/hour is a sensitive measure of adequacy of circulating volume to other vital areas of the body.)
- Administer cardiac glycosides, diuretics, vasodilators, anticoagulants, and antibiotics as ordered.
- Administer oxygen as ordered.

Table 11-1   Hemodynamic Pressure Readings

	Normal Pregnancy	Low	High
CVP (measures right ventricular end-diastolic pressure when tricuspid valve is open and therefore right atrium and ventricle are common chambers)	1–10 mm Hg	Reflects inadequate circulatory volume from: Hemorrhage Third spacing Extreme vasodilation	Reflects: Increased preload High pulmonary resistance Poor cardiac contractility
Systolic PAP (reflects pressure in pulmonary artery when right ventricle is contracting and pulmonary valve is open)	15–25 mm Hg	Reflects a decreased venous return to heart from: Hemorrhage Third spacing Extreme vasodilation	Reflects: Increased blood volume Pulmonary arteriole constriction in response to increased P_{CO_2} and decreased P_{O_2} Increased blood pressure with pulmonary disease such as embolus or edema
Diastolic PAP (reflects left heart when pulmonary valve is closed and left valves are open)	8–10 mm Hg		
PAWP (reflects only pressure from left side of heart)	3–10 mm Hg	Results from: A low circulating volume Extreme vasodilation	Reflects: Increased preload Poor contractility Increased afterload Increased P_{CO_2}

CVP, central venous pressure; *PAP*, pulmonary artery pressure; *PAWP*, pulmonary arterial wedge pressure.

- Administer salt-poor intravenous fluids as ordered for maternal hydration to run only at a specifically ordered rate via infusion pump.
- Prepare for delivery. If vaginal birth is to be attempted, prepare for epidural anesthesia and shorten second-stage labor with forceps. If cesarean birth is planned, prepare for epidural anesthesia.
- Notify the level III nursery.

Postpartum Nursing Interventions

- Continue postpartum hemodynamic monitoring for a minimum of 24 to 72 hours.
- Assess blood pressure and apical and radial pulses after central invasive monitoring is discontinued.
- Auscultate lung fields every 1 to 4 hours as indicated by status of recovery and stabilization. The first several hours are critical as fluid shifts during remobilization of the increased pregnancy volume.
- Assess for presence of chest pain, shortness of breath, general anxiety, and edema.
- Provide adequate pain relief to prevent increased cardiac workload.
- Reevaluate feeding method for infant, especially if breastfeeding was strongly desired and fatigue during recovery phase and after discharge may become a risk to the mother.
- Provide photographs of delivered infant to mother; encourage early family contact.
- Refer to nursing specialists for critical care assistance.
- Refer to social service representative or chaplain for psychosocial or spiritual assistance.
- Encourage family participation in newborn visits and care.
- Facilitate and encourage exploration of feelings regarding maternal and newborn outcomes.
- Refer to intensive care nursery parent support group.
- Refer to social services for assistance with home care.
- Refer to and assist with follow-up with physician specialists.
- Provide education for medication and medical follow-up.
- Provide counseling to the woman and her partner about contraception because choices may be limited and risks and hazards of more common methods may need to be explored. Oral contraceptives are contraindicated if she is on anticoagulation because of thromboembolic potential (Johnson, 1997). If the sexual partnership is not a stable one, an IUD may not be a good choice because of the risk for infection, sepsis, and bacterial endocarditis if the mother has a prosthetic valve (Koszalka, 1997; Blanchard and Shabetai, 2004).

CONCLUSION

The primary goal of nursing care for the pregnant woman and her family when cardiac disease complicates the pregnancy is to reduce potential risks for complications. This is accomplished by education of the woman and her partner; routine assessment of all systems involved; referral to appropriate nursing, nutritional, social, and medical experts; and facilitation of patient participation in decisions. Identification of fears and solutions helps the family to maintain desired control of care. Anticipatory guidance assists in preliminary planning for potential problems and their solutions. The nurse is often in the best position to advocate for the family and coordinate the multidisciplinary team.

BIBLIOGRAPHY

Anthony J: Critical care of the obstetric patient. In James D and others, editors: *High risk pregnancy: management options,* ed 3, Philadelphia, 2005, Saunders.

Blanchard D, Shabetai R: Cardiac diseases. In Creasy R, Resnik R, and Iams J, editors: *Maternal-fetal medicine: principles and practice,* ed 5, Philadelphia, 2004, Saunders.

Chan W, Anand S, and Ginsberg J: Anticoagulation of pregnant women with mechanical heart valves: a systematic review of the literature, *Arch Intern Med* 160(2):191–196, 2000.

Chang J and others: Pregnancy-related mortality surveillance—United States 1990–1999, *MMWR Morb Mortal Wkly Rep* 52(SS02):1, 2003.

Emery S: Anticoagulation in pregnancy: Q&A on low molecular weight heparin, *OBG Management Online,* 2004. Retrieved from *http://www.obgmanagement.com/content*

Ginsberg J and others: Anticoagulation of pregnant women with mechanical heart valves, *Arch Intern Med* 163(6):694–698, 2003.

Johnson R: Thromboembolic disease complicating pregnancy. In Foley M, Strong T, editors: *Obstetric intensive care,* Philadelphia, 1997, Saunders.

Klein L, Galan H: Cardiac disease in pregnancy, *Obstet Gynecol Clin N Am* 31:429, 2004.

Koszalka M: Cardiac disease in pregnancy. In Foley M, Strong T, editors: *Obstetric intensive care,* Philadelphia, 1997, Saunders.

National Guideline Clearinghouse (NGC): Expert consensus document: management of cardiovascular diseases during pregnancy, *Eur Heart J* 24(8):761, 2004. Retrieved from *http://www.guideline.gov*

Nassar A and others: Pregnancy outcome in women with prosthetic heart valves, *Am J Obstet Gynecol* 191(3):1009–1013, 2004.

Tan J: Cardiovascular disease in pregnancy, *Curr Obstet Gynaecol* 14(3):155, 2004.

Tomlinson M: Cardiac disease. In James D and others, editors: *High risk pregnancy: management options,* ed 3, Philadelphia, 2005, Saunders.

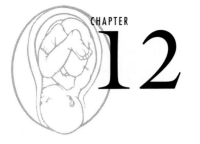

12

Renal Disease

Of the various physiologic alterations in pregnancy, those affecting the urinary tract are the most striking. Improvements in our knowledge related to pregnancy care have meant better care for pregnant women with renal disease. This chapter focuses on urinary tract infection (UTI), chronic renal disease, pregnancy in the dialysis patient, and acute renal failure in pregnancy.

INCIDENCE

Infection

Asymptomatic Bacteriuria

Asymptomatic bacteriuria occurs in 2% to 11% of the pregnant population (Gibbs, Sweet, and Duff, 2004). During pregnancy, if the bacteriuria is left untreated, 40% of women will develop symptoms of UTI. Approximately 25% of women with untreated asymptomatic bacteriuria will develop pyelonephritis during pregnancy (Williams, 2004).

Symptomatic Bacteriuria

Symptomatic bacteriuria occurs in another 1% to 1.5% of pregnancies. Women with a history of previous UTI and current bacteriuria are 10 times more likely to develop symptoms during pregnancy than women without either feature (Davison and Lindheimer, 2004).

Acute Renal Failure

Acute renal failure rarely occurs during pregnancy, but it can be triggered by various complications of pregnancy.

Renal Disease

The incidence of renal disease in pregnancy varies depending on the form it takes.

Renal Calculi

Renal calculi rarely occur in pregnancy. Less than 1 in 1000 pregnancies require surgery to correct this problem.

Lupus

Lupus, a multisystem disease that frequently effects the kidneys, exacerbates during pregnancy in 40% of women who are affected by the disease. If, before the pregnancy, renal involvement was present, the renal status may deteriorate during or immediately after the pregnancy.

Acute Glomerulonephritis

Acute glomerulonephritis during pregnancy is extremely rare, occurring in 1 of 40,000 pregnancies. This is attributed to the usual failure to ovulate in women with the disease.

Diabetic Nephropathy

Diabetic nephropathy is seen more frequently now that better control can be established and since it is known that pregnancy does not adversely affect diabetes.

Polycystic Kidney Disease

Because polycystic kidney disease does not generally become evident until after age 40 years, it is rarely seen in pregnancy. It is associated with autosomal dominant genetic transmission. Therefore there is a 50% chance of its transmission to each child born to a parent before the disease manifests itself.

After Renal Transplant

In the past, pregnancy after kidney transplant was extremely rare, not only because of the woman's renal status but also because of her age by the time of transplant. Reports of women successfully completing pregnancy while on continuous ambulatory peritoneal dialysis began in the 1980s (Hou, 1987). Today greater than 50% of pregnancies progress to term in the face of a 30% incidence of preeclampsia. The greatest loss is in the first trimester (Davison and Lindheimer, 2004). Immunosuppressive drug therapy must be considered antenatally and postpartum (Davison and Lindheimer, 2004; Williams, 2004).

ETIOLOGY

Infection

The cause of bacteriuria is often bacteria from the gastrointestinal tract contaminating the perineal area. Often, the organism implicated is *Escherichia coli*. It is common when contaminants from the rectal area are brought forward across the urethral meatus during perineal hygiene. It can also occur from trauma to the meatus during sexual intercourse, forcing perineal contaminants into the urethra. Bacteria may migrate from the urethra into the bladder and proliferate before the next urination. Bacteria may also pass into the dilated ureters during pregnancy and migrate into the kidney itself, causing inflammation of the tubules. Occasionally, other perineal organisms, such as yeast, are introduced into the bladder and cause infection.

Staphylococcal or streptococcal bacteria can enter the blood in the kidney and result in renal tissue reaction to the organism or to its toxins. However, these organisms rarely cause infection during pregnancy.

Acute Renal Failure

Acute renal failure can be precipitated by hemorrhagic shock caused by placenta previa, abruptio placenta, uterine rupture, operative trauma, or postpartum uterine atony. Endotoxic shock in the cases of chorioamnionitis, pyelonephritis, or puerperal sepsis can also precipitate acute renal failure. Urinary tract obstruction is another cause. Polyhydramnios, ureter calculi, pelvic or broad ligament hematoma, or damage to the ureters can cause a urinary obstruction during a cesarean delivery.

Renal Disease

Renal disease can be caused by a UTI before or during pregnancy, can be the result of other diseases such as diabetes, or can occur in pregnancy from complications such as hypertensive disorders of pregnancy.

NORMAL PHYSIOLOGY

The kidneys fulfill several functions essential for the body. They excrete water, electrolytes, and nitrogenous waste products. They perform a major function in acid-base balance and are active in the renin-angiotensin-aldosterone system. The kidney also produces erythropoietin, which aids in stimulating red blood cell production.

The kidneys have the largest blood supply of any organ in the body. Renal blood flow accounts for 20% to 25% of the cardiac output. The blood to each kidney is supplied by a renal artery, which branches finally into the afferent arteriole, leading into the glomerulus. From the glomerulus, the efferent arteriole leads out via branches into the renal vein.

Filtration of the blood through the glomerulus is the result of four forces acting on the capillaries: the permeability of the capillary walls, the hydrostatic pressure in the glomerular capillaries, the hydrostatic pressure in the glomerular capsule, and the osmotic pressure of the circulating plasma proteins. It is the pressure within the glomerular capillaries that determines the filtration rate. Glomerular filtration produces a protein-free filtrate of plasma. The glomeruli act as ultrafilters with microscopic pores. The microscopic pores do not normally allow the larger protein or glucose molecules through but rather send them along the circulatory route to the tubules. The major excretory product into urine is sodium. The tubules act on the glomerular filtrate to produce urine. Substances are reabsorbed from the glomerular filtrate either actively or passively. Substances such as water passively follow sodium that is actively reabsorbed into the urine. Urea, a nitrogenous waste product, diffuses passively. Glucose is actively reabsorbed against the concentration gradient after being freely filtered in the glomerulus.

The tubule cells also secrete a number of substances, such as potassium, hydrogen, ammonium (NH_4^+), and organic anions and cations. As the glomerular filtrate flows through the proximal tubule, sodium is actively reabsorbed and chloride follows passively. Water follows with the change in osmotic pressure. As it reaches the loop of Henle in the tubule, the fluid volume is reduced by 80%. As the fluid flows through the thin, descending loop of Henle, water is removed passively because of the hypertonicity of the interstitial tissues. As the fluid enters the distal convoluted tubules, it becomes hypotonic.

If circulating antidiuretic hormone is elevated, the distal tubule is permeable to water and the urinary fluid then becomes isotonic to the interstitial fluid. Chloride, sodium, and passive osmotic diffusion of water further reduce the urinary fluid volume as it enters the collecting duct, where it changes from an isotonic to a hypertonic fluid. The urinary fluid and sodium removed in the loop of Henle return to the general circulation.

If the antidiuretic hormone level is low, the distal tubule is not permeable to water and the urinary fluid remains hypotonic. It loses its solutes and increases its hypotonicity. The ultimate outcome is that the urine is both dilute and increased in volume.

The kidney regulates acid-base balance by maintaining plasma bicarbonate between 26 and 28 mEq/L in response to the respiratory system's maintenance of carbonic acid at 1.3 to 1.4 mEq/L. Organic anions in the urine accept hydrogen ions, producing carbonic acid, which is in turn broken down into water and carbon dioxide. Ammonia (a combination of nitrogen and three hydrogen ions) takes on another hydrogen ion and becomes NH_4^+ and then is excreted in the urine. In this way, the kidney serves as an efficient buffering mechanism.

During pregnancy, a number of alterations occur in renal function. Secondary to prostaglandin E_2, renal blood flow increases, vascular resistance decreases, and glomerular filtration rate increases 30% to 50% over that in the nonpregnant state. Because of this increased filtration rate, nitrogenous waste products such as creatinine, urea, and uric acid are cleared in greater quantities. Therefore urine clearance levels are higher and serum levels are lower than in nonpregnant women.

As the filtrate enters the tubules, considerable changes in the mechanisms controlling salt and water excretion occur. Progesterone normally causes increased salt loss. In pregnancy, this is countered by a rise in aldosterone to two to three times the nonpregnant levels. As a result, sodium is actually retained in the tissues in larger amounts, thus aiding in the necessary volume expansion of pregnancy.

The healthy pregnant woman also excretes larger amounts of sugar in her urine. This is not related to the blood glucose levels but rather to an intermittent tubular failure to reabsorb glucose.

Amino acid excretion is known to be increased in pregnancy. This is thought to be caused by a partial failure of the normal reabsorptive mechanisms. The increased excretion of amino acids is related to high levels of cortisol in pregnancy. Plasma albumin levels are normally lower.

Water-soluble vitamins, such as ascorbic acid, nicotinic acid, and folates, are also excreted at higher levels in the urine during pregnancy. This increased excretion is caused by failure of the tubules to reabsorb and can be serious when folate and protein intake are marginal.

Another important consideration of the high nutrient content of the urine is acknowledging its value as a culture medium for bacteria. Progesterone enhances the potential for UTI by relaxing the musculature of the bladder and the ureters. The dilation of the ureters, especially on the right side, is further compromised by the obstruction of the gravid uterus. All these factors contribute to the likelihood of urinary stasis of a fluid rich in nutrients, which substantially increases the potential for ascending UTI.

During pregnancy, the kidneys produce increased amounts of erythropoietin, and renin. Erythropoietin increases the RBC mass; however, with the increase plasma volume greater then the increase RBC mass, hemoglobin normally is lower. Renin acts to form angiotensin, which in turn increases the production of aldosterone. The aldosterone increase preserves sodium and facilitates blood volume expansion. The sensitivity to the pressor effects of renin-angiotensin is low during pregnancy, and normally the blood pressure does not rise.

PATHOPHYSIOLOGY

When infection from urinary bacteria ascends the urinary tract, the renal tubules can become inflamed. The inflammatory process leads to a decrease in tubular function. Reabsorption of sodium into the urinary fluid and secretion of buffering substances are affected adversely if large localized areas become inflamed. Sodium is then retained in body tissues, and water remains compartmentalized in tissues or in the intravascular space, which can cause edema or increased cardiac afterload (Bernasko and Alvarez, 1997; Asrat and Nageotte, 2005).

Secretion of buffering substances may also be reduced. When buffering substances such as potassium, ammonia, and organic ions are deficient in quantity, free hydrogen ions cannot be absorbed. The blood pH will reflect the increased carbonic acid with a tendency toward acidemia. Concurrent conditions such as diabetes can complicate potential acidemia because of nephropathy or metabolic failures inherent in the disease (Bernasko and Alvarez, 1997).

Hypertensive renal disease, diabetic nephropathy, pregnancy-induced hypertension, and glomerulonephritis can be differentiated by the specific histology of the lesion in the kidneys. Lesions can be either in the glomeruli or in the tubules. Some affect the vasculature surrounding or comprising the glomeruli and tubules; others affect the cells within the glomeruli or tubules. When the vasculature of the renal tissues is damaged and blood supply to the kidneys is compromised, renin activity increases and blood pressure rises. Pregnancy sometimes initially improves the blood pressure because of the vasodilating effect of progesterone. However, this may be counteracted by a continuation of sensitivity to the pressor effect, and preeclampsia may become superimposed (Williams, 2004).

If the glomeruli are damaged, filtration rate cannot increase to meet the demands of pregnancy. Nitrogenous waste cannot be removed from the bloodstream in sufficient quantities and builds up in abnormal amounts in the bloodstream. Creatinine, uric acid, and urea levels rise in the serum and fall in the urine (Bernasko and Alvarez, 1997).

Increased excretion of nitrogenous waste into the sweat and saliva can produce a characteristic ammonia odor. This can also cause itching and irritation of the skin (Bernasko and Alvaraez, 1997; Asrat and Nageotte, 2005).

If tubular cells or the surrounding vasculature is damaged, the primary tubular functions are affected. Because the tubules serve as the major sodium pump, it is this function that is dramatically decreased. Sodium cannot be pulled into the urine fluid in the proximal tubule; therefore water cannot follow. Urine output then reflects this in a reduced volume, with sodium remaining elevated in the blood and water increasing in the intravascular space. Sodium and water will therefore be increased in the tissues and result in edema (Asrat and Nageotte, 2005).

If proteins are lost into the glomerular filtrate because of damage to the micropores, osmotic pressure changes and fluid is lost from the intravascular space into the tissue more readily. Because pregnancy favors increased spillage of protein, a marginal kidney function can cause greater likelihood of spillage of large quantities of protein into the urine (Bernasko and Alvarez, 1997; Asrat and Nageotte, 2005).

SIGNS AND SYMPTOMS
Infection
Acute Cystitis Infection
Frequency, dysuria, and urgency of urination or suprapubic or low back pain may herald bladder infection.

Kidney Infection
Pyelonephritis is usually present when fever, chills, nausea, vomiting, malaise, and flank pain occur.

Renal Disease
Chronic renal disease from other origins can be associated with generalized edema and proteinuria, increased blood pressure, and decreased urinary volume. These symptoms rarely worsen during pregnancy unless hypertensive disorders of pregnancy are superimposed on an impaired renal function.

Nitrogenous Waste
Symptoms of increased nitrogenous waste products in the bloodstream include mental confusion, apathy, and itchy skin. Urinary output may be diminished, and the specific gravity is low.

Electrolyte Imbalance

Potassium excess occurs when the plasma potassium is higher than 5.6 mEq/L. Signs include tachycardia and later bradycardia, electrocardiogram changes with a high T wave and depressed ST segment, and oliguria, abdominal distention, or diarrhea.

- Potassium deficit occurs when the plasma potassium is below 4 mEq/L. Signs include anorexia, abdominal distention, muscle weakness, hypotension, and dysrhythmias. Severe hypokalemia can cause heart block.
- Sodium excess occurs when the plasma sodium is greater than 147 mEq/L. Signs include a urine specific gravity above 1.03; restlessness; dry, sticky mucous membranes; oliguria; hypertension; tachycardia; and edema. Severe hypernatremia can cause convulsions.
- Sodium deficit does not occur.
- Calcium excess occurs when plasma calcium levels are above 5.5 mEq/L. Signs include drowsiness, headaches, irritability, muscle weakness, hypertension, anorexia, and flank pain. Severe hypercalcemia may cause heart block.
- Calcium deficit occurs when plasma calcium levels are lower than 4.5 mEq/L. Signs include irritability, twitching around the mouth, numbness, muscle spasms, hypotension, dysrhythmias, and diarrhea. Severe hypocalcemia may cause convulsions.
- Primary base bicarbonate deficit can occur because of the inability of the tubules to secrete buffers. Metabolic acidosis may develop. Signs include urine pH below 6.0, plasma pH below 7.35, disorientation, and shortness of breath or deep, rapid breathing.

Fluid Imbalance

If renal tissues are severely damaged from hypertensive lesions, diabetic nephropathic lesions, or infectious processes, the loss of intravascular osmotic pressure can produce systemic and pulmonary edema. Signs and symptoms of pulmonary edema are sudden in onset and include shortness of breath, crackles, frothy sputum, and decreased Po_2.

Other Signs of Severe Renal Damage

Other signs of severe renal damage include serum potassium excess, which can lead to cardiac dysrhythmias, dilation of the myocardium, and cardiac arrest. Serum calcium levels may also be low, with similar cardiac effects. Loss of buffering can lead to signs of metabolic acidosis, including a compensatory increase in respiratory rate.

MATERNAL EFFECTS

Infection in the urinary tract may predispose a woman to preterm labor. The exact mechanism is not clear, and the cause-and-effect relationship is controversial (Gibbs, Sweet, and Duff, 2004). Certainly, repeated UTIs increase the likelihood of the same organisms infecting the fetal membranes.

Renal disease with preserved renal function usually causes minimal kidney deterioration and most often leads to a positive pregnancy outcome. The more impaired the renal function and the more associated complications, the greater the likelihood of renal deterioration and an adverse pregnancy outcome (Davison and Lindheimer, 2004).

FETAL AND NEONATAL EFFECTS

Because of the loss of water from the plasma volume, circulation to the uterus can be diminished. The fetus can suffer nutritionally from the resultant deficiency. Intrauterine growth retardation is common in the fetus of a woman with renal disease. If hypertension is also present, arterial resistance to blood flow into the intervillous space can cause chronic hypoxemia of the fetus. Depending on the severity and chronicity of hypoxia, the fetus can suffer central nervous system damage and face potential demise.

DIAGNOSTIC TESTING

Infection

Obtaining a clean-catch urine specimen and doing a quantitative urine culture make the diagnosis of asymptomatic or symptomatic bacteriuria. A bacteria count of the same species greater than 105 ml of urine is significant. A presumptive diagnosis can be made on urinalysis with bacteria greater than 20 ml in centrifuged urine or white blood cells greater than 5 to 10 ml on high-powered field when symptoms are present. All pregnant women should be screened for asymptomatic bacteriuria with a quantitative urine culture early in their prenatal care.

Significant bacteriuria may represent either bladder or kidney infection. The differentiation is made by the symptoms presented. However, asymptomatic pyelonephritis can occur, just as bladder infection can be asymptomatic. Asymptomatic pyelonephritis should be suspected when urine cultures detect recurrent or persistent infection despite antibiotic therapy. For this reason, urine cultures should be repeated after a course of antibiotic therapy.

Renal Disease

When disease or complications of pregnancy exist and there is renal impairment, renal function studies are usually done to ascertain the degree of impairment. It is therefore common to do renal function studies for baseline data in pregnant women who have class D or greater diabetes, have systemic lupus, have a history of chronic renal disease or chronic hypertension, or develop pregnancy-induced hypertension. Such laboratory studies include 24-hour urine collection for creatinine clearance, serum creatinine, serum uric acid, blood urea nitrogen (BUN), and total urinary protein. Laboratory values differ in pregnancy beginning as early as 8 to 10 weeks of gestation. This should be considered when interpreting the results (Davison and Lindheimer, 2004; Asrat and Nageotte, 2005). Table 12-1 describes differences between nonpregnant and pregnant normal values.

Table 12-1   Renal Function Studies

Study	Nonpregnant Normal Value	Pregnant Normal Value
BUN	10–16 mg/dl	8.7 ± 1.5 mg/dl
Serum creatinine	0.67–1.2 mg/dl	0.6–1.28 mg/dl
Uric acid	4.2 ± 1.2 mg/dl	3 ± 0.17 mg/dl
Urinary creatinine clearance	100 mg/dl	140 mg/dl
24-hr urinary protein	Not different	Not greater than 260 mg/24 hr

Modified from Good Samaritan Regional Medical Center Laboratory Manual, Phoenix, 1989.
BUN, Blood urea nitrogen.

Renal biopsy to diagnose a specific renal lesion is contraindicated during pregnancy because of the increased blood flow to the kidney. Increases in capillary pressures predispose the kidney to greater potential for hemorrhage, which can lead to further kidney damage.

Other diagnostic studies, such as renal ultrasound, can aid in the diagnosis of obstruction of the ureters or pyelonephritis. Radiographic studies, such as the intravenous pyelogram, are rarely used in pregnancy since the advent of sophisticated ultrasonic examinations.

USUAL MEDICAL MANAGEMENT AND PROTOCOLS FOR NURSE PRACTITIONERS

General Management

Treatment of renal disease in pregnancy depends on the nature of the disease.

Infection

The most common causative organism of UTI during pregnancy is *Enterobacteriaceae*. Asymptomatic bacteriuria and symptomatic bacteriuria are treated primarily with nitrofurantoin, cefazolin, cephalexin, ceftriaxone, and gentamicin (Le, 2004). Antibiotic therapy must be continued in maximum doses for 7 days. High doses are required during pregnancy because of increased excretion caused by greater renal blood flow. If reculture demonstrates continued bacterial growth, the course of antibiotics must be reinstituted for 6 weeks. Reculture is again done, and if it is positive, an antimicrobial such as nitrofurantoin can be continued for the duration of the pregnancy (Gibbs, Sweet, and Duff, 2004). If infection has been recurrent during the pregnancy or if acute pyelonephritis occurs, a postpartum intravenous pyelogram is often done to rule out an obstruction in the urinary tract (see Chapter 24).

Acute Renal Failure

Treatment of sudden, acute renal failure in the pregnant woman resembles that of the nonpregnant population. The aim of treatment is to retard the development of uremic symptoms and restore acid-base balance, electrolyte balance, and volume homeostasis. The choice of hemodialysis or peritoneal dialysis depends on the experience of staff and the availability of staff consultation. If acute renal failure occurs during pregnancy, termination of the pregnancy is usually necessary for the mother's safety (Bernasko and Alvarez, 1997).

Chronic Renal Disease

The treatment for chronic renal disease is more complicated. The hypertension that is frequently associated with the disease requires control with an antihypertensive drug. The urinary output and fluid intake must be closely monitored to prevent fluid overload. Salt solutions must be administered with great caution because of the inability to excrete large quantities of salt and the potential for overwhelming edema, especially in the lungs. Diuretics can be used to aid in excretion of retained fluid, and electrolyte balance must then be closely monitored. If acidosis occurs, lack of an adequate buffering system in the kidneys can create further problems when salt solutions must be administered for their alkalinizing effects. Because the production of erythropoietin is suppressed in chronic renal failure, it is not uncommon to find an associated anemia in pregnancy. Coupled with the tendency for hemodilution on hemoglobin measurement, the anemia can be quite severe, causing shortness of breath, easy fatigue, and failure of fetal growth. These signs may be initially overlooked and attributed to other causes. Increased folic acid and iron supplementation assist normal physiology and counteract some pathologic findings.

The effects of hypertension, loss of protein, and retention of sodium and water can create a life-threatening situation for the mother. If the fetus has little chance of surviving, the choice for termination of the pregnancy should be offered to the mother. If the maternal condition is likely to deteriorate, the risks and benefits of continuing the pregnancy should be discussed with the woman and her family. For the pregnancy that continues, fetal evaluation is ordered. Ultrasound examinations may be done every 2 weeks from 24 weeks of gestation on. Nonstress tests (NSTs) and contraction stress tests are usually done weekly after 26 weeks of gestation. Daily fetal activity charts are also kept.

End-Stage Renal Disease

Most patients with end-stage renal disease who become pregnant do so accidentally and without the advantage of preconceptual management considerations. Therefore both surgical termination of pregnancy and spontaneous fetal loss probably cause fetal loss rates to be artificially high. Attempts at managing pregnancy complicated by end-stage renal disease with hemodialysis or peritoneal dialysis have provided improved success in pregnancy outcome (Davison and Lindheimer, 2004). However, these patients must be monitored closely for anemia, hemorrhage, infection, and preterm labor. Iron and erythropoietin should be given as serum iron and hemoglobin levels indicate.

Drug Therapy

Antihypertensive Agents

Perinatal outcomes are improved by controlling hypertension in the pregnant woman with renal disease (see Chapter 21).

Diuretics

Diuretics are often used if fluid retention is contributing to hypertension. They also help to prevent pulmonary edema. Any diuretic can cause electrolyte imbalance. The pregnant woman especially should be instructed to report signs of potassium deficit and to help prevent this condition with an increased dietary intake of potassium. Bananas and citrus fruits are high in potassium.

Antimicrobials

Antimicrobials are prescribed for UTIs. It is important, for maintenance of blood levels, to administer them at evenly spaced intervals. The woman should be instructed to drink more fluids and to take the entire prescription. In the hospital setting, when antimicrobials are given intravenously, the site should be inspected for an inflammatory reaction. The site should also be changed every 48 hours to prevent phlebitis (see Chapter 25).

Tetracyclines are contraindicated for use in pregnancy because of rare maternal acute fatty liver necrosis. In addition, they bind with calcium orthophosphates and cause a permanent yellow staining of the fetal dentition. Chloramphenicol is not used in pregnancy because of the fatal gray syndrome that occurs in infants born of mothers receiving the drug. Sulfonamides and nitrofurantoin are contraindicated somewhat in the last trimester because of their potential for increasing levels of fetal bilirubin.

NURSING MANAGEMENT

Prevention

Prevention of symptomatic UTIs is greatly aided by nursing interventions. Pregnant women should be educated to practice correct perineal hygiene and to report any indication of vaginitis or UTI. Routine evaluation of the urine should be carried out at each office visit. The voided specimen should be fresh, not saved from home, and should be evaluated for protein, nitrites, or leukocyte esterase, which are produced in increased amounts when bacterial growth is significant. If the protein level is 1 or more in the absence of pregnancy-induced hypertension or if nitrites are evident, a clean-catch or sterile catheterized specimen should be obtained for urinalysis, culture, and sensitivity studies. The pregnant woman should be encouraged to drink at least 3000 ml of fluid every 24 hours.

Tertiary prevention of complications from existing renal disease is also important. A careful history should include questions regarding repeated bacteriurias, hypertension when not pregnant, and renal function studies if hypertension, diabetes, or connective tissue disorders have been previously diagnosed. This information helps in screening those women at risk for complications such as preeclampsia, pulmonary edema, uteroplacental insufficiency, and progression of existing renal disease.

Nursing Interventions for Renal Disease

- Assess for risk for fluid overload.
- In the presence of renal failure, fluid intake should be carefully monitored and intake should equal output unless the patient is febrile. If the patient is febrile, 100 ml of additional fluid is needed for every degree Celsius of elevation from 38° C.
- Evaluate the degree of edema.
- When drug therapy is prescribed, teach the patient about the purpose, dosage schedule, and potential side effects.
- Discuss the importance of nutritional modifications and make referrals to a registered dietitian when necessary. This is especially relevant if sodium or protein intake is decreased or there is a need for increased protein, iron, or potassium.
- Teach the patient or family to do home blood pressure monitoring.
- Instruct the patient and family about the importance of recognizing and reporting signs of fluid or electrolyte imbalance, medicine-induced side effects, and superimposed preeclampsia or HELLP (*h*emolysis, *e*levated *l*iver enzymes, and *l*ow *p*latelet count) syndrome.
- Modify home activities to reduce onset of dangerous hypertension and avoid added fatigue factors.
- Teach the patient how to avoid infections.
- Teach the patient the signs and symptoms of preterm labor and when to report it if it becomes regular (four painless contractions per hour unrelieved by 1 hour of rest).
- Avoid using urinary catheters in the presence of renal disorders to prevent introduction of new bacteria into the urinary tract. Avoid indwelling catheters without triple lumen because they are intended for irrigation with antibacterial agents.
- Always run a clean catch urine specimen with a 48-hour culture and sensitivity before beginning the first dose of antimicrobial therapy. (It is not necessary to have results first, but they should be reviewed within 3 days of sending the specimen to select the appropriate antimicrobial.)
- Perform dipstick urine test for protein, nitrites, and leukocyte esterase at each antepartum office visit and at least weekly for hospitalized patients.
- Ask the patient at each visit whether she has symptoms of burning, frequency, and flank pain and assess whether she presents with signs of preterm labor.
- Educate the patient about the importance of drinking a variety of fluids (avoid high acid, carbonated, or caffeinated beverages), at least 8 to 10 ounces every waking hour.
- Instruct the patient to empty her bladder at least every 2 hours while awake and to void after intercourse.
- Tell the patient to perform perineal hygiene front to back.
- Educate the patient about the importance of reporting signs of kidney or bladder infections immediately.

- Educate the patient regarding prophylactic antibiotic therapy if she has a history of pyelonephritis.
- Start fetal surveillance with electronic fetal monitoring, biophysical profile (BPP), NSTs, AFV, or some combination of testing by 28 to 32 weeks of gestation.
- After 24 weeks of gestation, evaluate for fetal intrauterine growth restriction every 4 to 6 weeks by ultrasound.
- See Chapter 2 for interventions for fear, ineffective coping, and altered parenting; Chapter 3 and 4 for assessment of fetal health; Chapter 5 for alternative and complementary therapies; and Chapter 7 for perinatal anticipatory or actual loss.

Critical Care for Acute Renal Failure*

- Carefully evaluate intake and output of any high risk patient.
- Assess for hypertensive disorders of pregnancy or disseminated intravascular coagulation.
- Evaluate laboratory and diagnostic data such as BUN and serum creatinine levels. (These are frequently the earliest signs of acute kidney failure.)
- Assess for signs of superimposed preeclampsia by evaluating blood pressure at each antepartum visit or daily if hospitalized.
- Assess for signs of hemorrhage and coagulopathy.
- Assess respirations and breath sounds if there is a possibility of renal compromise.
- Assess for signs of fluid, electrolyte, and acid-base imbalances.
- Prevent acute renal failure by assisting in replacement of blood and fluids in the event of massive hemorrhage.
- Report early signs of an infection.
- If acute renal failure develops, be prepared to use invasive hemodynamic monitoring to assess intravascular volume (see Chapter 11) and kidney dialysis.
- Report any signs of preeclampsia or fluid, electrolyte, or acid-base imbalances to the attending physician.
- Report abnormal blood chemistries to the attending physician.
- Perform dialysis as ordered.
- Weigh the patient at each dialysis exchange.
- Report any signs of abnormal fluid retention if the patient is on dialysis.
- Administer appropriate salt-poor intravenous fluids if pyelonephritis or signs of renal failure are present.
- Refer the patient to a nurse clinician or specialist for education regarding dialysis.

*Gonik and Foley, 2004; Asrat and Nageotte, 2005; Maresh and others, 2005.

CONCLUSION

The primary aim for care of the pregnant woman with bacteriuria is prevention of symptomatic UTI and preterm labor. Prophylactic administration of antibiotics with instructions for increased oral fluids and proper perineal hygiene are most effective.

Prompt treatment of renal tract infection and medical response to maternal renal failure can prevent life-threatening events for the mother and intrauterine growth restriction or intrauterine fetal death. In the presence of mild renal impairment, pregnancy does not affect renal function. In the presence of moderate-to-severe renal impairment, pregnancy outcomes can be significantly affected (Williams, 2004). Pregnancy after renal transplant has been quite successful if the original medical condition is stabilized and carefully monitored.

BIBLIOGRAPHY

Asrat T, Nageotte P: Renal disease. In James D and others: *High risk pregnancy: management options,* ed 3, London, 2005, Saunders.

Bernasko J, Alvarez M: Acute renal failure in the obstetric intensive care patient. In Foley M, Strong T: *Obstetric intensive care,* Philadelphia, 1997, Saunders.

Davison J, Lindheimer M: Renal disorders. In Creasy R, Resnik R, and Iams J, editors: *Maternal-fetal medicine: principles and practice,* ed 5, Philadelphia, 2004, Saunders.

Gibbs R, Sweet R, and Duff W: Maternal fetal infectious disorders. In Creasy R, Resnik R, and Iams J, editors: *Maternal-fetal medicine: principles and practice,* ed 5, Philadelphia, 2004, Saunders.

Gonik B, Foley M: Intensive care monitoring of the critically ill obstetric patient. In Creasy R, Resnik R, and Iams J: *Maternal-fetal medicine: principles and practice,* ed 5, Philadelphia, 2004, Saunders.

Hou S: Peritoneal and hemodialysis in pregnancy, *Clin Obstet Gynecol* 1:1009, 1987.

Le J and others: Urinary tract infections during pregnancy, *Ann Pharmacother* 38(10): 1692–1701, 2004.

Maresh M, James D, and Neales K: Critical care of the obstetric patient. In James D and others: *High risk pregnancy: management options,* ed 3, London, 2005, Saunders.

Roberts J: Pregnancy related hypertension. In Creasy R, Resnik R, and Iams J, editors: *Maternal-fetal medicine: principles and practice,* ed 5, Philadelphia, 2004, Saunders.

Williams D: Renal disease in pregnancy, *Curr Obst Gynaecol* 14(3):166, 2004.

CHAPTER

13

Autoimmune Diseases

utoimmune diseases can occur during pregnancy because 70% of
patients with an autoimmune disease are women of childbearing age
(Beeson, 1994). These diseases result from the body's immune system
inability to distinguish "self" from "nonself." When this inability occurs, the
body manufactures T cells and antibodies directed against its own cells. This
immunologic defect may be cellular or humoral in nature. Examples of cell-
mediated autoimmune diseases are rheumatoid arthritis (RA) and multiple
sclerosis. Frequently, pregnancy has no effect or may improve these diseases.
Humoral autoimmune diseases result from abnormal antibody formation. Examples of these disorders are systemic lupus erythematosus (SLE) and acquired
thrombophilias such as antiphospholipid syndrome (APS). These autoimmune
diseases worsen or are associated with pregnancy loss or placental insufficiency.
Table 13-1 summarizes the effects of some common autoimmune disorders
related to pregnancy. The remainder of the chapter focuses on SLE and APS,
two autoimmune disorders that have serious consequences for pregnancy.

INCIDENCE

Systemic Lupus Erythematosus

According to some sources (Porter and Branch, 2005), the incidence of SLE in
women from their late 20s to early 40s may be as high as 1:1000, with more
than 500,000 cases diagnosed each year. The prediction in the 1970s and early
1980s of an incidence of 6:100,000 has been changed dramatically because of
the improved ability to diagnose SLE by radioimmune assays. Women are
affected 10 times more often than men. Because childbearing is frequently
postponed in professional, educated women, their incidence of being diagnosed
with SLE before having children is higher.

Whether a woman is pregnant or not, SLE may be characterized by
exacerbations and remissions. Survival after exacerbation is 90% in the first 5
years and 80% after 10 years. Survival generally depends on the degree of
cardiac and renal involvement and the extent of multisystem insult.

Table 13-1   Common Autoimmune Disorders and Pregnancy

Autoimmune Disorder	Effect of Pregnancy on Disease	Effect of Disease on Pregnancy	Effect of Disease on Fetus
Graves' disease	Improved during pregnancy Exacerbation during postpartum	No significant effect	Intrauterine growth restriction (IUGR) Neonatal thyrotoxicosis
Myasthenia gravis	Variable with no change, or exacerbations during pregnancy and postpartum	Increased fatigue Potential respiratory difficulties in late pregnancy Preterm labor	Transient neonatal myasthenia
Rheumatoid arthritis (RA)	Variable • Over 50% disease improves • 25% experience no change • Small number disease worsens (Porter and Branch, 2005)	No significant effect	No significant effect Teratogenic risk for medications
Systemic sclerosis	Exacerbation • 20% disease worsens (Steen, 1997; 1999) • 33% experience exacerbations during postpartum (Steen, 1999)	Preterm labor Preeclampsia Renal failure	Intrauterine growth restriction (IUGR)

Antiphospholipid Syndrome (APS)

The incidence of patients with antiphopholipid antibodies is 2% to 8% of the general population. Of patients with SLE, 30% to 50% are positive for antiphopholipid antibodies.

ETIOLOGY

The exact causes of SLE and APS are unknown. Evidence indicates that causes may be interrelated with immunologic, environmental, hormonal, and genetic factors (Warren and Silver, 2004; Porter and Branch, 2005). Predisposing factors include viral infections, physical or psychologic stress, sunlight, immunization, and pregnancy.

NORMAL PHYSIOLOGY

See discussion of normal physiologic adaptations in pregnancy described by systems and functions in Chapter 1 and by the coagulation cascade in Chapter 19.

PATHOPHYSIOLOGY

In SLE and APS, the body is unable to distinguish "self" from "nonself." An immunologic deficit allows antibodies to be formed that attack the body's own cells and proteins. More than 50 autoantibodies and antigen-antibody complexes collectively have been identified in the serum of affected individuals.

Systemic Lupus Erythematosus

The autoimmune responses in SLE cause suppression of the body's normal immunity and damage to body tissue. The autoimmune response may initially involve one organ system or every organ system. The most common organ systems are skin, joints, kidneys, lung, cardiac, and nervous system. In pregnancy, inflammation of the connective tissue of the decidua can result in problems of placental implantation and functioning.

Antiphospholipid Syndrome (APS)

The antiphopholipid antibodies that are characteristic of APS are formed against normal plasma proteins that are involved in the coagulation cascade and disrupt the phospholipids-dependent anticoagulant process leading to a procoagulant state. These same antibodies can have a direct toxic effect on the trophoblast tissue impeding uteroplacental blood flow. They also interfere with the prostacyclin thromboxane balance by interfering with prostacyclin production.

SIGNS AND SYMPTOMS

Systemic Lupus Erythematosus

Clinical manifestations depend on the system(s) being attacked by the auto-antibodies. The most common symptoms are fever, malaise, fatigue, weight loss, skin rashes, and polyarthralgia. Table 13-2 gives clinical manifestations specific to various systems involved in SLE.

Antiphospholipid Syndrome (APS)

The presence of antiphospholipid antibodies does not product symptoms until a clot is precipitated. Therefore the common secondary signs and symptoms are:

- Superficial thrombophlebitis
- Deep vein thrombophlebitis
- Thrombosis (arterial or venous)
- Pulmonary embolism
- Septic pelvic thrombophlebitis

APS may be suspected when a patient gives a strong family history, has an unproven suspicious personal history, or has repeated spontaneous abortions when other underlying conditions have been ruled out.

Table 13-2   Clinical Manifestations of Systemic Lupus Erythematosus

System	Clinical Manifestations
General	Malaise
	Fatigue
	Fever
	Weight loss
Integumentary	Skin rashes, butterfly rash
	Mucous membrane ulcers
Musculoskeletal	Arthralgia
Cardiovascular	Pericarditis
	Myocarditis
	Endocarditis
	Tachycardia
Respiratory	Pleuritis
	Dyspnea
	Pneumonitis
Renal	Urinary tract infection
	Nephrotic syndrome characterized by:
	• Hematuria
	• Proteinuria
	• Urine sediment and cellular casts
	Glomerular nephritis
	May progress to total kidney failure
Central nervous system	Emotional instability
	Seizure disorders
	Psychosis
	Headaches
	Irritability
	Depression
Gastrointestinal	Mucosal ulcers of mouth
	Anorexia
	Nausea and vomiting
	Diarrhea
	Constipation
Hematologic	Chronic anemia
	Thrombocytopenia
	Leukocytopenia
	Lupus anticoagulant
Ocular	Conjunctivitis
	Photosensitivity

MATERNAL EFFECTS
Systemic Lupus Erythematosus

If the SLE has been in remission for at least 6 months before conception and renal function is normal, optimal pregnancy outcome is as high (Warren and Silver, 2004). If SLE is active at the time of conception, exacerbation of the disease is common, especially involving the renal, and central nervous systems (Warren and Silver, 2004). Disease flares are common during pregnancy. It is unknown if pregnancy increases the number of flares (Warren and Silver, 2004)

Complications such as, preeclampsia, HELLP (*h*emolysis, *e*levated *l*iver enzymes, and *l*ow *p*latelet count) syndrome in association with preeclampsia (see Chapter 21), and preterm labor are the most common. The risk for disease deterioration during pregnancy or postpartum is high if the patient has severe renal insufficiency before becoming pregnant.

Antiphospholipid Syndrome (APS)

APS may lead to a life-threatening event for the mother, especially thrombosis or stroke. A pregnant woman with an acquired thrombophilia such as APS is at greater risk for abruption, severe preeclampsia before 34 weeks of gestation, iatrogenic preterm labor, antenatal or postpartum deep vein thrombophlebitis, and pulmonary embolism (Lockwood and Silver, 2004). These patients should be screened for anemia, thrombocytopenia, and underlying renal disease.

FETAL AND NEONATAL EFFECTS
Systemic Lupus Erythematosus

SLE affects pregnancy by increasing the risk for spontaneous abortion by 8% to 40% (Warren and Silver, 2004), depending on the severity of exacerbations and the length of remission before conception. The risk for a spontaneous abortion is directly related to maternal renal involvement.

After spontaneous abortion risk, early intrauterine growth restriction with a high risk for stillbirth remains the next major risk to the fetus/newborn. The risk is primarily the result of the malformation of the placenta and placental insufficiency in serving the nutritional and respiratory functions for the fetus. The placenta has connective tissue as part of its makeup. Microangiopathic changes take place in the placenta, resulting in disruption of normal functioning. Premature labor and potential preterm birth presents a third major risk to the newborn (see Chapter 22). In addition, the connective tissue inflammation and the anti-DNA in the mother can affect the fetus and the newborn. The manifestations of connective tissue degradation can cause fetal heart block through disruption or destruction of the connective tissue in the fetal heart and can cause fetal developmental abnormalities. The neonate may exhibit a transient lupus complex with problems requiring up to 10 to 12 months of treatment before disappearing.

Antiphospholipid Syndrome (APS)

APS significantly increases pregnancy loss. It is estimated that 90% of women with APS experience at least one fetal loss. The high loss rate of the pregnancy through recurrent spontaneous abortions and unexplained second or third trimester fetal death may be related to an incompletely diagnosed acquired thrombophilia problem in the mother or failure to understand family history factors that may have been related to undiagnosed thrombophilia in family members. (Porter and Branch, 2005). In viable fetuses, the risks of intrauterine growth restriction related to uteroplacental insufficiency, chronic abruption, chronic abruption oligohydramnios (CAOS), preterm labor, and preterm delivery are increased. There also appears to be an increased risk for cardiac or neurologic anomalies in the fetus of a mother with MTHFR mutation or low homocysteine levels. When these factors are correctly and more completely diagnosed, a management plan can be developed and significantly decrease the loss rate and improve prognosis for outcomes.

MEDICAL DIAGNOSIS
Systemic Lupus Erythematosus
The American College of Rheumatology (Tan and others, 1982; Hochberg, 1997) has identified the following 11 criteria for the classification of SLE, 4 or more of which must be present to confirm the diagnosis:
- Malar rash (butterfly rash)
- Discoid rash
- Photosensitivity
- Oral ulcers (usually painless)
- Arthritis (involving two or more joints)
- Serositis (pleuritis or pericarditis)
- Renal disorder (persistent proteinuria over 0.5 g /day)
- Neurologic disorder (seizure or psychosis)
- Hematologic disorder (hemolytic anemia, leucopenia, lymphopenia, or thrombocytopenia)
- Immunologic disorder (anti-DNA, anti-Sm, or a false positive serologic test for syphilis for 6 months)
- Antinuclear antibody (abnormal ANA titer)

During pregnancy, if the fetus is diagnosed with congenital heart block and the mother has not previously been diagnosed with lupus, she should have a complete SLE workup. In addition, certain clinical manifestations indicate a need to investigate a pregnant woman's predisposition for SLE and the lupus anticoagulant:
- Recurrent fetal losses
- Connective tissue disorder
- Thrombotic events
- Prolonged coagulation studies
- Positive autoantibody tests
- Thrombocytopenia

Antiphospholipid Syndrome (APS)
According to the International Consensus Statement (Wilson and others, 1999), APS is defined by certain laboratory and clinical criteria.
Clinical Criteria
- Vascular thrombosis
  - Venous
  - Arterial (stroke)

- Pregnancy morbidity
  - One or more unexplained fetal deaths beyond 10 weeks of gestation
  - One or more premature births before 34 weeks of gestation
  - Three or more unexplained consecutive spontaneous abortions without hormonal or chromosomal abnormalities0

Laboratory Criteria
- Anticardiolipin antibody (aCL)
- Lupus anticoagulant (LA)

One clinical and one laboratory criterion must be present to confirm the diagnosis.

USUAL MEDICAL MANAGEMENT AND PROTOCOLS FOR NURSE PRACTITIONERS

Systemic Lupus Erythematosus

General Management

Women with SLE should be counseled about the:
- Medical and obstetric risks of miscarriage, fetal death, fetal growth restriction, preeclampsia, preterm labor, and neonatal lupus
- Planning pregnancy
- Importance of being at least 6 months in remission before conception

After conception, a pregnancy complicated with SLE or other autoimmune disease requires close supervision of both the woman and the fetus. These patients will need frequent visits to assess SLE status and to screen for obstetric risks. They should be evaluated for evidence of anemia, thrombocytopenia, renal disease, and thrombophilias.

Other Management

Other methods of treatment and management depend on clinical manifestations. For example, if the major threat to maternal health stems from cardiac problems related to valvular problems, a cardiology consultation may be sought. Medical management is directed at treatment and stabilization. If the primary clinical characteristics are arthritic in nature, a rheumatologist may be consulted. If pulmonary problems, hypertension, coagulation defects, or renal problems are the presenting complications, a pulmonologist, cardiologist, hematologist, or nephrologist should be consulted (see Chapters 10, 11, 12, 18, 19, and 21).

Drug Therapy for Systemic Lupus Erythematosus

The four most common categories of drugs used in the general treatment of SLE are NSAIDs and aspirin, corticosteroids, antimalarials, and cytotoxic agents such as azathioprine, methotrexate, and cyclophosphamide (Cytoxan).

During pregnancy in the patient with SLE, the goal is to keep drug therapy to a minimum. Patients who have a mild form of the disease or who are experiencing a remission require minimal to no medication. The usual drug therapy, when indicated, includes an antiinflammatory drug, especially predni- sone or low-dose aspirin. NSAIDs (except low-dose aspirin) and cytotoxic agents should be discontinued prior to pregnancy. Long-term use of NSAIDs during pregnancy is associated with decreased fetal urine output, oligohydram- nios, and neonatal renal insufficiency. An antimalarial drug, hydroxychloro- quine is currently being considered as first-line therapy for SLE in pregnancy. This drug does not appear to increase the risk for fetal eye or ear deformities (Warren and Silver, 2004; Porter and Branch, 2005).

When corticosteroids and hydroxychloroquine are inadequate in managing severe exacerbations, cyclosporine, Plaquenil, or azathioprine are sometimes considered when the benefits outweigh the risks.

Antiphospholipid Syndrome (APS)
General Management
The three goals of current medical treatment for APS are as follows:
- Thrombosis prevention with low-dose aspirin (81 mg) plus heparin (cur- rently the most common treatment)
- Improvement of placenta blood flow by decreasing thromboxane to pros- tacyclin ratio with low-dose aspirin
- Immune system suppression with prednisone and intravenous immuno- globulin (IVIG) (used less frequently today because of the side effects of steroids)

Heparin Therapy for APS
Unfractionated heparin. Heparin may be delivered intravenously, subcutaneously by pump, or two or three times a day with subcutaneous injections. When delivered through a pump, it is given at continuous levels. When the drug is given in multiple injections, it is important to give it at regular intervals. Levels are best measured by an anti-factor Xa activity.

There are some risks associated with heparin therapy, which must be addressed with patients. Long-term therapy carries a risk for contributing to loss of bone density. Therefore additional calcium should be supplemented daily. When given in multiple dose subcutaneous injections, it must be given using an atraumatic technique. Using ice before and after the injection helps alleviate bruising.

Pregnant women are advised to use the abdomen for injection because the absorption rate is less likely to be affected and because the abdomen has a large fatty "apron" providing good subcutaneous tissue. The concentration of heparin also affects the amount of bruising. Whenever possible, the most concentrated form should be used to deliver no more than 0.5 ml per injection. Heparin comes in 5000 units/ml, 10,000 units/ml, 20,000 units/ml, and 40,000 units/ ml. The latter two are difficult to obtain. Because dosing may vary from 5000 units two times daily to greater than 10,000 units three times daily, concentra- tions can be problematic. There is also the risk for localized tissue reactions.

If this occurs, it may be necessary to switch to LMWH, such as enoxaparin sodium, until before delivery.

Low-molecular-weight heparin. LMWH is given subcutaneously or intravenously once or twice daily. Because of the increase drug clearance during pregnancy, twice a day dosing may be necessary to obtain therapeutic levels. Usually, it is not necessary to check levels of bleeding times at frequent intervals. However, during pregnancy because the coagulable state changes from trimester to trimester, it may be necessary to check the levels every 1 to 2 weeks at initiation of LMWH therapy and then trimester by trimester thereafter. LMWH is more expensive than unfractionated heparin and may only be measured by an anti-factor Xa activity level. It has a longer half-life than heparin and therefore may not be used just before the intrapartum period, especially if an epidural or spinal regional anesthetic is planned for pain relief or cesarean birth.

Heparin dosing. The dosing of heparin depends on whether the patient has a positive history for thromboembolism. The full-dose anticoagulation dosing is used if the patient has a positive history, whereas the thromboprophylaxis dosing is used if the patient has a negative history for thromboembolism (Table 13-3).

Intrapartum and Postpartum Management of Patients on Heparin

- For patients on full-dose anticoagulation with unfractionated heparin for thromboembolic diagnosis, artificial heart valve, or chronic atrial fibrillation, change to intravenous heparin to take advantage of its short half-life (1½ hours). Patients can then be changed postpartum to warfarin (Coumadin). Both must be overlapped during the first 4 days postpartum until INR has reached the 2.0 to 3.0 range. Coumadin creates a rapid decrease in protein C. Therefore overlapping with heparin is important to prevent paradoxical thromboembolism.
- Other patients requiring full-dose anticoagulation may be managed with prophylactic doses of heparin during the labor and delivery period.
- Patients on prophylactic heparin anticoagulation should be instructed to withhold their heparin injections at the onset of labor.
- The safety of epidural anesthesia and daily dosing of LMWH is of concern and should be withheld for 24 hours after the last injection.
- Epidural anesthesia appears to be safe in women taking unfractionated, prophylactic heparin if the partial thromboplastin time (PTT) is normal.
- Heparin can be resumed following a vaginal delivery within 4–6 hours and 12 hours after a cesarean. If the patient is switched to Coumadin, there must be an overlap with heparin for the first 4 days. An International Normalized Ratio (INR) measures therapeutic or prophylactic levels. For therapeutic dosing, an INR of 2 to 3 is desired. For prophylactic dosing, an INR of 1 to 2 is desired. Anticoagulants should be continued for at least 6 weeks following delivery related to the increase risk for embolic formation. With a history of any thrombolic event, lifelong anticoagulation is indicated (Porter and Branch, 2005).
- Coumadin is safe during breastfeeding.

Table 13-3   Heparin Dosing for APS During Pregnancy

Heparin Type	Dosing
Thromboprophylaxis Dosing Protocols	
Standard unfractionated heparin	First trimester: 5000 units twice a day
	Second trimester: 7500 units twice a day
	Third trimester: 10,000 units twice a day (all based on measuring levels before and after changing doses)
Low-molecular-weight heparin (LMWH)	Enoxaparin (Levenox) 40 mg once a day or 30 mg every 12 hours
	or
	Dalteparin (Fragmin) 5000 units once a day or every 12 hours (to achieve a level of anti-factor Xa of 0.2 to 0.4 units/ml)
Full-Dose Anticoagulation Dosing Protocols	
Standard unfractionated heparin	Subcutaneous injections every 8–12 hours or continuous heparin pump to achieve a level of anti-factor Xa of 0.4 to 0.7 units/ml
Low-molecular-weight heparin (LMWH)	Weight adjusted:
	Enoxaparin 1 mg/kg every 12 hours or
	Dalteparin 200 units/kg every 12 hours
	Intermediate dose:
	Until 16 weeks gestation: Enoxaparin 40 mg or dalteparin 5000 units once daily
	After 16 weeks gestation: Enoxaparin 40 mg or dalteparin 5000 units every 12 hours

Data from Porter T, Branch D: Autoimmune diseases. In James D and others, editors: *High risk pregnancy: management options*, ed 3, London, 2005, Saunders; Weiner C, Buhimschi C: *Drugs for pregnant and lactating women*, Philadelphia, 2004, Churchill Livingstone.

NURSING MANAGEMENT
Secondary and Tertiary Prevention

Preventive nursing care focuses on early recognition and reporting of signs of SLE flare, recognition and evaluation for any of the thrombophilias, and avoidance of the common pregnancy complications precipitated by SLE and the thrombophilias. In an effort to do that, the family members and the pregnant woman need adequate information for her care. Collaboration with the medical management plan includes reinforcing preconceptual counseling, interpreting clinical information in lay terms, and being vigilant in physical and psychosocial assessments for the family and the pregnant woman.

Prenatal Nursing Interventions for Systemic Lupus Erythematosus

- Discuss the importance of having good control over SLE before the woman becomes pregnant.

- Discuss the possible effects of SLE or the thrombophilias on pregnancy and the possible risk for exacerbations of SLE during pregnancy.
- Assess for evidence of anemia, thrombocytopenia, and thrombophilias.
- Be prepared to assess for thrombophilia by doing a complete thrombophilia workup as described in standard medical management and nurse practitioner protocols. This assessment is needed to determine whether anticoagulation is necessary and whether prophylactic or therapeutic dosing is needed. If needed, instruct the patient in administration.
- Assess for underlying renal disease by checking urine for protein and specific gravity that measures retention of urea solutes, serum creatinine, and 24-hour urine for total protein and creatinine clearance.
- Monitor for signs or symptoms of SLE flare.
- Emphasize the importance of frequent prenatal visits to early detect preeclampsia, preterm labor, and SLE exacerbations.
- Discuss implications of all drug therapies. Teach the patient and family about the self-administration of all prescribed medications.
- Assess for signs of infection at each prenatal visit, especially urinary tract and upper respiratory infections because prednisone drug management can mask signs of infection and lower resistance.
- Assess weight gain.
- Measure the blood pressure in the same arm and in the same position each visit; determine the mean arterial pressure.
- Emphasize the importance of a balance between activity and adequate rest as well as adequate nutrition.
- Teach prevention and recognition of preterm labor.
- Provide emotional support as needed.
- Instruct regarding skin care such as washing with a mild soap, avoiding sun exposure, using sunscreens, and avoiding products that cause side effects.
- Assess fetal surveillance with some combination of nonstress tests, contraction stress tests, biophysical profiles, or placental Doppler flow studies.
- Evaluate fetal growth by ultrasound every 3 to 4 weeks after 24 weeks of gestation. Measure fundal height between ultrasound evaluations.
- Instruct in the importance of counting fetal movements beginning at 24 weeks of gestation.
- Refer to the Lupus Foundation of America and to a high risk pregnancy support group such as Sidelines.
- Assess family coping styles and ability to cope with the effects of chronic illness. Refer for psychosocial evaluation and support as needed.

Postpartum Nursing Interventions for Systemic Lupus Erythematosus

- Assess for early signs of maternal infection by checking temperature every 4 hours.
- Assess breath sounds for early evidence of pneumonia.
- Assess for hematoma formation and lack of wound healing (episiotomy or cesarean incision).

- Monitor for SLE exacerbation.
- Be prepared to restart maintenance therapy.
- Provide adequate information about true chances for survival of fetus or newborn.
- Make appropriate grief referrals (see Chapter 7).
- Discuss the importance of birth control and the effects of various birth control methods on the disease. Oral contraceptives may stimulate drug-induced SLE. An IUD may increase the risk for an infection. Therefore the barrier methods carry the least risk to the patient.

Prenatal Nursing Interventions for Antiphospholipid Syndrome (APS)

- Discuss medical and pregnancy risks associated with this condition such as fetal loss, thrombosis or stroke, preeclampsia, intrauterine growth restriction, and preterm labor.
- Assess for evidence of anemia, thrombocytopenia, and underlying renal disease.
- Emphasize the importance of frequent prenatal visits.
- Screen for preeclampsia and preterm labor.
- Discuss implications of all drug therapies. Teach the patient and family about the self-administration of all prescribed medications.
- If heparin is used in thromboprophylaxis, discuss the importance of 1000 mg of calcium daily, vitamin D, and weight-bearing exercises to decrease the risk for osteoporosis.
- Prepare patients for the importance of fetal surveillance every 3 to 4 weeks starting around 17 to 18 weeks of gestation to monitor fetal growth impairment and oligohydramnios and to evaluate uteroplacental perfusion with serial ultrasounds. Around 30 weeks of gestation, daily fetal movement counts, biophysical profiles or nonstress test with amniotic fluid volume measurements are usually added.
- Teach prevention and recognition of preterm labor.
- Refer to a high risk pregnancy support group such as Sidelines.

Intrapartum Nursing Interventions for Antiphospholipid Syndrome (APS)

- Monitor closely for preeclampsia and uteroplacental insufficiency with continuous electronic fetal monitoring.
- Monitor closely for bleeding. Be prepared to hold or adjust the anticoagulant during labor as ordered.
- If patient has been on an anticoagulant, spinal and epidural blocks increase the risk for spinal hematoma. According to the American Society of Regional Anesthesia (ASRA), regional anesthesia should not be used until 24 hours after the last injection for patients on full-dose anticoagulation dosing, or 12 hours if the patient is on unfractionated heparin thromboprophylaxis dosing, or 24 hours if the patient is on LMWH thromboprophylaxis dosing.

Postpartum Nursing Interventions for Antiphospholipid Syndrome (APS)

- Provide adequate information about true chances for survival of fetus or newborn.
- Make appropriate grief referrals (see Chapter 7).
- Be prepared to resume anticoagulant therapy (refer to Intrapartum and Postpartum Management of Patients on Heparin above).
- Discuss the importance of birth control and the effects of various birth control methods on the disease. Oral contraceptives containing estrogen is contraindicated. An IUD may increase the risk for an infection. Therefore the barrier methods carry the least risk to the patient.

Intrapartum Critical Care Interventions for Systemic Lupus Erythematosus or Antiphospholipid Syndrome (APS)

- Evaluate cardiac function by assessing for signs of congestive heart failure, blood pressure, and pulse rate for dysrhythmias; ECG monitoring and invasive monitoring may become necessary.
- Evaluate renal function by assessing urinary output, specific gravity, and proteinuria every 4 hours in the presence of hypertension (see Chapter 12).
- Evaluate pulmonary function by assessing breath sounds every 4 hours and determining whether chest pain develops. If tocolytics are used or if the patient has a positive history of pulmonary, cardiac, or renal involvement, the pulmonary assessment should be done more often (see relevant chapters for cardiac, renal, and hypertension critical care).
- Evaluate the hematologic function by assessing for signs of disseminated intravascular coagulation.
- Observe closely for late-onset preeclampsia.
- If there is a positive history of central nervous system involvement, evaluate the central nervous system function by assessing for seizure activity, unexpected mood swings, or transient changes in level of consciousness.
- If either cardiac or renal complications are severe or if preeclampsia is superimposed, prepare for invasive hemodynamic monitoring.
- If noninvasive monitoring is ordered instead, use ECG and conventional blood pressure monitoring to assess the hemodynamic status (see Chapters 11 and 21).
- Initiate prompt treatment of early pulmonary problems with antibiotics, bronchodilators, intravenous heparin, or diuretics as appropriate (see Chapter 14).

CONCLUSION

Autoimmune disease greatly complicates management of both the disease and the pregnancy. The complications, although not insurmountable, require close supervision. The keys to a successful outcome for mother and baby include the following:

- Accurate diagnosis of the specific disease, the systems involved, or the thrombophilic abnormalities identified

- Preconceptual counseling to attempt pregnancy only after at least 6 months of remission
- Vigilance during the pregnancy for progression of the disease, effects on the fetus, and development of pregnancy-related maternal complications

With better, more accurate diagnostic laboratory evaluations available through radioimmune assays and a greater number of coagulopathies being identified through laboratory testing for various factors, closer and more adequate follow-up can now be provided. Nursing care must be directed at early detection of signs and symptoms, education of the mother and involved family members, and careful evaluation of the fetal status. If the pregnancy fails despite good care, grief support and referrals can aid the family affected by maternal connective tissue disorders and thrombophilias. Because autoimmune diseases, including SLE and APS, are multisystem disorders, see the relevant chapters for specific nursing care related to effects on each system.

BIBLIOGRAPHY

Beeson P: Age and sex asssociations of 40 autoimmune diseases, *Am J Med* 96:457–462, 1994.

Branch D, Khamashta M: Antiphospholipid syndrome: obstetric diagnosis, management, and controversies, *Obstet Gynecol* 101(6):1333–1344, 2003.

Carp H: Antiphospholipid syndrome in pregnancy, *Curr Opin Obstet Gynecol* 16(2): 129–135, 2004.

Esplin M: Management of antiphospholipid syndrome during pregnancy, *Clin Obstet Gynecol* 44(1):20–28, 2001.

Geis W, Branch W: Obstetric implications of antiphospholipid antibodies: pregnancy loss and other complications, *Clin Obstet Gynecol* 44(1):2–10, 2001.

Gharavi A and others: Mechanisms of pregnancy loss in antiphospholipid syndrome, *Clin Obstet Gynecol* 44(1):11–19, 2001.

Hochberg M: Updating the American College of Rheumatology revised criteria for the classification of systemic lupus erythematosus, *Arthritis Rheum* 40(9):1725, 1997.

Lash A, Mertens D, and Okumus H: Antiphospholipid antibody syndrome and pregnancy loss: management in primary care settings, *Adv Nurse Pract* 9(6):58–65, 2001.

Lockwood C, Silver R: Thrombophilias in pregnancy. In Creasy R, Resnik R, and Iams J, editors: *Maternal-fetal medicine: principles and practice,* ed 5, Philadelphia, 2004, Saunders.

Porter T, Branch D: Autoimmune diseases. In James D and others, editors: *High risk pregnancy: management options,* ed 3, London, 2005, Saunders.

Steen V: Pregnancy in women with systemic sclerosis, *Obstet Gynecol* 94(1): 15–20, 1999.

Steen V: Scleroderma and pregnancy, *Rheum Dis Clin North Am* 23(1):133–147, 1997.

Tan E and others: The 1982 revised criteria for the classification of systemic lupus erythematosus, *Arthritis Rheum* 25(11):1271–1277, 1982.

Warren J, Silver R: Autoimmune disease in pregnancy: systemic lupus erythematosus and antiphospholipid syndrome, *Obstet Gynecol Clin North Am* 31(2):345–372, 2004.

Weiner C, Buhimschi C: *Drugs for pregnant and lactating women,* Philadelphia, 2004, Churchill Livingstone.

Wilson W and others: International Consensus Statement on Preliminary Classification Criteria for Definite Antiphospholipid Syndrome: report of an international workshop, *Arthritis Rheum* 42(7):1309–1311, 1999.

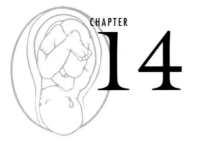

Pulmonary Disease and Respiratory Distress

P
regnancy complicated by pulmonary disease can be dangerous to both maternal well-being and fetal outcome. Understanding alterations in pulmonary physiology and the additional changes in immune responses that occur during pregnancy can help the health care provider anticipate problems and prevent complications in patients with chronic and acute pulmonary disease. This chapter reviews the management of cystic fibrosis, asthma, respiratory infections, and respiratory emergencies, such as acute respiratory distress syndrome (ARDS), pulmonary embolism, and anaphylactoid syndrome of pregnancy in the pregnant patient.

INCIDENCE

Pulmonary diseases have become more prevalent in the general population and in pregnant women.

Cystic Fibrosis

Thick, viscid secretions that lead to multisystem dysfunctions such as chronic pulmonary disease, malabsorption, insufficient pancreatic enzymes, nasal polyps, sinusitis, and elevated sweat chloride concentrations characterize cystic fibrosis, an autosomal recessive disease. This disease is caused by mutations in the cystic fibrosis transmembrane regulator (CFTR) gene. It occurs most often (1:2500) in the white European and Ashkenazi Jewish ethnic groups, with a carrier rate of 1:29. Because women with cystic fibrosis now live longer and have improved quality of life, they face the new complication of pregnancy. The median age of survival of women with cystic fibrosis is about 29 years, and the disease occurs in 1 of 2000 births. Because of abnormally dense cervical mucus, women with cystic fibrosis are thought to have lower fertility (Whitty and Dombrowski, 2004).

Asthma

Reversible airway obstruction and bronchial hyperresponsiveness characterize asthma, a chronic inflammatory disorder of the tracheobronchial airways.

Asthma is the most common medical condition to complicate pregnancy (NAEPP, 2005), occurring in 4% to 6% of the general population and occurring in pregnancy at the same rate (Kwon, Belanger, and Bracken, 2003; Dombrowski and others, 2004).

Respiratory Infections

Respiratory infections that may have a significant effect on pregnancy outcome include bronchitis, pneumonia, and tuberculosis. Bronchitis progressing to pneumonia complicates 0.1% to 1.0% of all pregnancies. It is important to distinguish bronchitis from pneumonia because pneumonia is more dangerous. Tuberculosis, once considered rare in the United States, is now increasing in women of childbearing years. In endemic areas around the world, tuberculosis may occur in 0.1% of pregnancies. Endemic areas include countries with high tuberculosis prevalence or long-term facilities, such as prisons or mental health facilities.

Respiratory Emergencies

Respiratory emergencies are rare in pregnancy and include pulmonary embolism, anaphylactoid syndrome of pregnancy (formerly called *amniotic fluid embolism*), and ARDS. Respiratory emergencies are generally secondary to other physiologic complications. Patients may have acute asthmatic exacerbation or, through drug exposure, be at risk for respiratory alkalosis, acidosis, or infections. Pulmonary embolism may occur in as many as 24% of patients with untreated or inadequately treated deep vein thromboses (DVTs), or it may occur as a complication of septic pelvic thrombophlebitis. More rarely, it may be caused by ovarian vein thrombosis (Smith, 1997; Gates, Brocklehurst, and Davis, 2002; Doyle and Monga, 2004). It is the leading cause (46%) of pregnancy-related deaths (Cox, Kilpatrick, and Geller, 2004).

Anaphylactoid syndrome of pregnancy is an obstetric catastrophe and occurs rarely. However, when it does occur, there is a reported 60% maternal mortality and of the 40% that survive, 25% will have resulting neurologic damage (Anthony, 2005).

ARDS in pregnancy is also very rare. The outcome for mother and fetus is variable and depends on the underlying cause and the extent of other organ or system involvement.

ETIOLOGY

Infections are frequently identified as being caused by viruses, influenza, *Haemophilus*, *Streptococcus*, *Mycoplasma*, *Chlamydia*, or tuberculosis. These infections may also cause respiratory complications in women already compromised by asthma or cystic fibrosis. The etiology of pulmonary emboli is usually DVT, whereas the etiology of amniotic fluid emboli is unknown. ARDS is often preceded by respiratory sepsis, aspiration pneumonia, or severe trauma or injury (Powrie, 2005).

NORMAL PHYSIOLOGY

In pregnancy, the following alterations in respiratory anatomy and physiology occur:

- The lower ribs flare out, and the subcostal angle and transverse diameter of the chest increase.
- The diaphragm rises by approximately 4 cm.
- Progesterone stimulates the respiratory centers to produce hyperventilation and a sensation of dyspnea.
- Because of hyperventilation, there is a decrease in alveolar tension and Pco_2 relative to respiratory alkalosis.

To understand respiratory function as it relates to pregnancy, it is important to understand some of the following basic terminology:

- *Functional residual capacity.* The most important parameter for the health care provider to understand. It is the volume of the lungs at the end of a normal exhalation. It is affected by several factors:
  - Supine position
  - Obesity
  - Pregnancy
  - Impaired chest wall mechanics
  - Thoracoabdominal splinting
  - Ascent of the diaphragm (as with abdominal distention)
  - Increased airway resistance
  - Atelectasis
  - Decreased removal of secretions
  - General anesthesia
  - Pulmonary edema
- *Vital capacity.* The volume of air expired with maximal inspiration. It is the effective working volume of the lungs and correlates well with deep breathing and effective coughing. It decreases in patients with restrictive lung diseases such as asthma, cystic and pulmonary fibrosis, massive ascites, pneumothorax, pleural effusion, and pregnancy.
- *Tidal volume.* The volume of gas that moves in and out of the lungs during normal, quiet breathing. It decreases with weaker lung compliance, lessened respiratory muscle strength, and anesthesia; it increases in pregnancy.
- *Closing capacity.* The lung volume at which small airways begin to close. Normally, functional residual capacity is greater than closing capacity.
- *Dead space.* The anatomic area where gas exchange does not occur. In pulmonary embolism there is dead space.

PATHOPHYSIOLOGY

Infections of the respiratory system, asthma, and cystic fibrosis can all lead to obstruction of the airway and alveoli. Obstruction causes an inability to clear CO_2 and results in hypercarbia. Patients with obstructive pulmonary disease may also be unable to breathe in sufficient amounts of oxygen. Hypoxia is the major threat to the fetus because the maternal-fetal placental unit depends on a passive system of oxygen uptake and the fetus grows in a lower Po_2 than its host, the mother.

Infectious agents invade and inflame the respiratory structures and mucous membranes. Inflammation of these structures causes the body to increase mucus production in an effort to repair itself. The mucus contains protein and other substrates and provides a good medium for bacterial or viral growth. As respiratory effort increases, there is a concomitant loss of moisture through increased breathing. The loss of moisture in turn causes the mucus to become drier and more viscous, thus obstructing the airways (ACOG, 1996).

Intrapulmonary shunting describes a phenomenon in which a fraction of the blood goes through the lungs without being oxygenated. The resultant hypoxemia cannot be corrected with supplemental oxygen. Carbon dioxide moves more readily than oxygen. Hence it is easier for carbon dioxide to build up than for oxygenation to improve (Smith, 1997).

Some causes of hypoxemia are the following:

- High altitude
- Hypoventilation, as in decreased respiratory drive secondary to central nervous system depressants
- Diffusion impairment, such as seen with severe pulmonary fibrosis and thickened alveolar capacity membrane
- Ventilation-perfusion mismatch
- Shunting, as seen in alveoli that are collapsed or filled with blood, pus, or edema

SIGNS AND SYMPTOMS
General Signs of Respiratory Distress
Dyspnea

Most women experience dyspnea at some time during a normal pregnancy. It may be a normal response to the anatomic pressure of the gravid uterus against the diaphragm and the conscious awareness of an increase in respiratory rate. Dyspnea is also a classic symptom of respiratory disease and distress, especially when coupled with prolonged expiratory phase hypoxemia.

Because respiratory physiology in a normal pregnancy tends toward respiratory alkalosis, hypoxemia is initially not accompanied by a corresponding increase in CO_2 (hypercarbia). Hypercarbia generally occurs in severe hypoxemia.

Leukocytosis

The complete blood cell count may show an increase in leukocytes, with a left shift on differential if there is a bacterial infection. If mycoplasmal pneumonia is present, an increase in the sedimentation rate is common also. Hemoconcentration may also be seen.

Cough

A productive cough may be seen in cystic fibrosis as a normal part of the disease. If it produces thick, dark, bloody, or rusty-colored sputum, infection is probably superimposed. Productive cough in an asthmatic pregnant woman should be treated as an infection in the respiratory tract. Any thick or colored mucus that is produced with coughing is presumed to be a sign of infection.

Other Signs

Other signs and symptoms of respiratory distress include the following:
- Fever
- Sudden onset of chills
- Chest pain, pleuritic pain
- Bronchial breath sounds
- Chest dullness
- Decreased breath sounds
- Rales, crackles
- Egophony, whispered pectoriloquy

A chest radiographic film may show infiltration and either segmental or lobar consolidation.

Asthma Exacerbations Signs

Clinical manifestations of asthma exacerbation are progressively worsening symptoms of cough, wheezing, shortness of breath, chest tightness, and sputum production (NAEPP, 2005). These symptoms occur on a continuum ranging from mild persistent to severe life-threatening.

MATERNAL EFFECTS
Cystic Fibrosis

The physiologic changes of pregnancy are not tolerated as well by the patient with cystic fibrosis, which increases the risk for respiratory decompensation and therefore increases maternal mortality. If the patient has pulmonary hypertension, maternal mortality is significantly increased. Labor is an especially vulnerable time, with risk for possible heart failure.

Asthma

Asthma seems to have no consistent effect on pregnancy. The severity of the disease is unchanged in 33% of pregnant women with asthma, is improved in 33%, and is worsened in 33% (Revan, Sun, and McMorris, 2002). If it worsens, the more severe symptoms usually occur during gestational weeks 24 to 36. A pregnancy factor that may promote asthma improvement is the fact that pregnancy hormones—progesterone and prostaglandins—have a natural bronchodilator effect. Factors that may exacerbate asthma during pregnancy are:
- Pulmonary refractoriness to cortisol
- Increased susceptibility to respiratory infection related to immune system changes
- Increased risk to gastroesophageal reflex disease (GERD).

Respiratory Infections

Bronchitis poses little threat to pregnant women except that it may more readily progress to pneumonia and therefore must be differentiated from pneumonia (ACOG, 1996). Pneumonia frequently is accompanied by a productive cough. Because of the anatomic accommodations to the respiratory system in pregnancy, forceful coughing to raise sputum may be more difficult. It is also more likely to cause painful separation of the cartilage between ribs and occasionally a spontaneous pneumothorax (Whitty and Dombrowski, 2004).

Respiratory Emergencies

Pulmonary embolism is the leading cause of maternal mortality with an approximately 15% risk for maternal death in the presence of a pulmonary emboli (Gates, Brocklehurst, and Davis, 2002).

ARDS can be the final result of several different obstetric complications, including inhalation of gastric contents during anesthesia and disseminated intravascular coagulation, as seen in preeclampsia, eclampsia, abruptio placentae, dead fetus syndrome, anaphylactoid syndrome of pregnancy, and acute exacerbation of asthma. All of these can be fatal to the mother.

FETAL EFFECTS

The greatest fetal threat is hypoxemia secondary to any condition that leads to acute respiratory emergencies. Chronic respiratory disease, such as asthma and cystic fibrosis (CF), can result in uteroplacental insufficiency and intrauterine growth restriction. A true respiratory emergency, such as pulmonary embolism or anaphylactoid syndrome of pregnancy, may necessitate emergency cesarean delivery at the same time that maternal resuscitation is being attempted. If maternal hypoxia and respiratory acidosis occur, the fetal brain is vulnerable to the resultant fetal hypoxia. Depending on the degree of hypoxia and the timing of the event in fetal gestational age, the fetus may suffer some degree of irreversible brain damage or death.

DIAGNOSTIC TESTING

Cystic Fibrosis

In 2001, the American College of Obstetricians and Gynecologists (ACOG), the American College of Medical Genetics (ACMG), and the National Institutes of Health (NIH) initiated carrier screening protocols for cystic fibrosis (Shulman and Elias, 2001) for the following individuals:

- Adults with a positive family history of CF
- Partners of individuals with CF
- White couples of European and Ashkenazi Jewish heritage planning a pregnancy or seeking prenatal care

The 25 ACMG/ACOG panel is used (The Reference Laboratory at the Cleveland Clinic, 2004).

Table 14-1   Comparison of Pulmonary Values in Pregnant and Nonpregnant Women

Definition of Terms	Nonpregnant	Pregnant	Clinical Significance
V_T = amount of air moved in one normal respiratory cycle	450 ml	600 ml	
RR = number of respirations per min	16/min	Slight increase	
Minute ventilation = volume of air moved per min; $V_T \times RR$	7.2 L	9.6 L	Increased O_2 available to fetus
FEV_1	80%–85% of vital capacity	Unchanged	Valuable to measure because there is no change
PEF		Unchanged	Valuable to measure because there is no change
FVC = maximum amount of air that can be moved from maximum inspiration to maximum expiration	3.5 L	Unchanged	If over 1 L, pregnancy usually tolerated well
RV = amount of air that remains in lung at end of a maximal expiration	1000 ml	Decreases to approximately 800 ml	Improves gas transfer from alveoli to blood (Smith, 1997)

FEV_1, Forced expiratory volume in 1 second; *PEF*, peak expiratory flow; *FVC*, forced vital capacity; *RR*, respiratory rate; *RV*, residual volume; *Vt*, tidal volume.

Asthma

People with asthma have airways that are hyperresponsive to stimuli such as allergens, viruses, air pollutants, exercise, and cold air. The hyperactivity is manifested by bronchospasm, mucosal edema, and mucus plugging in the airways, with hyperinflation of the lungs. Because of the inflammation in airway mucosa, forced expiratory volume measured with a spirometer or peak expiratory flow rate measured with a peak flow meter (Table 14-1) can help to objectively quantify the degree of obstruction. Measurement of these two values is also useful in monitoring the effectiveness of treatment (NAEPP, 2005).

Diagnostic Testing for Respiratory Compromise

Diagnostic testing is the same for pregnant women as for nonpregnant women. The following tests are routine when respiratory compromise is evident:
• Complete blood cell count
• Sputum culture
• Chest radiograph with abdominal shield

Table 14-2   Arterial Blood Gas Values in Pregnant and Nonpregnant Women

	pH	Po$_2$ (mm Hg)	Pco$_2$ (mm Hg)
Pregnant	7.4	100–105	30
Nonpregnant	7.4	93	35–40

Data from National Institutes of Health Expert Panel Report 2: *Guidelines for the diagnosis and management of asthma*, Publication No. 97-4051, Washington, DC, 1997, NIH. Retrieved from *http://www.nhibisupport.com/asthma/index.html*

- Arterial blood gases (Table 14-2)
- Pulmonary function tests (see Table 14-1)

In addition, if DVT is suggested, compression ultrasonography is the preferred test. When pulmonary embolism is suspected, chest x-ray with lead apron fetal shielding, spiral computed axial tomography, and a D-dimer assay may be obtained (Farquharson and Greaves, 2005). If an anaphylactoid syndrome of pregnancy is suggested, coagulation blood studies are ordered during the critical care recovery, after initial resuscitation (Anthony, 2005).

Blood Gas Interpretation

Interpretation of blood gases should be done in a systematic fashion, beginning with the pH. Normal adult pH is 7.35 to 7.45. A pH of less than 7.35 indicates acidemia. Next, it is important to understand whether the pH is primarily respiratory or metabolic (i.e., from respiratory failure or from kidney failure) or whether it is mixed, stemming from both problems.

To sort out the blood gases, both the pH and the pulmonary arterial carbon dioxide (Paco$_2$) must be evaluated in relationship to the relative change in the pH. If the following three scenarios are examined, it is possible to determine the degree of acidosis:

- Paco$_2$ is high, but pH is relatively low: *simple respiratory acidosis*
- Paco$_2$ is high, but pH is lower than expected: *mixed metabolic and respiratory acidosis*
- Paco$_2$ and pH are both low: *simple metabolic acidosis*

A pH of greater than 7.45 indicates alkalemia. To sort out whether the cause is respiratory, metabolic, or mixed, consider the following (Smith, 1997):

- Paco$_2$ is high, and pH is also relatively high: *simple metabolic alkalosis*
- Paco$_2$ is low, but pH is higher than expected: *mixed respiratory and metabolic alkalosis*
- Paco$_2$ is low, but pH is high: *simple respiratory alkalosis*

USUAL MEDICAL MANAGEMENT AND PROTOCOLS FOR NURSE PRACTITIONERS

Cystic Fibrosis

- Provide preconceptual counseling to enable the patient to be in optimal physical condition.
- Provide genetic counseling and carrier testing of the father.

- Perform pregnancy screen for such risk factors as severe lung disease, pulmonary hypertension using echocardiogram, poor nutritional status, or liver/pancreatic diseases.
- Consult with a pulmonary specialist or, ideally, a specialist in cystic fibrosis.
- Obtain a baseline and ongoing pulmonary function using forced vital capacity, FEV_1, lung volumes, and pulse oximetry.
- Closely monitor nutritional status with ongoing diagnostic screens of total protein, serum albumin, prothrombin time related to vitamin K deficiency, and fat-soluble vitamins A and E.
- Provide dietary consultation; an increased caloric intake (20%–50% above normal recommendation) is necessary because of decreased digestive enzymes.
- Closely monitor weight gain.
- Closely monitor for pulmonary infection.
- Treat pulmonary infections promptly and vigorously with antibiotics, fluids, and respiratory therapy to include physical therapy and bronchial drainage.
- Provide early screening for diabetes because it frequently occurs in women with cystic fibrosis.

Asthma

Asthma must be as aggressively treated during pregnancy as at any other time because the benefits of asthma control far outweigh the risks associated with the medications. Almost all common asthma medications are considered safe during pregnancy and lactation (Dombrowski and others, 2004; NAEPP, 2005). According to the NAEPP (2005), the following four management components are recommended for managing asthma during pregnancy:

- Ongoing monitoring of the disease, noting signs and symptoms, pulmonary function studies with a spirometer and peak expiratory meter, and history of asthma exacerbations.
- Avoidance of triggers such as allergens, tobacco smoke, and pollutants/irritants.
- Pharmacologic therapy using the stepwise approach (Table 14-3). Table 14-4 provides a summary of the most commonly used asthma medications during pregnancy.
- Education to promote self-management in collaboration with health care provider, correct use of inhalers, and management plan of acute exacerbations using the NAEPP (2005) algorithm.

Respiratory Infections

Viral Bronchitis or Upper Respiratory Infection

The most common respiratory infections during pregnancy are viral bronchitis and the common cold. These should never be treated with antibiotics. The best care is supportive: keep track of fever, contact health care provider if fever is higher than 102°F, increase fluids, use guaifenesin liberally (tablet form, 600 mg

Table 14-3 Stepwise Treatment Approach to Asthma During Pregnancy

	Step 1 Mild Intermittent	Step 2 Mild Persistent	Step 3 Moderate Persistent	Step 4 Severe Persistent
Peak expiratory flow	80%–100% of personal best	≥80% of personal best	60%–80% of personal best	<60% of personal best
Signs and symptoms	(≤2 times/week)	>2 time/wk but <1 time/day	Daily	Frequently
Exercise tolerance	Good	May not be affected	Diminished	Poor
Nocturnal waking	≤2 times/mo	>2 times/mo but <1 time/wk	>1 time/wk	Nightly
Work attendance	Good	May not be affected	Diminished	Poor
Treatment	Quick relief: Short-acting inhaled beta$_2$-agonist (Albuterol) Daily long-term control: None	Quick relief: Short-acting beta$_2$-agonist (Albuterol) Daily long-term control preferred treatment: low-dose inhaled corticosteroid budesomide or Daily long-term control alternative treatment: Leukotriene receptor antagonist (montelukast or zafirlukast), mast cell stabilizer (cromolyn), or sustained-release theophylline	Quick relief: Short-acting beta$_2$-agonist (Albuterol) Daily long-term control: medium-dose inhaled corticosteroid budesomide or inhaled corticosteroid (low dose) and add a long-acting beta$_2$-agonist such as long-acting inhaled beta$_2$-agonist or sustained-release theophylline or long-acting beta$_2$-agonist tablet	Quick relief: Short-acting beta$_2$-agonist (Albuterol) Daily long-term control: high-dose inhaled corticosteroid budesomide and long-acting inhaled beta$_2$-agonist and oral corticosteroids tablets or syrup if needed while making repeated attempts to reduce systemic steroids and maintain control with high dose inhaled steroids

Data from National Asthma Education and Prevention Program (NAEPP): Managing asthma during pregnancy: recommendations for pharmacologic treatment—2004 update, *J Allergy Clin Immunol* 115(1):34–46, 2005. Retrieved from http://www.nhlbi.nih.gov/health/prof/lung/asthma/practgde.htm

Table 14-4 Summary of Common Medications for Asthma During Pregnancy

Drug Class	Drug Action	Medication	Dose
Quick-Relief Medications Short-acting beta$_2$-agonists	Bronchodilators; relax smooth muscle of the bronchioles	Albuterol (Proventil)	MDI 2–4 puffs q20min up to 4 h; then q1–4h, then prn Use spacer
Long-Term Control Medications Inhaled corticosteroids	Antiinflammatory agents decrease edema and mucus secretions in the bronchioles by inhibiting the synthesis of leukotrienes and activation of inflammatory cells; use with a bronchodilator	Budesonide (Pulmicort)	Dry powder inhaler 200 mcg/inhalation Low daily dose: 200–600 mcg Medium daily dose: 600–1200 mcg High dose: more than 1200 mcg
Mast-cell stabilizes	Mild-to-moderate antiinflammatory agent that inhibits the degranulation of mast cells, blocking eosinophil chemotaxis and activation, improving asthma	Cromolyn sodium	MDI 2–4 puffs tid/qid

secretion, and vascular permeability

Sustained-release theophylline — Methylxanthines and various generic drugs (Theo-Dur, Slo-bid); theophylline blood levels may be followed with the use of this drug — 100, 200, 300, or 450 mg bid

Zafirlukast (Accolate) — 20 mg po bid

Mild-to-moderate bronchodilator used primarily with inhaled corticosteroids to prevent nocturnal asthma symptoms

Oral (systemic corticosteroids) — Use of systemic steroids during pregnancy increases the risks for congenital malformation, preeclampsia, and preterm delivery; however, for severe asthma, the benefits still outweigh the risks

Data from National Asthma Education and Prevention Program (NAEPP): Managing asthma during pregnancy: recommendations for pharmacologic treatment-2004 update, J Allergy Clin Immunol 115(1):34–46, 2005. Retrieved from http://www.nhlbi.nih.gov/health/prof/lung/asthma/practqde.htm; National Asthma Education and Prevention Program (NAEPP): Expert Panel Report guidelines for the diagnosis and management of asthma: update on selected topics 2002, Publication No. 02-5075, Bethesda, Md, National Heart, Lung, and Blood Institute, National Institute of Health. Retrieved from http://www.nhlbi.nih.gov/guidelines/asthma/asthrpdt.htm

MDI, Metered-dose inhaler.

twice daily), use nasal saline spray, use humidifiers at bedtime, and occasionally use a nasal corticosteroid (no more than twice daily).

Nasal congestion is often more pronounced during pregnancy because of the hormonal influences on mucosal swelling. Treating nasal congestion also treats the cough, frequently because the cough is caused by postnasal discharge. This symptom is generally worse at night and may benefit from nighttime guaifenesin or codeine phosphate with promethazine HCl (Phenergan with Codeine) cough syrups. No adverse pregnancy outcomes have been noted with the use of these drugs at any stage of pregnancy (Weiner and Buhimschi, 2004).

If an antihistamine is necessary, chlorpheniramine and tripelennamine are the antihistamines of choice during pregnancy even though they are more sedating than the second-generation antihistamines, according to ACOG and the American College of Allergy, Asthma, and Immunology (2000). Whenever possible, avoid all oral decongestants during the first trimester.

Pneumonia

Pneumonia is an inflammation of the lower respiratory tract, including the alveoli and bronchioles. It may be caused by bacterial or viral invasion or chemical contact with the respiratory tract. Coinfection with HIV or tuberculosis may worsen the prognosis for mother and fetus.

Careful consideration should be given to such possible differential diagnoses as pulmonary embolism, asthma, and pulmonary edema prior to diagnosing pneumonia in pregnancy. A chest radiograph and both blood and sputum cultures are usually obtained to diagnose the extent of infection and identify the organism(s) responsible. If atypical bacterial infection is suspected, cold agglutinins are used to test for mycoplasma pneumonia (ACOG, 1996; Powrie, 2005).

Usually, therapy is started with a broad-spectrum antibiotic; then, once the specific causative organism or organisms are detected and reported with sensitivity, more specifically directed antibiotic therapy is used. For gram-negative and *Staphylococcus aureus* infection, a combination third-generation cephalosporin with aminoglycoside is usually used. For mycoplasmal pneumonia, the erythromycins are used. Antibiotic therapy in pregnancy usually requires high doses because of increased blood volume and dilution.

For viral pneumonias, the course may be complicated by a secondary bacterial infection. Although broad-spectrum antibiotics such as cephalosporins may work for the secondary infection, antivirals such as amantadine are not used in pregnancy except in fulminant respiratory failure. Amantadine is both embryotoxic and teratogenic in animal studies and is therefore reserved for life-threatening disease in the pregnant woman. Acyclovir is currently recommended for varicella pneumonia in pregnant women.

According to the recently revised CDC guidelines, prepregnancy care should include advice about routine influenza vaccination with the inactivated vaccine if the pregnancy occurs during the influenza season (CDC, 2004). Pneumococcal vaccine is recommended before, but not during, pregnancy for high risk patients with conditions such as asthma, chronic pulmonary or cardiac disease, diabetes mellitus, or immune compromise disease (CDC, 2002).

Tuberculosis

Treatment regimens for tuberculosis include the following:

- Absence of active disease with less than 2 years converted PPD (purified protein derivative [tuberculin]) status is treated with 300 mg/day of isoniazid, starting after the first trimester and continuing for 6 to 9 months.
- Women younger than 35 years with an unknown duration of positive PPD result should receive 300 mg/day of isoniazid for 6 to 9 months postpartum.
- Women older than 35 years do not receive isoniazid unless they have active disease.
- Women with active disease in pregnancy are treated immediately with dual-agent therapy for a full 9 months. The standard regimen is isoniazid, 300 mg/day, combined with rifampin, 600 mg/day. If resistance to isoniazid is identified, ethambutol, 2.5 g/day, is substituted and the treatment period extends to 18 months.
- Pyridoxine (vitamin B_6), 50 mg/day, is an essential supplement for all patients.

Although isoniazid, ethambutol, and rifampin have been used in pregnancy with no adverse fetal effects, antituberculous agents that may not be used include streptomycin, kanamycin, ethionamide, capreomycin, cycloserine, and pyrazinamide (ACOG, 1996).

Antituberculous agents should not be used concurrently in the newborn if the mother is being treated and is breastfeeding. Antituberculous agents cross into breast milk; if the mother is being treated, these agents will reach sufficient levels in the newborn and infant for the duration of breastfeeding (Whitty and Dombrowski, 2004).

NURSING MANAGEMENT

Prevention

Pregnant women with chronic diseases, such as cystic fibrosis and asthma, should be counseled before becoming pregnant about the importance of having their disease under good control, continuing good management, and avoiding exposure to environmental agents that may exacerbate or trigger disease response.

Pregnant women should be counseled during early pregnancy to avoid exposure to crowds of people during influenza season and during other acute respiratory disease outbreaks and to avoid exposure to people infected with HIV and tuberculosis. Because of the depressed immune response in normal, healthy pregnant women, they are more susceptible to contracting infections than are nonpregnant women.

Nursing Interventions for Respiratory Infections

- Discuss the risks of exposure to respiratory infections with the woman and her family.
- Encourage early treatment of upper respiratory signs and symptoms.
- Encourage health-promoting behaviors such as the following:
  - Avoid crowds during high infection incidence.
  - Use a cool mist humidifier at night to help the respiratory tract stay healthy.
  - Drink at least 8 oz of nutritious liquid or water each hour of the day while awake.
- Respond to detected or reported signs and symptoms, chest radiograph, and sputum and blood cultures, as warranted.
- Treat with appropriate oral or intravenous antibiotics, when necessary.
- Have baseline function studies in early pregnancy available for comparison of disease states.
- Seek and keep referrals and collaborate with pulmonary specialists.
- Use small volume nebulizers (SVNs) as needed in the acute phase if the woman is hospitalized; otherwise, an inhaler with spacer should be used with beta-agonists, antiinflammatories, and corticosteroids, as needed. There are actually two categories of medications to use:
  - *Rescuers.* These are beta-agonists such as albuterol and should be used only on an outpatient basis in conjunction with controllers (described next). If rescuers are used on an outpatient basis more than four times a day or more than three times a week, several areas need to be evaluated: the patient's usage technique, the appropriate dosage of controllers, and any acute illness in the patient that would benefit from inpatient care.
  - *Controllers.* These are corticosteroids, which may be taken orally or in inhaler form, and antihistamines, which are generally taken orally. Both may be used during pregnancy and in combination with each other, especially when there is an allergic component to the disease and resultant infection (see Tables 14-1, 14-3, and 14-4).
- Teach women with chronic respiratory tract disease how to self-detect and prevent preterm labor.

Antepartum Nursing Interventions for Pregnancy Complicated with Asthma

- Discuss the importance of maintaining asthma control during pregnancy. Inadequate asthma management increases the risk for adverse maternal and fetal outcomes. Systematic review of various asthma medications indicates the safety (with no increase in congenital abnormalities) of the following drugs: albuterol; Pulmicort Turbuhaler (budesonide inhalation powder), an inhaled corticosteroid; cromolyn; and leukotriene modifiers (montelukast and zafirlukast) (Dombrowski and others, 2004; NAEPP,

2005). Oral corticosteroids are associated with an increased risk for isolated cleft lip if taken during the first trimester, as well as an increased risk for preeclampsia and preterm delivery. However, for severe asthma, the benefits of oral corticosteroids still outweigh the risks.

- Assess for complementary alternative medicine use and advise accordingly. Emphasize that alternative healing methods are no substitute for prescribed pharmacologic therapy (Perlman and Serbin, 2001; NAEPP, 2005).
- Collaborate management with the obstetric team and asthma and allergy specialists.
- Explain the difference between asthmatic and normal airways and what happens during an asthma attack.
- Reinforce the importance of not smoking, because smoking contributes to asthma.
- Teach the importance of avoiding environmental triggers, which include the following: inhalant allergens such as pollens and molds; dust mites; cockroach antigens; irritants such as cigarette smoke, spray cleaners, and colognes; nonspecific stimuli such as infections; foods such as wine, shellfish, wheat, eggs, nuts, or dairy products; and medicines such as aspirin and some nonsteroidal antiinflammatory drugs (NAEPP, 2005).
- Teach the importance of continuing all needed medications to control asthma without exacerbation or activity limitation. The benefits of medication have been shown to far outweigh the risks. Uncontrolled asthma is a more dangerous risk to both mother and baby than medication-controlled asthma.
- Teach correct use of inhalers with a spacer.
- Instruct the patient in the use of a peak flow meter; provide parameters for concern and increased use of rescuers, based on the patient's weight and height.
- Instruct the patient in the use of controllers and rescuers.
- Develop and explain the individualized asthma action plan for when and how to take rescue actions based on the stepwise treatment approach to asthma outlined in Table 14-3.
- Demonstrate how to use the peak flow meter and explain that it should be used with moderate and severe persistent asthma or to help regulate medicine changes.
- Emphasize the importance of having an ultrasound during the first trimester to confirm the accuracy of the due date and having repeat ultrasounds during the second and third trimesters to follow fetal growth.
- Be prepared to implement fetal surveillance tests such as fetal movement counts and biophysical profiles with nonstress tests by 32 weeks of gestation.
- Teach to self-detect signs of preterm contractions.
- Teach the importance of adequate calories and nutrients. Make appropriate referrals to a dietitian, the WIC (Women, Infants, and Children) program, and specialists in high risk pregnancy.

- Access educational materials from the following Internet sites:
  - National Asthma Education Program: *Teach Your Patients About Asthma: A Clinician's Guide (http://www.meddean.luc.edu/lumen/MedEd/ medicine/Allergy/Asthma/asthtoc.html)*
  - National Heart, Lung, and Blood Institute: *Practical Guide for the Diagnoses and Management of Asthma (http://www.nhlbi.nih.gov/ health/prof/lung/asthma/practgde.htm)*

Intrapartum Nursing Interventions for Asthmatics

- Instruct the patient to continue her routine asthma medications.
- Assess PEFR at time of admission and every 12 hours.
- Maintain adequate maternal oxygenation. A pulse oximetry may be used to evaluate maternal oxygenation status. Normal is greater than 95%.
- Maintain adequate hydration during labor.
- Monitor fetal well-being according to hospital protocol.
- Avoid the use of histamine-releasing narcotics such as meperidine (Demerol) or morphine to manage pain.
- If labor induction or augmentation is medically indicated, oxytocin is the preferred agent because prostaglandin E_2 preparations have been shown to cause bronchospasms (Whitty and Dombrowski, 2005).
- If the patient was on chronic oral corticosteroid therapy during pregnancy for more than 1 month, parenteral steroids are used during labor to prevent adrenal suppression.
- If cesarean delivery is indicated, general anesthesia should be used only as a last resort.

Postpartum Nursing Interventions for Asthmatics

- Assess the patient carefully for hemorrhage and respiratory distress.
- Discuss the importance of continuing the same asthma medications during breastfeeding. To decrease the medication in breast milk, instruct the patient to take asthma medications 15 minutes after breastfeeding (Peters, 1999).
- Educate how to decrease the chances of the infant developing asthma by breastfeeding for at least the first 6 months (Schmierer, 2001), introducing solid foods gradually at 6 months of age, feeding the infant no eggs or homogenized milk for the first year of life, feeding the child no peanut products for the first 2 years of life, and preventing cigarette smoke exposure (Kramer, 2000).

Nursing Interventions for Acute Exacerbation of Asthma

- Obtain a good history, if possible, of similar attacks and effective therapy.
- Ascertain how the patient is using a peak flow meter to monitor signs before initiating rescue medication because it is easy to confuse the shortness of breath that is normal during pregnancy with the shortness of breath that signals exacerbation of asthma.

- Evaluate the patient's understanding of how to use inhalers with a spacer. Perform an objective physical examination that includes auscultation of breath signs and addresses the following questions:
  - General appearance: is the patient cyanotic?
  - Can she complete sentences without shortness of breath?
  - Can she walk across a room?
  - Is she using accessory muscles?
- Obtain some or all of the following additional data:
  - Temperature, pulse, and respiratory rate
  - Laboratory values for forced expiratory volume or peak expiratory flow rate (repeat after bronchial dilation treatment)
  - Pulse oximetry monitoring
  - Breath sounds with auscultation of all lung fields
  - Chest radiograph
  - Arterial blood gas levels (see Table 14-2), cardiac monitoring, and electronic fetal monitoring after point of viability
- Treat an acute exacerbation based on lung function (FEV_1 or PEF), oxygen saturation, and symptoms following the NAEPP algorithm—*Management of asthma exacerbation during pregnancy and lactation: home* and *Management of asthma exacerbation during pregnancy and lactation: emergency department and hospital-based care* (NAEPP, 2005). Albuterol, a short-acting inhaled beta$_2$ agonist, via nebulizer or MDI, is the initial treatment medication. Be prepared to give corticosteroids as well.
- If infection is present, treat infection (see actual respiratory infection assessment and interventions).
- If the weeks of gestation are equal to or greater than 24 weeks, monitor the fetus during the acute phases, initially by 12 to 24 hours of electronic fetal monitoring and then by nonstress tests twice weekly when stable after 28 to 32 weeks of gestation. The fetus is also evaluated by ultrasound for growth rate every 3 to 4 weeks. If the woman is hypoxemic, she is monitored for contractions twice daily during the acute phase and is taught self-palpation and home monitoring for preterm labor during ambulatory care and home care.

Critical Care Interventions for Respiratory Emergencies
Management of Acidosis
- Blood gases to evaluate initial status (see Table 14-2)
- Chemistry profile to determine electrolytes and other multisystem potential causes
- Chest radiograph and other radiologic studies as determined by initial assessment
- Adequate oxygenation, ventilation-perfusion pressure, and oxygen delivery
- Treatment of underlying cause
- For pH lower than 7.2, give sodium bicarbonate, using this formula: give one half of the total base deficit (TBD = base excess × 0.2 of kg body weight)

Management of Alkalosis

- Perform a drug screen to evaluate for cause of alkalosis.
- Draw blood gases to evaluate initial status and every 6 to 12 hours to evaluate therapy (see Table 14-2).
- Correct underlying pathophysiology.
- Correct the ongoing acid loss.
- Attempt a trial of NaCl or KCl if urinary chloride is lower than 10 nmol/L.
- Possibly use a carbonic anhydrase inhibitor (acetazolamide).

Management of Severe Alkalosis

- Diluted HCl infusion via central line
- Oral arginine HCl
- Ammonium chloride infusion (not done in presence of hepatic dysfunction)
- Hemodialysis (Smith, 1997; Gonik and Foley, 2004)

Critical Care Interventions of Acute Pulmonary Edema and Pulmonary Embolism

- Chest radiograph
- Magnetic resonance image or computed tomographic scan
- Contrast dye studies, if embolism
- Elevation of head of bed
- Oxygen therapy via nonrebreather at 10 L or continuous positive airway pressure
- Nitroglycerine
- Continuous pulse oximetry and cardiac monitoring
- Furosemide
- Fetal heart and maternal blood pressure monitoring
- Digoxin as clinically indicated
- Anticoagulant therapy with heparin for therapeutic levels for embolism (see related Chapters 11, 13, and 19); therapeutic levels will be necessary for the remainder of the pregnancy or for a minimum of 3 to 6 months after the pregnancy
- Cardioversion as clinically indicated
- Continuous electronic fetal heart rate monitoring
- In the presence of anaphylactoid syndrome of pregnancy, cardiac output is increased with crystalloid fluids to replenish intravascular volume, and a vasopressor to treat acute hypotension and congestive heart failure (Gonik and Foley, 2004)

CONCLUSION

Respiratory disease can complicate a pregnancy, and pregnancy can complicate the management of acute or chronic respiratory disease. These complications require early health-promoting activities, prompt response and supervision, and close collaboration with pulmonary specialists.

BIBLIOGRAPHY

American Academy of Family Physicians (AAFP): *Pregnancy: respiratory infections*, Leawood, Kan, 2001, AAFP. Retrieved from *http://www.familydoctor.org/handouts/582.html*

American College of Obstetricians and Gynecologists: Pulmonary disease in pregnancy, *ACOG Technical Bulletin*, No. 224, Washington, DC, 1996, ACOG.

American College of Obstetricians and Gynecologists and American College of Allergy, Asthma, and Immunology: The use of newer asthma and allergy medications during pregnancy, *Ann Allergy Asthma Immunol* 84(5):475–480, 2000.

Anthony J: Critical care of the obstetric patient, In James D and others, editors: *High risk pregnancy: management options*, ed 3, Philadelphia, 2005, Saunders.

Burton J, Reyes M: Breath in, breath out: controlling asthma during pregnancy, *AWHONN Lifelines* 5(1):24–30, 2001.

Centers for Disease Control and Prevention (CDC): *Guidelines for vaccinating pregnant women. Recommendations of the Advisory Committee on Immunization Practices (ACIP)*, Atlanta, Ga, 2002, Centers for Disease Control and Prevention.

Centers for Disease Control and Prevention (CDC): Prevention and control of influenza: recommendations of the Advisory Committee on Immunization Practices (ACIP), *MMWR Recomm Rep* 53(RR–6):1–40, 2004.

Cousins L: Fetal oxygenation, assessment of fetal well-being, and obstetric management of the pregnant patient with asthma, *J Allergy Clin Immunol* 103(2 Pt 2):S343–S349, 1999.

Cox S, Kilpatrick S, and Geller S: Preventing maternal deaths, *Contemporary Ob Gyn*, Sept 1, 2004.

Dombrowski M and others: Asthma during pregnancy, *Obstet Gynecol* 103(1):5–12, 2004.

Doyle N and Monga M: Thromboembolic disease in pregnancy, *Obstet Gynecol Clin N Am* 31:319–344, 2004.

Farquharson R, Greaves M: Thromboembolic disease. In James D and others, editors: *High risk pregnancy: management options*, ed 3, Philadelphia, 2005, Saunders.

Gates S, Brocklehurst P, and Davis L: Prophylaxis for venous thromboembolic disease in pregnancy the early postnatal period, *Cochrane Database Syst Rev* 2: 2002: CD001689.

Gonik B, Foley M: Intensive care monitoring of the critically ill pregnant patient. In Creasy R, Resnik R, Iams J, editors: *Maternal-fetal medicine: principles and practice*, ed 5, Philadelphia, 2004, Saunders.

James A: Asthma, *Obstet Gynecol Clin North Am* 28(2):305–320, 2001.

Kramer M: Maternal antigen avoidance during pregnancy for preventing atopic disease in infants of women at high risk, *Cochrane Database Syst Rev* 2:CD000133, 2000.

Kwon H, Belanger K, and Bracken M: Asthma prevalence among pregnant and childbearing-aged women in the United States; estimates from national health surveys, *Ann Epidemiol* 13(5):317–324, 2003.

National Asthma Education and Prevention Program (NAEPP): Managing asthma during pregnancy: Recommendations for pharmacologic treatment–2004 update, *J Allergy Clin Immunol* 115(1):34–46, 2005. Retrieved from *http://www.nhlbi.nih.gov/halth/prof/lung/asthma/practgde.htm*

National Asthma Education and Prevention Program (NAEPP): *Expert Panel Report guidelines for the diagnosis and management of asthma: update on selected topics 2002*, Publication No. 02–5075, Bethesda, MD, 2002, National Heart, Lung, and Blood Institute, National Institute of Health. Retrieved from *http://www.nhlbi.nih.gov/guidelines/asthma/asthrpdt.htm*

Perlman A, Serbin J: Complementary and alternative medicine: does it have a role in treating asthma? *Womens Health Prim Care* 4:282, 2001.

Peters S: Under control: managing asthma and diabetes in pregnancy, *Adv Nurse Pract* 7(11):73–74, 1999.

Powrie R: Respiratory disease. In James D and others, editors: *High risk pregnancy: management options*, ed 3, Philadelphia, 2005, Saunders.

Revan V, Sun E, and McMorris M: Management of asthma in pregnancy, *The Female Patient* 27(9):18, 2002.

Schatz M and others: The safety of asthma and allergy medications during pregnancy, *J Allergy Clin Immunol* 100:301–306, 1997.

Schmierer T: Setting the stage: pregnancy is the ideal time for preventing allergies and asthma, *Adv Nurse Pract* 9(1):71–72, 2001.

Shulman L, Elias S: Metabolic and genetic screening, *Clin Perinatol* 28(2): 2001.

Smith H: Respiratory emergency during pregnancy. In Foley M, Strong T: *Obstetric intensive care,* Philadelphia, 1997, Saunders.

The Reference Laboratory at the Cleveland Clinic: Cystic fibrosis carrier screen for pregnant or pre-pregnant couples, 2004. Retrieved from *http://www.clevelandclinic.org/pathology/uploads/TechnicalBriefs-Oct2004-CF.pdf*

Weiner C, Buhimschi C: *Drugs for pregnant and lactating women,* Philadelphia, 2004, Churchill Livingstone.

Whitty J, Dombrowski M: Respiratory diseases in pregnancy. In Creasy R, Resnik R, and Iams J, editors: *Maternal-fetal medicine: principles and practice,* ed 5, Philadelphia, 2004, Saunders.

Complications in Pregnancy

V arious complications can develop during the course of a pregnancy and can affect the health and well-being of the mother and fetus, as well as the outcome of the pregnancy. With early recognition and today's advanced technology, the incidence of maternal and perinatal mortality and morbidity resulting from complications is declining. To continue to reduce maternal mortality and further decrease maternal morbidity related to complications, the perinatal nurse needs an in-depth understanding of complications of pregnancy.

The next 10 chapters present a physiologic and pathologic basis for the most common complications of pregnancy. Nursing care, which provides a basis for early recognition and effective management, is discussed.

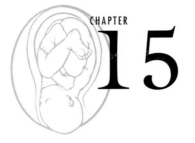

15

Spontaneous Abortion

Spontaneous abortion (SAB) is a natural termination of pregnancy before the fetus has reached viability. A fetus of less than 20 weeks of gestation and weighing less than 500 g is not considered viable. SAB is further divided into early and late. An *early abortion* occurs before 12 weeks of gestation, and a *mid-trimester* or *late abortion* occurs between 12 and 20 weeks of gestation. An SAB is commonly referred to as a *miscarriage*. This term is preferred in talking with patients because the word *abortion* is frequently associated with induced abortions.

INCIDENCE

SAB occurs in approximately 10% to 30% of all clinically apparent pregnancies, with a recurrence loss of 25% to 47% (ACOG, 2001; Dawood, Farquharson, and Quenby, 2004).

ETIOLOGY

Sporadic Abortions

Nonrecurring Genetic Abnormality

Early abortions are likely to be caused by a nonrecurring genetic abnormality of the embryo (Cunningham and others, 2005). Studies substantiate the fact that approximately 60% of most early abortions (before 12 weeks of gestation) have a chromosomal abnormality (Stern and others, 1996; Cunningham and others, 2005). The majority of these chromosomal abnormalities are related to numeric error occurring during meiotic cell division of the ovum or sperm or early mitotic cell division of the zygote or blastocyst.

Teratogenic Agents

Exposure to various teratogenic agents, such as high-dose radiation (Cunningham and others, 2005), chemicals, cytotoxic drugs (Hill, 2004), cocaine (Brent and Beckman, 1994), alcohol (Pietrantoni and Knuppel, 1991), smoking

(Brent and Beckman, 1994; Floyd and others, 1999), moderate-to-heavy caffeine consumption (Cnattingius and others, 2000), and heavy decaffeinated coffee consumption (Fenster and others, 1997), can cause placental vascular compromise and embryonic damage, leading to an SAB. These teratogenic agents act in a dose-dependent manner (ACOG, 2001).

Systemic Infections

Any severe viral or bacterial infection that causes viraemia or bacteraemia can cause congenital malformations and stimulate abortions. There is an increased risk for a spontaneous abortion with a first-trimester varicella infection (AAP and ACOG, 2002). However, rubella, cytomegalovirus, coxsackievirus, herpesvirus, toxoplasmosis, and listeria do not cause a severe enough infection to cause a sporadic SAB (Matovina and others, 2004; RCOG, 2003).

Uncontrolled Systemic Diseases

Systemic diseases that are not well controlled, such as diabetes, systemic lupus erythematosus, sickle cell anemia, hypertensive cardiovascular disease, phenylketonuria, and thyroid imbalance can cause an SAB.

Obesity

Obesity has been associated with increased risk for a sporadic abortion (Lashen, Fear, and Sturdee, 2004).

Environmental Factors

A relationship has been shown between stressful life events and working the night shift with an increased risk for SAB (Axelsson, Ahlborg, and Bodin, 1996; Neugebauer and others, 1996). Exposure to certain organic solvents has been linked to an increased SAB risk (Sharara, Seifer, and Flaws, 1998).

Recurrent Abortions

Chromosomal Disorders

Parental structural chromosome abnormalities account for approximately 2% to 5% of recurrent abortions (ACOG, 2001; RCOG, 2003).

Maternal Age

There appears to be a significantly increased risk for SAB in women older than 36 years (Nybo, Anderson, and others, 2000).

Uterine Anomalies

Structural uterine defects that interfere with the growth and development of the embryo or fetus may elicit an abortion. The uterine defect may be the result of a congenital defect or an acquired defect secondary to diethylstilbestrol (DES) exposure.

Antiphospholipid Syndrome

Antiphospholipid syndrome is one example of an autoimmune-mediated pregnancy loss. This disorder is characterized by presence of antiphospholipid antibodies. Two of the most common of these antibodies are lupus anticoagulant and anticardiolipin antibody. They both cause vascular endothelium damage and block the release of prostacyclin. Placental thrombosis and vascular insufficiency occur, causing subsequent fetal death (Meroni and others, 2004).

Inherited Thrombophilic Defect

Thrombophilia, an inheritable hypercoagulable condition, is most commonly the result of activated protein C resistance caused by mutations of the Factor V Leiden (FVL) gene, prothrombin gene (G20210A), protein C or S deficiency, antithrombin III, or hyperhomocysteinaemia (MTHFR C677T, the gene causing folate deficiency) (ROCG, 2003; Kovalevsky and others, 2004; Sheiner and others, 2005). The hypercoagulable state causes systemic thrombosis and uteroplacental insufficiency, which result in recurrent abortions.

Incompetent Cervix

An incompetent cervix is a weak, structurally defective cervix that spontaneously dilates around 16 weeks of gestation.

NORMAL PHYSIOLOGY

Embryo and Placenta Development

The gametes (sperm and ovum) undergo developmental changes before fertilization. During the gamete maturation process, the number of chromosomes is reduced to 23, which is half the original number. This process is called *meiosis.*

When fertilization takes place and a mature sperm enters the mature ovum, the 23 chromosomes from each gamete pair up to form a new cell with 46 chromosomes called the *zygote.* This new cell begins mitotic cell division. When the zygote has developed into a solid ball of cells, it is called a *morula.* As maturation continues, the morula develops into a *blastocyst.* At this stage, an outer layer of cells called the *trophoblast,* which will form the placenta and fetal membranes, and an inner cluster of cells called the *embryoblast,* which will form the embryo, are present.

On approximately the sixth day after fertilization, the blastocyst is ready to implant into the endometrium of the uterus. This is accomplished as the trophoblast cells begin to secrete a proteolytic enzyme that digests an opening a few cells wide and burrows its way into the uterine lining. A small amount of blood may be lost at this time, which can cause mild vaginal spotting. The opening is closed by a blood clot at first and later by regenerated epithelium.

After the blastocyst is implanted into the endometrium of the uterus, the endometrium is called the *decidua.* The decidua is usually divided into three parts. The part of the decidua lying directly beneath the implanted blastocyst is called the *decidua basalis.* This is where the placenta primarily grows. The part of the decidua that covers the buried blastocyst is called *decidua capsularis,* and the remainder of the decidua that is not in direct contact with the blastocyst is called *decidua vera*.

After ovulation, when the mature ovum is released from the ovary, the ovary enters its luteal phase. During this time it excretes high levels of progesterone and some estrogen to prepare and maintain the endometrium for the fertilized ovum. Both hormones stimulate the glandular cells of the endometrium to secrete mucus and glycogen and increase the blood supply to the endometrium to facilitate an adequate nutritional environment for the implanted blastocyst, embryo, or fetus. Progesterone also facilitates the maintenance of pregnancy by keeping the myometrium quiet so that implantation can take place. For the corpus luteum to continue its production of progesterone and estrogen, the trophoblastic tissue must secrete human chorionic gonadotropin (hCG) until the placenta is mature enough to take over the production of hormones. This hormone maintains the corpus luteum for about the first 8 weeks of gestation.

Placental Immunology

The mother's body does not reject the blastocyst, which remains a mystery. On the surface of all body cells are structural antigens. The lymphocyte white blood cells are able to identify these antigens as either familiar or unfamiliar (foreign), and these white blood cells manufacture antibodies to destroy the antigens if they are identified as foreign. Because the antigens are determined genetically, half the antigens on fetal cells come from each parent. Therefore half the antigens should be foreign to the mother's body.

Currently, it is unknown what mechanism or mechanisms prevent the rejection of the fetus. Some recent research suggests that the immunologic interaction between mother and fetus appears to be beneficial for fetal and placental growth and development and limits trophoblast invasion. This is the result of immunotolerance and immunosuppression. First, the placental tissue (syncytiotrophoblast) that contacts with maternal tissue lacks the ability to activate the immune system. Second, the placenta tissue (cytotrophoblast) does not stimulate major histocompatibility complex (MHC) antigen formation because of the presence of human leukocyte antigen G (HLA-G). Therefore the mother creating immunotolerance (Silver, Peltier, and Branch, 1999) does not normally produce harmful antipaternal antibodies. Certain cytokines (transforming growth factor-beta [TGF-β] and interleukin 10), prostaglandin E_2, hCG, and steroid hormones appear to have immunosuppressive activity in normal gestational tissue. Progesterone is also important in maintaining the pregnancy throughout the nine months by inhibiting myometrial activity and preventing T cell-mediated rejection (Ragusa and others, 2004).

Cervical Changes

An important structure that facilitates pregnancy continuation is the cervix. The cervix must resist the forces of gravity and intrauterine pressure for 9 months and then become soft and distensible, allowing the fetus to pass through to the vagina. The pregnancy is maintained primarily because of the formation of a sphincterlike structure that forms at the internal cervical os (Iams, 2004). This develops because of the distending muscular isthmus above and the cervix below, which is composed primarily of connective tissue (ground substance) plus collagen with scattered smooth muscle fibers (Huszar and Walsh, 1991).

During pregnancy, collagen fibers are laid down in an orderly fashion among the connective tissue, which gives the cervix strength to remain firm and closed. At the end of pregnancy, rearrangement of the collagen fibers takes place so that the fibers become more separable, promoting softening of the cervix (Cabrol, 1991). Numerous cervical glands line the cervical canal. During pregnancy, hypertrophy and hyperplasia of the cervical glands occur as well, forming the mucus plug.

PATHOPHYSIOLOGY

Embryo, Fetal, Placental Effect

Death of the embryo or failure of the embryo or placenta to develop normally is usually the first step in the sequence of events that lead to an SAB. Hemorrhage into the decidua basalis results, which causes necrotic changes at the site of implantation. Infiltration of leukocytes follows. Because of the absence of functioning fetal circulation, the chorionic villi often become edematous and resemble a hydatidiform mole. At the same time, hormonal levels of progesterone and estrogen drop, causing decidual sloughing, which results in vaginal bleeding. The uterus becomes irritable, and uterine contractions result.

Cervical Incompetence

An incompetent cervix contains more smooth muscle than a normal cervix (Iams, 2004); the collagen concentration is also less than normal. Cervical resistance is lowered because collagen fibers give the cervix strength to remain firm and closed. This is usually caused by one of three factors: a congenital defect, past cervical trauma, or hormonal factors.

Congenital Defect

With a congenital defect, the lower genital tract is structurally abnormal. A genetic inherited short cervical length can increase the risk for cervical incompetence. Exposure to DES can affect the lower uterine segment, increasing the risk as well (Kaufman and others, 2000).

Cervical Trauma

Cervical trauma is usually the result of mechanical trauma such as excessive dilation for curettage, cervical biopsy, or cervical lacerations acquired during a previous delivery.

Hormonal Factors

Increased amounts of relaxin, the effects of exogenous estrogen and progesterone, and multiple gestations all increase the risk for cervical incompetence.

Relaxin, a hormone secreted by the corpus luteum, causes connective tissue remodeling, which affects the collagen concentration. Levels of relaxin are increased in multiple gestations.

SIGNS AND SYMPTOMS
Vaginal Bleeding

The classic sign of an SAB is vaginal bleeding. At first, the bleeding usually appears as dark spotting related to the decreased hormonal levels of progesterone and estrogen that cause the decidua (endometrium) to begin to slough. It may progress to frank, bright red bleeding as the products of conception begin to separate, opening up uterine blood vessels.

Abdominal Pain

Pain may be manifested in different ways. It may be rhythmic or persistent, and it may present as a low backache or as pelvic pressure or tenderness over the uterus.

Incompetent Cervix

A woman with an incompetent cervix commonly presents with complaints of pelvic pressure, increased vaginal discharge, or light spotting. Spontaneous cervical dilation is painless and unaccompanied by contractions, amniotic fluid leakage, or signs of infection.

CLASSIFICATION

SABs are classified into seven clinical types: threatened, inevitable, complete, incomplete, missed, septic, and recurrent (Fig. 15-1). Table 15-1 lists signs and symptoms manifested by each type.

MATERNAL EFFECTS

The major contributions to maternal death surrounding an SAB are related to two potential complications that rarely occur today: hemorrhage and infection. Hemorrhage may be related to a delay in seeking medical treatment or to perforation of the uterus during surgical treatment. Infection may be related to a delay in diagnosing a septic abortion or to inappropriate use of antibiotics.

FETAL EFFECTS

Death of the fetus always occurs as the result of an SAB. In fact, it may be the actual cause of the abortion.

DIAGNOSTIC TESTING
Spontaneous Abortion

When vaginal bleeding occurs during the first 20 weeks of pregnancy, careful evaluation must be made to determine whether the bleeding is a threatened

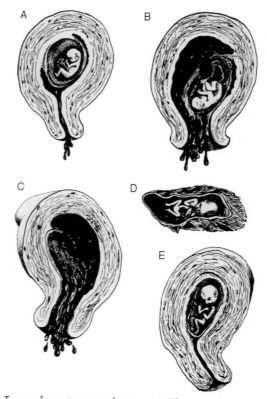

Figure 15-1 Types of spontaneous abortions. **A,** Threatened. **B,** Inevitable. **C,** Incomplete. **D,** Complete. **E,** Missed. (From Lowdermilk D, Perry S: *Maternity and women's health care,* ed 8, St Louis, 2004, Mosby.)

abortion or is related to another cause. About 20% of all patients experience some vaginal bleeding during the first trimester, and only about half of these women actually have SABs (Cunningham and others, 2005). Therefore consideration must be given to other possible causes of vaginal bleeding, which may be related to one of the following:

- Normal implantation of the blastocyst into the endometrium
- Lesions of the cervix or vagina or cervical polyps that bleed because of increased vascularity of the vagina and cervix during pregnancy
- Cervicitis or vaginitis
- Hydatidiform mole
- Ectopic pregnancy
- Carcinoma of the cervix

The evaluation to differentiate among the various possible causes of vaginal bleeding usually includes inspecting the vagina and cervix by a speculum examination to rule out vaginal or cervical lesions or cervical polyps, along with a Pap smear to rule out carcinoma. Vaginal ultrasound is usually done to determine whether there is an intrauterine gestational sac. This rules out an

Table 15-1   Clinical Classification of Spontaneous Abortions

Classification	Definition	Manifestations
Threatened	Condition in which continuation of pregnancy is in doubt	Vaginal bleeding or spotting, which may be associated with mild cramps of back and lower abdomen Closed cervix Uterus that is soft, nontender, and enlarged appropriate to gestational age
Inevitable	Condition in which termination of pregnancy is in progress	Cervical dilation Membranes may be ruptured Vaginal bleeding Mild-to-painful uterine contractions
Complete	Condition in which products of conception are totally expelled from uterus	
Incomplete	Condition in which fragments of products of conception are expelled and part is retained in uterus	Profuse bleeding because retained tissue parts interfere with myometrial contractions
Missed	Condition in which embryo or fetus dies during first 20 weeks of gestation but is retained in uterus for 4 weeks or more afterward	Amenorrhea or intermittent vaginal bleeding, spotting, or brownish discharge No uterine growth No fetal movement felt Regression of breast changes
Septic	Condition in which products of conception become infected during abortion process	Foul-smelling vaginal discharge
Recurrent	Condition in which two or more successive pregnancies have ended in spontaneous abortion	

ectopic pregnancy. A gestational sac, if present, should be identifiable with ultrasound by 6 weeks after the last menstrual period. Real time ultrasound can be used to document lack of heart movement, which indicates fetal death. Quantitative beta-hCG assays and progesterone levels are helpful in determining the state of the fetus. Serial doubling of quantitative beta-hCG assays every 36 to 48 hours between gestational weeks 3 and 10 and progesterone levels greater than 15 ng/ml strongly indicates a healthy pregnancy. See Table 16-3 for a summary of diagnostic tests.

If the patient presents with signs of an inevitable abortion, tests are not usually necessary to make the diagnosis. Any patient with a history of cervical trauma or painless second trimester abortion should be examined weekly during the second trimester for an incompetent cervix.

Box 15-1 provides a nurse practitioner workup summary.

Incompetent Cervix

In an incompetent cervix, a vaginal examination indicates cervical softening, but dilation of the cervix typically occurs later. Transvaginal ultrasound measuring of the length of the cervix is the best diagnostic tool to detect early cervical changes. Incompetent cervix is diagnosed if the cervix shortens below 20 to 25 mm or below 25 to 30 mm in the presence of a funnel or beak (effacement at the internal os moving to the external os). Zilianti and others (1995) suggested a useful acronym to describe the presence of effacement seen on transvaginal ultrasound: TYVU. A normal cervix without any funneling is a T. As the cervix begins to efface at the internal os moving to the external os, it first looks like a Y, with further shortening toward the external os as a V, and finally to a fully effaced cervix as a U.

USUAL MEDICAL MANAGEMENT AND PROTOCOLS FOR NURSE PRACTITIONERS

Most often, when vaginal bleeding is definitely related to an SAB, treatment centers on determining the cause (if possible), keeping the couple informed, and providing emotional support instead of attempting to sustain the pregnancy. This protocol is based on the following factors:

- In an early threatened abortion, the embryo or fetus is usually dead before the bleeding begins.
- Approximately 60% of all early abortions are associated with chromosomal anomalies and are nature's way of preventing the birth of a genetically defective child.
- In late abortions, after 12 weeks of gestation, maternal factors are usually the cause, and death does not usually precede the vaginal bleeding. However, if the pregnancy is maintained, the bleeding itself can increase perinatal mortality or the risk for developing congenital abnormalities.
- Controlled studies have also failed to prove that bedrest, hormones such as progesterone, or sedatives have any effect on the outcome of a threatened abortion.
- Administration of medications during organogenesis (weeks 3–8) exposes the embryo to possible teratogenic effects.

Threatened Abortion

When a threatened abortion is diagnosed, an assessment is done to determine the probable outcome. Prompt evacuation of the uterus must be carried out if any of the following findings are present:

- Bleeding has become excessive.
- Any part of the products of conception has been lost.
- Cervix shows signs of dilation.
- Signs and symptoms of an intrauterine infection are present.

Box 15-1   Nurse Practitioner Workup Summary

- **Evaluation of amount of blood loss**
  - **Subjective report**
  - **Vital signs**
  - **Orthostatic blood pressure.** Check orthostatic blood pressure if condition permits. To do this, take the patient's blood pressure and pulse while she is supine. Retake these vital signs after the patient has been standing for 5 minutes. A decrease in systolic blood pressure of 10 mm Hg or an increase in the pulse rate of 10 beats per min or more is interpreted as an indication of significant blood loss.
  - **Pulse pressure.** The *diastolic blood pressure* reflects the amount of systemic vasoconstriction present; the *pulse pressure* (difference between systolic and diastolic pressure) indicates stroke volume; the *systolic blood pressure* denotes the interrelationship between the level of vasoconstriction and the stroke volume. A narrowing of the pulse pressure (normal 30 to 40 mm Hg) is an early sign of hypovolemia.
  - **Hypothenar refilling.** Squeeze the hypothenar area of the hand (the fleshy elevation of the ulnar side of the palm) for 1 to 2 seconds. Normal blood volume is indicated by initial blanching with return to the normal pink coloration within 1 to 2 seconds. A blood volume deficit of 15% to 25% is indicated by delayed refilling.
- **Menstrual history. Last normal menstrual period, frequency, duration, and flow.**
- **Gynecologic history**
  - **Contraceptive history**
  - **Sexually transmitted disease**
- **Obstetric history**
- **Coagulation disorder history**
- **Physical examination**
  - **Abdominal examination**
  - **Auscultation**
  - **Percussion**
  - **Palpation (tender area last)**
  - **Rebound tenderness**
  - **McBurney point**
  - **Iliopsoas**
  - **Obturator test**
  - **Murphy sign**
- **Vaginal speculum examination** to determine the following:
  - **Source of the bleeding.** Rule out cervical or vaginal causes such as polyps, cervical or vaginal lesions, vaginal infection, vaginal trauma, cervical pregnancy, cervical cancer, or pelvic inflammatory disease.
  - **Amount of vaginal bleeding**
  - **Cervical status: opened or closed**
  - **Presence of tissue at the cervix**
- **Bimanual vaginal examination**

Continued

Box 15-1   Nurse Practitioner Workup Summary—cont'd

- **Uterine examination.** Determine uterine size, and determine the presence of an adnexal mass or tenderness.
- **Diagnostic data**
  - **Quantitative serum human chorionic gonadotropin (hCG)**
  - **Progesterone levels**
  - **Hemoglobin and hematocrit with complete blood cell count**
  - **Blood type, platelet count, and antibody screen**
  - **Vaginal ultrasound**
  - **Urine for culture and sensitivity**

- Definite diagnosis of a dead fetus is made with ultrasound.

To assess for the presence of one of these negative findings, a medical workup is done that usually includes the following:

- Pelvic examination to determine signs of dilation.
- Blood count for red blood cells, hemoglobin, and hematocrit to aid in the determination of the amount of blood lost and the presence or absence of anemia.
- Blood count for white blood cells to determine whether an infection is present.
- Vaginal ultrasound, serial serum quantitative beta-hCG assays, and serum progesterone values to determine whether the fetus is alive. (Indicators of fetal well-being include a well-formed gestational ring with central echoes from the embryo, serum progesterone greater than 10/15 ng/ml, and serial doubling of quantitative beta-hCG assays.)

If the assessment does not reveal a negative finding, the patient is usually managed as an outpatient. She has frequent physician's visits and is instructed to limit her activity, abstain from intercourse, and save any passed tissue. If an IUD is in place and the string is visible, it is usually removed. Further treatment depends on the signs and symptoms that develop.

Inevitable, Complete, or Incomplete Abortion

Once the cervix begins to dilate, there is no hope for pregnancy continuation and an abortion becomes inevitable. If part of the products of conception is lost, the abortion becomes incomplete; if all of the products of conception are lost, the abortion is complete.

From the time an abortion becomes inevitable until it becomes complete, naturally or with surgical intervention, there is a high risk for complications such as hemorrhage or an infection. The risk for hemorrhage usually correlates with the gestational age of the pregnancy. For the first 6 weeks, the placenta is very tentatively attached to the decidua of the uterus. Therefore if an SAB occurs before 6 weeks of gestation, the bleeding usually takes the form of a heavy menstrual period.

Between 6 and 12 weeks of gestation, the chorionic villi of the placenta begin to grow into the decidua of the uterus, and by week 12 or shortly after, the chorionic villi have deeply penetrated into the decidua. If an SAB occurs after the placenta has completed its penetration process (week 12), the fetus is usually expelled before placental separation. Bleeding is usually held in check by the placenta until it separates from the uterus and then by uterine contractions if the separation is complete. Therefore the most severe bleeding is seen between 6 and 12 weeks of gestation because the placenta can detach before expulsion of the fetus. Severe bleeding can result after 12 weeks of gestation if the placenta does not separate completely and parts are retained. If the gestational age is known, the risk for bleeding can be more easily estimated.

The risk for infection usually depends on many factors, such as the nutritional state of the patient, perineal hygiene, and whether anything other than a sterile speculum entered the vagina after dilation began.

If all the embryonic or fetal and placental tissue can be identified and there are no signs of bleeding or infection, the abortion is complete and no surgical intervention is necessary. If the abortion is incomplete, according to Nielsen and Hahlin (1995), expectant management to allow spontaneous resolution (maximum 3 days) was found to be just as safe a treatment plan for first trimester SAB as was immediate surgery. Complications were similar between the two treatment groups with less incidence of pelvic inflammatory disease in the expectant management group.

However, prompt evacuation of the uterus may be indicated in the presence of excessive cramping, heavy bleeding, or emotional instability. According to the Cochrane Review (Forna and Gülmezoglu, 2001), vacuum aspiration is preferred over sharp curettage. It is safe, quick, and less painful than sharp curettage. *Vacuum aspiration* is the removal of the products of conception with a vacuum aspirator suction curet that is inserted through the dilated cervix after the patient is anesthetized. The vacuum aspirator is moved gently over the surface of the uterine wall in a systematic pattern to cover all the uterine cavity, and the products of conception are collected in a vacuum container.

This procedure is done primarily in an outpatient setting. The woman is hospitalized only if severe bleeding or signs of infection are present. If time permits, a history and physical examination are usually performed and a complete blood count is done. A tube of blood is usually held for typing and cross-matching in case a transfusion becomes necessary. A dilute solution of intravenous (IV) oxytocin is often started before the surgery to reduce blood loss and to decrease the risk for uterine perforation by causing the uterus to contract and thicken. A preoperative medication of 5 to 10 mg of diazepam (Valium) may be ordered. The procedure can be done with a paracervical block, especially if the procedure is performed on an outpatient basis, or with the patient under a light general anesthesia. If the procedure is done with the patient under local anesthesia, the patient may experience some cramping sensations during the procedure.

If the bleeding is severe, the patient's vital signs must be stabilized before surgery. This is usually accomplished by infusing 1 to 2 L of a crystalloid solution such as IV lactated Ringer's solution with 30 units of oxytocin per 1000 ml. If lactated Ringer's solution with oxytocin is used, the infusion rate is usually set at 200 ml/hr or more. This large dose of oxytocin is needed during the first half of pregnancy because the uterus is less sensitive to oxytocin at this time because of the low levels of estrogen present to potentiate its effect. If oxytocin is not effective, an erythrocyte infusion or another appropriate blood component may be used. If signs of infection are present or develop, antibiotic therapy is usually initiated.

If the cervix is not partially dilated, dilation is usually accomplished slowly by placing *Laminaria* dilators or a prostaglandin suppository or gel in the cervix before the evacuation procedure. *Laminaria* tents, such as *Laminaria digitata* or *Laminaria japonica*, are natural cervical dilators made from seaweed, the stems of which have been peeled, dried, and sterilized. Synthetic alternatives are being used more frequently. Dilapan, a hygroscopic cervical dilator, and Lamicel, an alcohol polymer sponge impregnated with 450 mg of magnesium sulfate and compressed into a tent, are two commonly used synthetic dilators.

Inserted into the full length of the cervical canal, the dilators absorb cervical fluids and swell, dilating the cervix slowly (Fig. 15-2). The patient may experience cramping, which is easily controlled with a mild analgesic. Then, at the time of surgery or before the evacuation procedure, the *Laminaria* dilators are removed. Serial applications of prostaglandin gel or vaginal suppositories placed in the cervix can accomplish the same result. Because both methods dilate the cervix slowly, they decrease the risk for cervical trauma, which can occur with mechanical dilators.

Missed Abortion

Most missed abortions terminate spontaneously. However, if there are no signs of an SAB at the time a missed abortion is diagnosed, the physician usually evacuates the uterus as soon as possible because of the following potential problems:
- Psychologic stress related to carrying a dead fetus
- Sepsis
- Disseminated intravascular coagulopathy, a coagulation defect with hypofibrinogenemia, increased fibrin, and decreased platelets, which occur because the dead products of conception release thromboplastin into the maternal circulation, stimulating this process (see Chapter 19)

The techniques used for the evacuation usually depend on the length of pregnancy. Pregnancies up to 16 weeks of gestation are usually terminated by prostaglandin E1 vaginal suppositories or dilation and evacuation by curettage or vacuum aspiration. Vacuum aspiration is preferable to curettage during the first 10 weeks of gestation; there is less chance of perforation, bleeding, or infection. After 16 weeks, the likelihood of uterine perforation, cervical lacerations, hemorrhage, incomplete removal of the products of conception, and infection are the usual reasons given for not using curettage or vacuum aspiration. Various prostaglandin preparations are used from 16 to 20 weeks of gestation.

Prostaglandins can be administered orally, parenterally, into the amniotic sac, or as a vaginal suppository. The oral method is not used because of the

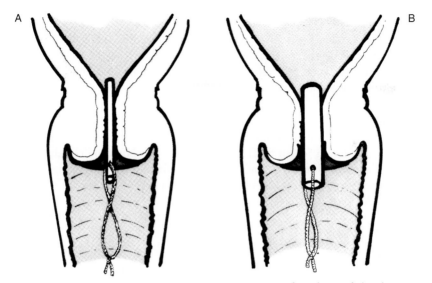

Figure 15-2 A, Properly inserted laminaria. **B,** Laminaria after 8 hours of absorbing cervical fluid, causing it to swell and dilate cervix gradually. (Illustration by Vincenza Genovese, Phoenix, Ariz.)

extremely uncomfortable side effects, such as severe gastrointestinal distress. All other routes are used to induce contractions and cause the uterus to expel the products of conception. Possible side effects are nausea, vomiting, diarrhea, fever, dizziness, headache, and hypertension. Rare side effects are bronchospasm, cardiac dysrhythmias, chest pain, and hyperventilation.

Intraamniotic injection of hypotonic saline is rarely used because of the reduced volume of amniotic fluid, which makes the procedure too difficult. The hypertonic saline solution can also further increase the risk for developing a coagulation defect.

Dilation of the cervix should take place before any of these methods of evacuation. A *Laminaria* tent or intravaginal prostaglandins is usually the treatment of choice to dilate the cervix without risk for injury.

Recurrent Spontaneous Abortion

Some recurrent abortions occur by chance; others are related to a maternal or paternal cause. Treatment should focus on identifying the cause and treating it accordingly. The current suggested screening and treatment methods after a recurrent SAB are outlined next. According to the American College of Obstetrics and Gynecology (2001), it is not necessary to routinely screen for endocervical bacteria or viruses or to test for glucose intolerance, thyroid abnormalities, paternal human leukocyte antigen status, or maternal antipaternal antibodies after recurrent pregnancy loss. After unexplained recurrent SAB, the couple should be encouraged by the 35% to 85% successful pregnancy rate without treatment (ACOG, 2001).

Chromosomal Disorder

When a couple repeatedly loses an embryo or fetus early in gestation, a chromosomal disorder of the father or mother may be the cause. A genetic history should be taken, karyotyping is recommended, and genetic counseling should follow as indicated.

Uterine Anomalies

Uterine defects are occasionally the cause of late recurrent SABs. During vacuum aspiration for an SAB, the uterine cavity should be closely examined for any abnormalities. If a double uterus is noted, a hysterosalpingography or hysteroscopic evaluation and reparative surgery have been shown to be therapeutic (ACOG, 2001).

Endocrine Factors

A luteal phase defect (LPD) occurs in approximately 35% of recurrent spontaneous abortions. However, there is no reliable method to diagnose LPD (Bukulmez and Arici, 2004). The benefits of supplemental natural progesterone suppositories are unproved (ACOG, 2001). If used, the usual dose is 100 mg twice per day. To be most effective, the progesterone should be started at the time of ovulation and continued until 10 to 12 weeks of gestation (Hill, 2004).

In patients with polycystic ovary syndrome (PCOS), a hyperandrogenic disorder, metformin therapy throughout the pregnancy is being studied (Glueck and others, 2001). Hypothyroidism is treated with thyroid replacement medication. The dosage is titrated to maintain normal TSH levels.

Immunologic Factors: Antiphospholipid Syndrome

A patient who tests positive for a lupus anticoagulant or an anticardiolipin antibody on two different occasions, 6 weeks apart, should be placed on thromboprophylaxis during the next pregnancy. Therapeutic recommendations are aspirin, 81 mg/day, followed by unfractionated or low-molecular-weight heparin (LMWH). Refer to Box 13-2 for heparin dosing guidelines. Weight-bearing exercise and calcium and vitamin D supplementation are encouraged to lower the risk for osteoporosis. According to the American College of Obstetrics and Gynecology (2001), mononuclear cell immunization and intravenous immunoglobulin (IVIG) are not effective in preventing a recurrent SAB (see Chapter 13).

Incompetent Cervix

Treatment for recurrent abortions caused by an incompetent cervix is usually cerclage, a surgical procedure in which a purse-string suture is placed around the cervix to reinforce it. Preoperative vaginal cultures are obtained and appropriate treatment instituted for group B streptococcus, *Neisseria gonorrhoeae*, and *Chlamydia*. This surgical procedure is considered in three different circumstances, described in the following paragraphs.

Prophylactic Cerclage. The prophylactic cerclage is usually performed based on a positive obstetric history around 10 to 14 weeks of gestation, before cervical dilation, effacement, or shortening takes place and before any bleeding or cramping is present. After the procedure, prophylactic antibiotics, such as penicillin for 5 days, are given. Instruct the patient to abstain from intercourse, not to stand for prolonged periods of more than 90 minutes, and not to lift anything heavy.

Therapeutic Cerclage. The therapeutic cerclage is placed when transvaginal ultrasound reveals signs of funneling or beaking (beginning effacement at the internal os moving to the external os) and shortened cervical length, in the absence of other discernible causes. After the procedure, prophylactic antibiotics, such as penicillin for 5 days, are given. Instruct the patient to abstain from intercourse, not to stand for prolonged periods of more than 90 minutes, and not to lift anything heavy. If the transvaginal cervix length is less than 25 mm, the patient is encouraged to stop working. If the cervix length is less than 20 mm the patient is told to limit her activity.

Rescue Cerclage. The rescue cerclage is placed when the transvaginal ultrasound reveals advanced cervical dilation, shortened cervical length, or bulging or hourglass membranes. Amniocentesis may be performed to reduce the bulging and obtain cultures. After the procedure, prophylactic antibiotics and indomethacin are usually prescribed. These patients are on bedrest with bathroom privileges only until stabilized with no further evidence of preterm labor changes.

NURSING MANAGEMENT

Prevention

Because teratogenic agents increase the risk for an SAB, preventive measures should be taken to avoid this area of risk. These measures should be instituted before pregnancy. The woman should maintain a healthful lifestyle, including eating a nutritious diet, not smoking, not drinking alcoholic beverages, and receiving available immunizations against infectious diseases. When pregnancy is diagnosed, instructions given to the expectant mother include ways she can decrease her chance of contracting infections, such as by eating nutritiously, avoiding fatigue, and avoiding people with infections. She is also instructed that if she eats meat, to cook it well; if she has a pet cat or bird, to leave the cleaning of the litter area to someone else; and if she works in the yard, to use gloves to avoid contact with the toxoplasmosis virus. She is instructed to avoid radiographs and medications, especially nonprescription ones, unless they are ordered by her obstetrician.

Nursing Interventions for Hemorrhage Management

- Obtain a history of onset, duration, amount, color, and consistency of bleeding.
- Obtain a history of associated symptoms, prior bleeding episodes, and physical activity at onset of bleeding.

- Record visual blood loss in cubic centimeters of blood stained on pad in a certain period of time, or weigh saturated pads, linen protectors, or linen (1 g × 1 ml).
- Record blood pressure, pulse, and respirations as indicated (depends on severity).
- Observe for passage of tissue or clots.
- Observe for signs of shock.
- Keep an accurate record of intake and output.
- Refer to laboratory data such as hemoglobin level, hematocrit level, and red blood cell count.
- Determine gestational age by estimated date of delivery.
- Save all expelled tissue and clots for examination.
- If bleeding is severe or the hemoglobin or hematocrit level is low, start an IV line with an 14-gauge intracatheter and normal saline to be prepared for blood component therapy or blood administration as ordered. Start another IV line to administer a crystalloid solution such as lactated Ringer's solution as ordered, usually 1.5 to 2 liters given through a warming device (Anthony, 2006). Prepare for type and cross-match, and have oxytocin available. Usual dose of oxytocin is 10 units in 500 ml of 0.9% (normal) saline or D_5W solution to infuse at a rate to control uterine atony (Weiner and Buhimschi, 2004).
- Notify physician if the blood pressure drops, pulse or respirations increase, more than one pad is saturated with blood in 1 hour, urinary output drops below 30 ml/hr or 120 ml/4 hr, or the hematocrit level is less than 30% or hemoglobin level less than 11 g. Be prepared to intervene based on percentage of blood loss. See Table 18-3 for guidelines for blood component replacement.
- Assist with medical management based on diagnosis.

If no signs of an inevitable, incomplete, or missed abortion are found, the following interventions apply:
- Provide discharge instructions that include the importance of limiting activity, abstaining from intercourse, and returning for a reevaluation appointment.
- Instruct as to the importance of notifying the physician immediately if bleeding becomes heavier than a period or persists, if cramps develop, or if a fever develops.
- Encourage patient to continue to take prenatal vitamins and eat foods high in protein, iron, and fiber.

If signs of an inevitable, incomplete, or missed abortion are present, the following interventions apply:
- Prepare for surgical or medical intervention as applicable.
- Explain procedure to patient.
- Surgically prepare patient.

If vacuum aspiration is to be used, the following interventions apply:
- Have patient empty bladder before procedure.

- Be prepared to start an IV line so that oxytocin can be administered to facilitate uterine contractions during or after the procedure.
- If cervix is not dilated, be prepared to assist with some form of cervical dilation.
- Administer an antiemetic or analgesic as ordered.
- Explain sensations that may be experienced during the procedure.
  If prostaglandins are used, the following interventions apply:
- Observe for side effects such as nausea and vomiting, diarrhea, drug-related fever, or a blood pressure change.
- If intraamniotic prostaglandins are used, be prepared for and assist with amniocentesis.
- If a prostaglandin vaginal suppository or gel is used, be prepared to assist with insertion.
- Assess for uterine contractions.
- Provide comfort measures.

Postsurgical Nursing Interventions to Prevent Complications or to Provide Early Detection of Signs of Hemorrhage, Infection, and Anemia

- Be prepared to give methylergonovine maleate (Methergine), 200 mg orally every 6 hours for six doses if bleeding is heavy.
- Check the vital signs according to protocol.
- Check vaginal discharge according to protocol.
- Refer to laboratory data such as white blood cell count.
- Teach the importance of perineal care after each voiding, and encourage to change perineal pads often.
- If signs of an infection develop, be prepared to administer antibiotics as ordered.
- Discharge instructions include appropriate perineal care: shower (no baths) for first 2 weeks; no using tampons, douching, or having sexual intercourse for 2 weeks; and notify physician if an elevated temperature or a foul-smelling vaginal discharge develops.
- Determine mother's blood type and Rh factor.
- If mother is Rh-negative, be prepared to administer Rho (D) immune globulin. The usual dose is Rho (D) immune globulin Standard dose (RhoGAM; HypRho-D) IM 300 microgram if the gestational age is greater than 12 weeks or Rho (D) Globulin Microdose (HypRho-D MiniDose, MicRhoGAM) IM 50 microgram for a gestation of 12 weeks or less.
- Refer to laboratory data, such as hemoglobin, to rule out anemia.
- Provide discharge instructions as to the importance of eating foods high in iron and protein to promote tissue repair and red blood cell replacement. Foods high in iron include meat, legumes, dried fruits, whole grains, and green, leafy vegetables. Iron from plant-based foods is less well absorbed by the body, but absorption can be improved by eating these foods along with a food high in vitamin C.

Nursing Interventions for Anticipatory Grieving

- Assess the significance of the loss to all family members. According to Hutti and others (1998), parents experience more intense grief if they perceive the pregnancy and baby as real, if the actual miscarriage experience was not congruent with their expectations, and if they felt unable to influence their experience.
- Acknowledge, permit, and help individual family members identify feelings of relief, sadness, distress, or neutrality toward the loss.
- Encourage the patient and her family to express their individual levels of satisfaction and control regarding the actual miscarriage experience.
- Give the parents choices and opportunities for decision making.
- Provide physical care such as back rubs or nourishment as needed.
- Consider any significant cultural beliefs or values. Refer to a pastor, priest, or chaplain based on family's request for spiritual assistance to work through their grief.
- Refer to a support group such as Resolve Through Sharing or Compassionate Friends, if available.
- Refer to psychologic support or counseling if indicated.
- Provide family with a list of helpful publications, including the following:
  - *Understanding Miscarriage: Coping With the Loss* (Krames Communication, 800-333-3032)
  - *When Pregnancy Fails* (Susan Borg and Judith Lasker)
  - *Death of a Dream* (Donna and Rodger Ewy)
  - *After a Loss in Pregnancy* (Nancy Barezin)
  - *Ended Beginnings* (Claudia Panuthos and Catherine Romeo)
  - *Empty Arms: Coping After Miscarriage, Stillbirth and Infant Death* (Ilse Sherokee and Arlene Appelbaum)

  See Chapter 7 for more information about this topic.
- Discuss with the family the importance of grieving the loss before becoming pregnant again. Many parents try to lessen their grief by quickly planning and becoming pregnant. According to Frost and Condon (1996), another pregnancy too soon inhibits mourning and delays resolution.

Nursing Interventions to Decrease Risk for Recurrence

- Discuss with the couple the cause, if known, or otherwise explain possible reasons for an SAB.
- If this is a second or third SAB, the couple should be encouraged to have a diagnostic and genetic workup to attempt to determine the cause. This might include the following:
  - Karyotyping of abortus
  - Karyotyping of parents
  - Pelvic ultrasound to rule out uterine anomaly
  - Ruling out autoimmune disease with tests for lupus anticoagulant or anticardiolipin (aCL) antibodies
  - Thyroid panel and fasting blood sugar, only if symptoms indicate

Cervical Competence

- If the couple asks, discuss the prognosis of a subsequent abortion (35% risk after the initial abortion with a 55% risk with consecutive abortions [Cole, 1995]).
- Teach the couple the importance of using contraception except for Depomedroxyprogesterone acetate (Depo-Provera) through two normal menstrual periods, at least, to allow time for the woman's body to recover. After an abortion, the woman usually ovulates during the next cycle, but there is a significantly increased risk for endometrial abnormalities for the next two cycles.
- Develop and consistently use a self-administered, matter-of-fact, nonjudgmental questionnaire to ascertain lifestyle behaviors such as patterns of smoking, alcohol consumption, caffeine intake, recreational drug use, nonprescription medication use, and occupation.
- Analyze the responses for potential risk.
- Motivate the family to make lifestyle changes to improve health-related behaviors by providing them with information about health risks and possible effects on pregnancy outcome.
- Provide supportive counseling to aid the family in making changes and help them to build self-esteem and overcome feelings of guilt. Avoid using threatening statements that make them feel guilty.
- Assess patient's immunization record and encourage immunization for rubella if rubella titer is less than 1:10.
- Provide instructions regarding ways to decrease the chance of contracting an infection, such as eating nutritiously, preventing fatigue, avoiding people with infections, cooking meat well, and leaving the cleaning of the litter area of any pet cats or birds to someone else to avoid contact with the toxoplasmosis virus.
- Instruct the pregnant woman to avoid radiographs and medications, especially nonprescription drugs, unless ordered by her obstetrician.
- Make appropriate community referrals to resources that enable implementation of family's goals.

CONCLUSION

Many times, an SAB is nature's way of eliminating a fetus with chromosomal defects. These defects can be caused by an unpreventable, nonrecurring genetic abnormality or by a preventable teratogenic agent. The nurse can lower the incidence of SAB by implementing an education program. This program should include educating about the effects of alcohol, smoking, infections, radiographs, cocaine, and other teratogenic agents on the developing fetus. In these cases and in cases in which the cause is unpreventable, the nurse provides emotional support so that the parents are not left with emotional scars because of anxiety or guilt over their failure to maintain the pregnancy to term.

In some cases, the cause is related to a maternal defect. The nurse should work with the health care team to recognize these cases and then make appropriate referrals to facilitate treatment so that a recurrent abortion does not occur.

BIBLIOGRAPHY

American Academy of Pediatrics (AAP) and American College of Obstetricians and Gynecologists (ACOG): *Guidelines for perinatal care,* ed 5, Washington, DC, 2002. Author.

American College of Obstetricians and Gynecologists: *Management of recurrent early pregnancy loss,* ACOG Practice Bulletin, No. 24, Washington, DC, 2001, ACOG.

Anthony J: Major obstetric hemorrhage disseminated intravascular coagulation. In James D and others, editors: *High risk pregnancy: management options,* ed 3, Philadelphia, 2006, Saunders.

Axelsson G, Ahlborg G Jr, and Bodin L: Shift work, nitrous oxide exposure and spontaneous abortion among Swedish midwives, *Occup Environ Med* 53(6):374–378, 1996.

Brent R, Beckman D: The contribution of environmental teratogens to embryonic and fetal loss, *Clin Obstet Gynecol* 37(3):646–670, 1994.

Bukulmez O, Arici A: Luteal phase defect: myth or reality, *Obstet Gynecol Clin North Am* 31(4):727–744, 2004.

Cabrol D: Cervical distensibility changes in pregnancy, term, and preterm labor, *Semin Perinatol* 15(2):133–139, 1991.

Carter S: Overview of common obstetric bleeding disorders, *Nurs Pract* 24(3):50, 1999.

Cnattingius S and others: Caffeine intake and the risk of first-trimester spontaneous abortion, *N Engl J Med* 343(25):1839–1845, 2000.

Cole K and others: Pregnancy loss through miscarriage or stillbirth. In O'Hara M and others, editors: *Psychological aspects of women's reproductive health,* New York, 1995, Springer.

Cunningham F and others: *Williams' obstetrics,* ed 22, New York, 2005, McGraw-Hill.

Dawood F, Farquharson R, and Quenby S: Recurrent miscarriage, *Curr Obstet Gynaecol* 14:247, 2004.

Fenster L and others: Caffeinated beverages, decaffeinated coffee, and spontaneous abortion, *Epidemiology* 8(5):515–523, 1997.

Floyd R, Decoufle P, and Hungerford D: Alcohol use prior to pregnancy recognition, *Am J Prev Med* 17(2):101–117, 1999.

Forna F, Gülmezoglu AM: Surgical procedures to evacuate incomplete abortion, *Cochrane Database Syst Rev* Issue 1, 2001.

Frost M, Condon J: The psychological sequelae of miscarriage: a critical review of the literature, *Aust N Z J Psychiatry* 30(1):54–62, 1996.

Glueck C and others: Continuing metformin throughout pregnancy in women with polycystic ovary syndrome appears to safely reduce first trimester spontaneous abortion: a pilot study, *Fertil Steril* 75(1):46–52, 2001.

Hill J: Recurrent pregnancy loss. In Creasy R, Resnik R, and Iams J, editors: *Maternal-fetal medicine: principles and practice,* ed 5, Philadelphia, 2004, Saunders.

Huszar G, Walsh M: Relationship between myometrial and cervical functions in pregnancy and labor, *Semin Perinatol* 15(2):97–117, 1991.

Hutti M and others: A study of miscarriage: development and validation of the Perinatal Grief Intensity Scale, *J Obstet Gynecol Neonatal Nurs* 27(5):547–555, 1998.

Iams J: Abnormal cervical competence. In Creasy R, Resnik R, and Iams J, editors: *Maternal-fetal medicine: principles and practice,* ed 5, Philadelphia, 2004, Saunders.

Kaufman R and others: Continued follow-up of pregnancy outcomes in diethylstilbestrol-exposed offspring, *Obstet Gynecol* 96(4):483–489, 2000.

Kovalevsky G and others: Evaluation of the association between hereditary thrombophilias and recurrent pregnancy loss, *Arch Intern Med* 164(5):558–563, 2004.

Lashen H, Fear K, and Sturdee D: Obesity is associated with increased risk of first trimester and recurrent miscarriage: matched case control study, *Hum Reprod* 19(7):1644–1646, 2004.

Lowdermilk D, Perry S: *Maternity and women's health care,* ed 8, St Louis, 2004, Mosby.

Matovina M and others: Possible role of bacterial and viral infections in miscarriages, *Fertil Steril* 81(3):662–669, 2004.

Meroni P and others: Antiphospholipid antibodies as cause of pregnancy loss, *Lupus* 13(9):649–652, 2004.

Naef R, Morrison J: Transfusion therapy in pregnancy, *Clin Obstet Gynecol* 38(3):547–557, 1995.

Neugebauer R and others: Association of stressful life events with chromosomally normal spontaneous abortion, *Am J Epidemiol* 143(6):588–596, 1996.

Nybo, Andersen A and others: Maternal age and fetal loss: population based register linkage study, *BMJ* 320(7251):1708–1712, 2000.

Pietrantoni M, Knuppel R: Alcohol use in pregnancy, *Clin Perinatol* 18(1):93–111, 1991.

Ragusa A and others: Progesterone supplement in pregnancy: an immunologic therapy? *Lupus* 13(9):639–642, 2004.

Rogers J, Davis B: How risky are hot tubs and saunas for pregnant women? *MCN Am J Matern Child Nurs* 20(3):137–140, 1995.

Royal College of Obstetricians and Gynaecologists (RCOG): *The investigation and treatment of couples with recurrent miscarriage,* Guideline No. 17, London, 2003, RCOG Press. Retrieved from *http://www.rcog.org.UK/index.asp?PageID=1042*

Sharara F, Seifer D, and Flaws J: Environmental toxicants and female reproduction, *Fertil Steril* 70(4):613–622, 1998.

Sheiner E and others: Pregnancy outcome following recurrent spontaneous abortions, *Eur J Obstet Gynecol Reprod Biol* 118(1):61–65, 2005.

Silver R, Peltier M, and Branch D: The immunology of pregnancy. In Creasy R, Resnik R, and Iams J, editors: *Maternal-fetal medicine: principles and practice,* ed 5, Philadelphia, 2004, Saunders.

Stern J and others: Frequency of abnormal karyotypes among abortuses for women with and without a history of current spontaneous abortion, *Fertil Steril* 65(2):250–253, 1996.

Weiner C, Buhimschi C: *Drugs for pregnant and lactating women,* Philadelphia, 2004, Churchill Livingstone.

Zilianti M and others: Monitoring the effacement of the uterine cervix by transperineal sonography: a new perspective, *J Ultrasound Med* 14(10):719–724, 1995.

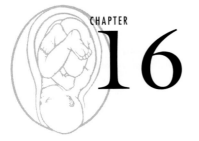

Ectopic Pregnancy

An ectopic pregnancy develops as the result of the blastocyst implanting somewhere other than in the endometrium of the uterus. Sites of an ectopic pregnancy (Fig. 16-1) are the fallopian tube, ovary, cervix, or abdominal cavity. The majority of ectopic pregnancies (95%) are located in the fallopian tube, with 0.5% located on an ovary, 0.3% on the cervix, and 1.5% in the abdominal cavity (Attar, 2004).

Of all tubal ectopic pregnancies, 55% are located in the *ampulla,* or largest portion of the tube. The next most common site is the *isthmus,* or the narrow part of the tube that connects the interstitium to the ampullar portion. Three percent of ectopic pregnancies are located in the *interstitium,* which is the muscular portion of the tube adjacent to the uterine cavity. Rarely does the ectopic pregnancy locate in the *fimbria* or terminal end of the tube (Cunningham and others, 2005; Lozeau and Potter, 2005). The outcome and gestational length of the tubal ectopic pregnancy are influenced by its location in the fallopian tube.

INCIDENCE

The incidence of ectopic pregnancy in the general population is approximately 2% of all pregnancies (Lozeau and Potter, 2005). In a high risk population, the incidence is approximately 1 of every 30 pregnancies (Tenore, 2000). Indicators of high risk are associated with fallopian tube scarring or impaired tubal mobility.

ETIOLOGY
Previous Tubal Infections

Previous pelvic infections caused by certain sexually transmitted diseases such as chlamydia or gonorrhea, postpartum endometritis, and postabortal uterine infections can predispose a woman to tubal infection (ACOG, 1998; Tenore, 2000). A tubal infection can damage the mucosal surface of the fallopian tube, causing intraluminal adhesions and scarring that interfere with tubal motility.

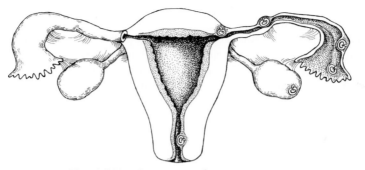

Figure 16-1 Common sites for an ectopic pregnancy.

Previous Tubal or Pelvic Surgery

During surgery, if blood is allowed to enter the fallopian tubes, tubal adhesions can result from the irritation of the mucosal surface. Therefore previous tubal surgery and previous pelvic surgery can cause tubal pregnancies.

Hormonal Factors

Altered estrogen and progesterone levels or inappropriate levels of prostaglandins, oxytocin, or catecholamines can interfere with normal tubal motility of the fertilized ovum.

Contraceptive Failure

Intrauterine devices (IUDs) are 99% effective in decreasing the risk for all pregnancies, including ectopic pregnancies. However, in the event of a pregnancy occurring while an IUD device is in place, there is an increased risk for an ectopic pregnancy. The cause is unknown but may be related to altered tubal motility or a tubal infection.

There does not seem to be an increased risk for ectopic pregnancy with the use of progestin-only contraceptives. However, any pregnancy that occurs due to contraceptive failure is more likely to be ectopic (Hatcher and others, 2004). When the morning-after pill is used and fails, the risk for ectopic pregnancy increases 10 times because the pill has a high estrogen level, which interferes with tubal motility (Cunningham and others, 2005). Of women who become pregnant after tubal ligation, 60% experience an ectopic pregnancy (Marchiano, 2004).

Assisted Reproduction

There is an increased incidence of ectopic pregnancy associated with ovulation-stimulating drugs such as human menopausal gonadotropin and clomiphene citrate. These drugs alter the estrogen and progesterone levels in the woman's body, which can affect tubal motility. There is an increased risk, as well, of an ectopic pregnancy with in vitro fertilization or gamete intrafallopian transfer because underlying tubal damage is frequently one of the factors predisposing a woman to require this type of infertility treatment.

Behavioral Factors

Maternal cigarette smoking at the time of conception has an independent and dose-related effect on the risk for ectopic pregnancy (Attar, 2004). It is thought to affect the ciliary action in the fallopian tubes. Research has also found an increased risk for ectopic pregnancy of six times if a woman has douched for 10 years or more (Kendrick and others, 1997; Pisarska and Carson, 1999; Cunningham and others, 2005).

Transmigration of Ovum

Migration of the ovum from one ovary to the opposite fallopian tube can occur by an extrauterine or intrauterine route. This can delay transportation of the fertilized ovum to the uterus. In this case, trophoblastic tissue is present on the blastocyst before it reaches the uterine cavity; therefore the trophoblastic tissue implants itself on the wall of the fallopian tube.

NORMAL PHYSIOLOGY

The fallopian tube wall is muscular and narrow and contains few ciliated cells at the interstitial area. In the ampullar area, the fallopian tube becomes less muscular, the luminal size increases, and the ciliated cells are more abundant.

The fimbriated end of the fallopian tube serves to pick up the ovum when it is released from the ovary. Then the fallopian tube has the unique function of moving the ovum and sperm in opposite directions almost simultaneously, by *peristaltic* (muscular) contractions and ciliated activity. Two or more adjacent pacemakers in the ampullar and isthmic areas of the fallopian tube initiate this tubal activity by sending out myoelectrical activity in either direction.

The net directional movement in the fallopian tubes varies during the menstrual cycle. During menstruation, the net directional force is toward the uterus starting from the ampullar area to prevent menstrual blood reflux into the tubes (Pulkkinen and Talo, 1987). This is stimulated primarily by estrogen-induced prostaglandins. Just before ovulation, the directional force from the ampullar area is inward, to pick up the released ovum from the ovary and move it into the ampullar area of the fallopian tube. At the same time, the directional force from the uterine area is the opposite, to facilitate sperm mobility toward the ovum (Pulkkinen and Talo, 1987). This is influenced by estrogen primarily. After fertilization, the directional force varies in the ampullar area, which delays ovum transport. Approximately 5 days after ovulation, the net directional force from the middle of the ampullar area is inward through the isthmus, to transport the ovum to the uterus. This is influenced by increasing progesterone and prostaglandin E_2. Approximately 7 days after ovulation, the myoelectrical activity becomes variable again, moving in both directions from each of the pacemakers (Pulkkinen and Talo, 1987).

The fertilized ovum reaches the uterine cavity in 6 to 7 days—just about the time the trophoblast cells begin to secrete the proteolytic enzyme and start to develop the threadlike projections called *chorionic villi*, which initiate the implantation process.

The uterus is normally prepared by estrogen and progesterone to accept the fertilized ovum, now called a *blastocyst*. As the chorionic villi invade the endometrium, the villi are held in check by a fibrinoid zone. The uterus is also supplied with an increased blood supply capable of nourishing the products of conception.

PATHOPHYSIOLOGY
Tubal Ectopic Pregnancy

Because most ectopic pregnancies initially implant in a fallopian tube, the pathophysiology focuses on tubal ectopic pregnancies. The blastocyst burrows into the epithelium of the tubal wall, tapping blood vessels, by the same process as normal implantation into the uterine endometrium.

The environment of the tube, however, is quite different because of the following factors:

- Resistance to the invading trophoblastic tissue by the fallopian tube is decreased.
- Muscle mass lining the fallopian tubes is decreased; therefore their distensibility is greatly limited.
- The blood pressure is much higher in the tubal arteries than in the uterine arteries.
- Decidual reaction is limited; therefore human chorionic gonadotropin (hCG) is decreased and the signs and symptoms of pregnancy are limited.

It is because of these characteristic factors that termination of a tubal pregnancy occurs gestationally early by an abortion, spontaneous regression, or rupture, depending on the gestational age and the location of the implantation (Table 16-1). If the embryo dies early in gestation, spontaneous regression often occurs. If spontaneous regression fails to occur, usually an ampullar or fimbriated tubal pregnancy ends in an abortion and an isthmic or interstitial pregnancy ends in a rupture (Cunningham and others, 2005).

A tubal abortion (Fig. 16-2) occurs primarily because of separation of all or part of the placenta. This separation is caused by the pressure exerted by the tapped blood vessels or tubal contractions. With complete separation, the products of conception are expelled into the abdominal cavity by way of the fimbriated end of the fallopian tube, and unless there is an injured blood vessel, the bleeding stops. With an incomplete separation, bleeding continues until complete

Table 16-1   Tubal Pregnancy

Type	Duration (weeks)	Usual Method of Termination
Ampullar	6–12	Tubal abortion
Fimbriated	6–12	Tubal abortion
Isthmic	6–8	Tubal rupture
Interstitial	12–14	Tubal rupture startle response

separation takes place, and the blood flows into the abdominal cavity, collecting in the rectouterine cul-de-sac of Douglas.

Tubal rupture (Fig. 16-3) results from the uninterrupted invasion of the trophoblastic tissue or tearing of the extremely stretched tissue. In either case, the products of conception are completely or incompletely expelled into the abdominal cavity or between the folds of the broad ligaments by way of the torn tube.

The duration of the tubal pregnancy depends on the location of the implanted embryo or fetus and the distensibility of that part of the fallopian tube. For instance, if the implantation is located in the narrow isthmic portion of the tube, it ruptures early, within 6 to 8 weeks; the distensible interstitial portion may be able to retain the pregnancy up to 14 weeks. An ampullar or fimbriated tubal pregnancy is usually lost between 6 and 12 weeks of gestation.

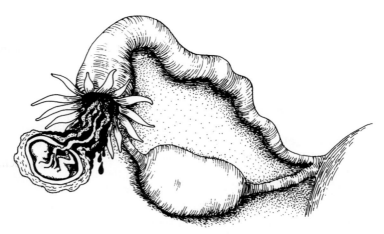

Figure 16-2 Tubal abortion.

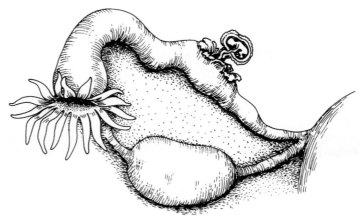

Figure 16-3 Tubal rupture.

The outcome of the pregnancy at the time of the interruption depends on the age of the embryo or fetus and whether the rupture is complete or incomplete. In rare cases, when the abortion occurs very early in the pregnancy and the placenta is initially separated completely from the tubal wall, the trophoblastic tissue reimplants in the abdominal cavity and the placenta and embryo or fetus will continue to grow. This leads to the development of a secondary abdominal pregnancy. Usually only a small amount of blood is lost at this time.

If the rupture is incomplete, in rare cases, the ruptured part of the placenta reattaches to some surrounding abdominal tissue. This leads to the development of a tuboabdominal, tuboovarian, or broad ligament pregnancy. In most instances, however, the embryo or fetus dies at the time of the abortion or rupture. If not surgically removed, it can be absorbed if small or, if too large to be absorbed, it can mummify or calcify. When the bleeding is slight, no problems result. However, in most cases blood vessels are torn open and bleeding is profuse. This blood and the lost products of conception collect in the cul-de-sac of Douglas, causing severe pain and hypovolemia. A real emergency is present, which can end in maternal death if the bleeding is not quickly stopped.

Abdominal Ectopic Pregnancy

An abdominal pregnancy almost always results from an implantation secondary to a tubal rupture or abortion through the fimbriated end of the fallopian tube. In these cases, the placenta continues to grow after attachment to some abdominal structure, usually the surface of the uterus, broad ligaments, or ovaries. However, it can be any abdominal structure, including the liver, spleen, or intestines. Because the invading trophoblastic tissue is not held in check, it can erode major blood vessels at any time and cause severe bleeding. Fetal movements are also painful because they are not cushioned by the myometrium.

Cervical Ectopic Pregnancy

In very rare cases, the fertilized ovum bypasses the uterine endometrium and implants itself in the cervical mucus. Accelerated migration of the blastocyst through the uterus caused by an intrauterine device or changes in the endometrial lining as the result of prior curettage or endometrial inflammation are possible contributing factors (Leeman and Wendland, 2000). Because the uterine artery gains entry to the uterus by way of the cervix, there is an abundant blood supply to a cervical ectopic pregnancy and tremendous bleeding can ensue when removal is attempted.

SIGNS AND SYMPTOMS
Before Rupture

Currently, most ectopic pregnancies are diagnosed before rupture based on the three most classic symptoms: abdominal pain, delayed menses, and abnormal vaginal bleeding (spotting) that occurs 6 to 8 weeks after the last normal menstrual period.

Abdominal Pain

Abdominal pain occurs nearly 100% of the time. It is usually first manifested by a dull, lower quadrant, unilateral pain caused by tubal stretching; this is followed by a sharp, colicky tubal pain caused by further tubal stretching and stimulated contractions. It progresses to a diffuse, constant, severe pain generalized throughout the lower abdomen (Lipscomb, Stovall, and Ling, 2000).

Delayed Menses

A history of a period that is delayed approximately 1 to 2 weeks or a lighter than usual or irregular period is reported by 75% to 90% of the patients (Della-Giustina and Denny, 2003).

Abnormal Vaginal Bleeding

Mild to intermittent dark red or brown vaginal discharge occurs in 79% of the cases related to uterine decidual shedding secondary to decreased hormones such as progesterone and hCG (Tay and others, 2000).

Absence of Common Signs of Pregnancy

Absence of common signs of pregnancy is secondary to decreased pregnancy hormonal levels frequently occurs (Cahill and Wandle, 2006).

Abdominal Tenderness

Abdominal tenderness occurs in more than 91% of the cases (Tay and others, 2000).

Palpable Pelvic Mass

A pelvic mass is palpable in approximately 20% of the cases (Cunningham and others, 2005).

Tubal Rupture

Exacerbation of the pain occurs during tubal rupture in an ectopic pregnancy.

After Tubal Rupture

Generalized, Unilateral, or Deep Lower Quadrant Acute Abdominal Pain

Abdominal pain is caused by blood irritating the peritoneum.

Referred Shoulder Pain

Referred shoulder pain is related to diaphragmatic irritation from blood in the peritoneal cavity.

Faintness and Dizziness

Faintness and dizziness occur in the presence of significant bleeding.

Signs of Shock

Shock is related to the severity of the bleeding into the abdomen.

Afebrile State

In the beginning, usually no signs of an infection are present.

MATERNAL EFFECTS

Ectopic pregnancies account for 10% to 15% of all pregnancy-related maternal deaths (Della-Giustina and Denny, 2004; Cunningham, 2005). They are the leading cause of maternal mortality, but they are the number-one cause of maternal mortality in the first trimester of pregnancy (CDC, 2000). Hemorrhage is the major cause of death and occurs most frequently with a cervical or abdominal ectopic pregnancy. Infection and anesthesia complications are infrequent causes of death.

FETAL AND NEONATAL EFFECTS

Death is almost certain for the fetus in an ectopic pregnancy. About 5% of abdominal ectopic pregnancies reach viability (Tasnim and Mahmud, 2005). However, it is not recommended to continue an abdominal pregnancy if it is diagnosed early because of the extreme risk for hemorrhage at any time during the pregnancy. The risk for fetal deformity is also high related to pressure deformities caused by oligohydramnios.

DIAGNOSTIC TESTING

Diagnosis before extrauterine rupture or abortion can minimize tubal damage, decrease maternal mortality from hemorrhage, and simplify management of an ectopic pregnancy. However, because this condition mimics other diseases (Table 16-2) and no one diagnostic tool is specific for detecting an early ectopic gestation, early diagnosis is difficult.

A pertinent history and physical examination are the foundations for initiating an appropriate diagnostic workup that results in the accurate and timely diagnosis of an ectopic pregnancy. Physical findings can include a normal or slightly enlarged uterus, palpable adnexal mass in 50% of tubal ectopic pregnancies, and cervical motion tenderness 50% of the time as well. The most important diagnostic tools are serial hCG levels, and transvaginal ultrasound (TVU). For a summary of the diagnostic test results and interpretation, see Table 16-3.

Serial Serum Beta-Human Chorionic Gonadotropin Levels

The fertilized ovum and the chorionic villi produce hCG, which maintains the corpus luteum to produce progesterone and estrogen. This maintains the pregnancy until the placenta is mature enough to assume that role at around 10 weeks of gestation. In a normal pregnancy, hCG is present in detectable

Text continued on p. 371

Table 16-2   Pelvic Pain: Differential Diagnosis

	Appendicitis	Cholelithiasis During Pregnancy	Ectopic (Unruptured or Ruptured*)	Ovarian Cyst	Pelvic Inflammatory Disease	Spontaneous Abortion
Chief complaint	Abdominal pain	Abdominal pain Associated flatulence	Abdominal pain	Lower abdominal or pelvic pain	Lower abdominal and pelvic pain	Cramping with or without vaginal bleeding
Workup of associated symptoms						
P: Provoked What causes the symptoms? What makes symptoms better or worse?		Pain associated with high-fat meal	Sex and activity increase symptoms	Increased with movement, especially when standing or stooping		
Q: Quality or Quantity How does the pain feel?	Steady ache or colicky	Lancinating, cramping, colicky, or steady up to 1 hr	Dull pain/*deep acute abdominal pain*	Dull	Tender	Crampy
R: Region or Radiation Where are the symptoms? Do symptoms spread?	Usually generalized or unilateral RLQ	Originating in midportion of epigastrium, radiating to back, chest, shoulders	Unilateral or bilateral lower quadrant/ *generalized deep/ referred shoulder pain related to diaphragmatic*	Unilateral	Lower bilateral abdominal or pelvic pain radiating to lower back or down one or	Pressure pain, generalized or localized in the lower abdomen

			severe			
How severe are the symptoms?						
T: Timing When did the symptoms begin? Associated with menses?	Sudden onset	Abrupt onset pain	Continuous or intermittent		Frequently after onset or cessation of menses	
Review of symptoms (ROS)	Anorexia N/V preceded by pain Low-grade fever (100.2°–100.6°F)	Flatulence, bloating/ indigestion Anorexia N/V Pain associated with high-fat meals	Delayed menses/ amenorrhea Absence of common signs of pregnancy Urinary frequency After rupture: vertigo/ fainting Decreased BP and increased pulse, if bleeding is continuous and rapid	N/V Amenorrhea Possible fever	Possible vaginal discharge, dysuria, dyspareunia, menstrual abnormality Anorexia N/V Possible high fever Positive signs of high risk sexual behaviors	Vaginal bleeding Any sign of shock equal to obvious bleeding

Continued

Table 16-2   Pelvic Pain: Differential Diagnosis—cont'd

	Appendicitis	Cholelithiasis During Pregnancy	Ectopic (Unruptured or Ruptured*)	Ovarian Cyst	Pelvic Inflammatory Disease	Spontaneous Abortion
Complete physical examination	RLQ tenderness at McBurney's point Abdominal guarding/ muscular rigidity on palpation Rebound tenderness Positive iliopsoas and obturator test	Localized abdominal tenderness on palpation Positive Murphy sign	Lower abdominal tenderness on palpation *After rupture: severe generalized abdominal tenderness*		**Lower abdominal bilateral tenderness with deep and light palpation	No abdominal tenderness
Pelvic examination	No vaginal discharge Rectal examination may increase pain		Dark red or brown vaginal discharge Cervix and uterus slightly soft to palpation Positive CMT Positive adnexal mass	Tenderness with pelvic examination Enlarged ovaries palpated 50% of the time Unilateral adnexal mass with tenderness	Positive BUS Purulent vaginal discharge Cultures may be increased for gonorrhea/ Chlamydia **Positive CMT **Positive adnexal tenderness Palpable adnexal if abscess is	Cervix closed or dilated Vaginal bleeding mild to severe Negative CMT Negative adnexal mass

polymorphonuclear leukocytosis

May use high-resolution, real-time ultra-sonography

phosphates elevated

Abdominal ultrasound may indicate stones

ultrasound to reveal ectopic mass or a uterine sac

Positive hCG levels that do not double in 48 hr

Progesterone levels less than 8 mg/ml

transvaginal ultrasound should demonstrate the cyst

C-reactive protein elevated

WBC elevated with left shift

Pelvic or transvaginal ultrasound

CT scan may indicate a thickened fluid-filled tube

Endometrial biopsy

Laparoscopy

ultrasound

Quantitative hCG

*Signs and symptoms of ruptured ectopic pregnancy are in *italics*.

**Minimum criteria for diagnosis.

BP, Blood pressure; *BUS,* Bartholin, urethral, scene glands; *CBC,* complete blood count; *CMT,* cervical motion tenderness; *ERS,* erythrocyte; *N/V,* nausea and vomiting; *RLQ,* right lower quadrant; *RUQ,* right upper quadrant; *WBC* white blood cells.

Table 16-3   Diagnostic Tests

Test	Results	Interpretations
Serum progesterone	Greater than 25 ng/ml	Normal intrauterine pregnancy (except after ovarian stimulation)
	Greater than 5 ng/ml but less than 25 ng/ml	Undetermined viability
	Less than 5 ng/ml	Nonviable; may indicate ectopic pregnancy or a spontaneous abortion
Beta-hCG	Detected in the serum 8–10 days after fertilization	Normal intrauterine pregnancy
	Levels normally double every 36–48 hours for the first 5–8 weeks after conception	
	Levels at about 4.5 weeks (50–250 mIU/ml)	
	Levels at about 6.5 weeks (10,000 mIU/ml)	
	Levels peak at 8–10 weeks (100,000–150,000 mIU/ml)	
	After 10-week start, decreasing sharply	
	Prolonged doubling time of hCG levels may indicate an ectopic pregnancy or a spontaneous abortion	May indicate an ectopic pregnancy or a spontaneous abortion
	Levels plateau at around 6 weeks	Predictive of ectopic pregnancy
	Extremely high levels	Hydatidiform mole or multiple gestation
Transvaginal ultrasound	Visible intrauterine fetal sac after hCG levels are greater than 1500–2000 mIU/ml	Normal intrauterine pregnancy, 5–6 weeks of gestation
	Pulsating fetal heart within the intrauterine sac	Normal intrauterine pregnancy, 6.5–7.0 weeks of gestation
	No fetal heart action within the intrauterine sac after 7 weeks	Spontaneous abortion
	Absence of intrauterine sac with hCG greater than 1500–2000	Ectopic pregnancy
	Pseudogestational sac without fetus found in uterus or fetal sac found in tubes	Ectopic pregnancy

hCG, Human chorionic gonadotropin.

levels (greater than 2 mIU/ml) in the maternal serum 8 to 10 days after fertilization. Levels normally double every 48 hours for the first 5 to 8 weeks after conception, rising well above 100,000 mIU/ml and then gradually decreasing after 10 weeks. In an ectopic or spontaneous abortion, hCG levels rise slower than normal and usually plateau at about 6 weeks below 6000 mIU/ml (Lipscomb, Stovall, and Ling, 2000). A consistently decreasing hCG level indicates a nonviable pregnancy (ACOG, 1998). Thus serial hCG levels 48 hours apart aid in the differentiation between a normal and an abnormal pregnancy.

Transvaginal Ultrasound

The usefulness of ultrasound in the diagnosis of an ectopic pregnancy is increasing continuously. In the past, ultrasound was useful only in diagnosing an intrauterine pregnancy, which would rule out an ectopic pregnancy. One exception was in the case of an advanced abdominal pregnancy. In these cases, ultrasound would show a fetal head outside the uterus.

TVU is becoming an important diagnostic tool in diagnosing ectopic pregnancy before rupture because the probe can be placed closer to the pelvic structures. With the more sophisticated real-time equipment and an expert technician, all normal pregnancies should be seen by TVU by 3 to 4 weeks after fertilization. When hCG levels are 1500 to 2000 mIU/ml or greater, a normal intrauterine pregnancy should be visible with TVU (Lemus, 2000). Therefore when hCG levels are greater than 1500 mIU/ml with no visible intrauterine pregnancy, ectopic pregnancy is very likely (Lozeau and Potter, 2005). With TVU, the location of the gestational sac of an early ectopic pregnancy can be visualized only 20% of the time (Sherbahn, 2001). If an ectopic sac is identified, it is measured for size and attempts are made to determine any fetal cardiac activity. This determines which therapy is used.

In 10% to 20% of ectopic pregnancies, a "pseudosac" produced by decidual reaction in the uterus is seen and can be confused with an intrauterine gestation. A corpus luteum cyst can be confused as an adnexal mass indicating an ectopic pregnancy as well. Any mass seen on ultrasound must contain a yolk sac, fetal pole, or fetal cardiac activity to indicate a pregnancy (Lipscomb, Stovall, and Ling, 2000).

Serum Progesterone Levels

Serum progesterone levels are used in combination with hCG levels and TVU to determine who needs further testing. In a normal pregnancy, the corpus luteum produces an increased amount of progesterone for the first 8 to 10 weeks. Then the placenta takes over the production of progesterone. Serum progesterone levels above 25 ng/ml most often indicate a normal intrauterine pregnancy. In an ectopic pregnancy, progesterone levels are usually decreased to lower than 5 ng/ml (Buster and Heard, 2000). Values between 5 and 25 ng/ml are not conclusive and indicate the need for further testing (Buster and Heard, 2000). If the woman had medication-induced ovarian stimulation, these values may not be applicable.

Curettage

There is no research evidence to support the use of curettage as a diagnostic tool (McCollum, 2001; Tulandi and Sammour, 2000).

USUAL MEDICAL MANAGEMENT

Tubal Ectopic Pregnancy Before Rupture

Surgical Treatment

The type of surgical management depends on the location and cause of the ectopic pregnancy, the extent of tissue involvement, and the patient's wishes for future fertility. The choice of treatment for an unruptured tubal pregnancy is a laparoscopic salpingostomy, in which a longitudinal incision is made over the pregnancy site and the products of conception are gently and very carefully removed to prevent or control the bleeding (Hajenius and others, 2001). The fallopian tube incision is allowed to close by secondary intention.

To rule out persistent trophoblastic growth, follow-up treatment includes serial hCG levels. Usually, hCG is undetectable by the twelfth postsurgical day.

Nonsurgical Medical Treatment

A well-studied medical therapy in the treatment of an ectopic pregnancy is methotrexate. Methotrexate, a type of chemotherapy, is a folic acid antagonist that interferes with DNA synthesis and cell multiplication, causing dissolution of the ectopic mass (Lipscomb and others, 1999; Tulandi, 1999; Lozeau and Potter, 2005). Criteria for its use follow:

- Hemodynamically stable with no signs of severe abdominal pain, weakness, dizziness, syncope, orthostatic hypotension, tachycardia, or falling hematocrit
- Ectopic sac smaller than 3 to 5 cm in diameter
- Fetus not alive as indicated by any cardiac activity
- Serum hCG levels lower than 5000 mIU/ml
- Liver function studies within normal limits
- Normal kidney function as indicated by normal serum creatinine and blood urea nitrogen (BUN)
- No evidence of peptic ulcer disease or ulcerative colitis
- No evidence of leukopenia (blood leukocytes greater than 3500/mm^3)
- No evidence of thrombocytopenia (platelet count greater than 100,000/mm^3)
- No evidence of AIDS due to additive immunosuppressive effects
  Protocols for methotrexate therapy include single-dose and multiple-dose regimens.
- Single-dose method: Methotrexate 50 mg per square meter of body surface intramuscularly. Repeat dose if beta-hCG levels have not dropped at least 15% between day 4 and day 7.
- Multiple-dose method: methotrexate, 1 mg/kg intramuscularly every other day (even days) and leucovorin, 0.1 mg/kg intramuscularly every other day (odd

days), until beta-hCG levels drop at least 15% in a 48-hour period; or maximum of four doses each (Lozeau and Potter, 2005). Hajenius and others (2001) concluded, on the basis of a Cochrane Review, that medical treatment with systemic methotrexate in a multiple-dose intramuscular regimen is as effective as laparoscopic surgery for a small, unruptured ectopic pregnancy.

Mifepristone, an antiprogesterone, used with methotrexate is being studied (Barnhart, Gosman, Ashby, and Sammel, 2003). Follow-up continues until β-hCG levels are nondetectable. Average resolution of the ectopic pregnancy is 7 weeks, but it can take anywhere from 35 to 109 days.

Surgical intervention may be necessary if any of the following occurs to the patient:
- Experiences worsening abdominal pain indicating tubal rupture
- Becomes hemodynamic unstable
- β-hCG levels increase, plateau, or fail to decline 15% by day 7

Tubal Ectopic Pregnancy After Rupture

After a ruptured tubal pregnancy, a *laparotomy salpingectomy* (removal of the affected fallopian tube) is the most common surgical treatment. Occasionally, a *salpingo-oophorectomy* (removal of the affected fallopian tube and adjacent ovary) is performed if the blood supply to the ovary is affected or if the ectopic pregnancy involved the ovary. Otherwise, preservation of the ovary is recommended. If the couple does not wish to have more children, a hysterectomy may be done if the woman's condition is stable.

Abdominal Ectopic Pregnancy

For an abdominal pregnancy, hemorrhage is a serious possibility because the placenta can separate from its attachment site at any time. Abdominal surgery to remove the embryo or fetus is usually done as soon as an abdominal pregnancy is diagnosed. Unless the placenta is attached to abdominal structures that can be removed, such as the ovary or exterior of the uterus, or the blood vessels that supply blood to the placenta can be ligated, the placenta is left without being disturbed (Daiter, 2001). If the placenta were removed, large blood vessels would be opened and there would not be a constricting muscle such as the uterus to apply a sealing pressure.

If the placenta is left intact, the body usually absorbs it, although it may cause such complications as infection, abscesses, adhesions, intestinal obstruction, paralytic ileus, postpartum preeclampsia, and wound dehiscence. However, these complications are less life-threatening than the hemorrhage that could result if the placenta were removed. Medical treatment can be used as primary or supplementary treatment for residual placental tissue.

Cervical Ectopic Pregnancy

Because of the risks of uncontrollable hemorrhage and urinary tract injury, surgical management is the last alternative treatment for a cervical ectopic pregnancy. Methotrexate is being successfully used. The agent is injected directly into the gestational sac or given systematically as outlined earlier (Leeman and Wendland, 2000). If methotrexate is contraindicated and surgical management is necessary, several methods are used to diminish the risk for hemorrhage. Such treatments include a cerclage and local injection of vasopressin before evacuation, inflation of a 30 ml Foley catheter bulb in the cervix, and vaginal packing after curettage, or potassium chloride injection into the gestational sac (Lemus, 2000).

NURSING MANAGEMENT

Prevention

An ectopic pregnancy is closely associated with tubal scarring. Preventing tubal scarring is the key to prevention of an ectopic pregnancy. Discussing safe sex practices that prevent sexually transmitted infection should be a routine part of well-woman care. Screening for chlamydia and gonorrhea should be included in the yearly gynecologic examination for at-risk women because they often have no symptoms. A sexually transmitted infection should be treated to prevent pelvic inflammatory disease (PID). If PID does develop, rapid treatment can decrease the chance of tubal scarring. When a woman chooses an IUD, descriptions of the signs of PID should be included in the teaching.

If pregnancy occurs while the woman has an IUD in place, ectopic pregnancy should be considered because it is more likely to occur. Because a correlation exists between cigarette smoking and an increased risk for an ectopic pregnancy, women during their childbearing years should be encouraged to avoid smoking. If an elective abortion is desired, only medically prepared professionals should perform it. These measures decrease the chance of tubal defects and thereby decrease the incidence of an ectopic pregnancy. Because of the increasing incidence of ectopic pregnancy, health professionals should consider the possibility in any woman who presents with any type of abdominal discomfort during her childbearing years.

Assessment

Because of the high maternal mortality associated with an ectopic pregnancy that goes undiagnosed until after rupture or tubal abortion, it is essential for nurses to be alert to signs and symptoms of this pregnancy complication. Therefore any woman in her childbearing years who experiences irregular vaginal spotting associated with a dull, aching pelvic pain, with or without signs of pregnancy, should be evaluated for a possible ectopic pregnancy. The following areas should be explored:

Risk Factors

A history of any PID, previous ectopic pregnancies, elective abortions, or prior infertility disorders is determined; these conditions can increase the patient's risk for a tubal defect.

Pain

If an ectopic pregnancy is suspected, a detailed history includes questions regarding the type of abdominal pain. The pain caused by an unruptured ectopic pregnancy can be a unilateral, cramplike pain related to tubal distention by the enlarging embryo or fetus. At the time of tubal rupture, many patients experience a sudden, sharp, stabbing pain in the lower abdomen. Blood in the peritoneum can cause a dull aching or severe, generalized pain. If the blood touches the diaphragm, it usually causes referred shoulder pain. Many times, movement of the body aggravates the pain.

Vaginal Bleeding

Assess for vaginal bleeding, and obtain a menstrual history. Vaginal bleeding is usually related to the sloughing of the endometrial lining related to decreasing progesterone and estrogen levels and can be continuous or intermittent in small or large quantities. It usually differs from the patient's normal period. Pad counts should be kept to determine the amount and type of vaginal bleeding.

Syncope

Assess for the presence of any signs of syncope. When an ectopic pregnancy ruptures or aborts, blood is lost into the peritoneal cavity. At this time, the patient can experience a feeling of faintness or weakness related to hypovolemia. If the bleeding is not continuous, the depleted blood volume is restored to near normal in 1 or 2 days by hemodilution, and the faint or weak feeling subsides. If the bleeding is profuse, the patient can go into shock quickly.

Vital Signs

To assess the amount of intraperitoneal blood loss, the patient's vital signs should be checked as frequently as the situation indicates.

Nursing Interventions to Allay Fear Regarding Possible Diagnosis

- Assess family's anxiety over maternal well-being because 10% to 15% of pregnancy-related deaths are caused by ectopic pregnancy (Della-Giustina and Denny, 2003).
- Assess family's level of guilt (e.g., their feeling as to what they did to cause this to happen).
- Assess family's coping strategies and resources.
- Explain all diagnostic and treatment modalities and reasons for each in understandable terms.
- Prepare patient for serial beta-hCG levels, progesterone levels, or TVU. If a TVU diagnostic procedure is ordered, have patient empty her bladder before the procedure.
- Prepare patient for the medical or surgical procedure.

Postoperative Nursing Interventions

- Tell patient that the incidence of persistent trophoblastic tissue growth following laparoscopic salpingostomy is 5% to 10% (Daiter, 2001).

- Prepare patient for weekly hCG levels until results are negative. If levels increase or plateau, be prepared for methotrexate therapy.
- Validate with the couple that this is a loss of a pregnancy and it is acceptable to grieve over the loss.
- If mother is Rh-negative and unsensitized, be prepared to administer Rho (D) immune globulin. The usual dose is Rho (D) immune globulin Standard dose (RhoGAM; HypRho-D) IM 300 microgram if the gestational age is greater than 12 weeks or gestation unknown; for a gestation of 12 weeks or less, the usual dose is Rho (D) Globulin Microdose (HypRho-D MiniDose, MicRhoGAM) IM 50 microgram.

NURSING INTERVENTIONS FOR MEDICAL MANAGEMENT

- Review how the medication or medications work. Be prepared to discuss the risks and benefits of this type of management. Benefits include a 80% to 90% success rate (Weiner and Buhimschi, 2004), cost effectiveness, noninvasive outpatient management, and 83% preservation of tubal patency. Risks include long resolution time (average time 7 weeks, but range between 35 and 109 days), limitations in physical functioning, less energy, possible discomfort, and possible tubal rupture.
- Prepare patient for possible increase in adnexal discomfort or pain related to tubal absorption or tubal distention caused by the formation of a hematoma, which usually lasts 4 to 12 hours, sometime between 5 and 10 days after initial dose of medication. Tubal rupture, however, must be considered and ruled out in the presence of severe or significant change in discomfort.
- Teach the patient appropriate pain management, such as ibuprofen 800 mg every 6 hours. Advise patients to avoid using aspirin and some antiinflammatory drugs such as ibuprofen (Motrin), naproxen (Aleve; Naprosyn), and indomethacin; they worsen the gastrointestinal side effects of the treatment.
- Explain that side effects such as nausea, vomiting, transient stomatitis, oral ulcers, and diarrhea occur in about 5% of cases.
- Provide emotional support for patient and her family.
- Be prepared to obtain baseline levels such as a complete blood cell count and chemistry profile with liver enzymes and renal function studies including BUN and creatinine, platelet count, blood type, and Rh factor.
- Prepare patient as to the importance of follow-up that includes hCG titers until they reach zero because of continued inflammation of the ectopic site until resolution of the ectopic pregnancy is complete.
- Teach patient the importance of refraining from alcohol consumption, vitamin supplements with folic acid (including prenatal vitamin), and sexual intercourse until the ectopic pregnancy is resolved to decrease the risk for medication side effects or exacerbating the rupture of the ectopic pregnancy.
- Teach patient to report signs of ectopic rupture immediately, such as severe, sharp, stabbing, unilateral abdominal pain.

- Encourage patient to avoid sun exposure related to the photosensitivity of the drug during treatment.
- Validate with the couple that this is a loss of a pregnancy and that it is acceptable to grieve over the loss.

Nursing Interventions for Anticipatory Grieving

- Assess level of loss and desire for future childbearing.
- Encourage the patient and her family to express their feelings and concerns openly.
- Discuss with the patient and family the chances of recurrence (15%) and infertility problems (40% to 50%) (Sherbahn, 2001).
- Teach the couple the importance of using a contraceptive for at least three menstrual cycles to allow time for the woman's body to recover.
- Refer to a support group, such as Resolve Through Sharing, if available (a comprehensive, passionate Internet resource can be found at *http://www.ectopicpregnancy.com*).
- Refer to a pastor, priest, or chaplain per family's request for spiritual assistance.
- See Chapter 7 for additional interventions.

CONCLUSION

The ultimate goal for nursing intervention is prevention of complications that can cause tubal or uterine defects. These complications set the stage for an ectopic pregnancy. If an ectopic pregnancy develops, the goal is to prevent complications during the treatment. Therefore efforts are best directed at prevention of future impairment of fertility through patient education. Education should include information for self-detection of signs of infections contributing to ectopic pregnancy. Efforts should also be directed at detecting and reporting early signs of an ectopic pregnancy so that diagnosis before a rupture or abortion can be made. Thus the complication of hemorrhage, which is the major cause of maternal death, can be prevented.

BIBLIOGRAPHY

American College of Obstetrics and Gynecology (ACOG): *Medical management of tubal pregnancy,* Practice Bulletin, No. 3, Washington, DC, 1998, ACOG.

Atrash H and others: Maternal mortality in the United States, 1979–1986, *Obstet Gynecol* 76(6):1055–1060, 1990.

Attar E: Endocrinology of ectopic pregnancy, *Obstet Gynecol Clin North Am* 31:779–794, 2004.

Barnhart K and others: The medical management of ectopic pregnancy: a meta-analysis comparing "single dose" and "multidose" regimens, *Obstet Gynecol* 101(4):778–784, 2003.

Buster J, Heard M: Current issues in medical management of ectopic pregnancy, *Curr Opin Obstet Gynecol* 12(6):525–527, 2000.

Cahill D, Wardle P: Bleeding pain in early pregnancy. In James D and others, editors: *High risk pregnancy: management options,* ed 3, Philadelphia, 2006, Saunders.

Centers for Disease Control and Prevention: *Fact sheet: risk of ectopic pregnancy after tubal sterilization,* Washington, DC, 2000, CDC. Retrieved from *http://www.cdc.gov/nccdphp/drh/mh_ectopic.htm*

Cunningham F and others: *Williams' obstetrics,* ed 22, New York, 2005, McGraw-Hill.

Daiter E: Ectopic pregnancy: overview, *OBGYN.net Publications*, 2001. Retrieved from *http://www. obgyn.net*.

Della-Giustina D, Denny M: Ectopic pregnancy, *Emerg Med Clin North Am* 21:565–584, 2003.

Eddy L, Hricko J: Introduction to differential diagnosis in management of abdominal pain across the life span, *Am J Nurse Pract* 5(3):10, 2001.

Hajenius P and others: Interventions for tubal ectopic pregnancy (Cochrane Review). In *The Cochrane Library*, Issue 4, 2001, Oxford, Update Software.

Hatcher R and others: *Contraceptive technology*, ed 18, New York, 2004, Irvington Publishers.

Kendrick J and others: Vaginal douching and the risk of ectopic pregnancy among black women, *Am J Obstet Gynecol* 176(5):991–997, 1997.

Leeman L, Wendland C: Cervical ectopic pregnancy: Diagnosis with endovaginal ultrasound examination and successful treatment with methotrexate, *Arch Fam Med* 9(1):72–77, 2000.

Lemus J: Ectopic pregnancy: an update, *Curr Opin Obstet Gynecol* 12(5):369–375, 2000.

Lipscomb G, Stovall T, and Ling F: Nonsurgical treatment of ectopic pregnancy, *N Engl J Med* 343(18):1325–1329, 2000.

Lipscomb G and others: Predictors of success of methotrexate treatment in women with tubal ectopic pregnancies, *N Engl J Med* 341(26):1974–1978, 1999.

Lozeau A, Potter B: Diagnosis and management of ectopic pregnancy, *Am Fam Physician* 72(9):1707–1714, 2005.

Marchiano D: Medical Encyclopedia: ectopic pregnancy, *MedlinePlus*, Washington, DC, 2004, American Accreditation Health Care Commission.

McCollum J: Diagnostic curettage in the evaluation of ectopic pregnancy, *Am Fam Physician* 63(2):220–225, 2001.

Pisarska M, Carson S: Incidence and risk factors for ectopic pregnancy, *Clin Obstet Gynecol* 42(1):2–8, 1999.

Pulkkinen M, Talo A: Tubal physiologic consideration in ectopic pregnancy, *Clin Obstet Gynecol* 30(1):164–172, 1987.

Royal College of Obstetricians and Gynaecologists (RCOG): *The management of tubal pregnancy*, Guideline, No. 21, London, 2004, RCOG Press. Retrieved from *http://www.rcog.org.uk/index. asp?PageID=1042*

Sherbahn R: *Ectopic pregnancy*, Gurnee, Ill, 2001, Advanced Fertility Center of Chicago. Retrieved from *http://www.advancedfertility.com/ectopic.htm*

Tasnim N, Mahmud G: *Evidence based report: advanced abdominal pregnancy—a diagnostic management dilemma*, PIMS, Islamabad, 2005, Department of Obstetrics and Gynacology. Retrieved from *http://www.cpsp.edu.pk/jcpsp/ARCHIEVE/Aug2005Article10pdf*

Tay J, Moore J, and Walker J: Ectopic pregnancy, *West J Med* 173(2):131–134, 2000.

Tenore J: Ectopic pregnancy, *Am Fam Physician* 61(4):1080–1088, 2000.

Tulandi T: Current protocol for ectopic pregnancy, *Contemp Obstet Gynecol* 44:42, 1999.

Tulandi T, Sammour A: Evidence-based management of ectopic pregnancy, *Curr Opin Obstet Gynecol* 12(4):289–292, 2000.

Weiner C, Buhimschi C: *Drugs for pregnant and lactating women*, Philadelphia, 2004, Churchill Livingstone.

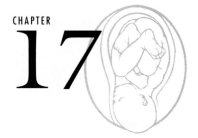

CHAPTER

17

Gestational Trophoblastic Disease

G
estational trophoblastic disease is a spectrum of pregnancy-related trophoblastic proliferative disorders without a viable fetus. The benign hydatidiform mole represents the beginning of the disease continuum, and metastatic gestational trophoblastic neoplasia (GTN) is at the end of the continuum. Malignant nonmetastatic (invasive) GTN is somewhere in the middle when the trophoblastic invades the myometrium only.

HYDATIDIFORM MOLE

A hydatidiform mole is a benign proliferative growth of the trophoblast in which the chorionic villi develop into edematous, cystic, avascular, transparent vesicles that hang in a grapelike cluster (Fig. 17-1). There are two categories of hydatidiform moles: complete and partial.

Complete Moles

- Generalized areas of the chorionic villi become hyperplastic, edematous, and avascular.
- There is no embryo or fetus and amniotic sac.
- A diploid karyotype is present that is most often a 46,XX chromosomal pattern of paternal origin; a sperm with 23,X chromosomes duplicates itself because it fertilizes an ovum that contains no genetic material or the genetic material is inactive (ACOG, 2004). Occasionally (6% to 10% of the time) the karyotype is 46, XY. In these cases, two sperm have fertilized an ovum without genetic material (Bentley, 2003; ACOG, 2004).

Partial Moles

- Localized areas of chorionic villi become hyperplastic, edematous, and avascular.
- There is an embryo or fetus and an amniotic sac, usually with multiple congenital anomalies.
- A triploid karyotype of 69,XXY, 69,XXX, or 69,XYY chromosomes is present in most of the cases: one set of chromosomes of maternal origin

379

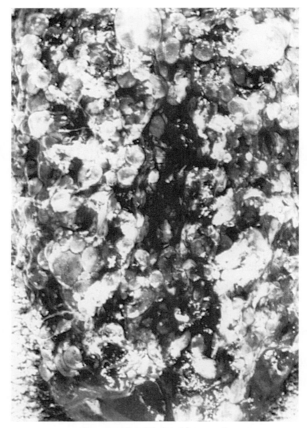

Figure 17-1 Hydatidiform mole.

and two sets of paternal origin. In these cases, two sperm have fertilized an apparently normal ovum (Bentley, 2003; ACOG, 2004).

Incidence

The incidence of hydatidiform mole in the United States is 1 per 1500 pregnancies (Berkowitz and Goldstein, 2005). In many other countries, especially in southeast Asia and the Far East, the incidence is 1 of every 120 pregnancies (Cohn and Herzog, 2000). There is a 1% to 2% increased risk for a repeat occurrence of hydatidiform mole (Hurteau, 2003).

Etiology

The cause of a hydatidiform mole is unknown, but it is theorized that an ovular defect, stress, or a nutritional deficiency (especially in carotene) may contribute to its development. Maternal age older than 35 years might be a factor as well because older oocytes are more susceptible to abnormal fertilization (Ngan, 2003). In rare cases, a hydatidiform mole is related to an abnormal genetic predisposition (Fallahian, 2003).

Normal Physiology

Normally, one sperm fertilizes one ovum and each contributes 23 chromosomes to form a new cell called a *zygote*. The zygote begins to grow immediately by undergoing a series of rapid mitotic cell divisions to form a solid mass of cells called a *morula*. As cellular activity continues, fluid begins to form in the center of the morula and causes the cells to rearrange until there is one single layer of cells lining the periphery and an inner cluster of cells. The single layer of cells, called the *trophoblast*, grows and develops into the placenta, and the inner cluster of cells, called the *embryoblast*, develops into a fetus. The umbilical cord eventually connects the two structures.

The trophoblast cells send out threadlike projections termed *chorionic villi* into the endometrium of the uterus primarily under the embryo to form the placenta. As the chorionic villi grow, they erode areas of the endometrium, forming intervillous spaces that fill with maternal blood. Invasion is normally held in check by the endometrium. Inside the chorionic villi, blood vessels and connective tissue begin to form. These blood vessels connect with the blood vessels inside the umbilical cord.

Pathophysiology

What actually causes the proliferation of the placenta is unknown. In any case, the trophoblastic tissue absorbs fluid from the maternal blood. Fluid then begins to accumulate in the chorionic villi because of inadequate or absent fetal circulation. As the pooling of fluid continues, vesicles are formed out of the chorionic villi.

Signs and Symptoms: Complete Mole

Characteristic symptoms of a complete hydatidiform mole are described in the following paragraphs.

Abnormal Uterine Bleeding

Abnormal uterine bleeding, which is intermittent or continuous (usually not profuse) and often brownish in color, occurs in approximately 75% of cases (Ngan, 2003). This is usually related to the lack of circulatory integrity of molar tissue. When the molar tissue starts separating from the uterus, bright red bleeding may result.

Variable Uterine Size

A uterus larger than expected for the estimated gestational age occurs in approximately 50% of the cases of complete mole (ACOG, 2004).

Ovarian Enlargement

Bilateral ovarian enlargement caused by theca lutein cysts occurs in 50% of patients with complete mole and may cause abdominal pain. This enlargement is usually related to the elevated levels of human chorionic gonadotropin (hCG) (Ngan, 2003).

Absence of Fetus

Inability to detect a fetal heart rate (FHR) after 10 to 12 weeks of gestation is an indication for ultrasound to be used to rule out a molar or other complication of pregnancy.

Other Signs and Symptoms

The following traditional signs and symptoms are rarely seen today because of the earlier diagnosis (Coukos and others, 1999; Ngan, 2003):

- Hyperemesis gravidarum
- Anemia
- Preeclampsia signs such as proteinuria, hypertension, and edema before 24 weeks of gestation
- Hyperthyroidism
- Passage of vesicles or grapelike structures
- Respiratory distress related to a trophoblastic pulmonary embolus
- Coagulopathy

Signs and Symptoms: Partial Mole

A partial mole does not exhibit the preceding clinical symptoms as often. It may present with signs of an incomplete or missed abortion, which include irregular vaginal bleeding, no FHR, or a uterus that is small for the estimated delivery date.

Maternal Effects

Maternal effects of hydatidiform mole, if not diagnosed early, include the following:

- Preeclampsia
- Bleeding
- Anemia
- Hyperemesis gravidarum
- Intrauterine infection or sepsis
- Uterine rupture
- Rupture of ovarian cysts
- Trophoblastic embolism
- Emotional trauma
- GTN

After surgical evacuation of a complete mole, there is a 20% risk for developing a persistent GTN (Ngan, 2003). This risk increases 40% to 50% if there was marked trophoblastic proliferation before evacuation, as evidenced by a high serum hCG level, excessively enlarged uterus, or theca lutein cysts (Ngan, 2003). After a partial mole, there is only a 2% to 4% risk for developing a nonmetastatic GTN (Cohn and Herzog, 2000).

Fetal Effects

The embryoblastic tissue of the complete hydatidiform mole never develops into a fetus. The embryoblastic tissue of the partial hydatidiform mole is always abnormal and never matures. A living child can be delivered from a hydatidiform molar pregnancy. These are twin gestations, and only one of the gestational sacs is affected by the molar changes.

Diagnostic Testing

Diagnostic tests used to validate a hydatidiform mole include transvaginal ultrasound and serum hCG. Transvaginal ultrasound is the most accurate tool for diagnosing the presence of a mole. A characteristic pattern of multiple diffuse echogenic, intrauterine masses, or "snowstorm pattern" is shown in place of, or along with, an embryo or a fetus.

The trophoblast tissue starting at about the time of implantation secretes hCG hormone. In a normal pregnancy, hCG levels gradually increase until around 10 weeks of pregnancy; then the levels plateau at approximately 60,000 to 140,000 mIU/ml. Between 10 and 12 weeks of gestation, the levels begin to decline sharply. In a molar pregnancy, the hCG titers are persistently high or rising beyond the normal peak (Cunningham and others, 2005).

Usual Medical Management

Immediate Evacuation

The uterus is usually emptied by suction evacuation because sharp curettage increases the risk for uterine perforation (ACOG, 2004). If the patient is no longer interested in childbearing, however, an abdominal hysterectomy might be performed. Even if the ovaries are enlarged or cystic, they do not have to be removed; they usually regress spontaneously when the hCG levels decline.

The four primary complications of surgical evacuation of the uterine contents are hemorrhage, perforation of the uterus, infection, and respiratory insufficiency. Oxytocin infusion is started at the beginning of surgery to promote myometrial contractions, which will decrease bleeding and thicken the uterine wall to reduce the risk for perforation of the uterus. It is contraindicated to start the oxytocin or administer prostaglandins before surgery because of the increased risk for trophoblastic embolization with uterine contractions in the presence of a molar pregnancy. Dilation of the cervix is usually accomplished while the patient is under general anesthesia unless the cervix is long and closed; then one of the cervical ripening methods may be used to dilate the cervix.

RhD-negative women may become sensitized after the evacuation of a hydatidiform mole. Therefore they should receive D immune globulin within 72 hours after the surgery to prevent D isoimmunization.

Follow-Up Assessment

Because of the existing risk for development of a GTN, these patients should be instructed regarding the importance of follow-up assessment. When the patient obtains this assessment, early detection of a tumor is possible and treatment is most effective. The follow-up assessment may include the following:

- Baseline hCG determination level 48 hours after evacuation, chest radiograph, and ultrasound scan of the abdomen; repeat hCG in 48 hours
- Weekly serum hCG values until the hCG level drops to normal and remains normal for 3 consecutive weeks, then every two weeks for three months, then monthly for 6 to 12 months
- Regular pelvic examinations to assess uterine and ovarian regression and to observe changes in the vagina that would indicate GTN
- Regular chest radiographs to detect pulmonary metastasis
- Assessments for symptoms such as dyspnea, cough, and pleuritic pain (may indicate pulmonary metastasis); dull headache, behavioral change, or dizzy spells (may indicate cerebral metastasis); right upper quadrant pain or jaundice (may indicate liver metastasis); and vaginal bleeding (may indicate vaginal metastasis)
- Recommendation that the patient use a contraceptive to avoid becoming pregnant during the follow-up assessment period, which usually lasts about 1 year, because the hCG of the GTN cannot be distinguished from the hCG of pregnancy

Interpret the hCG levels according to the criteria standardized by the International Federation of Gynecologists and Obstetricians (FIGO) in consensus with the Society of Gynecologic Oncology, the International Society for the Study of Trophoblastic Disease, and the International Gynecologic Cancer Society (Kohorn, 2001):

- A plateau of the hCG for 3 weeks or longer (days 1 to 21)
- Rise of hCG over a 2-week period from days 1 to 14
- Persistence of detectable hCG for 6 or more months

Prophylactic Chemotherapy

Some obstetricians recommend prophylactic chemotherapy, but its use is controversial. There is no evidence that such therapy improves long-term prognosis, and it may cause toxicity that occasionally leads to death. Gestational trophoblastic neoplasia may reoccur, requiring increasing amounts of chemotherapy (ACOG, 2004).

Co-Existing Hydatidiform Mole with a Normal Fetus

An amniocentesis is usually performed to determine the fetal karyotype of a fetus that coexists with a hydatidiform mole. If the karyotype is normal and the woman's condition is stable, continuation of the pregnancy may be attempted. If the karyotype of the fetus is abnormal, uterine evacuation is recommended (Bruchim and others, 2000).

When continuation of the pregnancy is planned, the patient is usually placed on a regimen of limited activity to minimize vaginal bleeding and then closely monitored for pregnancy-induced hypertension, HELLP (hemolysis, elevated liver enzymes, and low-platelet count in association with preeclampsia) syndrome, preterm labor, anemia, and pulmonary edema (Bruchim and others, 2000; ACOG, 2004). The patient has an increased risk for persistent GTN as well.

GESTATIONAL TROPHOBLASTIC NEOPLASIA

GTN is persistent trophoblastic proliferation. It may develop after a hydatidiform mole, an abortion, or an ectopic or normal pregnancy. GTN is divided into nonmetastatic, metastatic low risk, and metastatic high risk disorders (Cohn and Herzog, 2000). Common metastasis sites are lungs (80%), vagina (30%), pelvis (20%), liver (10%), and brain (10%) (Cohn and Herzog, 2000).

Etiology

Approximately 50% to 60% of these tumors follow a hydatidiform mole. The risk for occurrence after an ectopic pregnancy or a spontaneous abortion is approximately 25%. A GTN can occur after an apparently normal term pregnancy (Soper, 2003).

Signs and Symptoms

After any type of delivery, the following signs may indicate a GTN:

- Irregular bleeding—continuous or intermittent irregular bleeding related to uterine subinvolution caused by the presence of trophoblastic tissue
- Metastatic vaginal or vulvar tumors
- Bloody sputum related to pulmonary metastasis
- Intraperitoneal hemorrhage caused by perforation of the uterus as the result of continuous trophoblastic growth throughout the uterus

Maternal Effects

There is virtually a 100% cure rate after nonmetastatic and low risk metastatic GTN if treated early and appropriately. The risk for maternal mortality is 10% to 15% after high risk metastatic GTN (ACOG, 2004), usually the result of hemorrhage or pulmonary insufficiency. When metastasis occurs to the brain or liver, the prognosis is poorer (Ngan, 2003).

Diagnostic Testing

During the intense follow-up program after a hydatidiform mole or anytime abnormal postdelivery bleeding occurs, persistent or rising hCG levels in the absence of another pregnancy indicates GTN. Once a diagnosis is made, the stage of the tumor must be established to determine the tumor severity and the appropriate initial therapy. The International Federation of Gynecologists and Obstetricians (FIGO) along with the Committee of the International Society for the Study of Trophoblastic Diseases (ISSTD), the International Society for Gynecological Cancer (IGCS), and the World Health Organization (WHO) have provided a universal standardized scoring system that considers the stage and risk factors for GTN (Table 17-1). First, any patient diagnosed with GTD is allocated a stage from I-IV. Secondly a risk factor score is determined from the sum of the risk factors as outlined in the table. This is written by first indicating the stage as a roman numeral, followed by a colon, and then the risk factor number (example II:4). A risk score of 0–6 is classified as the low risk category. A score of 7 or higher is classified as the high risk group (Kohorn, 2001).

Table 17-1   Revised FIGO Stage and Risk Factor Scoring System for GTN

Stage	Description
Stage I	Disease confined to the uterus
Stage II	GTN metastasis outside of the uterus to the genital structures
Stage III	GTN metastasis to the lungs, with or with metastasis to the genital structures
Stage IV	Metastasis to the brain, liver, spleen, kidney

Risk Factor Score	0	1	2	4
Age	Less than 40 years	40 years or more	—	—
Antecedent pregnancy	Hydatidiform mole	Abortion	Term pregnancy	—
Interval from index pregnancy (months)	Less than 4	4–6	7–12	More than 12
Pretreatment hCG level (mIU/mL)	Less than 1,000	1,000–10,000	Greater than 10,000–100,000	Greater than 100,000
Largest tumor size including uterus (cm)	—	3–4 cm	5 cm or larger	—
Site of metastases	Lung, vagina	Spleen, kidney	Gastrointestinal tract	Brain, liver
Number of metastases identified	0	1–4	5–8	More than 8
Previous failed chemotherapy	—	—	Single drug	2 or more drugs
Total				

Modified from Kohorn E: The new FIGO 2000 staging and risk factor scoring system for gestational trophoblastic disease: description and clinical assessment, *Int J Gynecol Cancer* 1(1):73–77, 2001.

To employ the scoring system, the following workup is essential:
- Complete blood count (CBC), platelet determination, clotting function studies, blood type and antibody screen
- Renal and liver function tests
- Pretreatment hCG titer
- Pelvic ultrasonography
- Chest radiograph
- Computed tomographic scan or magnetic resonance imaging of brain, lungs, liver, and pelvis to determine presence or level of metastasis

Usual Medical Management

Refer to an oncologic specialist for treatment for GTN with chemotherapy whenever the serum level of hCG rises or plateaus for more than 3 consecutive weeks or when signs of metastasis are detected during examinations. The initial treatment plan is dependent on tumor staging and risk factors as described above and in Table 17-1 or the less complicated clinical classification of gestational trophoblastic neoplasia (Table 17-2).

Nonmetastatic Gestational Trophoblastic Neoplasia

Single-agent chemotherapy such as methotrexate or actinomycin D is usually effective (Schorge and others, 2000).

Low Risk Metastatic Gestational Trophoblastic Neoplasia

Treatment for low risk metastatic GTN usually starts with methotrexate, a single-agent chemotherapy that is 90% effective (Cohn and Herzog, 2000). Alternative single-agent regimens such as etoposide or dactinomycin are usually

Table 17-2   Clinical Classification of Gestational Trophoblastic Neoplasia

Type	Description
Nonmetastatic	Neoplasm confined to uterus
	Cure rate virtually 100%
Metastatic	Neoplasm has spread outside uterus
Low risk; good prognosis	Neoplasm present less than 4 months
	No liver, brain, or peritoneal metastases
	Metastases limited to lungs or vagina
	No prior chemotherapy
	Cure rate virtually 100%
High risk; poor prognosis	Serum hCG level less than 40,000 ml units/ml
	Liver, brain, or peritoneal metastases
	Failed prior chemotherapy
	Neoplasm after term pregnancy
	Cure rate 75% depending on type of chemotherapy used

Modified from Cohn D, Herzog T: Gestational trophoblastic diseases: new standards for therapy, *Curr Opin Oncol* 12(5):492–496, 2000.

effective and well tolerated in the other 10% (Dobson and others, 2000). Combination chemotherapy, such as methotrexate, actinomycin D, and cyclophosphamide, is rarely necessary in patients with low risk metastatic GTNs.

High Risk Gestational Trophoblastic Neoplasia

Multiagent chemotherapy, which includes the most preferred combination of etoposide, methotrexate, actinomycin D, cyclophosphamide, and vincristine (EMA-CO regimen); or methotrexate, etoposide, and dactinomycin (MEA regimen), has been found to be most effective in cases of high risk GTN. Multiagent chemotherapy is tolerated well and does not appear to affect future fertility (Dobson and others, 2000; Schorge and others, 2000; Ngan, 2003).

Follow-Up

After the initial treatment, serum hCG levels are evaluated every 1 to 2 weeks. As long as the hCG level is regressing, further chemotherapy is withheld. A plateau or rise in the level indicates a need for additional chemotherapy. When hCG is undetectable for 3 consecutive weeks, remission has occurred. Serial hCG levels are usually checked monthly for 1 year. To check the serial hCG levels accurately, the patient should avoid becoming pregnant during the follow-up period.

NURSING MANAGEMENT

Prevention

Because the cause of a hydatidiform mole is unknown, there is no known prevention. However, malnutrition and stress might play parts in influencing its development; therefore instructions should be given to all patients who are planning a pregnancy regarding the importance of stress management and a balanced diet high in protein and vitamin A.

Assessment

Hydatidiform Mole

Transvaginal ultrasound is used on any pregnancy not progressing normally in order to detect a hydatidiform mole early. Signs such as uterine bleeding, small or large uterine size for dates, hyperemesis gravidarum, preeclampsia before 24 weeks of gestation, passage of grapelike vesicles, or inability to detect FHR using Doppler FHR device after 10 to 12 weeks of gestation should be evaluated immediately.

Gestational Trophoblastic Neoplasia

Because a GTN may develop after a normal delivery, an ectopic pregnancy, or an abortion, all patients should be taught the importance of reporting any unusual bleeding after any reproductive event. In these cases, hCG levels should be determined to detect a GTN early.

Nursing Interventions for Evacuation of Mole

- Monitor for evidence of hemorrhage such as abnormal vital signs, abdominal pain, uterine status, and vaginal bleeding.
- Start intravenous infusion with an 18-gauge intracatheter.
- Prepare for surgery according to preoperative protocol, and type and cross-match 2 to 4 units of packed red blood cells as ordered.
- Avoid using oxytocin or prostaglandins before beginning surgery because of the risk for trophoblastic embolization with uterine contractions in the presence of a molar.

Postevacuation Nursing Interventions

- Monitor for postoperative complications such as the following: hemorrhage; respiratory compromise; congestive heart failure precipitated by anemia, hyperthyroidism, or iatrogenic fluid overload; and altered urinary elimination related to the antidiuretic effect of oxytocin.
- Initially continue any added postoperative intravenous infusions of oxytocin to facilitate uterine contractions and decrease uterine bleeding.
- Do not massage a boggy uterus if ovaries are enlarged, because the massage can cause ovarian rupture related to the theca lutein cysts stimulated by the high hCG levels.
- Do not use methylergonovine maleate (Methergine) postoperatively, because it can precipitate a hypertensive crisis.
- If the patient is RhD-negative and unsensitized, be prepared to administer Rho (D) immune globulin (RhoGAM; HypRho-D). The usual dose is 1 vial, which equals approximately 300 mcg.

Nursing Interventions to Allay Fear

- Provide time for the patient and her family to express their concerns regarding the possible outcome and inconvenience to the mother and family during the treatment and long-term follow-up assessment period. Encourage them to vent any feelings, fears, and anger they may be experiencing.
- Assess family's support system and coping mechanisms.
- Provide information to the family regarding the disease process, plan of treatment, and risk for the patient.
- Explain all treatment modalities and reasons.
- Keep patient informed of health status and results of tests.
- Discuss risk for a GTN based on whether the patient had a partial or complete mole.
- Reassure patient that she can anticipate normal future reproduction even if she was treated for persistent GTN (Hurteau, 2003).
- Refer to social services for financial concerns if the family is without health benefits.

Anticipatory Grieving Nursing Interventions

- Assess significance of the loss to all family members and level of guilt or blame.
- Assess family's communication pattern and support systems.
- Reaffirm with the family their losses, and let them know you are aware that these are real.
- Provide physical care such as a back rub or nourishment as needed.
- Consider any significant cultural beliefs or values.
- Spiritual assistance might help the family work through their grief. Refer to the chaplain or family's own clergy.
- Refer to psychiatric services when deemed necessary.

Follow-Up Nursing Interventions for Early Detection of Gestational Trophoblastic Neoplasia

- Assess the patient's and family's understandings of the disease and of the risks of an ongoing GTN.
- Explain the disease and plan of treatment.
- Educate about the importance of the follow-up assessment for early detection of a GTN because it is almost 100% curable.
- Educate about the importance of avoiding pregnancy during the follow-up assessment to prevent masking the hCG rise of a GTN and to obtain better future pregnancy outcome.
- Teach that any effective contraceptive method may be used except an IUD because of bleeding irregularities associated with the IUD. Oral contraceptives are the preferred method because they are highly effective (ACOG, 2004).
- Explain the treatment program if a GTN develops.
- Facilitate future family planning by reassuring the couple that even after chemotherapy, they can anticipate a normal reproductive outcome in the future with no increased risk for congenital fetal malformations. The risk for a repeat molar pregnancy is 1% to 2%. After two molar pregnancies, the risk is about 20% (Hurteau, 2003).

CONCLUSION

The goals of the nurse in treating patients who have had a hydatidiform mole are twofold. First, the nurse must emphasize the importance of the follow-up assessment. To determine whether a GTN is going to occur, serum hCG levels should be checked closely. The hCG levels should progressively decline and by 10 to 12 weeks be nondetectable. Second, the nurse must help the patient work through the loss of an expected baby, a defective pregnancy, the fear of the development of proliferative trophoblastic disease, and the fear of recurrence in subsequent pregnancies.

The goal of GTN management is early detection because there is an almost 100% cure rate with appropriate treatment. To detect all GTNs early, keep in mind that they may occur after any reproductive event; therefore any abnormal bleeding should be evaluated as a possible indication of this disorder.

BIBLIOGRAPHY

American College of Obstetricians and Gynecologists (ACOG): *Diagnosis and treatment of gestational trophoblastic disease,* Practice Bulletin No. 53, 2004. Author.

Bentley R: Pathology of gestational trophoblastic disease, *Clin Obstet Gynecol* 46(3): 513–522, 2003.

Berkowitz R, Goldstein D: Gestational trophoblastic diseases. In Hoskins W and others, editors: *Principles and practice of gynecologic oncology,* Philadelphia, 2005, Lippincott, Williams & Wilkins.

Bruchim I and others: Complete hydatidiform mole and a coexistent viable fetus: report of two cases and review of the literature, *Gynecol Oncol* 77(1):197–202, 2000.

Cohn D, Herzog T: Gestational trophoblastic diseases: new standards for therapy, *Curr Opin Oncol* 12(5):492–496, 2000.

Coukos G and others: Complete hydatidiform mole. A disease with a changing profile, *J Reprod Med* 44(8):698–704, 1999.

Cunningham F and others: *Williams' obstetrics,* ed 22, New York, 2005, McGraw-Hill.

Dobson L and others: Persistent gestational trophoblastic disease, *Br J Cancer* 8(9): 1547–1552, 2000.

Fallahian M: Familial gestational trophoblastic disease, *Placenta* 24(7):797–799, 2003.

Hurteau J: Gestational trophoblastic disease: management of hydatidiform mole, *Clin Obstet Gynecol* 46(3):557–569, 2003.

Kohorn E: The new FIGO 2000 staging and risk factor scoring system for gestational trophoblastic disease: description and clinical assessment, *Int J Gynecol Cancer* 1(1): 73–77, 2001.

Ngan H: Gestational trophoblastic disease, *Curr Obstet Gynaecol* 13:95, 2003.

Omura G: Chemotherapy of gestational trophoblastic disease, *J Clin Oncol* 18(10):2187, 2000.

Schorge J and others: Recent advances in gestational trophoblastic disease, *J Reprod Med* 45(9): 692–700, 2000.

Soper J: Staging and evaluation of gestational trophoblastic disease, *Clin Obstet Gynecol* 46(3):570–578, 2003.

Tidy J and others: Gestational trophoblastic disease: a study of mode of evacuation and subsequent need for treatment with chemotherapy, *Gynecol Oncol* 78(3 Pt 1):309–312, 2000.

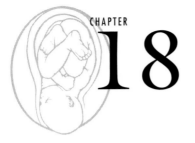

Placental Abnormalities

pproximately 5% of all pregnant women experience some type of vaginal bleeding during their third trimester of pregnancy (Morgan and Arulkumaran, 2003). The major causes of this bleeding are abruptio placentae and placenta previa (MacMullen, Dulski and Meagher, 2005). This chapter focuses on these two main causes and contrasts the treatments of both. Other causes of third trimester bleeding are heavy bloody show, cervical carcinoma, polyps, cervical or vaginal infection, cervical trauma, varicosities, invasive placenta, and vasa previa. Invasive placenta and vasa previa are briefly covered in this chapter as well.

ABRUPTIO PLACENTAE

An *abruptio placentae* is the premature separation, either partial or total, of a normally implanted placenta from the decidual lining of the uterus after 20 weeks of gestation. It is normally classified into one of three categories: mild, moderate, or severe (Table 18-1). Some medical personnel refer to grade 1, 2, or 3 instead. Mild abruptio placentae is a grade 1; moderate, a grade 2; and severe, a grade 3. Maternal bleeding in any class can be marginal, concealed, or both (Fig. 18-1), depending on whether it is trapped in the uterus.

Maternal bleeding is classified as one of the following:

- *Marginal or apparent.* The separation is near the edge of the placenta, and the blood is able to escape.
- *Central or concealed.* The separation is somewhere in the center of the placenta, and the blood is trapped.
- *Mixed or combined.* Part of the separation is near the edge, and part is concealed in the center area.

Incidence

Abruptio placentae occurs in approximately 1% of pregnancies (Salihu and others, 2005). There is a ten times greater risk in a subsequent pregnancy (Morgan and Arulkumaran, 2003).

Table 18-1   Comparison of Three Classifications of Abruptio Placentae

	Mild: Grade 1	Moderate: Grade 2	Severe: Grade 3
Definition	Less than 1/6 of placenta separates prematurely	From 1/6 to 1/2 of placenta separates prematurely	More than 1/2 of placenta separates prematurely
Incidence	48%	27%	24%
Signs and symptoms	Total blood loss less than 500 ml	Total blood loss 1000–1500 ml	Total blood loss more than 1500 ml
	Dark vaginal bleeding (mild to moderate)	15%–30% of total blood volume	More than 30% of total blood volume
	Vague lower abdominal or back discomfort	Dark vaginal bleeding (mild to severe)	Dark vaginal bleeding (moderate to excessive)
	No uterine tenderness	Gradual or abrupt onset of abdominal pain	Usually abrupt onset of uterine pain described as tearing, knifelike, and continuous
	No uterine irritability	Uterine tenderness present	Uterus boardlike and highly reactive to stimuli
		Uterine tone increased	
Hypovolemia	Vital signs normal	Mild shock	Moderate-to-profound shock common
		Normal maternal blood pressure	Decreased maternal blood pressure
		Maternal tachycardia	Maternal tachycardia significant
		Narrowed pulse pressure	Narrowed pulse pressure
		Orthostatic hypotension	Orthostatic hypotension severe
		Tachypnea	Significant tachypnea
DIC	Normal fibrinogen of 450 mg/dl	Early signs of DIC common	DIC usually develops unless condition is treated immediately
		Fibrinogen 150–300 mg/dl	Fibrinogen less than 150 mg/dl
Fetal effects	Normal FHR pattern	FHR shows nonreassuring signs of possible fetal distress	FHR shows signs of fetal distress and death can occur

DIC, Disseminated intravascular coagulation; *FHR,* fetal heart rate.

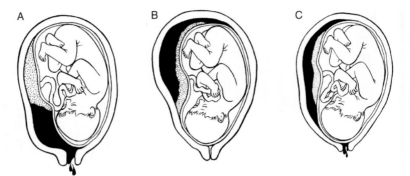

Figure 18-1 Classification of abruptio placentae. **A,** Marginal or apparent. **B,** Central or concealed. **C,** Missed or combined.

Etiology

The actual cause of an abruptio placenta is unknown. Conditions frequently associated with abruptio placentae are listed below:

- *Pregnancy-induced or chronic hypertension.* This is the most common cause of an abruption and is more likely than the other causes to result in a severe abruption (Cunningham and others, 2005).
- *Previous abruption.* There is a 10% increased risk for recurrence after one abruption and a 25% increased risk for recurrence after two abruptions (Cunningham and others, 2005).
- *Trauma.* A placental abruption may result from a direct blow to the abdomen, most commonly as the result of a motor vehicle collision or maternal battering.
- *Cigarette smoking.* Smoking causes approximately 40% of abruptions by vasoconstriction of the spiral arteriole, which can lead to decidual necrosis (Morgan and Arulkumaran, 2003).
- *Cocaine abuse.* Cocaine causes vasoconstriction and hypertension, which can interfere with placental adherence to the uterine wall (Addis and others, 2001; Morgan and Arulkumaran, 2003).
- *Preterm premature rupture of membranes.* A 5% risk for developing an abruptio placentae after premature rupture of membranes exists (Morgan and Arulkumaran, 2003).
- *Hyperhomocysteinuria.*

Normal Physiology

The blastocyst normally implants into the endometrium, now called the *decidua,* by sending out threadlike projections called *chorionic villi* from the trophoblast cells. These villi open up intervillous spaces, which fill with maternal blood. These spaces are supplied by the spiral arteries. At the same time, the trophoblast cells send out anchoring cords to attach themselves to the uterus.

Pathophysiology

An abruptio placentae is theoretically thought to be caused by degeneration of the spiral arterioles that nourish the decidua (endometrium) and supply blood to the placenta, causing decidua basalis necrosis. When this process takes place, rupture of that blood vessel occurs and bleeding quickly results because the uterus is still distended and cannot contract sufficiently to close off the opened blood vessels.

Separation of the placenta takes place in the area of the hemorrhage. If the tear is at the margin of the placenta or if it separates the membranes from the decidua, vaginal bleeding is evident. Otherwise, the blood is concealed between the placenta and the decidua. If it is concealed, enough pressure can build up for blood to be forced through the fetal membranes into the amniotic sac or into the myometrial muscle fibers, which is called *Couvelaire uterus*. This increases uterine tone and irritability. Clotting occurs simultaneously with the hemorrhage because the decidual tissue is rich in thromboplastin. This leads to the formation of a retroplacental or a subchorionic hematoma, causing the release of large quantities of thromboplastin into the maternal circulation. This can lead to disseminated intravascular coagulopathy (DIC).

Signs and Symptoms

Classic Manifestations

The classic manifestations of an abruptio placenta follow:
- Dark vaginal, nonclotting bleeding (80%)
- Abdominal or low back pain (50%)
- Uterine hypertonus (17%)
- Uterine contractions (17%)
- Uterine tenderness
- Fetal distress signs or fetal death
- Signs of hypovolemia beyond those expected on the basis of observed external blood loss

The presence and degree of each sign are related to the amount of concealed blood trapped between the placenta and the decidua and the degree of separation. If the separation occurs at the margin of the placenta, the blood usually tears the membranes away from the decidua and escapes externally. The blood appears dark because it has had time to begin clotting. If the separation is in the center of the placenta, blood is trapped between the placenta and the decidua.

Concealed blood causes pressure and myometrial contractions, and this results in abdominal pain and uterine tenderness. With no way to escape, pressure builds up and can force blood into the myometrial tissue of the uterus, causing increased uterine irritability. Increasing uterine size and decreasing serial hematocrits are other signs of concealed bleeding. If some of this trapped blood is forced through the fetal membranes into the amniotic cavity, the amniotic fluid is bloody.

Mild Abruptio Placentae: Grade 1

Mild forms of abruptio placentae usually develop gradually and produce mild to moderate dark vaginal bleeding without uterine tenderness. Signs of fetal distress are absent, and the mother's vital signs remain stable. There are no signs of DIC. This type of abruption can be self-limiting or can progress into a more advanced form.

Moderate Abruptio Placentae: Grade 2

A moderate abruptio placenta can develop gradually or abruptly and produce persistent abdominal pain accompanied by visible dark vaginal bleeding. The uterus may be tender on palpation and may remain firm between contractions if the mother is in labor. This can make auditory appraisal of the fetal heart rate (FHR) difficult. Fetal distress may be present depending on the extent of placental separation and the amount of maternal blood loss. Signs of shock may be present.

Severe Abruptio Placentae: Grade 3

A severe abruptio placentae usually develops suddenly, causing excruciating, unremitting abdominal pain often referred to as *knifelike* or *tearing*. The uterus is often boardlike and tender and fails to relax. Profuse bleeding results, although it may not be evident vaginally if the blood is trapped behind the placenta. In situations in which the blood is trapped, the uterus shows signs of enlarging. Shock can ensue, although the signs of shock may not be in proportion to the amount of visible blood loss. Signs of fetal distress are usually evident, and fetal death may result.

Posteriorly Implanted Abruptio Placentae

In a few instances, when an abruptio placenta occurs in a posteriorly implanted placenta, no signs of uterine tenderness or pain are manifested. In these cases, the classic signs are only vaginal bleeding and backache.

Complications

Shock

Shock results as the body attempts to protect the vital organs, especially the brain and heart, from a reduction of effective circulating blood volume. When blood is lost from the vascular system, venous return is diminished and cardiac output is consequently reduced. Physiologic compensatory mechanisms are then activated. The decrease in arterial pressure initiates powerful sympathetic reflexes that stimulate vasoconstriction of the arterioles and venules in the kidneys, liver, lungs, gastrointestinal tract, muscles, skin, and uterus. Blood is then redistributed to the heart and brain from these areas.

The heart and respiratory rates increase in an attempt to compensate by delivering increased volume and better oxygenated blood to the vital organs. A slower compensatory mechanism is activated that stimulates the absorption of fluid from the intestinal tract and stimulates the kidneys to increase reabsorption of sodium and water. Therefore the results are classic signs of hypovolemic shock, which include hypotension; oliguria; rapid, thready pulse; shallow, irregular respirations; cold and clammy skin; pallor; syncope; and thirst. Should severe bleeding continue, the compensatory mechanisms cannot keep up with tissue needs, and cardiac deterioration, loss of vasomotor tone, and release of toxins by ischemic tissue result; cellular death ensues.

Because of the normally increased maternal blood volume during pregnancy, the classic signs of shock are not always present until after the fetal circulation is affected. During pregnancy, signs of shock usually do not present until after 25% to 30% of maternal blood volume is lost. Shunting of blood away from the placenta occurs before this 25% to 30% blood loss. Table 18-2 lists the manifested symptoms of blood loss.

Disseminated Intravascular Coagulation

An abruptio placenta is the most common cause of DIC. This coagulation defect results because of placental tissue fragments (thromboplastin) being forced into the circulatory system. These substances activate widespread intravascular clotting. Soon, the coagulation factors are consumed. Therefore the platelet count is usually decreased, fibrinogen is low, and circulating fibrin degradation products (FDPs) are increased (see Chapter 19).

Other Complications

Renal failure can develop as a result of hypoxia if shock, vascular spasms, or DIC have occurred. Pituitary necrosis (Sheehan syndrome) occasionally results from the same conditions that cause renal failure. In the presence of pituitary necrosis, lactation does not occur because pituitary hormones regulate lactation.

Maternal Effects

In fewer than 1% of cases, maternal death occurs from hemorrhagic shock. This low maternal mortality is mainly due to the availability of blood replacement therapy. However, maternal morbidity is significant. Because of the potential for massive bleeding, the patient is at high risk for developing shock and DIC at any time before delivery. In rare cases, a fetal-to-maternal hemorrhage may occur, which can cause the Rh-negative mother to become sensitized.

During the postpartum period, mothers who had experienced an abruptio placentae are at an increased risk for anemia, development of an infection related to prolonged separation of the placenta, postpartum hemorrhage related to a poorly contracted uterus caused by blood infiltrating the uterus, and DIC. Other complications that can develop as a result of ischemia are renal failure and anterior pituitary necrosis (Sheehan syndrome). Because of increase blood flow to the pituitary gland during pregnancy, it is more sensitive to hypoxia during pregnancy.

Fetal and Neonatal Effects

Perinatal mortality is approximately 14 in 1000, depending on the degree of abruption, causing 12% of all third trimester stillbirths (Salihu and others,

Table 18-2 Manifested Symptoms of Blood Loss

Percentage of Blood Loss	Manifested Symptoms	Treatment
15% = 900 ml	Minimal tachycardia Normal blood pressure Normal pulse pressure Normal respiratory rate Normal capillary refill	Stabilize with crystalloid
20%–25% = 1200–1500 ml	Tachycardia Tachypnea (rate doubles) Increased blood pressure, especially diastolic Narrowing pulse pressure Delayed hypothenar refilling Orthostatic blood pressure changes	Usually successful when stabilized with crystalloid
30%–35% = 1800–2100 ml	Significant tachycardia (30–50 bpm) Decreased blood pressure especially systolic Decreased pulse pressure Significant tachypnea (30–50 breaths/min) Classic shock signs of cold, clammy extremities	Infuse 1–2 L of a crystalloid solution Infuse blood component therapy, such as packed RBCs 40% or greater
40% or greater 2400 ml or greater	Marked tachycardia Significant depression of blood pressure Narrow pulse pressure Significant tachypnea Oliguria Syncope, shortness of breath, headaches, chest pain Skin cold and pale	Infuse 1–2 L of crystalloid solution Then infuse blood component therapy Whole blood Infuse platelets and fresh frozen plasma after several units of whole blood

Data from Benedetti T: Obstetric hemorrhage. In Gabbe S, Niebyl J, and Simpson J: *Obstetrics: normal and problem pregnancies,* ed 4, New York, 2002, Churchill Livingstone.

2005). In surviving infants, the most common causes of morbidity are fetal hypoxia, neonatal prematurity, intrauterine growth restriction neurologic defects. These conditions result when approximately 50% of the placental surface has separated or maternal blood loss is 2000 ml or greater.

Fetal Hypoxia

Fetal hypoxia is caused by uteroplacental insufficiency resulting from placental separation or decreased uterine perfusion resulting from maternal hypovolemia, uterine hypertonus, or less often, fetal hemorrhage. Total anoxia may develop.

Neonatal Prematurity

The neonate is frequently premature because of early delivery necessitated by fetal distress or preterm labor.

Intrauterine Growth Restriction

Even if the bleeding and separation stop, the decreased placental surface area that remains intact may not be adequate to meet the increased needs of the growing fetus.

Neurologic Defects

The infant who survives is at increased risk for a neurologic defect such as cerebral palsy (Cunningham and others, 2005).

Diagnostic Testing

Diagnosis usually is made on the basis of presenting symptoms and a physical assessment. Severe abruptio placentae and moderate abruptio placentae are easier to diagnose; a patient presents with one or more of the classic symptoms. A mild abruptio placenta is more difficult to diagnose; it is easily confused with a placenta previa because vaginal bleeding may be the only presenting symptom. Therefore ultrasound is usually used to rule out a placenta previa and is accompanied by a clinical examination to rule out other less common causes of third trimester bleeding. However, at present, no diagnostic method is available to determine the degree of placental separation.

Usual Medical Management and Protocols for Nurse Practitioners

Treatment of an abruptio placenta depends on the severity of blood loss, fetal maturity, and fetal well-being.

Expectant Management

If the abruptio placenta is mild and there are no signs of hypovolemia or anemia, gestational age of the fetus is determined first. With an immature fetus of less than 36 weeks of gestation without signs of fetal distress, expectant management is usually the treatment. The components of expectant management follow:

- Hospitalize in a facility that can immediately intervene by cesarean delivery because the placenta may further separate at any time and, very quickly, seriously compromise the fetus unless cesarean delivery can be performed immediately. Corticosteroids to accelerate fetal lung maturity may be part of the plan.
- Closely observe for signs of concealed or external bleeding.
- Do continuous FHR monitoring until 72 hours have passed without bleeding, hypertension, or abnormal FHR pattern.
- Monitor for preterm uterine contractions, which can be stimulated by prostaglandin release from placental separation. Tocolytic therapy is usually

contraindicated. If a tocolytic agent is used, magnesium sulfate is the drug of choice (Cunningham and others, 2005). Beta-sympathomimetics can cause maternal tachycardia and thereby falsely indicate hemorrhage. Calcium channel blockers can cause hypotension and thereby adversely affect maternal perfusion of the uterus.

- Obtain baseline laboratory data such as complete blood cell count, coagulation studies, abnormal bleeding panel, serum electrolytes panel, and renal function studies such as serum blood urea nitrogen and serum creatinine.

Emergency Management

If the abruptio placenta is moderate to severe, the following are the objectives of treatment:

- Monitor maternal volume status continuously.
- Restore blood loss quickly.
- Continuously monitor the fetus.
- Correct coagulation defect if present.
- Expedite delivery.

Maternal volume status must be monitored continually with (1) an indwelling Foley catheter to determine urine output and (2) serial hematocrits every 2 to 3 hours. If urine output drops below 30 ml/hr despite vigorous volume replacement, Swan-Ganz monitoring is needed to determine intravascular volume status.

Fluid replacement is usually accomplished with a crystalloid solution, such as lactated Ringer's, and blood component therapy as soon as it is available. Intravenous (IV) lactated Ringer's solution and blood are usually administered at a rate adequate to maintain the hematocrit at 30% or greater and urinary output at 30 ml/hr or greater. In rare instances, the patient's blood loss is rapid and massive, leading to severe shock. In these cases, volume expanders or immediate transfusions with type O, Rh-negative blood may be given until matched blood is available. Oxygen should be administered with facemask because it increases oxygen tension and increases oxygen delivery to end-organs.

The fetus must be monitored continuously until delivery takes place. Keep in mind that a maternal heartbeat may be picked up through the fetal scalp electrode in the event of fetal death. Therefore the FHR should be compared with the maternal pulse.

If a coagulation defect develops (fibrinogen level, 150 mg/dl), replacement of the clotting factors is the usual treatment. This can be accomplished by administering cryoprecipitate or fresh frozen plasma to replace fibrinogen and a platelet transfusion if the platelet count is below 50,000/mm^3. Heparin was once used to treat DIC in the presence of an abruptio placentae, but it is no longer an acceptable treatment. Within 24 hours after delivery, the coagulation defect normally corrects itself. The platelet count may not return to a normal level for 2 to 4 days. Table 18-3 lists guidelines for blood component replacement.

Table 18-3   Guidelines for Blood Component Replacement

Conditions	Blood Component	Volume per Unit	Dose	Effect	Administration
Acute blood loss	Volume expansion with crystalloid solutions (lactated Ringer's and NS) Other volume expanders: albumin, hydroxyethyl starch, dextran, purified protein fractions	1000 ml	Depends on amount of blood lost		If bleeding stops and BP rises after 1–2 L, blood components may not be necessary
Hgb 7 g/dl or less Hct 21% or less • Syncope • Shortness of breath • Chest pain • Oliguria • Tachycardia	Packed RBCs to restore oxygen-carrying capacity	240 ml	Depends on Hgb/Hct levels and amount of continued bleeding	1 unit will increase Hgb 1 g/dl and Hct 3%	Packed RBCs have an Hct of 70% and therefore increased viscosity; if need to infuse rapidly, mix with 200 ml of NS per unit
Deficiency in clotting factors (II, V, VII, IX, XI) indicated by PT or PTT 1.5 × normal or greater • PT > 18 sec • PTT >55sec	FFP	250 ml	Normal dose: 2 bags	1 unit will increase each clotting factor by 2%–3%	

Continued

Table 18-3 Guidelines for Blood Component Replacement—cont'd

Conditions	Blood Component	Volume per Unit	Dose	Effect	Administration
Platelet count less than 50,000/mm^3 with active bleeding or surgery	Platelet transfusions	50 ml	1 unit × 10 kg of body weight Minimum of 6 units	1 unit will increase platelet count 5000/mm^3	Do not use a platelet count RBC leukocyte-depleting filter because most of the platelets will also be removed
Abnormal function as indicated by normal platelet count with bleeding time more than 9 min					Approximately 0.5 ml of RBCs are present in platelet transfusions; if ABO and CBE (Rh) type-specific platelets are not available, a D-negative woman can be sensitized with D-positive platelets; administer RhoGAM (one vial needed for every

more of the following clotting factors: • Fibrinogen (less than 200 mg/dl) • Factor VIII or XIII von Willebrand factor	contains factors VIII and XIII, fibrinogen, fibronectin, von Willebrand factor	frozen	1 bag × 5 kg of body weight	increase fibrinogen 10 mg/dl
Total blood loss exceeds 25% of total blood volume	Packed RBCs and FFP or Whole blood	250 ml 500 ml		All blood products should be administered through a Y-type blood administration set with a filter designed to remove debris; only NS should be infused through the same line

Data from Cunningham G and others: *Williams' obstetrics*, ed 22, New York, 2005, McGraw-Hill.

BP, Blood pressure; *FFP*, fresh frozen plasma; *Hct*, hematocrit; *Hgb*, hemoglobin; *NS*, normal saline; *PT*, prothrombin time; *PTT*, partial thromboplastin time; *RBCs*, red blood cells.

Delivery

Delivery should be started if the abruption is moderate to severe, if the fetus is older than 36 weeks, or at any time fetal distress is noted. If the fetus is mature and in a cephalic presentation, a vaginal delivery may be attempted with continuous fetal monitoring in an environment where a cesarean delivery can be performed immediately. If the woman is not in labor and nonreassuring signs of fetal stress are absent, vaginal delivery can be initiated by an amniotomy or a labor stimulant such as oxytocin, provided that the patient is in a tertiary care center in which rapid emergency measures can be initiated if further abruption occurs with contractions. If the fetus is not in a cephalic presentation or if, during the induction of labor, bleeding increases, the uterus fails to relax between contractions, fetal distress occurs, or labor fails to progress actively, a cesarean delivery is performed.

In the presence of a severe abruptio placenta, if the fetus is alive, a cesarean delivery should be performed as soon as possible. If the fetus is dead, a vaginal delivery is preferred unless bleeding cannot be controlled.

PLACENTA PREVIA

Placenta previa occurs when the placenta attaches to the lower segment of the uterus, near or over the internal os, instead of in the body or fundal segment of the uterus. It is normally classified into one of three categories, depending on the degree of coverage of the cervix (Fig. 18-2):

1   *Marginal.* The placenta lies within 2 to 3 cm of the internal os.
2   *Partial.* The placenta implants near and partially covers the internal os.
3   *Total.* The placenta completely covers the internal os.

The placenta is referred to as *low lying* when the exact relationship of the placenta to the internal os is not known.

Incidence

The incidence of placenta previa is 0.33% with a 4% to 8% recurrence risk (Martin and others, 2002).

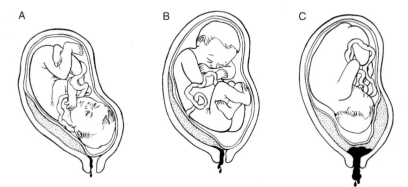

Figure 18-2 Classifications of placenta previa. **A,** Marginal. **B,** Partial. **C,** Total.

Etiology

The actual cause of placenta previa is unknown. However, damage to the endometrium or myometrium or any process that interferes with placental migration increases the risk for a placenta previa. Women of Asian descent who are living in the United States have an increased risk as well. Therefore it is frequently associated with endometrial scarring, impeded endometrial vascularization, and increased placental mass.

Endometrial Scarring

Endometrial scarring can result from a previous placenta previa, an abortion, a cesarean delivery, an increased parity 4 or greater, or closely spaced pregnancies (Gesteland and others, 2004). Subsequent pregnancies, after a cesarean delivery, have a 1.5% greater likelihood of a placenta previa complication (Morgan and Arulkumaran, 2003).

Impeded Endometrial Vascularization

Factors that interfere with adequate blood supply to the endometrium, such as hypertension or diabetes, uterine tumor, drug usage (e.g., cocaine), cigarette smoking, or advancing maternal age can cause placenta previa (Clark, 2004).

Increased Placental Mass

A multiple pregnancy leads to more than one placenta and therefore increases the risk for placenta previa.

Normal Physiology

The blastocyst normally implants into the upper anterior portion of the uterus, where the vascular blood supply is rich. After implantation of the blastocyst, the trophoblastic tissue sends out threadlike projections, chorionic villi, which grow into the decidua (endometrium). At first, these chorionic villi surround the blastocyst; however, soon after, the portion of the chorionic villi in contact with the decidua basalis proliferates to form the placenta, and the villi, in contact with the decidua capsularis, atrophies.

The chorionic villi are of two types. One type opens up intervillous spaces, which fill with maternal blood to form an area of exchange between the embryonic and maternal circulatory systems. Another type of villi forms anchoring cords to stabilize the placenta and embryo in the uterus. The chorionic villi growth is normally confined to the endometrium because of the fibrinoid layer of Nitabuch, which separates the decidua from the myometrium and stops chorionic villi growth.

Pathophysiology

With placenta previa, the blastocyst implants itself in the lower uterine segment, over or very near the internal os. A large percentage, approximately 90%, of placentas that initially implant low migrate upward. In the presence of more than a 2-cm placental cervical overlap, migration is rare (Oppenheimer and others, 2001). There are two current theories as to why placental migration takes place. According to the first theory, the growth of the lower uterine segment from 0.5 to 5.0 cm causes movement of the placenta away from the cervical os (Clark, 2004). The second theory postulates that the chorionic villi have the ability to grow in one area and to remain dormant in another (Lockwood, 1990; Bhide and Thilaganathan, 2004).

The decidua basalis is less developed in the lower segment of the uterus. The fibrinoid layer of Nitabuch, which stops chorionic villi growth, may be absent. Therefore placental tissue may come into direct contact with the myometrium and a placenta accreta, increta, or percreta may develop.

Signs and Symptoms

The two classical presentations of placenta previa are antepartum hemorrhage and fetal malpresentation in later pregnancy (Neilson, 2001).

Painless, Bright Red, Vaginal Bleeding

Normally, during the latter half of pregnancy, the lower uterine segment elongates as the fundal segment of the uterus hypertrophies. Toward the end of the pregnancy, the cervix begins to efface and dilate. When the placenta is implanted in the lower uterine segment over or around the internal cervical os, separation or tearing of portions of the placenta can occur with subsequent bleeding. Usually, the greater the percentage of placenta covering the os, the earlier the first episode of bleeding occurs. Because the normal uterine changes occur gradually until labor begins, the initial bleeding episode is usually slight, presents commonly in the third trimester, and ceases spontaneously as clot formation occurs. This is not always the case, however. The bleeding is usually painless and bright red in color without associated uterine tenderness because the blood is not trapped behind the placenta. In about 20% of the cases, uterine contractions accompany the bleeding (Carter, 1999). Recurrence is unpredictable and can take place at any time.

Fetal Malpresentation

The presenting part of the fetus usually remains high even in late pregnancy because the placenta occupies the lower uterine segment. For this same reason, the risk for malpresentations, such as transverse, oblique, or breech, increases.

Maternal Effects

The incidence of maternal mortality is less than 1% (Clark, 2004). The most common morbidity factors follow:

- *Hemorrhage and hypovolemic shock.* Placenta previa can cause maternal hemorrhage and hypovolemic shock in the antepartum, intrapartum, and postpartum periods. Puerperal hemorrhage can occur even in the presence of a firmly contracted uterus. This is because the lower uterine segment does not have the contractility of the upper uterine segment, and as a consequence, there is less compression of the open vessels, resulting from the removal of the placenta. This risk for hemorrhage is further increased by the larger than normal surface area denuded by the removal of the placenta.

- *Invasive placenta (includes accreta, increta, and percreta).* The risk for invasive placenta is 5% to 10% with any placenta previa, and if the woman had a previous cesarean delivery, the risk is 10% to 25% (Clark, 2004). The risk for invasive placenta can be more than 50% in a pregnancy after multiple cesarean deliveries and a history of placenta previa (Clark, 2004).
- *Septicemia.* The opened blood vessels are near the cervical os and can become infected easily.
- *Thrombosis.*
- *Renal failure.*
- *D-sensitization.* An RhD-negative woman can become sensitized during any antepartum bleeding episode (ACOG, 1999).
- *Postpartum anemia.* Puerperal anemia is the result of increased blood loss.

Fetal and Neonatal Effects

Risk for perinatal mortality is less than 10% with a placenta previa (Ananth, Smulian, and Vintzileos, 2003). However, there is an increased risk for stillbirth. There is also a greater risk for neonatal morbidity. Such effects include the following:

- *Prematurity.* Prematurity is the greatest cause of mortality (Morgan and Arulkumaran, 2003).
- *Malpresentation.* The risk for malpresentation is increased with placenta previa.
- *Intrauterine growth restriction.* Intrauterine growth restriction occurs if the placental exchange is chronically compromised (Morgan and Arulkumaran, 2003).
- *Fetal anemia.* Anemia is in proportion to maternal blood loss and, if the anemia is severe, it may predispose to fetal hypoxia and death (Crane and others, 1999).

Diagnostic Testing

Determining Placental Location

When any pregnant woman complains of vaginal bleeding after 20 weeks of gestation, placenta previa is considered. To diagnose a placenta previa, the location of the placenta must be determined. Both transabdominal and transvaginal ultrasonography facilitate diagnosis; however, transvaginal is more accurate and just as safe (RCOG, 2004).

Ruling Out Other Causes of Bleeding

A speculum examination is usually done to rule out other causes of bright red vaginal bleeding such as cervicitis, cervical polyps, heavy show, or cervical carcinoma.

Determining Gestational Age

An amniocentesis may be included in the diagnostic workup to determine fetal lung maturity. If the lecithin/sphingomyelin (L/S) ratio is 2:1 or phosphatidyl glycerol is present, indicating fetal pulmonary lung maturity, delivery is probably the treatment of choice.

Early Diagnosis of Placenta Previa

An asymptomatic placenta previa, which is identified before the latter half of the third trimester, has a 90% chance of changing to a normal placenta (Oppenheimer and others, 2001).

Usual Medical Management and Protocols for Nurse Practitioners

Expectant Management

Treatment of placenta previa depends on the gestational age and the extent of bleeding. If the gestational age is less than 36 weeks, the fetus has a reassuring FHR tracing, the bleeding is mild (less than 250 ml) and stops, the patient is not in labor, and a cesarean delivery can be performed immediately when indicated, the treatment of choice is expectant management. The purpose is to allow the fetus time to mature to lessen the chance of perinatal mortality from prematurity and perhaps allow time for placental migration. When expectant management is chosen, it usually includes the following:

- Hospitalize initially, and use clinical judgment to consider outpatient management once a bleeding episode has occurred. During the third trimester, inpatient management is advocated (RCOG, 2004).
- Initiate bedrest with bathroom privileges with the intent of improving blood flow to the uterus and increasing fetal growth. Complete bedrest is almost never necessary. To decrease bedrest complications while improving uterine blood flow, bathroom privileges can be interpreted as allowing the woman to be up to use the bathroom and shower and move around the room for 15 to 30 minutes at a time, four times a day.
- Closely observe for signs of bleeding.
- Start IV infusions with a 14- to 16-gauge needle, unless bleeding is minimal; then a heparin lock may be left in place and changed as needed.
- Have a maternal blood sample available at all times in the blood bank for immediate type and cross-match for blood component therapy. If there are no antibodies on the antibody screen, blood does not need to be held. Periodic blood component therapy may be given to maintain hemoglobin at 8 or above. See Table 18-3 for a list of guidelines for blood component replacement.
- Establish continuous fetal monitoring to facilitate early detection of fetal distress during bleeding episodes; otherwise, assess every 4 hours with a Doppler FHR device or fetoscope.
- Perform a nonstress test (NST) with amniotic fluid index, a modified biophysical profile, twice weekly to determine fetal well-being because of the increased risk for stillbirth. Contraction stress tests are contraindicated.

- Use antepartum corticosteroids such as betamethasone (Celestone) or dexamethasone to enhance fetal pulmonary maturity between 24 and 34 weeks of gestation.
- Monitor for signs of preterm uterine contractions stimulated by prostaglandin release from placental separation. Tocolytic therapy, preferably magnesium sulfate for treatment of uterine activity, can be useful to slow cervical change (Morgan and Arulkumaran, 2003).
- Initiate antenatal iron supplementation to facilitate tolerance to mild and moderate blood loss (Morgan and Arulkumaran, 2003).
- Perform amniocentesis between 34 and 36 weeks of gestation to determine fetal lung maturity because risk for bleeding increases with increasing gestational age.

If the patient is allowed to return home after stabilization and after 72 hours without vaginal bleeding, the family should be informed about the potential for complications. She should be instructed to comply with the activity level of bedrest with bathroom privileges and pelvic rest. She must remain within 15 minutes of the hospital, have a telephone, have 24-hour access to transportation, and have close supervision by family in the home. Discharge is not the most desirable choice of care but may be necessary for social, financial, or insurance reasons. Fetal activity charts should be kept daily, and a modified biophysical profile should be done weekly or more often as indicated with weekly clinic visits.

Delivery

Expectant management is terminated as soon as the fetus is mature, excessive bleeding occurs, active labor begins, or any other obstetric reason to terminate the pregnancy develops, such as an intraamniotic infection.

If the bleeding is profuse, the gestational age is 36 or more weeks, the L/S ratio is 2:1, or phosphatidyl glycerol is present, immediate delivery is usually the treatment of choice. Cesarean delivery is the accepted method of delivery in almost all complete or partial placenta previa cases with careful attention for an invasive placenta. Only if the fetus is dead, the fetus has anomalies incompatible with life, or the delivery has already advanced with an engaged fetal head would vaginal delivery be attempted.

A marginal placenta previa may be allowed, and facilities are prepared for immediate cesarean if indicated at any time during the labor.

Table 18-4 compares placenta previa and abruptio placentae.

INVASIVE PLACENTA (PLACENTA CRETAS)

There are three types of invasive placenta: accreta, increta, and percreta. *Placenta accreta* is an uncommon condition in which the chorionic villi adhere to the myometrium. Its more advanced forms are placenta increta and placenta percreta. *Placenta increta* is invasion of the chorionic villi into the myometrium, and *placenta percreta* is growth of the chorionic villi through the myometrium. This causes the placenta to adhere abnormally to the uterus. The abnormal

Table 18-4   Comparison of Placenta Previa and Abruptio Placentae

Parameter	Placenta Previa	Abruptio Placentae
Description	Implantation of placenta in lower segment of uterus near or over internal os	Premature separation of normally implanted placenta after 20 weeks of gestation
Classification	Marginal: placenta implanted near but does not cover any part of internal os Partial: placenta implants near and partially covers internal os Total: placenta completely covers internal os	Mild: less than 1/6 of placenta is separated, mild-to-moderate bleeding, and no uterine tenderness; maternal vital signs of FHR normal Moderate: 1/6 to 1/2 of placenta is separated; abdominal pain; increased uterine tone; maternal vital signs may show mild hypovolemia; FHR may indicate distress Severe: more than 1/2 of placenta is separated; profuse bleeding; persistent and severe abdominal pain and increased tenderness; signs of shock or coagulopathy frequently present with fetal distress or death resulting
Etiology	Unknown: theoretic considerations include a defective vascularization of decidua resulting from uterine scarring or interference with adequate blood supply to endometrium; increased placental mass; early or late ovulation *Associated conditions* • Multiparity of more than five children • Previous placenta previa • Prior uterine scar related to history of suction curettage or previous cesarean birth • Smoking or drug addition • Uterine tumor	Unknown: theoretic considerations include degeneration of spiral arteriole, which causes rupture of involved blood vessels and bleeding; bleeding under placenta separates placenta from deciduas *Associated conditions* • Gestational hypertensive disorder • Previous abruption • Trauma from motor vehicle collision or maternal battering • Cigarette smoking • Cocaine use

Signs and symptoms	slight-to-moderate and ceases spontaneously Presenting part high or displaced Uterus soft and nontender During labor, uterus relaxes between contractions Blood usually clots normally	bleeding is slight to profuse and usually continues Presenting part engaged Uterus tender or rigid (moderate-to-severe abruption) During labor, uterus usually has increased resting tone Clotting defects may be present According to signs and symptoms
Diagnosis	Ultrasound No vaginal examination except under double setup	
Treatment	If initial bleeding episode is slight and gestational age is less than 37 weeks, expectant management is usual choice of treatment: • Close observation of fetal well-being and amount of bleeding • Limited physical activity • No douches, enemas, or sexual intercourse • Delivery when fetus is mature or hemorrhage dictates When bleeding is profuse, gestational age greater than 36 weeks, or L/S ratio 2:1 or greater, delivery is choice of treatment; if placenta previa is: • Marginal, a vaginal delivery may be attempted • Partial or complete, a cesarean delivery is performed	In presence of mild abruption placentae and gestational age is less than 36 weeks, expectant management is usual choice of treatment; close observation of fetal well-being and amount of bleeding Serial hematocrits to assess concealed bleeding Delivery when fetus is mature or hemorrhage dictates; in presence of mild abruptio placentae, with gestational age of 36 weeks or more, delivery is usual choice of treatment In presence of moderate-to-severe abruption placentae: • Restore blood loss • Correct coagulation defect if present • Facilitate delivery • Vaginal delivery is attempted if there is no evidence of fetal or maternal distress with fluid and blood replacement, fetus is in cephalic presentation, labor progresses actively, or fetus is dead

Continued

Table 18-4   Comparison of Placenta Previa and Abruptio Placentae—cont'd

Parameter	Placenta Previa	Abruptio Placentae
		• Cesarean delivery is indicated for severe abruption if fetus is alive, fetal or maternal distress develops with fluid and blood replacement, labor fails to progress actively, or fetal presentation is not cephalic
Maternal outcome	Less than 1% maternal mortality	Less than 1% maternal mortality
Maternal complications	Hemorrhage and hypovolemic shock	Hemorrhage and hypovolemic shock
	Placenta accreta/increta/percreta	DIC
	Premature rupture of membranes	D-sensitization
	D-sensitization	Couvelaire uterus
	Puerperal infection	Puerperal infection
	Puerperal anemia	Puerperal anemia
	Puerperal hemorrhage	Puerperal hemorrhage
		Puerperal DIC
		Renal failure
		Pituitary necrosis
Fetal outcome	Perinatal mortality 10.7 in 1000	Perinatal mortality 14.3 in 1000
Neonatal complications	Prematurity	Prematurity
	Intrauterine hypoxia	Intrauterine hypoxia
	Malpresentation	Small for gestational age
	Small for gestational age	Central nervous system malformations
	Congenital abnormalities	
	Velamentous inserted umbilical cord	
	Vasa previa	
	Neonatal anemia	

DIC, Disseminated intravascular coagulation; *FHR,* fetal heart rate; *L/S,* lecithin/sphingomyelin; *PROM,* premature rupture of membranes.

placental adherence may involve a single cotyledon (focal), a few cotyledons (partial adherence), or all the cotyledons (total adherence).

Incidence

In the presence of a placenta previa, there is a 5% to 10% risk for invasive placenta. The risk is 10% to 25% with a history of one cesarean delivery, increasing to 40% or 50% with a history of two or more cesarean deliveries (ACOG, 2002; Clark, 2004).

Etiology

Placenta accreta can occur if there is an inadequate or absent decidua basalis and fibrinoid layer of Nitabuch. Predisposing factors are those that contribute to an abnormal decidua (endometrium). These factors include prior uterine surgery such as cesarean delivery and women who have a current placenta previa.

Diagnosis

Antepartum

Usually, there is no clinical evidence until after delivery. Because of the increased risk in the presence of a placenta previa, ultrasonographic evaluation of all placenta previas for invasive placenta should be done. Ultrasound imaging or magnetic resonance imaging can confirm or exclude the presence of an invasive placenta (Clark, 2004). However, none of the diagnostic tests ensures 100% diagnostic accuracy (ACOG, 2002).

Postpartum

Placenta accreta is usually diagnosed soon after delivery when the placenta fails to normally separate from the uterine wall and spontaneously deliver. In a focal or partial adherence, the placenta may separate only partially, opening blood vessels while leaving part of the placenta attached. Profuse hemorrhage results because the uterus cannot contract. In a totally adhering placenta, there is no bleeding until attempts are made to manually remove it. Resulting tears in the placenta or partial removal then causes profuse hemorrhage.

Maternal and Fetal Effects

The fetus is rarely affected by this condition unless uterine rupture or extensive bleeding occurs during the pregnancy. The mother is at extreme risk for hemorrhage, infection, and pelvic organ damage. Shock and even death can occur. Maternal mortality is approximately 7% (ACOG, 2002).

Usual Medical Management

If there is any evidence of increased risk for invasive placenta, consideration of a cesarean hysterectomy should be discussed before delivery with the family. This surgery should take place at a facility with excellent blood banking capabilities. A team of physicians, including a surgeon who is skilled in pelvic surgery, should assist. Hypotensive anesthesia can reduce blood loss.

Unexpected invasive placenta treatment depends on the number of cotyledons involved and the depth of penetration. In a focal accreta, the one cotyledon can usually be gently removed from the myometrium. The increased bleeding that results is treated with massage and oxytocin. With more extensive involvement, treatment begins with immediate blood replacement therapy and, nearly always, prompt hysterectomy. Conservative treatment may be attempted in some cases if preservation of fertility is desired.

VASA PREVIA

Vasa previa is a rare developmental disorder of the umbilical cord that may occur with a *velamentous inserted umbilical cord*. Velamentous inserted umbilical cord is a condition in which the umbilical blood vessels are separated when they leave the placenta and are not protected with Wharton jelly as they course between the amnion and chorion before uniting to form the umbilical cord (Fig. 18-3). Vasa previa occurs when velamentous vessels cross the region of the internal os and occupy a position ahead of the presenting part. These vessels are easily compressed or ruptured, which causes immediate fetal distress or death.

Etiology

One postulated cause of vasa previa is that it is the result of the blastocyst failing to implant with the area of the embryonic disk first into the endometrium. This causes the umbilical cord and the placenta to lie opposite each other. Another possible cause may be the result of one side of the placenta growing toward the vascularized uterine fundus and the other side remaining dormant (Lockwood, 1990).

Maternal Effects

Vasa previa presents no danger to the mother because her circulatory system is not involved.

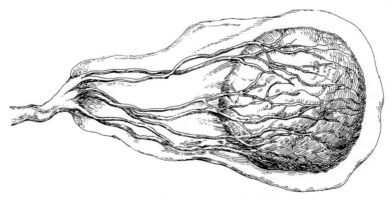

Figure 18-3 Velamentous inserted umbilical cord.

Fetal Effects
Death
The unprotected umbilical vessels are vulnerable to tearing. If one of the umbilical vessels ruptures, death is virtually certain. When the fetal membranes rupture, 75% to 90% of the time velamentous umbilical vessels will rupture as well (Clark, 2004).

Fetal Deformities
Umbilical vessels without Wharton jelly are easily compressed. Compression affects the blood flow to the fetus. Resultant chronic fetal hypoxia leads to fetal growth defects or fetal death in 75% of the cases (Clark, 2004).

Signs and Symptoms
Occasionally, the umbilical vessels may be felt in the membranes during a vaginal examination, and the vessels can be visualized directly with ultrasound. However, most often, the first sign of vasa previa is vaginal bleeding at the time the membranes rupture.

Diagnosis
Vasa previa should be considered if the FHR drops during a vaginal examination and then returns to baseline. In the presence of vaginal bleeding when vasa previa is indicated, a Kleihauer-Betke stain should be obtained to determine whether the blood is of fetal origin.

Management
Once vasa previa is confirmed in the presence of a live fetus, emergency cesarean delivery is carried out. If the fetus is dead, the woman should deliver vaginally.

NURSING MANAGEMENT
Prevention
Because inadequate blood supply to the decidua (endometrium) before implantation may be the underlying cause of a placenta previa and because inadequate blood supply to the decidua during pregnancy may be the underlying cause of an abruptio placentae, any condition that would decrease the uterine blood supply should be avoided if possible. Because cigarette smoking decreases uterine blood supply, the mother should not smoke.

Adequate contraceptive instructions should be given so that couples can plan the time and number of their children, preventing therapeutic abortions and closely spaced pregnancies. Hypertensive disorders of pregnancy are the most common causes of abruptio placentae. Use of cocaine is known to cause transient acute hypertensive episodes, which can initiate abruption of the placenta. For this reason and others, illicit drugs should be avoided altogether during pregnancy (see Chapter 26).

Assessment of Blood Loss

- Obtain a history of onset, duration, amount, color, and consistency of bleeding; obtain a history regarding associated symptoms, prior bleeding episodes, and activity at onset of bleeding.
- Visually record blood loss in cubic centimeters or by weighing saturated pads, linen protectors, or linen (1 g = 1 ml).
- Estimate blood loss related to manifested symptoms. Record blood pressure, pulse, and respiratory rate, determining pulse pressure (difference between systolic and diastolic pressures), orthostatic blood pressure changes, hypothenar refilling (by blanching the fleshy elevation of the ulnar side of the palm of the hand; normal refill is 1 to 2 seconds), skin temperature, and color of skin and mucous membranes. Vital signs may be misleadingly normal even in the presence of severe blood loss. This is related to the normal increase of 40% to 50% in the circulatory blood volume during pregnancy. In fact, after week 32 of gestation, the pregnant patient can lose 25% to 30% of her blood volume without exhibiting signs of shock. The blood supply to the placenta is affected before a 25% to 30% decrease in the maternal blood volume. See Table 18-2 for an interpretation of these symptoms.
- Monitor urinary output as indicated by severity. Because of increased peripheral resistance, cerebral and cardiac perfusion may be preserved, but renal blood flow is often jeopardized because it is sensitive to lack of perfusion. Therefore urinary output during pregnancy is the best noninvasive indicator of circulatory volume. Less than 30 ml/hr indicates decreased circulatory volume to the uterus.
- Monitor laboratory data such as complete blood count, electrolyte panel, renal function with serum creatinine and blood urea nitrogen, and coagulation factors such as bleeding time, fibrinogen, platelet count, FDPs, prothrombin time, and partial thromboplastin time. Serial hematocrits can facilitate early detection of concealed blood loss.
- Do a clot observation test for DIC if the bleeding is moderate to severe.
- Check for abdominal pain, uterine tenderness, or rigidity.
- Observe fundal height changes.
- Assess for fetal well-being and gestational age.
- Assess fetal presentation. Transverse or oblique position is common with a placenta previa because the placenta usually interferes with engagement.
- Assess level of consciousness.
- Obtain baseline breath sounds before starting fluid replacement.
- If the patient is hemodynamically unstable despite apparently adequate fluid replacement or has an underlying renal, cardiac, or pulmonary disease, a triple-lumen Swan-Ganz catheter may be placed for a more accurate assessment of central venous pressure, pulmonary capillary wedge pressure, and cardiac output.

Nursing Interventions for Mild Bleeding (Less Than 15% Blood Loss)

- Continue the assessment as indicated.
- Do not perform vaginal or rectal examinations and do not give enemas or douches in the presence of vaginal bleeding. If there is a placenta previa, enemas and douches can initiate further separation, and profuse bleeding would result. In the presence of an abruptio placentae, when delivery is not to be initiated immediately, no vaginal or rectal examinations should be carried out to avoid disturbing the injured placenta any further.
- Implement bedrest with bathroom privileges. To decrease bedrest complications while improving uterine blood flow, bathroom privileges can be interpreted as up to bathroom and shower, around the room for 15 to 30 minutes at a time, four time a day.
- Establish an IV access with a 14- or 16-gauge IV catheter to allow for fluid and blood component therapy if necessary. Once bleeding has stopped and the hematocrit level is within normal limits, a heparin lock may be placed.
- Have a maternal blood sample in the blood bank at all times for immediate type and cross-match for blood component therapy, and be prepared to transfuse to maintain hemodynamic stability.
- Prevent constipation and excessive stool straining by educating as to the importance of a high-fiber diet. Administer a stool softener as ordered.
- Decrease risk for anemia by teaching the importance of foods high in iron (e.g., whole grains, green leafy vegetables, legumes), vitamin C (e.g., citrus, strawberries, potatoes, broccoli), and protein. Administer ferrous gluconate as ordered between meals to facilitate the absorption of supplemental iron.
- Monitor for signs of preterm uterine contractions and administer tocolytic therapy, preferably magnesium sulfate, for treatment of uterine activity. Terbutaline is contraindicated if hemodynamically unstable because it relaxes vascular beds, decreasing the body's natural compensatory mechanism.

Nursing Interventions for Moderate (20% to 25% Blood Loss) to Severe Bleeding (30% to 35% Blood Loss)

- Complete bedrest in a quiet environment optimizes the outcome. Activity and sensory stimulation can increase the bleeding and elevate the basal metabolic rate, which increases oxygen consumption. Encourage the mother to lie on either side to prevent pressure on the vena cava and further compromise of the fetal circulation.
- Tilt the uterus to the left by placing a folded sheet under the patient's right hip to keep the gravid uterus off the vena cave, if for any reason the patient must be positioned on her back.
- Start an IV line immediately with a 14- or an 16-gauge intracatheter to allow for blood administration.

- Aim fluid therapy at maintaining an adequate circulating blood volume and a hematocrit of 30% or greater.
- Have blood available for type and cross-matching. Administer 2 units of packed red blood cells at the time of each bleeding episode. A lactated Ringer's solution can be administered until blood component therapy is available; it is a better volume expander than dextrose in water. Volume expanders can also be ordered while waiting for properly matched blood components. Prepare for blood component therapy as ordered by having 250 ml of normal saline available. Administer blood component therapy or volume expanders as ordered. See Table 18-4 for a list of guidelines for blood component replacement.
- Allow nothing by mouth unless otherwise ordered.
- Assess for fetal well-being. FHR is usually normal unless excessive blood loss, maternal shock, or major placental detachment compromises the placental exchange.
- Continue to assess for signs of bleeding as severity of condition indicates.
- Keep an accurate intake and output record, and assess urine specific gravity intermittently to determine kidney perfusion.
- Monitor oxygen saturation with pulse oximeter and blood gases as indicated. A maternal oxygen saturation of at least 95% and a PO_2 of at least 65 mm Hg are necessary for adequate fetal oxygenation.
- Observe for signs of hypovolemic shock.
- After stabilization of the patient with adequate blood component replacement, be prepared to facilitate delivery. Be prepared to assist with an amniotomy and administer a labor stimulant as ordered. Prepare patient for possible cesarean delivery.
- Treat postpartum hemorrhage with uterine massage, with direct compression, by ensuring no retained placental fragments and by using pharmacologic agents for uterine atony such as 10 to 20 units of oxytocin in 1000 ml of Ringer's lactate or normal saline at an infusion rate not to exceed 100 mU/min; methylergonovine maleate (Methergine) 0.2 mg intramuscularly in the deltoid every 1 to 2 hours for a maximum of five times (Weiner and Buhimschi, 2004). Rule out vaginal and cervical lacerations. Oxytocin can cause hypotension and has a marked antidiuretic effect when a dose of 20 to 40 mU/min is given. Methylergonovine maleate is contraindicated in hypertensive, increase intraocular pressure, hepatic dysfunction, or renal dysfunction patients.
- Report to the primary care provider any change in the patient's bleeding pattern, signs of shock, or failure to respond to treatment.

Critical Care Interventions for Hypovolemic Shock (40% Blood Loss or Greater)

- Restore the blood volume and oxygen-carrying capacity. Begin with lactated Ringer's solution while blood is being typed and cross-matched. It has a 3:1 replacement ratio, 3 ml of solution per 1 ml of estimated blood loss. O-negative packed red bloods cells follow as soon as possible until type-specific cross-matched blood is available. See Table 18-3 for guidelines for blood component replacement.

- Assess for risks caused by using blood and blood components such as hypothermia, dysrhythmias, acidosis, or electrolyte imbalance.
- Administer oxygen at 8 to 10 L/min by facemask to increase oxygen tension and increase oxygen delivery to end-organs.
- Improve autotransfusion by placing patient in modified Trendelenburg position (only elevate legs) to increase blood perfusion to vital organs until blood volume replacement is achieved without contributing to respiratory impairment.
- Always keep the uterus off the vena cava by using a wedge under the hip.
- Continuously monitor blood pressure to evaluate fluid replacement therapy.
- In the presence of a live fetus, continuously monitor FHR until delivery. Keep in mind that a maternal heart beat may be picked up through the fetal scalp electrode in the event of fetal death.
- Monitor input and output with a Foley catheter hourly. *Note:* 30 ml/hr or greater of urine indicates adequate organ perfusion and oxygenation.
- Treat the underlying cause of hemorrhage.
- Use invasive hemodynamic monitoring with a pulmonary artery catheter to evaluate fluid replacement therapy if the hypovolemic shock is unresponsive to initial volume resuscitation and to prevent fluid overload.
- Use the pulmonary artery catheter to obtain direct measurement of the heart rate, central venous pressure, pulmonary artery systolic and diastolic pressures, pulmonary capillary wedge pressure (PCWP), and cardiac output.
- Continuously monitor electrocardiograph as indicated.
- Assess for fluid overload with signs of pulmonary congestion, such as dyspnea, cough, or crackles, by auscultating lung fields every shift.
- Continue to monitor laboratory data as indicated.
- If fluid replacement is inadequate in restoring optimal cardiovascular function, vasopressor agents are indicated as the last resort. Administer dopamine hydrochloride as a continuous infusion starting at 2 to 5 mg/kg/min and titrate according to hemodynamic response. Remember that these agents decrease blood flow to the uterus while increasing maternal myocardial contractility, cardiac output, and systemic vascular resistance without effecting myocardial oxygen consumption. Norepinephrine and ephedrine are two other vasopressor drugs that are used.
- If hypovolemic shock occurred, assess for the possible development of pituitary necrosis (Sheehan syndrome) during postpartum by assessing for the onset of lactation. Instruct patient to notify physician if onset of lactation does not occur by the fifth postpartum day.
- Evaluate for urinary output greater than 30 ml/hr with clear breath sounds. If a Swan-Ganz catheter is in place, pulmonary capillary wedge pressure maintained between 10 and 15 mm Hg and central venous pressure between 12 and 15 cm.

Critical Care Interventions for Disseminated Intravascular Coagulation

- Observe for signs of DIC such as oozing of blood from the IV site, easy bruising, or petechiae.
- Monitor the DIC coagulopathy profile, which includes fibrinogen, platelet count, prothrombin time, partial thromboplastin time, fibrin split products, and fibrin degradation products (FDPs) with a D-dimer test. *Note:* The most sensitive test for diagnosis of abruptio-related DIC is the determination of FDP with a D-dimer test (Clark, 2004). Prothrombin time and partial thromboplastin time are late indicators because 50% or more of the clotting factors must be consumed before these tests are abnormal. It should be noted that normal measurements during pregnancy are bleeding time less than 4 minutes, fibrinogen levels of 400 to 650 mg/dl, platelets between 100,000 and 350,000/mm^3, prothrombin time 12 to 14 seconds, and partial prothrombin time between 14 and 36 seconds.
- Serial clot observation tests may be done at the bedside to assess for severe DIC. To carry this out, the nurse places 5 ml of venous blood in a test tube, hangs it in the room, and observes the time it takes to clot. If it does not form a clot within 6 to 8 minutes, a significant coagulation defect is usually present.
- Treat the underlying disease process and bleeding. Administer procoagulants such as platelets, clotting factors with fresh frozen plasma at 0.1 to 0.2 bags/kg, and factor VIII and fibrinogen with cryoprecipitate. Heparin is rarely needed. See Chapter 19 for management. *Note:* Minimal clotting factor levels for surgery are fibrinogen above 100 mg/dl and platelets greater than 50,000/mm^3.
- DIC usually resolves spontaneously after delivery.

Nursing Interventions for Antepartum Fetal Surveillance

- Assess FHR. It is usually normal unless excessive blood loss, maternal shock, or major placental detachment compromises the placental exchange.
- Determine gestational age.
- Monitor FHR as indicated (depending on severity).
- Evaluate FHR for tachycardia, bradycardia, late or variable decelerations, and loss of long- or short-term variability.
- During labor, check uterine contractions for duration, frequency, and uterine resting tone. Observe amniotic fluid for meconium staining.
- Prevent vena cava syndrome by keeping patient positioned on her left or right side; if she must be on her back, tilt uterus to the left by placing folded sheet under the right hip.
- Administer oxygen as indicated with facemask at 8 to 10 L/min.
- Prepare the patient for fetal well-being and maturity studies as ordered. Modified biophysical profiles, ultrasound, and amniocentesis are usually ordered on a frequent basis in an attempt to determine the optimal time for delivery.

- Antepartum corticosteroids such as betamethasone or dexamethasone are indicated to enhance fetal pulmonary maturity between 24 and 34 weeks of gestation.
- Be prepared to intermittently assess blood to determine whether it is of fetal origin by a Kleihauer-Betke analysis or APT (alum-precipitated toxoid) test because of the increased risk for a vasa previa associated with a placenta previa.
- If vaginal bleeding occurs immediately after rupture of membranes, vasa previa is suggested.
- Notify physician if a baseline or periodic FHR change is noted or if there is a nonreactive NST or amniotic fluid index less than 8.
- During a trial of labor, notify the physician of a hypertonic uterus, increased signs of bleeding, a labor that progresses abnormally slowly, or any signs of fetal stress.
- Once delivery is imminent, notify the intensive care nursery of a possible high risk infant.

Nursing Interventions to Manage Fear Related to Effect on Health Status and Threat of Fetal or Neonatal Death

- Assess level of maternal anxiety. Parents are usually very concerned about the health and well-being of the baby and the mother's safety. They may also be experiencing some common fears or worries such as wondering what they might have done to cause this to happen. Therefore the expectant parents should be encouraged to express their feelings and concerns. In this way, the nurse knows better how to individualize emotional support.
- Assess other family members' feelings of guilt, such as wondering what they might have done to cause this to happen.
- Assess the family's coping strategies and resources.
- Encourage expression of feelings, concerns, and labor experience.
- Clarify any misconceptions. Explain that the cause of the condition is unknown but it is not related to patient's activity at time of occurrence.
- Provide information to the patient and her family regarding the pregnancy complication, plan of treatment, and implications for mother and fetus in understandable terms. Discuss with the expectant parents the possibility of a cesarean delivery. The parents are then more prepared if the event arises.
- Explain all treatment modalities and reasons for each.
- Keep parents informed of health status, test results, and fetal well-being. Focus them on the positive signs of fetal well-being such as a normal FHR, fetal activity, and reactive NSTs.
- Compliment the patient for her cooperation in adhering to medical therapy.
- Refer to the social worker if inadequate coping is noted.
- Refer to pastor, priest, or chaplain per parents' request.
- Evaluate. The patient and her family will be able to communicate their fears and concerns openly.

Nursing Interventions for Altered Role Performance Related to Prolonged Hospitalization and Treatment with Bedrest

- Assess the patient's responsibilities to determine difficulties she will have in implementing prescribed bedrest.
- Teach importance of bedrest in the lateral position with bathroom privileges.
- Help the family problem solve if difficulties arise in implementing bedrest.
- Refer to Sidelines high risk support group.
- Make needed referrals, such as to social worker, if problems are identified.
- Encourage participation in her care and decision making as much as possible.
- Evaluate the patient's plan that will take care of all her work- and family-related responsibilities during her absence.

Diversional Activity for Therapeutic Management of Bedrest

- Assess patient's interest in various diversional activities within the activity limit.
- Provide activities such as crafts, reading, and puzzles that can be done in bed, or encourage patient to have these items brought in.
- Provide classes in preparation for childbirth by way of video, hospital television, or group classes that can be attended while reclining.
- Refer to a diversional therapist or volunteer to provide reading materials, handicrafts, or other interesting materials.
- Evaluate. Ask the patient to verbalize various appropriate activities she would like to do while maintaining bedrest.

Nursing Interventions to Prevent RhD Alloimmunization in a D-Negative Mother Carrying an Rh-Positive Fetus

- Monitor the RhD antibody titer with an antibody screen, indirect Coombs test at 28 weeks of gestation, and then again at the time of admission. An antibody titer may be repeated after any bleeding episode if a fetal-maternal bleed is suggested.
- Administer Rho (D) immune globulin (RhoGAM; HypRho-D) 300 mcg intramuscularly in the deltoid as ordered at 28 weeks, after any suspected fetal-maternal bleed, and within 72 hours postpartum.
- After any antepartum bleed, evaluate for fetal cells in the maternal circulation. If fetal cells are found, be prepared to order a Kleihauer-Betke stain to assess the amount of fetal blood in the maternal circulation. If the bleed is greater than 30 ml of fetal whole blood (15 ml packed RBC), administer additional Rho (D) immune globulin based on this formula: PRBC divided by 2; then divide by 15 = number of vials (Weiner and Buhimschi, 2004).

CONCLUSION

The ultimate goal of treatment for both an abruptio placenta and a placenta previa is early recognition and appropriate intervention to prevent hemorrhage and its resulting complications of shock, DIC, multisystem failure, and ultimately death of mother or fetus. At the same time, premature delivery must be avoided as long as intrauterine hypoxia is not present.

BIBLIOGRAPHY

Addis A and others: Fetal effects of cocaine: an updated meta-analysis, *Reprod Toxicol* 15:341, 2001.

American College of Obstetricians and Gynecologists (ACOG): *Placenta accreta,* Committee Opinion, No. 266, Washington, DC, 2002, ACOG.

American College of Obstetricians and Gynecologists: *Prevention of Rh D alloimmunization,* Practice Bulletin, No. 4, Washington, DC, 1999, ACOG.

Ananth C, Smulian J, and Vintzileos A: The effect of placenta previa on neonatal mortality: a population-based study in the United States, 1989 through 1997, *Am J Obstet Gynecol* 188(5):1299–1304, 2003.

Bhide A, Thilaganthan B: Recent advances in the management of placenta previa, *Curr Opin Obstet Gynecol* 16(6):447–451, 2004.

Carter S: Overview of common obstetric bleeding disorders, *Nurse Pract* 24(3):50–58, 1999.

Clark S: Placenta previa abruptio placentae. In Creasy R, Resnik R, and Iams J: *Maternal-fetal medicine: principles and practice,* ed 5, Philadelphia, 2004, Saunders.

Crane J and others: Neonatal outcomes with placenta previa, *Am Coll Obstet Gynecol* 93:541, 1999.

Cunningham G: *Williams' obstetrics,* ed 22, New York, 2005, McGraw-Hill.

Gesteland K and others: Rates of placenta previa and placental abruption in women delivered only vaginally or only by cesarean section, Abstract No 403, *J Soc Gynecol Investig* 11:208A, 2004.

Lockwood C: Placenta previa and related disorders, *Contemp Ob/Gyn* 35(1):47, 1990.

MacMullen N, Dulski L, and Meagher B: Red alert: perinatal hemorrhage, *MCN Am J Matern Child Nurs* 30(1):46–51, 2005.

Martin J and others: Births: final data for 2001. *National Vital Statistics Reports,* Vol 51, No 2, Hyattsville, MD, National Center for Health Statistics, 2002.

Morgan K, Arulkumaran S: Antepartum heamorrhage, *Curr Obstet Gynaecol* 13(2):81, 2003.

Neilson J: Interventions for suspected placenta previa (Cochrane Review). In *The Cochrane Library,* Issue 2, Oxford, 2001, Update Software.

Oppenheimer L and others: Diagnosis of low-lying placenta: can migration in the third trimester predict outcome? *Ultrasound Obstet Gynecol* 18(2):100–102, 2001.

Royal College of Obstetricians and Gynaecologists (RCOG): *Placenta praevia: diagnosis and management,* Guideline No. 27, London, 2004, RCOG Press. Retrieved from *http://www.rcog. org.uk/indes.asp?PageID=1042*

Salihu H and others: Perinatal mortality associated with abruptio placenta in singletons and multiples, *Am J Obstet Gynecol* 193(1):198–203, 2005.

Weiner C, Buhimschi C: *Drugs for pregnant and lactating women,* Philadelphia, 2004, Churchill Livingstone.

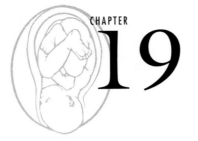

Disseminated Intravascular Coagulation

D isseminated intravascular coagulation (DIC) is not a primary disease but rather a secondary event activated by a number of severe illnesses. It occurs when a severe illness causes a generalized activation of the coagulation process. If coagulation factors are consumed faster than the liver can replace them, depletion occurs. At that point, the process of fibrinolysis is activated in response to coagulation. The result is rampant coagulation and simultaneous massive bleeding (Kilpatrick and Laros, 2004).

INCIDENCE

It is estimated that the incidence of DIC is 1 per 8,000 to 30,000 pregnancies (Moore and Ware, 2005).

ETIOLOGY

The following stimuli are known to activate the coagulation syndrome during pregnancy (Kalpatrick and Laros, 2004; Anthony, 2006):
- Infusion of tissue extract from injured tissue
- Severe injury to endothelial cells
- Red cell or platelet injury seen in hemolytic processes
- Bacterial debris or endotoxins
- Immune reactions
- Thrombocytopenia
- Chemical and physical agents
  Some of the conditions that commonly activate this process are listed (Furlong and Furlong, 2005):
- Greater than expected blood loss with inadequate crystalloid or colloid replacement
- Placental abruption
- Severe preeclampsia, eclampsia or the HELLP (hemolysis, elevated liver enzymes, and low-platelet count in association with preeclampsia) syndrome
- Sepsis
- Acute fatty liver of pregnancy

- Retained dead fetus
- Major trauma
- Amniotic fluid embolus or anaphylactoid syndrome of pregnancy

NORMAL PHYSIOLOGY

The processes of clot formation and clot breakdown (*fibrinolysis*) must be understood to comprehend DIC. Clot formation and fibrinolysis are intertwined with the activation of factors maintaining a homeostasis under normal circumstances.

Whenever blood vessels or tissues become damaged and bleeding occurs, several factors attempt hemostasis. First, central nervous system reflexes cause vascular spasms, reducing blood flow to the area. Second, platelets attempt to plug the break. Finally, clot formation occurs. Clot formation can be activated by intrinsic and extrinsic factors. The intrinsic factors exist within the vascular system and are activated with blood vessel damage. The extrinsic factors are within the tissue and are activated in response to tissue trauma. When either process is activated, prothrombin activator is formed. Prothrombin activator, along with calcium and phospholipids, acts as a catalyst to convert inactive plasma prothrombin into thrombin. The enzyme *thrombin* converts inactive plasma fibrinogen into fibrin. Fibrin, along with platelets, causes the red blood cells (RBCs) and plasma to mesh, and a clot is then formed (Fig. 19-1).

Fibrinolysis normally occurs simultaneously with clot formation as long as activators are present. Plasminogen, a plasma euglobulin, is activated into

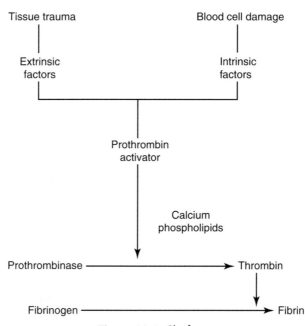

Figure 19-1 Clot formation.

plasmin. Plasmin then breaks fibrin down into fibrin split products and fibrinogen into fibrinogen split products. This process consumes factors V, VIII, and XII (intrinsic factors) and prothrombin. Anticoagulants, antithrombin III, and heparin also facilitate fibrinolysis. Antithrombin III neutralizes thrombin, plasmin, and factors VII, VII, X, and XII, which are intrinsic and extrinsic factors. Heparin greatly enhances the action of antithrombin III (Fig. 19-2) (Kilpatrick and Laros, 2004).

In pregnancy, fibrinogen, platelet adhesiveness, and factor VIII are increased. Antithrombin III and the activators for plasminogen are decreased. Plasminogen itself is increased. Therefore the equilibrium of coagulation and fibrinolysis is skewed toward procoagulation. Factors in pregnancy that can promote this include fetoplacental hormones, pregnancy-specific hormones, immunologic complexes, and entry of placental thrombin into maternal circulation through the vascular interfaces (Auerbach and Lockwood, 2006). See Chapter 13 for further description of clotting factors.

The listed clotting factors are the important ones for DIC (Chapter 13). See Chapter 18 for placental abnormalities and Chapter 21 for hypertensive disorders and their relationships to DIC.

PATHOPHYSIOLOGY

DIC occurs when factor consumption of the coagulation-fibrinolysis processes exceed the liver's capacity to produce factors. The coagulation process is stimulated by endothelial or tissue injury. When coagulation factors are depleted, equilibrium is disrupted and bleeding occurs because of deficient coagulation factors. The body continues to attempt clot formation in the presence of bleeding, which further depletes coagulation factors. Small clots can plug the small blood vessels and lead to organ ischemia (Kilpatrick and Laros, 2004).

Amniotic fluid embolism, also called *anaphylactoid syndrome of pregnancy*, causes an extravasation of amniotic fluid with vernix, squamous cells, and mucus into the maternal circulation. Maternal immunologic defenses attempt

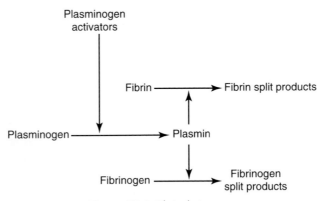

Figure 19-2 Fibrinolysis.

to wall off the huge quantities of these foreign substances, which leads to an anaphylactic-like response. This response is rapid and overwhelming, depending on the amount of amniotic debris sent into the maternal circulation (Anthony, 2006). The response initiates a cascade of activation of both the coagulation and the fibrinolysis processes, as well as simultaneous respiratory and cardiac arrest (Moore and Ware, 2005).

When the products of conception are retained after intrauterine fetal demise, thromboplastic material can seep into the maternal circulation. This infusion of tissue extract activates the overwhelming depletion of coagulation factors.

In preeclampsia and eclampsia, damage to vessel walls occurs secondary to oxidative stress and ischemic endotoxin substance released by the placenta. The vessel wall damage causes products of cellular breakdown to come in contact with the surface of the platelets, and the coagulation-fibrinolysis process occurs simultaneously. The process then consumes massive amounts of coagulation-fibrinolysis factors, and the liver is unable to replace factors as rapidly as is necessary (Anthony, 2006).

Hemorrhage and shock can also precipitate disequilibrium of coagulation-fibrinolysis. Hypovolemia causes decreased cardiac output, decreased arterial pressure, and decreased systemic blood flow. This results in decreased nutrition to the brain and vascular system. The hypoxic vascular endothelium triggers intravascular coagulation. Intravascular coagulation releases toxins that increase capillary permeability, further diminishing circulating volume. Brain anoxia results in cardiac depression and further compromises cardiac output.

SIGNS AND SYMPTOMS

Early symptoms of DIC include epistaxis, gingival bleeding, ecchymoses, and bleeding into the urine or at the site of an intravenous (IV) line. As DIC develops, these early signs may rapidly progress to the following severe signs of shock:

- Respirations progress from rapid and deep to rapid, shallow, and irregular and finally to barely perceptible.
- Pulse rate becomes rapid, weaker, irregular, and thready.
- Blood pressure may initially be normal but then begins falling until the systolic pressure is below 60 mm Hg or is not palpable.
- Skin color may then begin to pale and cool, progressing rapidly to being cold, clammy, and cyanotic.
- Urinary output initially remains stable and then quickly begins to decrease to less than 30 ml/hr.
- Level of consciousness changes from apprehension to increasing restlessness, lethargy, and finally coma.
- Central venous pressure and pulmonary artery wedge pressure drop.

Laboratory signs of DIC include decreased platelet count, fibrinogen, and antithrombin III levels, as well as increased fibrin split products, abnormal prothrombin fragment 1 and 2, abnormal fibrinopeptide A, and the presence of FDP/D-dimer.

MATERNAL EFFECTS

DIC can and often does result in maternal death. Maternal mortality from amniotic fluid embolism is approximately 80%, and fetal and neonatal mortality is approximately 70% (Moore and Ware, 2005). If it does not result in maternal death, few mothers survive neurologically intact. Damage ranges from relatively minor to very profound.

FETAL AND NEONATAL EFFECTS

DIC can result in fetal death or severe hypoxia. Possible neonatal sequelae to severe hypoxia are intracranial bleeding and brain death.

DIAGNOSTIC TESTING

The medical diagnosis is made based on a history of predisposing conditions, the early signs of ecchymosis formation, and bleeding from the IV site or urinary tract. Definitive diagnosis is made based on the laboratory data previously listed.

USUAL MEDICAL MANAGEMENT AND PROTOCOLS FOR NURSE PRACTITIONERS

When DIC occurs in the antepartum period, the initial treatment is to correct the underlying cause, which usually means emptying the uterus by the most expeditious means. To improve the circulatory volume, fluid replacement is essential. Blood replacement with packed cells, fresh frozen plasma (FFP), cryoprecipitate, and platelets may be necessary to replace volume and depleted coagulation factors. Simultaneously, the primary disease must be stabilized and corrected.

Blood Replacement

Red Blood Cell Transfusions

The main blood replacement is RBCs. These may come as packed RBCs, which contain RBCs and plasma—usually 250 ml of RBCs and 50 ml of plasma—and have a hematocrit level of approximately 80%. This replacement thus reduces the risk for fluid overload.

Platelet Concentrates

Platelets are separated from whole blood and suspended in small amounts of plasma and a small amount of serum-bound RBCs. Caution should be exercised in an Rh-negative woman.

Fresh Frozen Plasma (FFP)

FFP is extracted from whole blood within 6 hours of collection and then frozen. It contains 700 mg of fibrinogen. It is indicated to correct deficiencies of multiple clotting factors, including factors V, VIII, X, and XIII. It also increases fibrinogen level.

Cryoprecipitate

Cryoprecipitate is extracted from frozen whole blood, which has then thawed at a controlled, refrigerated temperature. FFP precipitates under these conditions and is then rich in Factor VIII and fibrinogen.

Supportive Measures

Supportive measures for monitoring fluid replacement and cardiac output are necessary. These include cardiac monitoring, hemodynamic monitoring, and blood pressure recordings every 5 to 15 minutes. Because clinical signs of DIC may be rapid in onset, the emergency initially threatens the mother's life and fetal considerations are excluded. Once factor replacement is instituted for the mother, the fetus is often delivered before continuous monitoring of the fetal heart rate (FHR) can be initiated. Fetal delivery may be accomplished simultaneously with resuscitation of the pregnant woman. Two teams, one for trauma response and one for perinatal response, are usually required for this approach.

Anticoagulants

Heparin and antithrombolytic therapy is rarely used unless clotting continues 4 to 6 hours after initiation of blood replacement therapy to decrease the risk for progressive renal failure and gangrene (Anthony, 2006).

NURSING MANAGEMENT

Secondary Prevention

When the mother has a condition that might predispose her to development of DIC, the nurse must be alert for early signs of ecchymosis: blood in the urine or bleeding from the gums, the IV insertion site, or other venous puncture sites. A simple test to confirm early signs of possible DIC is the clot retraction test, in which 5 ml of blood is drawn into a test tube, capped, and taped to the bedside wall. If a clot does not form and the serum does not separate from the cells within 8 to 10 minutes, DIC is possible and the physician should be notified. Late signs of disequilibrium are watched for as well. These signs include progressive changes in respiration, pulse, blood pressure, skin color, and urinary output, as well as indications of mild to moderate shock and acute renal failure (see Chapter 12).

Tertiary Prevention

During the recovery phase, care should include early detection and treatment of infection and transfusion hepatitis. Grief management is an important component of the recovery phase if maternal or fetal loss occurred. Maternal death occurs in approximately 75% to 85% of cases, and fetal loss occurs at a rate that is equally as high or higher. See Chapter 7 for information about perinatal loss and grief.

Critical Care Nursing Interventions for Disseminated Intravascular Coagulation

- Observe patients with complications precipitating DIC for early signs of shock.
- Evaluate vital signs for evidence of shock, that is, increased pulse rate preceding a drop in blood pressure (in fact, early signs may include a slight rise in blood pressure), restlessness, and loss of sensorium.
- Evaluate bedside clot retraction test by placing 5 ml of blood in test tube and observing after 8 to 10 minutes to see whether a clot has formed.
- Start an IV line with at least a 14-gauge angiocatheter and infuse physiologic saline solution.
- Notify laboratory trauma support personnel for possible need for uncrossed-matched blood and blood products.
- Prepare to transfuse rapidly with cryoprecipitate, packed cells, and FFP.
- Administer oxygen, 8 to 10 L/min by facemask.
- Position patient off her back, using a rolled towel under her right hip.
- Involve the intensive care or trauma team so that they can assist with fluid replacement and monitoring or refer.
- Assist with insertion of invasive hemodynamic lines.
- Monitor vital signs and hemodynamic data as indicated.
- Report vital signs, hemodynamic monitoring data, amount of continued bleeding, and laboratory data immediately to the physician in charge of fluid replacement therapy.
- Assess for the potential complication of acute renal failure.
- Institute fetal monitoring as soon as the intensive care team or trauma team begins managing the maternal emergency. Labor nurse's responsibility shifts to the fetus.
- Prepare for an emergent (agonal) cesarean birth if the mother is not immediately stabilized before delivery and the fetus is viable.
- Notify neonatal team.
- During postpartum recovery phase, monitor for signs of infection such as pneumonia, septic shock, or transfusion hepatitis.

Critical Care Interventions for Amniotic Fluid Embolism (Anaphylactoid Embolic Syndrome)

- Assess for signs such as acute hypotension, sudden respiratory and cardiac arrest (usually occur simultaneously), or sudden loss of consciousness.
- Call the code arrest team immediately to start cardiopulmonary resuscitation. Administer oxygen by facemask and then via pressure through an endotracheal tube when code team arrives to assume resuscitative efforts for the mother.
- Assemble all necessary obstetric and neonatal team members (anesthesiologist, obstetrician or perinatologist, neonatologist or pediatrician, and obstetric and neonatal nurses) for surgical delivery and neonatal resuscitation.

- Set up and be prepared to assist with an agonal-perimortem cesarean delivery.
- Prepare to use any and all of the blood replacement volume expanders and coagulation factors to treat shock and DIC.
- Have IV corticosteroids, histamine-1 agent diphenhydramine (Benadryl). and a histamine-2 agent ranitidine (Zantac) or famotidine (Pepcid) available for anaphylaxis therapy.
- Have pressor agents such as dopamine, norepinephrine, and ephedrine ready and available.
- Prepare to treat left ventricular failure with IV digoxin.
- Monitor cardiac output, afterload, and preload with central monitoring.
- Initially monitor maternal oxygen saturation with a pulse oximeter. Then, as the code team assumes responsibility, respiratory personnel monitor with respiratory ventilatory equipment.
- Assign a social worker, a chaplain, and/or a nurse with knowledge of grief support to the family while resuscitation efforts are underway.
- Manage grief of all involved family members by referring them to a qualified grief support team member who assists with recovery from probable traumatic and unexpected outcomes for either or both the mother and baby (see Chapter 7).
- Have mental health and grief support services available for involved staff members within 1 to 2 days after the events if maternal death is the outcome.

CONCLUSION

The primary goal of care of the pregnant woman with DIC is to prevent shock and its sequelae. Early recognition of conditions that predispose a woman to DIC can help prevent maternal death or unexpected long-term sequelae as well as promote a healthy newborn outcome. When a pregnant woman presents with a severe medical condition and has developed DIC, it is important to attempt rapid stabilization of the mother before attempting an emergency or agonal cesarean delivery.

BIBLIOGRAPHY

Anthony J: Major obstetric hemorrhage: disseminated intravascular coagulation. In James D and others, editors: *High risk pregnancy: management options*, ed 3, Philadelphia, 2006, Saunders.

Auerbach R, Lockwood C: Clotting disorders. In James D and others, editors: *High risk pregnancy: management options*, ed 3, Philadelphia, 2006, Saunders.

Furlong M, Furlong B: Disseminated intravascular coagulation, *eMedicine*, 2005. Retrieved from *http://www.emedicine.com/emerg/topic150.htm*

Kilpatrick S, Laros R: Maternal hematologic disorders. In Creasy R, Resnik R, and Iams J, editors: *Maternal-fetal medicine: principles and practice*, ed 5, Philadelphia, 2004, Saunders.

Moore L, Ware D: Amniotic fluid embolism, *eMedicine*, 2005. Retrieved from *http://www. emedicine.com/med/topic122.htm*

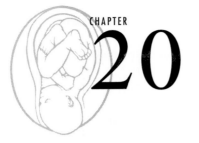

Hemolytic Incompatibility

H emolytic incompatibility occurs when a pregnant woman is sensitized to produce immunoglobulin G antibodies against fetal red blood cells usually from the CDE (Rh) or ABO blood group. The antibodies, returning to the fetal circulation, can cause erythrocyte destruction in the fetus and subsequent fetal anemia with liver failure and congestive heart failure (hydrops).

INCIDENCE

Despite routine use of postpartum anti-D immunoglobulin, Rh sensitization stills occurs in 7% of all live births according to the CDC (Martin and others, 2002). Although RhD incompatibility is the most common and usually the most serious, other hemolytic incompatibilities do occur. Hemolytic disease is seen in 10% of the ABO blood group incompatibilities. ABO and RhD incompatibilities account for 98% of all hemolytic disease in the fetus. Of the remaining 2%, rare antibodies, such as C, c, E, e, Kell, or Duffy antibodies, are implicated. The pathophysiologic processes for all incompatibilities are similar (Weiner, 2006).

ETIOLOGY

ABO incompatibility occurs when the mother's blood type is O and the fetal blood type is A, B, or AB. Compared with the CDE (Rh) system, the ABO system is weakly antigenic to its own factors for two reasons. First, A and B antibodies do not cross the placenta. Second, fewer A and B antigenic sites exist on fetal red cells. Therefore there is only a 5% risk for an ABO incompatibility, and it seldom causes hydrops fetalis.

Rh incompatibility occurs primarily when the mother is RhD-negative and the fetus is RhD-positive. However, it can also occur if the fetus has any antigen C, c, E, or e and the mother does not (Weiner, 2006).

NORMAL PHYSIOLOGY
Blood Type Genetics

Each father and mother, having received half of their blood type from each parent, can be said to be homozygous or heterozygous. Thus in the ABO system, combinations occur. All people with type O blood are homozygous. When the mother is type O, she is homozygous, having received an O from both parents. If the father is type O also, there are no antigenic possibilities for the fetal ABO system; the fetus must be type O. If the father is type A, he could be AO heterozygous or AA homozygous. If the father is type B, he could be BB homozygous or BO heterozygous. If the father is type AB, he is heterozygous. To understand the possible fetal blood types from heterozygous fathers with type A, B, or AB and homozygous O mothers or from homozygous type A or B fathers and homozygous O mothers, the following examples may be helpful:

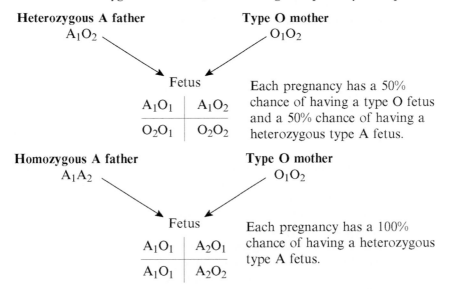

Heterozygous A father
A_1O_2

Type O mother
O_1O_2

Fetus

A_1O_1	A_1O_2
O_2O_1	O_2O_2

Each pregnancy has a 50% chance of having a type O fetus and a 50% chance of having a heterozygous type A fetus.

Homozygous A father
A_1A_2

Type O mother
O_1O_2

Fetus

A_1O_1	A_2O_1
A_1O_1	A_2O_2

Each pregnancy has a 100% chance of having a heterozygous type A fetus.

- The heterozygous type A fetus carried by a type O mother has antigen A that can evoke antibody formation in the type O mother. Type B works the same way.

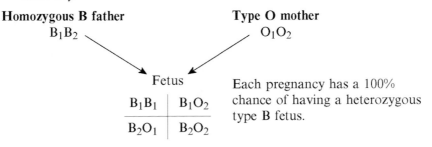

Homozygous B father
B_1B_2

Type O mother
O_1O_2

Fetus

B_1B_1	B_1O_2
B_2O_1	B_2O_2

Each pregnancy has a 100% chance of having a heterozygous type B fetus.

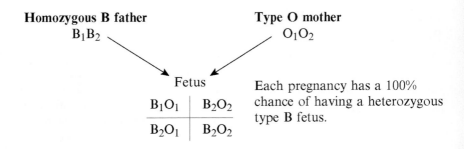

Homozygous B father
B_1B_2

Type O mother
O_1O_2

Fetus

B_1O_1	B_2O_2
B_2O_1	B_2O_2

Each pregnancy has a 100% chance of having a heterozygous type B fetus.

- The heterozygous type B fetus has the B antigen, which can evoke antibody formation in the type O mother.
- Type AB fathers are always heterozygous. Their children from a type O mother have the following chances:

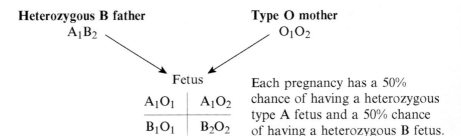

Heterozygous B father
A_1B_2

Type O mother
O_1O_2

Fetus

A_1O_1	A_1O_2
B_1O_1	B_2O_2

Each pregnancy has a 50% chance of having a heterozygous type A fetus and a 50% chance of having a heterozygous B fetus.

- Because type AB fathers having children with type O mothers always produce heterozygous A or heterozygous B children, each fetus has the potential of antigenic factors evoking antibody formation by the type O mother. All have antigenic factors that are relatively weak compared with the CDE blood system.
- If a mother is RhD-negative, she is always homozygous, having received the RhD-negative gene from both parents. The RhD-positive father may be RhD-positive heterozygous or RhD-positive homozygous. The following examples demonstrate this.

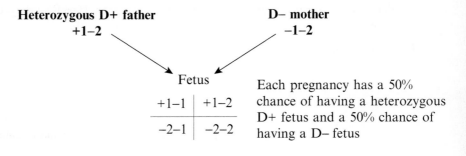

Heterozygous D+ father
+1–2

D– mother
–1–2

Fetus

+1–1	+1–2
–2–1	–2–2

Each pregnancy has a 50% chance of having a heterozygous D+ fetus and a 50% chance of having a D– fetus

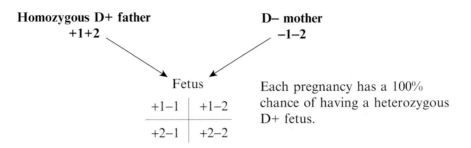

Homozygous D+ father
+1+2

D– mother
–1–2

Fetus

+1–1	+1–2
+2–1	+2–2

Each pregnancy has a 100% chance of having a heterozygous D+ fetus.

- The RhD fetus has a strong RhD antigen on the surface of each red blood cell. These antigens evoke antibody formation in the RhD mother. The degree of sensitivity to the fetal D antigen varies but is assumed to be related to the total number of RhD fetal red blood cells entering the maternal circulation (Moise 2004b; Weiner, 2006).

ABO Blood Group System

The ABO blood group system has the following antigens:
- A has antigen A.
- B has antigen B.
- AB has both antigens A and B.
- O has none.

The person who does not have the AB antigen probably has the antibody against the respective antigen.

CDE (Rh) Blood Group System

More than 400 red cell antigens have been identified. The person who lacks a specific red cell antigen and is exposed to that antigen can potentially produce an antibody against the antigen. It is fortunate that many of these red cell antigens are rare and many have low immunogenicity capability. The greatest immunogenicity capability is seen with the RhD (rhesus factor) antigen. If the mother is Rh-positive, she probably has the RhD antigen. If the mother is Rh-negative, she does not have the antigen and is extremely vulnerable to the formation of anti-D antibodies if she is exposed to the D antigen. However, recognition is growing of immunogenicity in the Rh system if factor E, c, C, or e (listed in order of frequency) is present (Weiner, 2006).

Placental Transport

The placenta provides a large area in which exchange of nutrients and waste can take place across the placental membrane. This membrane consists of fetal tissues that separate maternal and fetal blood. As the pregnancy advances, the placental membrane, which also serves as a barrier, becomes progressively thinner. Because of the thinning of this membrane, some fetal blood cells may pass into the maternal blood in the intervillous space. It has been established that small numbers of fetal erythrocytes pass into the maternal circulation normally throughout pregnancy. Typically, a greater amount enters at the time of delivery when the separation of the placenta traumatically forces entry of cells through the ciliated, open maternal vessels. However, small separations of the placenta can occur during pregnancy or with any potentially traumatic procedure such as amniocentesis. In most instances, the fetal-maternal transfusion is small enough to evoke no sensitivity or involves no incompatibilities from the CDE or ABO system.

PATHOPHYSIOLOGY

The pathophysiology for all the hemolytic incompatibilities is similar. D incompatibility, the most common type, is used here to describe the process of Rhesus alloimmunization. Alloimmunization occurs when the mother is sensitive to the fetal cells; thus it is also called *sensitization* (Weiner, 2006).

Fetal erythrocytes, with the paternal D antigen, gain entry across the placental membrane into the intervillous blood, which is made up entirely of maternal blood. The fetal erythrocytes mix with the maternal blood and are then carried into the mother's circulation.

The breakthrough of fetal erythrocytes carrying the RhD antigen into the maternal circulation requires certain conditions favorable to sensitization of the mother and antibody formation. The widely dilated uteroplacental vessels encouraging blood flow also facilitate this process. Maximum maternal blood volume increasing between 28 and 32 weeks of gestation further facilitates dilation of these vessels. Changes in fetal blood pressure are responsive to changes in blood flow in the maternal circulation and presumably could increase the chance of a few fetal erythrocytes, under increased pressure, breaking into the intervillous space. For this reason, the second most likely time for Rhesus alloimmunization to occur in the mother is at approximately 28 weeks of gestation.

The most likely time for fetal erythrocytes to escape into maternal circulation is at the time of delivery. The wide open vessels at the site of placental separation allow rapid back pressure as the uterus relaxes, and large numbers of fetal erythrocytes can escape into the maternal circulation.

The formation of antibodies is gradual in the mother. Conditions favoring small areas of placental separation such as placenta previa, marginal abruption, or trauma to the placenta during amniocentesis can also favor the entry of increased numbers of fetal erythrocytes carrying the D antigen into the maternal circulation.

SIGNS AND SYMPTOMS

Evidence of antibody formation in the RhD-negative woman can be detected with an indirect Coombs test and positive identification of the specific antibody on a screen. A titer of 1:4 or greater is significant and indicates maternal sensitization.

In the fetus, signs of anemia and impending hydrops include the following:
- A baseline heart rate of 180 beats per minute (bpm) or greater
- Late decelerations or loss of short-term variability with presence of regular sine-wave long-term variability (sinusoidal pattern) (Fig. 20-1)
- Decreased fetal activity
- Fetal ascites or congestive heart failure on ultrasound examination

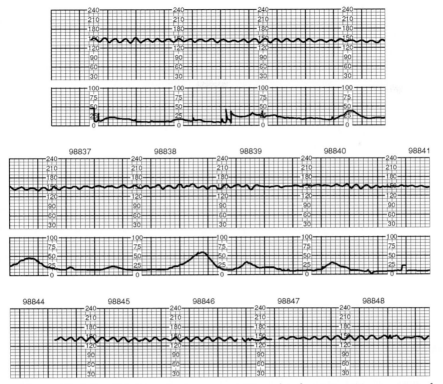

Figure 20-1 Top, D-isoimmunized woman at 30 weeks of gestation. Nonstress test after fourth amniocentesis. *Middle and bottom,* the following-day strip shows sinusoidal pattern. (Courtesy John P. Elliott, MD, Phoenix, Ariz.)

MATERNAL EFFECTS

There are no negative physiologic effects on the well-being of the mother other than discomfort if polyhydramnios occurs with fetal hydrops. If the mother is sensitized and desires future pregnancies, she may experience significant psychologic difficulties. The various feelings evoked depend on the circumstances leading to the Rhesus alloimmunization.

FETAL AND NEONATAL EFFECTS

Harmful effects of RhD alloimmunization of the mother are seen as hemolysis of fetal erythrocytes. If the sensitization process begins in one pregnancy, the effects will be seen in future pregnancies.

The current pregnancy may be in jeopardy if the process of sensitization is undetected. This can occur if minute placental tissue fragments enter maternal circulation during an amniocentesis, at 28 weeks of gestation or as a result of placenta previa or abruptio placentae. The current pregnancy may also be jeopardized because sensitization occurred inadvertently with a previous pregnancy.

Hemolysis of fetal erythrocytes can lead to various degrees of fetal anemia. When anemia becomes severe, large amounts of bilirubin, resulting from hemolysis of the erythrocytes, place an overwhelming burden on the fetal liver. As a result, swelling occurs in the liver and portal pressure increases, causing abdominal ascites and congestive heart failure. This phenomenon is called *hydrops fetalis* and can be fatal to the fetus if not corrected by intrauterine transfusion or by delivery so that exchange transfusion of the neonate can occur (Moise, 2004b).

Because of excessive bilirubin breakdown from rapid, increased hemolysis of fetal erythrocytes, the fetus attempts to excrete as much bilirubin as possible. It is excreted in abnormally large amounts into the amniotic fluid and gives it a characteristic yellow-brown appearance.

A fetal sign of hypoxia unique to hemolytic anemia or anemia from fetal-maternal hemorrhage is loss of short-term variability in the fetal heart rate (FHR). The pattern is that of regular smooth oscillations resembling a sine wave and is called a *sinusoidal pattern*. There are no accelerations or variations from the regular smooth oscillations around the baseline. A sinusoidal pattern (see Fig. 20-1), if left untreated, is terminal or may have serious consequences for neonatal outcome (Freeman, Garite, and Nageotte, 2003).

DIAGNOSTIC TESTING

Antibody Screen

Diagnosis of a hemolytic incompatibility is made by routine prenatal screening, which should be done in all patients, regardless of Rh factor, on the initial prenatal visit. The test that is used is an antibody screen or indirect Coombs test. The RhD-negative mother who is not sensitized at the beginning of the pregnancy is rescreened at 28 weeks because by this time, the placental membrane becomes thin enough for fetal red cells to cross (transplacental transfusion), making it the second most common time for sensitization to occur.

Severity of Fetal Bleed

In the event that a large fetal-maternal hemorrhage is suspected in the RhD-negative woman, a Kleihauer-Betke blood test is done on the mother. This test detects the number of fetal cells that have entered the maternal circulation. If more than 15 ml of fetal cells have entered the maternal circulation, the usual anti-D immunoglobulin dose of 300 mcg is not sufficient to prevent sensitization.

Severity of Disease

If the mother has been RhD-alloimmunized from a previous pregnancy, fetal erythroblastosis must be detected early to promote optimal fetal outcome by either early delivery or intrauterine transfusions (IUT). Unless previous obstetric history indicates earlier involvement, the fetal erythroblastosis is followed by serial maternal antibody titers beginning at 16 to 18 weeks of gestation. When the antibody titers are 1:16 or greater, serial ultrasounds for peak middle cerebral artery Doppler velocity or serial amniocenteses are begun.

Ultrasound for Peak Middle Cerebral Artery (MCA) Doppler Velocity

MCS Doppler velocity measures the fetal hemoglobin in order to detect fetal anemia. The cerebral artery can be easily visualized with color-flow Doppler. Pulsed Doppler is then used to measure the peak systolic velocity of the middle cerebral artery. In the presence of anemia the increased fetal output and a drop in blood viscosity causes an increased blood flow velocity in the cerebral artery (Moise, 2004a)

Amniocentesis

Bilirubin, a breakdown product of red blood cells, can be measured in the amniotic fluid. The breakdown product is identified as delta-OD 450. Liley, of Auckland, New Zealand, developed a graph for measuring the optical density of delta-OD in the amniotic fluid. He divided the levels of bilirubin optical density into "zones" of safety, based on gestation. Levels of delta-OD should decrease with increasing gestation. If the level of bilirubin optical density for delta-OD is increased, it indicates abnormal erythrocyte destruction (Moise, 2004b).

Cordocentesis

In cordocentesis, a direct fetal blood sample is obtained from the umbilical cord vessels to evaluate the fetal hemoglobin and hematocrit. An anemic fetus is indicative of abnormal erythrocyte destruction (Weiner, 2006). Currently, cordocentesis is not routinely used, related to the 1% incidence of fetal death and an increased chance of maternal sensitization (Moise, 2004a).

USUAL MEDICAL MANAGEMENT AND PROTOCOLS FOR NURSE PRACTITIONERS

Prevention

To prevent sensitization in unsensitized RhD-negative women, anti-D immunoglobulin is used. Anti-D immunoglobulin is a specially prepared gamma globulin that contains a specific concentration of D antibodies. These antibodies neutralize the RhD-positive fetal antigens that have entered the maternal circulation. For this reason, anti-D immunoglobulin cannot correct sensitization but can prevent it from occurring if given within 72 hours of the potential fetal-maternal red blood cell infusion (Crowther and Middleton, 1997; U.S. Preventive Services Task Force, 2004).

Because the antibody formation in the mother is gradual, it is also apparently effective in preventing sensitization during pregnancy. When anti-D immunoglobulin is given at 28 weeks of gestation to unsensitized women, the incidence of RhD alloimmunization has been further reduced (Crowther and Middleton, 1999). Anti-D immunoglobulin is also given any time a traumatic fetal-maternal bleed is likely to occur, such as after a genetic amniocentesis, a chorionic villi sampling, maternal abdominal trauma from MVA, abuse or fall, termination of an ectopic pregnancy or hydatidiform mole, spontaneous or induced abortion, placenta previa with bleeding, suspected abruption, or external cephalic version (Moise, 2004a; U.S. Preventive Services Task Force, 2004).

The usual dose of anti-D immunoglobulin is 300 mcg at 28 weeks of gestation, at the time of any amniocentesis or cordocentesis, and within 72 hours after delivery. Woelfer and others (2004) studied serum anti-D immunoglobulin levels in relationship to maternal weight. If the expectant mother's BMI is more than 27 kg per m^2, serum anti-D levels were significantly lower, indicating a possible need of a larger dosage of anti-D.

If a test such as the Kleihauer-Betke indicates that more than 30 ml of fetal blood or 15 ml of fetal red blood cells has entered the maternal circulation, a higher dose may be required to prevent sensitization. A first-trimester spontaneous or induced abortion, an ectopic pregnancy, or a chorionic villi sampling requires a minidose of 50 mcg within 72 hours (U.S. Preventive Services Task Force, 2004). There are no immunoglobulins for prevention of other blood group sensitization incompatibilities.

Treatment for Hemolytic Incompatibility

Follow-Up

If a hemolytic incompatibility is present, the usual medical management depends on the severity of fetal anemia. Two tests are currently being used to monitor for fetal anemia. The less invasive procedure measures by direct evaluation; the fetal hemoglobin and hematocrit method, by way of middle cerebral artery (MCA) Doppler velocity. An older alternative method measures bilirubin levels by optical density (Delta OD) in the amniotic fluid, which are obtained by serial amniocenteses. Testing is usually started around 19 weeks of gestation. When the level of bilirubin is low for a particular gestational age or the hemoglobin and hematocrit are normal, the test is repeated in 3 weeks. If the bilirubin level rises or the hemoglobin and hematocrit levels decrease, evaluation may be repeated in 1 to 2 weeks. Extremely abnormal levels for a particular gestation indicate a need for intrauterine transfusion in the very immature fetus. Cesarean delivery may be necessary when this occurs after 34 weeks of gestation (Moise, 2004a).

Fetal Surveillance

By 26 weeks of gestation, FHR monitoring should be started. A nonstress test may be done biweekly, a contraction stress test may be done weekly, or some combination of testing methods may be used. Between FHR monitorings, the mother should keep daily fetal activity charts.

Intrauterine Transfusions

If the fetus becomes anemic any time after 18 weeks of gestation, an intrauterine transfusion is indicated to allow more time for the immature or nonviable fetus to remain in utero (Moise, 2004a). The transfusion must be done by a skilled physician, usually a perinatologist, who has learned the procedure during postgraduate training in maternal-fetal medicine (see Chapter 4). The intra-uterine transfusion can be performed intravascularly or intraperitoneally (although the later is rarely used with current skills of perinatologists).

Intravascular Transfusion (IVT)

When an intravascular transfusion is performed, the fetal umbilical vein is used. The mother is medicated with a uterine relaxant and an antianxiety or tran-quilizer agent. The procedure is done under ultrasound direction. A 22-gauge spinal needle is guided through the mother's abdomen and the uterine wall into the umbilical vein at the site of placental insertion. Either washed, packed, leuko-reduced O RhD-negative blood or negative blood matched to the mother's blood type may be used (Moise, 2004a). Prophylactic antibiotics are given to the mother following the procedure.

Intraperitoneal Transfusion

Originally fetal alloimmune-induced hemolytic anemia was treated by intra-peritoneal transfusion. This practice has been replaced with the intravascular transfusion because a hemolytic anemic fetus absorbs transfused red cells poorly. If done, the procedure for intraperitoneal transfusion is performed under ultrasound direction. Approximately 50 to 150 ml of negative blood, cross-matched to the mother, is used. It is spun down to increase the hematocrit to 70% to 80%. Rh-negative blood from a donor must be used because it contains no antibodies to the fetal Rh-positive blood.

The mother is given a narcotic or tranquilizer to quiet the baby for the procedure. After an abdominal scrub of the amniocentesis site and with the direction of ultrasound, a large-gauge intracatheter is inserted through the maternal abdomen, into the uterus, and into the fetal abdomen, just under the fetal diaphragm. The intracatheter tubing, the attached intravenous tubing, and the syringe for the blood are all preflushed with normal saline. A small amount of normal saline can be injected to confirm placement on ultrasonic view. The syringe with the specially prepared blood is connected to an infusion pump designed for constant speed infusion via syringe. Depending on fetal gestation, 50 to 150 ml of blood is infused over a 1- to 2-hour period. The fetus is monitored before and during the procedure if greater than 26 weeks of gestation. If the fetus is less than 26 weeks, frequent auscultation of the FHR is usually done. During the next 3 to 4 days, the fetal diaphragmatic lymph system absorbs the blood, and improvement in fetal anemia can be expected.

Amniocentesis for Fetal Lung Maturity

Amniocentesis for fetal lung maturity is usually initiated at 35 weeks of gestation. If fetal lungs are mature, induction is the standard of care at 37 weeks of gestation. If fetal lungs are immature and fetal bilirubin is high, the mother is treated with 30 mg of oral phenobarbital 3 times a day for 1 week to accelerate fetal hepatic maturity and therefore enhance neonatal conjugation of bilirubin. If the fetal lungs are immature but fetal bilirubin is low, amniocentesis is usually repeated in 2 weeks.

Outcome

With intrauterine transfusions to prevent fetal alloimmune-induced hemolytic anemia, fetal survival rate is 85% to 90% (Moise, 2004a). Success of intrauterine transfusion generally depends on a number of factors. If the fetus is extremely immature or if there are significant liver and congestive heart failure, the potential for improved fetal well-being is less likely and death in utero can ensue in a few days. The earlier the transfusions must be started, the greater the number required for the fetus to gain maturity while maintaining well-being. This puts the fetus at higher risk for intrauterine infection or premature rupture of membranes and therefore interferes with the potentially successful outcome for the fetus.

NURSING MANAGEMENT

Prevention

The prenatal nurse caring for the pregnant woman must recognize the importance of antibody screening in all pregnant patients not only for D incompatibility but also for any blood system incompatibility. Education of the patient regarding necessary prenatal laboratory work should include the need for antibody screening. Patients can be given this information in early prenatal classes, as well as during early office visits.

To prevent RhD alloimmunization, all RhD-negative women should receive anti-D immunoglobulin at the following times:

- At 28 weeks of gestation
- Postnatally, within 72 hours, to unsensitized women who have given birth at any gestation to an RhD-positive or untyped fetus (Crowther and Middleton, 1997)
- In the event of a third-trimester bleed
- Following any procedure during pregnancy that may breach the integrity of the choriodecidual space and lead to a potential fetomaternal bleed (e.g., chorionic villus sampling, amniocentesis, cordocentesis, percutaneous fetal procedures, or external cephalic version)
- Even in situations in which the woman intends to undergo tubal ligation, the woman should be instructed regarding potential future problems should sterilization fail or should she ever choose to have a surgical reversal of the sterilization after becoming sensitized with this pregnancy. She also risks no longer being safe to receive uncrossed-matched universal donor blood should she experience a future emergent need for this blood.

Nursing Interventions for Administering Anti-D Immunoglobulin

Assess the RhD-negative woman's understanding of when sensitization can take place. Educate the patient in a reassuring manner regarding the use of anti-D immunoglobulin at all recommended times.

- At the initial prenatal visit, determine the mother's blood type and screen for the presence of antibodies by an indirect Coombs test (antibody screen). The RhD-negative unsensitized pregnant woman should be screened again at 26 to 28 weeks of gestation.
- Administer anti-D immunoglobulin intramuscularly.
- Prepare patient for such potential side effects as temporary soreness at the site of injection and a low-grade fever. In rare instances, an anaphylactic reaction occurs. For this reason, the patient should remain in the health care setting for 15 to 30 minutes following the injection.
- Fill out an identification card confirming the injection, and give it to the patient to keep. Instruct her to keep it with her identification papers. Of women who receive anti-D immunoglobulin antepartum prophylaxis, 15% to 20% will subsequently have passive acquired D antibodies at the time of delivery. This could lead to misinterpretation and withholding of eligible anti-D immunoglobulin. In the event of confusion, the mother should be instructed to present her identification card (PDR Drug Information, 2006).
- Fill out the blood bank form. Return the form and empty ampule or syringe to the blood bank. In the event of an allergic reaction, the blood bank needs the information these provide.
- Be prepared to discuss the issue of risk for transmission of HIV through anti-D immunoglobulin. According to PDR Drug Information (2006), the risk is eliminated because the preparing process is effective in removing any enveloped viruses such as HBV, HCV, and HIV.

Antepartum Nursing Interventions for Alloimmunization

- Obtain the patient's history to ascertain first day of last menstrual period, regularity of menstrual cycles, type of birth control used, date of a positive pregnancy test, and ultrasound to determine the estimated date of delivery. This will be invaluable in determining when necessary interventions should be instituted.
- Assess fetal growth with fundal height measurement. Concern for fetal growth should occur if fundal growth stops or decreases. If the fetus becomes anemic, the decreased oxygenation can lead to decreased growth rate. If the fetus becomes hydropic, fundal height can be abnormally large because of associated polyhydramnios.
- Assess FHR for tachycardia at each prenatal visit after 10 weeks.
- Monitor FHR during and after treatment for alloimmunization for evidence of sinusoidal FHR pattern or for nonreassuring features such as persistent late decelerations or loss of variability. Because of maternal sedation during intrauterine transfusion, baseline variability can be depressed (but without tachycardia, late decelerations, or a sinusoidal pattern) and should be compared with the strip before premedication and with the strip 1 hour after medication.
- Understand the importance of ultrasound examinations at least every 3 weeks after 20 weeks of gestation when alloimmunization has already occurred.

- Teach the mother to keep a daily fetal movement chart after 26 weeks of gestation. An active fetus is assumed to be adequately oxygenated.
- Explain special evaluation procedures and treatment.
- Assist with monitoring FHR during fetal evaluation by amniocentesis or PUBS. A baseline FHR should be determined before the procedure, and a 20- to 30-minute fetal monitoring strip should be run to assess FHR for signs of fetal compromise. Such signs include tachycardia, late decelerations, or absent long-term variability with the presence of short-term variability (sinusoidal pattern) (see Fig. 20-1).
- Assist with intrauterine fetal transfusion. During the initiation of the catheter insertion into the fetus, assist with ultrasound guidance and evaluation of the fetal well-being.
- Refer to a nurse specialist for patient education specific to tertiary level care and referral.
- Make appropriate referrals based on expressed psychosocial and financial needs.

Intrapartum Nursing Interventions for Alloimmunization

- Monitor FHR continuously with an electronic fetal monitor during labor for nonreassuring or preterminal patterns or events. If fetal anemia has developed, labor can further stress the fetus.
- Prepare the patient and her family for the possible necessity of a cesarean delivery if the fetus shows signs of hypoxia.
- Refer signs of fetal stress to the physician immediately because these fetuses are very sensitive.
- Assess the mother and her family for level of anxiety related to fear for the fetus or infant and potential outcome.
- Determine the family's support system. Assess the couple's support of each other.
- Keep the parents informed of the status of their fetus or neonate.
- Determine how the woman became sensitized. If the injection was overlooked or mistaken Rh results were reported with a previous pregnancy, anger may be unresolved. This can be true especially if the matter is under litigation. If the injection was omitted after a therapeutic abortion, guilt regarding the abortion may be overriding other feelings. When a previous pregnancy occurred before the routine use of anti-D immunoglobulin at 26 to 28 weeks of gestation, feelings of frustration over an event that could not be controlled and anxiety for the future or the present pregnancy will interact.
- If the neonate is sick or premature, assess the level of parental attachment behaviors such as frequent visitation, early touching and stroking, calling the infant by name, and attempting to establish eye contact.
- Encourage and facilitate early and close contact with the nursery personnel.

CONCLUSION

For the unsensitized RhD-negative woman, prevention is the primary goal. This can be accomplished (1) through antibody screening at the first prenatal visit; (2) through antibody screening at 26 to 28 weeks of gestation and by giving anti-D immunoglobulin by 26 to 28 weeks of gestation, after delivery, with potential placental accidents, and after an abortion. Education regarding indications for anti-D immunoglobulin and times of greatest risk can improve the future protection of RhD-negative women from unintentional Rhesus alloimmunization. As yet, there is no protective therapy for other hemolytic incompatibilities.

For the sensitized woman, the primary goal is to promote an optimal neonatal outcome through close monitoring of fetal well-being and through institution of therapy at the earliest safe time. High risk perinatal nurses should encourage the RhD-negative woman to seek information about new, proven methods of evaluation and treatment, such as those described in Chapter 4.

BIBLIOGRAPHY

Crowther C, Middleton P: Anti-D administration after childbirth for preventing Rhesus alloimmunisation, *Cochrane Database Syst Rev* Issue 2, 1997.

Crowther C, Middleton P: Anti-D administration in pregnancy for preventing Rhesus alloimmunisation, *Cochrane Database Syst Rev* Issue 2, 1999.

Freeman R, Garite R, and Nageotte M: *Fetal heart rate monitoring,* ed 3, Baltimore, 2003, Lippincott Williams & Wilkins.

Giancarlo M and others: Non-invasive diagnosis by Doppler ultrasonography of fetal anemia due to maternal red-cell alloimmunization, *N Engl J Med* 342(1):9–14, 2000.

Martin J and others: Births: final data for 2001, *Natl Vital Stat Rep* 51(2):1–102, 2002.

Moise K: Grand rounds: Rh disease: it's still a threat, *Contemporary OB/GYN* 49:34, 2004a.

Moise K: Hemolytic disease of the fetus newborn. In Creasy R, Resnik R, and Iams J, editors: *Maternal-fetal medicine: principles and practice,* ed 5, Philadelphia, 2004b, Saunders.

PDR Drug Information: *Rho (D) Immune globulin (Human),* Drugs.com, 2006. Retrieved from *http://www.drugs.com/pdr/rho__d__immune_globulin__human_.html*

U.S. Preventive Services Task Force: Screening for Rh(D) Incompatibility: Recommendation Statement, Rockville, MD, 2004, Agency for Healthcare Research and Quality. Retrieved from *http://ahrq.gov/clinic/3rduspstf/rh/rhrs.htm*

Weiner C: Fetal hemolytic disease. In James D and others, editors: *High risk pregnancy: management options,* ed 3, Philadelphia, 2006, Saunders.

Woelfer B and others: Postdelivery levels of anti-D IgG prophylaxis in D-mothers depend on maternal body weight, *Transfusion* 44(4):512–517, 2004.

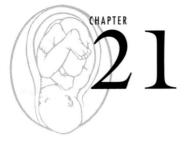

Hypertensive Disorders

T he specific terminology for hypertensive disorders of pregnancy is inconsistent. According to the National High Blood Pressure Education Program Working Group (2000), hypertensive disorders of pregnancy are classified into one of four disorders. Table 21-1 summarizes these classifications. Two of these disorders, gestational hypertension and preeclampsia/eclampsia, develop during pregnancy, labor, or the early postpartum period in a previously normotensive, nonproteinuric woman. The other two disorders, chronic hypertension and preeclampsia superimposed on hypertension, are related to a preexisting condition. This chapter first covers chronic hypertension and then focuses on preeclampsia. The primary pathophysiology of chronic hypertension is elevated blood pressure. Preeclampsia is a multisystemic, pregnancy-induced syndrome resulting from an endothelial cell dysfunction. Hypertension is a primary sign of the underlying disorder, most often developing after 20 weeks of gestation.

Both chronic hypertension and preeclampsia can be subclassified as either mild or severe. For chronic hypertension, subclassification is dependent on systolic and diastolic values. For preeclampsia, subclassification is dependent on the severity of end organ involvement. Severe forms of hypertension are HELLP syndrome and eclampsia. HELLP syndrome (**h**emolysis of red blood cells [RBCs], **e**levated **l**iver enzymes, and **l**ow **p**latelets) is a multisystem disease. Eclampsia is the development of seizures in the preeclamptic patient. Approximately 15% of patients with HELLP syndrome and 20% of patients who develop eclampsia are normotensive (c and Robson, 1999; Sibai, 2005a).

Gestational hypertension alone is usually benign and treated like mild preeclampsia (National High Blood Pressure Education Program Working Group, 2000).

INCIDENCE

Hypertension occurs in 7% to 9% of all pregnancies (ACOG, 2002). Preeclampsia accounts for about 80% of these cases and chronic hypertension for about 20% (von Dadelszen and Magee, 2005). The strongest risk factors for

Table 21-1   Classification of Hypertensive States of Pregnancy

Type	Description
Gestational hypertension	Development of mild hypertension during pregnancy in previously normotensive patient without proteinuria and with normal laboratory test Blood pressure returns to normal by 12 weeks postpartum
Preeclampsia	Development of hypertension and proteinuria in previously normotensive patient after 20 weeks of gestation or in early postpartum period; in presence of trophoblastic disease, it can develop before 20 weeks of gestation
Eclampsia	Development of seizures in the preeclamptic patient
Chronic hypertension	Hypertension occurring before pregnancy or a blood pressure 140/90 or higher before 20 weeks of gestation on two occasions 6 hours apart
Preeclampsia superimposed on chronic hypertension	Development of preeclampsia or eclampsia in patient with chronic hypertension

preeclampsia are a primigravida younger than 19 years or older than 40 years, a first pregnancy with a new father (Dekker and Sibai, 1999), or a history of severe preeclampsia (Al-Mulhim and others, 2003; Gudnasson, Dubiel, and Gudmundsson, 2004). Other factors associated with a higher-than-normal incidence of preeclampsia are as follows:

- Familial history
- Preexisting vascular disease such as diabetes, renal disease, chronic hypertension, or collagen disease
- Exposure to a superabundance of trophoblastic tissue, such as in multiple gestation and hydatidiform mole
- Antiphospholipid syndrome
- Obesity (increases the risk three-fold)
- Periodontal disease (Boggess and others, 2003)
- African-American descent (Flack and others, 2002)

CHRONIC HYPERTENSION

Chronic hypertension occurs in approximately 4% to 5% of all pregnancies, with 21% of these women developing superimposed preeclampsia (Walfisch and Hallak, 2006). Chronic hypertension in pregnancy is usually classified as to mild or severe (depending on the hypertensive stage) according to the staging system by Joint National Committee (JNC VII, 2003). Table 21-2 lists stages of hypertension.

Table 21-2   Stages of Hypertension

Blood Pressure Stages—JNC VII	Blood Pressure Reading
Prehypertension	Systolic 120–139 or diastolic 80–89
Stage 1 Hypertension	Systolic 140–159 or diastolic 90–99
Stage 2 Hypertension	Systolic above 160 or diastolic above 100

Reference: Joint National Committee (JNC) VII: *Prevention, detection, evaluation, and treatment of high blood pressure,* NIH Publication No. 03-5233, Bethesda, Maryland, 2003, U.S. Department of Health and Human Services. Retrieved from http://www.nhlbi.nih.gov/guidelines/hypertension/jncintro.htm

Preconception screening is ideal. During this visit, lifestyle changes are discussed, such as the DASH (Dietary Approaches to Stop Hypertension) diet with adequate potassium, calcium, and magnesium and sodium limited to 2.4 g; aerobic exercise until pregnant and then no exercise; no smoking or alcohol use; and if overweight, loss of weight before but not during pregnancy (Paruk and Moodley, 2005). The patient should be trained in home blood pressure monitoring. Baseline laboratory studies such as renal function and urinary protein excretion may be helpful for later comparison. Counseling should include review of pregnancy risk associated with hypertension. With mild chronic hypertension, 10% of the pregnant women went on to develop superimposed hypertension (Egerman and Sibai, 2001). The other 90% had favorable pregnancy outcomes. In the presence of severe chronic hypertension, there is increase risk for perinatal mortality starting in the first trimester and continuing throughout pregnancy related to superimposed preeclampsia, abruptio, or preterm delivery.

Current management should be evaluated and needed changes made for pregnancy. For stage 1 hypertension without complications such as left ventricular hypertrophy, peripheral arterial disease, renal disease, or retinopathy, the best therapy is periodic bedrest of 45 minutes in the middle of the day and 1 hour before the evening meal to promote uterine blood flow. A regimen of tapering and stopping hypertensive medication is usually tried (National High Blood Pressure Education Program Working Group, 2000).

When the diastolic blood pressure exceeds 100 mm Hg, systolic exceeds 160 mm Hg, left ventricular hypertrophy is present, drug therapy is usually initiated. The drug of choice continues to be methyldopa (Aldomet) (National High Blood Pressure Education Program Working Group, 2000). The usual dose of methyldopa is 750 to 2000 mg/day. The alternative drugs used to treat chronic hypertension during pregnancy are beta-blockers, such as atenolol (Tenormin), labetalol (Trandate, Normodyne), or pindolol (Visken), and calcium channel blockers, such as nifedipine. Table 21-3 lists common dosages of these hypertensive medications. The new angiotensin-converting enzyme inhibitors or angiotensin II receptor antagonists are contraindicated during pregnancy because they decrease uterine blood flow and may increase the chance of intrauterine growth restriction (IUGR) or fetal death (National High Blood Pressure Education Program Working Group, 2000). Diuretics are not used as

Table 21-3   Antihypertensive Medications for Chronic Hypertension
During Pregnancy

Medication	Drug Classification	Usual Dosage	Maximum Dosage
Methyldopa (Drug of choice: Aldomet)	Central-acting antiadrenergic agent	250 mg po bid or tid	2000 mg
Labetalol (Trandate)	Beta-blocker	Start at 100 mg po bid Increase 100 mg bid q 2–3 weeks	1200 mg
Pindolol (Visken)	Beta-blocker	5 mg po bid Increase by 10 mg/day q 3–4 weeks	60 mg
Nifedipine (Procardia)	Calcium channel blocker	10 mg po tid	180 mg

bid, Twice daily; *po,* orally; *q,* every; *tid,* three times daily.
Reference: Weiner C, Buhimschi C: *Drugs for pregnant and lactating women,* Philadelphia, 2004, Churchill Livingstone.

the first-line drug therapy because of their effect on plasma volume. If a diuretic is indicated, thiazide has the safest record. Furosemide is contraindicated because of its added risk for embryotoxicity. All pregnant patients with chronic hypertension should be monitored carefully for an abruption, as well as superimposed preeclampsia, renal failure, and disseminated intravascular coagulation (DIC). They have a 0.7% to 1.5% increased risk for an abruption and a 10%–25% chance of developing superimposed preeclampsia (Paruk and Moodley, 2005). Antepartum fetal assessment should begin at 28 to 30 weeks of gestation because the fetus is at greater risk for IUGR and fetal mortality increases 10-fold.

If renal failure occurs during pregnancy, volume overload may result, requiring sodium restriction, diuretic use, or dialysis. Magnesium sulfate is hazardous in the presence of renal failure and, if needed, dose is based on every 1- to 2-hour magnesium levels. Phenytoin may be a better alternative drug (National High Blood Pressure Education Program Working Group, 2000).

During postpartum recovery, monitor for such complications as pulmonary edema, renal failure, heart failure, and encephalopathy. If the mother is breastfeeding and in stage 1 or 2 hypertension, consider withholding any antihypertensive agent until cessation of breastfeeding. To women in stage 3 hypertension, give the lowest dose and monitor mother and infant. Methyldopa is the preferred drug. If a beta-blocker is indicated, labetalol or propranolol are preferred. There is no available evidence-based data about calcium-channel blockers. Angiotensin-converting enzyme inhibitors and angiotensin II receptor antagonists are contraindicated for the same reasons as during pregnancy. Diuretics may have a negative effect on milk production.

PREECLAMPSIA
Normal Physiology

Although the triggering factor of preeclampsia is unknown, much of the pathophysiology of the disease is understood. To understand the pathophysiology of preeclampsia, the nurse should be familiar with the normal physiologic changes of pregnancy, which are summarized in the following sections.

Cardiovascular System

Plasma blood volume is increased 30% to 50%; stroke volume and heart rates are increased as well. Increased plasma blood volume accounts for the 40% increase in cardiac output. There appears to be increased oxidative stress and an increase maternal antioxidant related to increase lipid peroxidation capacity (Spinnato and Livingston, 2005).

Renal Function

The normal glomerular filtration rate is increased by approximately 50% related to increase renal plasma flow. Serum creatinine normally decreases with an increase in creatinine clearance.

Fluid Balance

Renin, angiotensin II, and aldosterone levels are increased. These substrates, along with increasing estrogen, facilitate the normal expansion of the blood volume by 40% to 50% above nonpregnant levels (Baylis and others, 1998).

Placentation

Early in pregnancy, the muscular components of the uterine spiral arteries begin to be replaced by cytotrophoblast. To further increase fetoplacental blood flow, the trophoblast erodes the myometrial portions of the uterine spiral arteries so that they widen and lose their vasoconstrictive properties, increasing the diameter four to six times from their nonpregnant size.

Vasodilatory State

Angiotensin II is a potent pressor substance that stimulates a rise in blood pressure. In normal pregnancy, although the levels of angiotensin II are elevated, blood pressure does not rise. This is because healthy pregnant women have an increased resistance to the presser effects of angiotensin II (Baylis and others, 1998; Vedernikov, Saade, and Garfield, 1999; Walfisch and Hallack, 2006) related to increased levels of endothelial-derived vasodilator prostacyclin (PGI_2) and nitric oxide (Myatt and Miodovnik, 1999). The diastolic blood pressure normally drops 7 to 10 mm Hg during the first and second trimesters and returns to nonpregnant levels during the third trimester (National High Blood Pressure Education Program Working Group, 2000).

A delicate balance between vasodilator and vasopressor activity must be maintained during pregnancy to maintain a normotensive state. The placenta and intact endothelium that line the blood vessel walls produce prostacyclin.

Prostacyclin stimulates the renin-angiotensin-aldosterone cycle, which is important for fluid balance. Prostacyclin is a potent vasodilator because of its resistance to the presser effects of angiotensin II. It prevents platelet clumping and promotes increased uteroplacental blood flow as well. Nitric oxide is another vasodilator substance that is important to maintaining low basal blood vessel tone but at the same time weakening the action of vasoconstrictors (Ghabour and others, 1995) and inhibiting platelet aggregation (Lowenstein and others, 1994). Nitric oxide is derived from the endothelial blood vessel cells.

Active vasopressors are thromboxane, endothelins (endothelin-1), and increased lipid peroxides. Thromboxane is a vasoconstrictor, a stimulant of platelet aggregation, and a uterine-stimulating prostaglandin (Wang and others, 1991a, 1991b). Thromboxane is produced by the placenta and, in lesser amounts, by the platelets. Endothelin-1 production normally increases during pregnancy (Branch and others, 1991; Nova and others, 1991; Clark and others, 1992). In the event of endothelial damage, endothelin-1 is produced in abnormally increasing amounts, which causes inactivation of nitric oxide (Wang and others, 2004).

Fluid Shifts

Fluid moves from the intravascular space to the extracellular space in the dependent limbs. The fluid shift is related to plasma colloid osmotic pressure that decreases below 23 mm Hg secondary to the normal hemodilution of the blood. Fluid shift is also related to the increased venous capillary hydrostatic pressure in the dependent limbs secondary to the gravid uterus pressing on the inferior vena cava, interfering with the blood returning to the heart. The net result is physiologic edema in the dependent limbs during the last trimester of pregnancy. Physiologic edema should disappear after 8 to 12 hours of bedrest.

Pathophysiology

In preeclampsia it appears that the cytotrophoblastic tissue of the placenta fails to adequately migrate down the maternal spiral arteries and displace the musculoelastic structures of these arteries, *decreasing spiral artery remodeling* (Levine and Karumanchi, 2005). Therefore these arteries do not widen as they normally do, which means that the perfusion to the placental is suboptimal. This suboptimal perfusion is referred to as a *defective placentation* (Myatt and Miodovnik, 1999). Multiorgan system involvement results because of the ensuing *endothelial cell dysfunction* (van Beck and Peeters, 1998; Myatt and Miodovnik, 1999; Roberts, 2004). Endothelial cells line all blood vessels, providing blood vessel wall integrity, preventing intravascular coagulation, modulating smooth muscle contractility, and mediating immune and inflammatory responses. Fig. 21-1 presents a summary of the manifestations of damaged endothelial cells in preeclampsia.

It is currently postulated that endothelial cell dysfunction is caused by placental ischemia stimulating the release of a substance that is toxic to endothelial cells, an antiendothelial factors such as sFlt-1 (van Beck and Peeters,

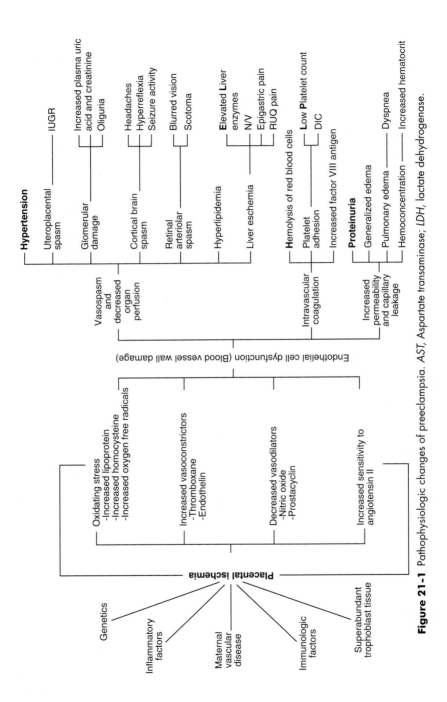

Figure 21-1 Pathophysiologic changes of preeclampsia. *AST,* Aspartate transaminase; *LDH,* lactate dehydrogenase.

1998; Var and others, 2003; Levine and others, 2004; Levine and Karumanchi, 2005), increasing oxidative stress response (Myatt and Miodovnik, 1999), and inflammatory released cytokines (tumor necrosis factor-alpha) (Taylor, 1997). Oxidative stress is the imbalance of pro-oxidants (homocysteine, low-density lipoprotein, hypertriglyceridemia, increased iron) and antioxidants (high-density lipoprotein and transferrin, a blood protein that binds with iron), leading to the formation of oxygen free radicals and lipid peroxides. Lipid peroxides and oxygen free radicals are directly toxic to the endothelial cells and increase the release of cytokines, which cause damage to the endothelial lining of blood vessel walls (Dekker, 2001; Cotter and others, 2003; Var and others, 2003; Roberts, 2004; Mignini and others, 2005).

With endothelial damage, there is significantly less production of vasodilators such as prostacyclin and nitric oxide (Myatt and Miodovnik, 1999; Var and others, 2003; Spinnato and Livingston, 2005), upsetting the delicate balance between prostacyclin and thromboxane (Mills and others, 1999). Decreased production of nitric oxide and increased production of thromboxane cause platelet adhesion to the surface of the trophoblast, resulting in intervillous thrombi (Ghabour and others, 1995), which further alters blood flow to the fetus. Damaged endothelial cells cause increased release of endothelin-1, which inactivates nitric oxide (Wang and others, 2004). Increased production of oxygen free radicals and lipid peroxides results, which further inactivates the vasodilator effect of nitric oxide (Myatt and Midovnik, 1999) and further damages endothelium.

Multiple-organ endothelial cell injury ensues (Hayman, 2004). Generalized vasospasm results, leading to poor tissue perfusion to all organ systems, increased total peripheral resistance with subsequent elevation of blood pressure, and increased endothelial cell permeability, which allows intravascular protein and fluid loss leading to decrease plasma osmotic pressure and plasma volume (Patrick and Roberts, 1999). Vascular endothelial cell injury may initiate coagulation pathways as well (Myatt and Miodovnik, 1999).

Resulting Pathophysiologic Changes

Other specific pathophysiologic changes result from preeclampsia; a discussion of these follows.

Uteroplacental Insufficiency

Uteroplacental perfusion is compromised, even before preeclamptic symptoms, related to pathologic spiral arteriole lesions and a deficiency of prostacyclin. The uteroplacental perfusion is further reduced as the disease progresses. The fetal blood flow is decreased related to constriction of umbilical vessels.

Renal Damage

In 70% of preeclamptic patients, glomerular endothelial damage, fibrin deposition, and resulting ischemia reduce renal plasma flow and glomerular filtration rate (National High Blood Pressure Education Program Working Group, 2000). Protein, mainly in the form of albumin, is lost into the urine. Uric acid, creatinine, and calcium clearance are decreased, and oliguria develops as the condition worsens. Therefore proteinuria and increased plasma uric acid levels are signs of preeclampsia, and oliguria is a sign of severe preeclampsia and kidney damage.

Fluid and Electrolyte Imbalance

Serum albumin is decreased as the result of serum protein lost into extracellular spaces and into the urine by way of damaged capillary walls. Decreased serum albumin causes a decrease in the plasma colloid osmotic pressure, an increase in intracellular edema, and failure of the normal expansion of the intravascular plasma volume (ACOG, 2002). Although there is intravascular hemoconcentration, the production of renin, angiotensin, and aldosterone decreases, resulting in an increased hematocrit.

Worsening Pathophysiologic Changes

As preeclampsia progresses, the following systemic changes, which are signs that the condition is worsening, may occur.

Pulmonary Involvement

Pulmonary edema may develop and is related to one of three factors. The most common factor is volume overload as a result of left ventricular failure caused by extremely high vascular resistance, excessive fluid infusion during treatment of the disease, or postpartum diuresis. The other two factors are related to a further decreased colloid osmotic pressure or an endothelial injury that increases pulmonary capillary permeability, resulting in a fluid leak or a noncardiogenic pulmonary edema.

Central Nervous System Involvement

Endothelial damage to the cortical region of the brain, resulting in fibrin deposition, edema, and cerebral hemorrhage, may lead to hyperreflexia and severe headaches and can progress to seizure activity (eclampsia) (National High Blood Pressure Education Program Working Group, 2000).

Ophthalmic Involvement

Visual changes, such as scotoma, photophobia, blurring, or double vision, can occur related to retinal arteriolar spasms caused by arteriolar narrowing (Walfisch and Hallak, 2006).

Hemodynamic Changes

Severe preeclampsia or eclampsia manifests with varying hemodynamic patterns related to the disease process. For example, elevated blood pressure may be related to increased vascular resistance or increased cardiac output. Pulmonary edema may result from volume overload and is the result of left ventricular failure from extremely high vascular resistance or excessive fluid infusion during treatment of the disease. Volume overload can also occur during the postpartum period when normal mobilization of the third-space fluid occurs.

The two other factors that can cause pulmonary edema are (1) further reduced colloid osmotic pressure and (2) increased pulmonary capillary permeability related to capillary wall damage. Oliguria is related to decreased renal blood flow as the result of intravascular volume depletion or severe vascular resistance, either of which can cause left ventricular failure. Occasionally, specific renal arteriospasms disproportionate to the systemic vasospasms can cause oliguria.

Coagulation Involvement

Endothelial damage causes activation of the clotting cascade. Fewer platelets are created. When platelets drop below 100,000 cells/mm^3, preeclampsia is severe. Abnormalities of blood coagulation sufficient to cause DIC are present in only about 10% of patients with preeclampsia.

Hepatic Involvement

Hepatic ischemia and fibrin deposition can cause anywhere from mild hepatocellular necrosis indicated by a mild increase in aminotransferase and lactate dehydrogenase to the ominous HELLP syndrome. In approximately 10% of these patients, hepatic involvement can lead to periportal hemorrhagic necrosis in the liver, which can cause a subcapsular hematoma (Williamson and Girling, 2006). Warning signs of hepatic involvement, such as right upper quadrant pain or epigastric pain, can indicate impending eclampsia.

HELLP Syndrome Development

In 5% of patients with preeclampsia, the HELLP syndrome, a severe form of preeclampsia characterized by hemolysis of RBCs, elevated liver enzymes, and low platelets, may develop (Weinstein, 1985; Martin and others, 1991; Sibai and others, 1993a; Roberts, 2004). This cascade of events is the result of systemic capillary endothelial cell damage exposing the basement membrane, which activates platelet adherence and fibrin deposition. Platelets are then decreased, and RBCs, which are torn trying to pass through the narrowed vessels, are deposited along with the fibrin. Activation of platelets results in release of more thromboxane, and endothelial damage leads to further reduction in prostacyclin production, thus setting up a vicious cycle (Walsh, 1990; Barton and Sibai, 2001). Hyperbilirubinemia *(jaundice)* may develop as a result of hemolysis of the RBCs. At the same time, endothelial damage and fibrin deposition in the liver may lead to impaired liver function and can result in hemorrhagic necrosis, indicated by right upper quadrant tenderness or epigastric pain, nausea, and vomiting (Phelan and Easter, 1990). Liver enzymes are elevated when liver tissue is necrotic. In rare cases, a subcapsular hematoma develops in the liver. Normal blood pressure is found in approximately 15% of the patients with HELLP syndrome (Anumba and Robson, 1999).

Eclampsia

Eclampsia is the occurrence of seizure activity in the presence of preeclampsia. Eclampsia is normally thought to be triggered by severe cerebral vasospasm, hemorrhage, ischemia, or edema. Occasionally, encephalopathy may trigger the seizure activity. Severe, persistent headache, visual disturbances, epigastric pain, and restlessness can be warning signs of impending eclampsia. Normal blood pressure is found in approximately 20% of patients with eclampsia (Anumba and Robson, 1999).

Etiology

The cause of preeclampsia remains unknown. Because of characteristic changes in the placental vessels, it is currently thought to be a placentation defect mediated by the interplay of three or more factors (Williamson, 2005).

Immunologic Maladaptation and Activation of Inflammatory Factors

The immunologic influence is supported by epidemiologic studies to be an impaired maternal immune response directed against the trophoblastic invasion and subsequently causing a defective placentation. This impaired immune response is postulated to be the result of decreased human leukocyte antigent (HLA) G protein normally produced to facilitate the mother's tolerance to the immunologically foreign placenta components (Harrison and others, 1997) or decreased formation of blocking antibodies to immunoprotect the immunologically partly foreign placenta (Cunningham and others, 2005). Repeated sperm exposure may prevent this impaired immunologic response, thus explaining the increased risk in primipaternity, use of barrier contraceptives, and donor insemination (Hayman, 2004).

This immune response or other variable may activate an inflammatory response. Oxidative stress caused by increased cytokines and interleukins damages the endothelial cells of the placenta, resulting in decreased nitric oxide and interfering with the thromboxane-to-prostacyclin balance (Var and others, 2003; Freeman and others, 2004; Wang and others, 2004).

Genetic Predisposition

There appears to be a familial tendency toward preeclampsia related to a single recessive gene (Chesley and Cooper, 1986), a dominant gene with incomplete penetrance (Dekker, 2001), or multifactorial inheritance (Hayman, 2004) that increase one's susceptibility to preeclampsia if other variables are present. Other research indicates that it might be the result of a growth-restricting effect on the daughter born to a woman with severe preeclampsia. A patient with a history of having a child who was IUGR is at considerable risk for hypertension, insulin resistance, and dyslipidemia later in life. Therefore the woman experiencing preeclampsia might have undiagnosed cardiovascular complications that increase her susceptibility to preeclampsia (Dekker and Sibai, 1999; Manten and others, 2005).

Vascular-Mediated Factors

The presence of a vascular defect caused by a disease such as diabetes, chronic hypertension, or collagen vascular disease or hidden abnormal metabolic factors such as the presence of anticardiolipin antibodies, hyperhomocystinemia, insulin resistance, metabolic syndrome, or obesity may interact with reduced placental perfusion to increase susceptibility to preeclampsia. It is postulated to influence the development of preeclampsia in one of three ways:

1 Defective placentation
2 Placental ischemia
3 Endothelial cell dysfunction

Maternal Effects

Preeclampsia is a very serious disease and is the second leading cause of maternal mortality (National High Blood Pressure Education Program Working Group, 2000; USDHHS, 2000), accounting for 16% to 18% of all maternal deaths (ACOG, 2002; Cox, Kilpatrick and Geller, 2004). If preeclampsia is treated early and effectively, maternal mortality is low. If the disease is allowed to progress to the HELLP syndrome or eclampsia, maternal mortality increases to as high as 24%, and morbidity levels are even higher. The most common causes of mortality or morbidity are related to abruptio placentae, pulmonary edema, stroke, renal or hepatic failure, myocardial infarction, DIC, and cerebral hemorrhage (Barton and Sibai, 2001; Sibai, 2005b). Women who receive no prenatal care are 12 times as likely to die from preeclamptic complications as women who do receive prenatal care (MacKay, Berg, and Atrash, 2001).

Fetal and Neonatal Effects

Perinatal mortality related to mild preeclampsia ranges from 1% to 8%, increasing to an overall average of 12% in severe preeclampsia, with a higher incidence found with early onset and lower incidence if the onset develops after 37 weeks of gestation (Sibai, 2005a). If the disease progresses into the HELLP syndrome or eclampsia or exists in the presence of preexisting chronic hypertension, perinatal mortality can be as high as 60% (Barton and Sibai, 2001). The majority of perinatal losses are related to placental insufficiency, which causes IUGR, prematurity associated with preterm delivery, or abruptio placentae (Odendaal, 2001).

Signs and Symptoms

Cardinal Signs

The cardinal signs of preeclampsia are hypertension and proteinuria (National High Blood Pressure Education Program Working Group, 2000). Except in the presence of a hydatidiform mole, these signs develop after 20 weeks of gestation. An elevated blood pressure is usually the first symptom in the early stages of this disease; therefore the disease may be diagnosed without the presence of proteinuria.

Hypertension

Hypertension is diagnosed if one of the following is present:
- Systolic blood pressure is 140 mm Hg or greater.
- Diastolic blood pressure is 90 mm Hg or greater.

Proteinuria

Proteinuria is diagnosed if one of the following is present:

- More than 3.0 g (300 mg/dl) of protein per liter of urine is found in a 24-hour urine collection.
- More than 0.3 g (30 mg/dl) of protein per liter is found in at least two random urine specimens collected on two or more occasions at least 6 hours apart when the specific gravity is 1.030 or less and the pH is less than 8. (This is indicated as 1 or greater on a dipstick.)

The following guidelines should be kept in mind when evaluating the urine for protein:

- Vaginal discharge, blood, amniotic fluid, and bacteria can contaminate the specimen and give a false-positive reading.
- The specimen should be obtained by either a voided midstream collection or catheterization to avoid contamination with vaginal discharge.
- Alkaline urine or very concentrated urine (specific gravity greater than 1.030) may give a false-positive reading (Davey and MacGillivray, 1988).
- Dilute urine (specific gravity less than 1.010) may give a false-negative reading.

Subjective Signs

Subjective signs of preeclampsia suggesting end-organ involvement include the following:

- Headaches
- Visual changes, such as blurred vision
- Rapid-onset edema of the face or abdomen or pitting edema in the feet or legs after 12 hours of bedrest
- Oliguria less than 500 ml/24 hours
- Hyperreflexia
- Nausea or vomiting
- Epigastric or right upper quadrant pain

HELLP Syndrome Signs

Signs of the HELLP syndrome follow:

- Vague symptoms before the onset of HELLP syndrome and increase in blood pressure develop
- Right upper quadrant tenderness or epigastric pain, which occurs in patients with HELLP syndrome and is related to obstructed hepatic blood flow because of fibrin deposition (O'Brien and Barton, 2005)
- Nausea or vomiting related to hepatic stretching occurs in 50% of patients
- Headache
- Influenza-like symptoms, such as malaise, occur 90% of the time
- Jaundice
- Hematuria
- One third of the time, HELLP syndrome develops in the postpartum period within 48 hours after delivery but may not be evident until the sixth day

Table 21-4   Comparison of Mild and Severe Preeclampsia

	Mild	Severe
Blood pressure		
Systolic	140–160 mm Hg	>160 mm Hg
Diastolic	90–110 mm Hg	≥110 mm Hg
Proteinuria (24 hr)	0.3–4.0 g	≥5 g
Dipstick	+2/+3	+4
Urinary output	>30 ml/hr	<20 ml/hr
	>650 ml/24 hr	<500 ml/24 hr
Pulmonary edema	Not present	Can be present
Subjective signs	Not present	Can be present
HELLP syndrome signs	Not present	Can be present

HELLP, hemolysis, elevated liver enzymes, and low platelet count in association with preeclampsia.

Comparison of Mild and Severe Preeclamptic Signs

Preeclampsia is usually categorized in grades of mild or severe for the purpose of treatment (Table 21-4).

Eclampsia

If coma or convulsions occur, preeclampsia is then classified as eclampsia. Severe persistent headaches, epigastric pain, hyperreflexia with clonus, and restlessness are warning signs of impending eclampsia. However, in the presence of only edema, some normal women have hyperreflexia.

In an eclamptic seizure, the convulsive activity begins with facial twitching followed by generalized muscle rigidity (Cunningham and others, 2005). During the convulsion, respiration ceases because of muscle spasms. Coma usually follows the seizure-like activity, and respiration naturally resumes.

Diagnostic Testing
Diagnostic Signs

The most easily diagnosed symptom of preeclampsia is a rise in blood pressure. To detect blood pressure diagnostic of early preeclampsia, one must consider two elements. First, the blood pressure, mainly the diastolic pressure, normally drops slightly during the second trimester of pregnancy and then gradually returns to its original baseline level during the third trimester. Second, the systolic blood pressure is more affected by cardiac output changes, whereas the diastolic blood pressure is more affected by peripheral vascular resistance changes (Foley, 2001). Therefore the diastolic blood pressure is the more diagnostic of the two.

Obtaining Accurate Blood Pressure Readings

To obtain an accurate blood pressure reading, the blood pressure cuff must cover approximately 80% of the upper arm. Because position can lead to variability in the blood pressure reading, blood pressure should be measured in the same arm and with the patient in a sitting position with arm at heart level (National High Blood Pressure Education Program Working Group, 2000). The blood pressure should be taken after a 10-minute rest period without caffeine or tobacco use for at least 30 minutes.

During pregnancy, Korotkoff phase V most accurately reflects intraarterial pressure (Brown and others, 1998). Therefore the National High Blood Pressure Education Program Working Group (2000) currently recommends that the Korotkoff phase V sound be used.

A second controversy exists as to the device used to take blood pressure. The question is whether blood pressure readings obtained by the standard mercury sphygmomanometer (manual) and the automated blood pressure device (electronic) can be used interchangeably. Brown and others (1998) found the auscultatory (manual) systolic pressures were 7 to 10 mm Hg lower than the oscillatory (electronic) values. Auscultatory diastolic pressures were 5 to 7 mm Hg higher than oscillatory values. Therefore use caution when interpreting blood pressure values taken with different devices (Green and Froman, 1996).

Diagnostic Tests

Tests that assist in the diagnosis of preeclampsia are found in Table 21-5. Diagnostic tests that can be helpful in diagnosing HELLP syndrome are summarized in Table 21-6.

Predictive Tests

Because the hypertensive disease process begins long before signs and symptoms appear, various researchers have attempted to develop a predictive test. More than 100 clinical biophysical and biochemical tests have been evaluated for predicting patients at risk for preeclampsia. Inconsistent and contradictory predictive abilities have limited their usefulness. According to the World Health

Table 21-5   Summary of Diagnostic Tests Used in the Diagnosis of Preeclampsia

Condition Evaluated	Diagnostic Test	Significant Finding
Hemoconcentration	Hematocrit	>35 and rising
Kidney involvement	Uric acid test	>4.5 mg
	BUN test	>10 mg/dl
	Serum creatinine test	>2 mg/dl
Coagulopathy	FSP test	>40 mg/ml
	Platelet count	<100,000/mm^3
Bleeding time prolonged	Fibrinogen levels	<300 mg/dl
Endothelial damage	Albumin levels	<2.5
	Fibronectin levels	Increased 2–3 times
Hepatic involvement	AST	>41 units/L
	ALT	>30 units/L

ALT, Alanine transaminase; *AST*, aspartate transaminase; *BUN*, blood urea nitrogen; *FSP*, fibrin split products.

Table 21-6   Summary of Diagnostic Tests Used in the Diagnosis of HELLP

Condition Evaluated	Diagnostic Test	Significant Finding
Hemolysis	Peripheral smear	Abnormal
		Schistocytes or burr cells present
	Bilirubin	>1.2 mg/dl
	LDH	>600 units/L
Hepatic involvement	Liver enzymes	
	AST (SGOT)	>72 units /L
	ALT (SGPT)	>50 units /L
	LDH	>600 international units /L
Thrombocytopenia	Platelet count	<100,000/mm^3

ALT, Alanine transaminase; *AST,* aspartate transaminase; *HELLP,* hemolysis, elevated liver enzymes, and low platelet in association with preeclampsia; *LDH,* lactate dehydrogenase; *SGOT,* serum glutamic oxaloacetic transaminase; *SGPT,* serum glutamic pyruvate transaminase.

Organization systematic review (Conde-Agudelo, Villar and Lindheimer, 2004), there is currently no ideal predictive test. A current study is evaluating the predictiveness of placental growth factor (P1GF) in urine (Levine and others, 2005).

USUAL MEDICAL MANAGEMENT AND PROTOCOLS FOR NURSE PRACTITIONERS

The only cure for preeclampsia is termination of the pregnancy. The goal of management is to prevent eclampsia and other severe complications while allowing the fetus to mature. Because fetuses are usually immature when the disease develops, the severity of the disease and the maturity of the fetus must be considered in determining when delivery should take place.

If the pregnancy has progressed 36 weeks or more or fetal maturity is confirmed by a lecithin/sphingomyelin (L/S) ratio of 2:1, delivery is the treatment of choice after the condition is stabilized. If the pregnancy is fewer than 36 weeks of gestation or the fetus is immature, interventions are instituted to attempt to arrest or improve preeclampsia and allow time for the fetus to mature. However, if the HELLP syndrome develops, signs of impending eclampsia are present, or symptoms manifest indicating the condition is worsening, immediate delivery is necessary at any gestational age.

Expectant Management

Medical interventions depend on the severity of the disease and gestational age. In mild preeclampsia when the gestational age is 36 weeks or greater, the patient is usually treated with intravenous (IV) magnesium sulfate and oxytocin to induce labor. In mild preeclampsia when the fetus is immature, the patient is usually hospitalized with decreased activity to attempt to arrest the disease or at least stabilize the disease to allow the fetus time to mature without jeopardizing the mother's health. If the patient becomes normotensive with no significant proteinuria (less than 500 mg/24 hours), research has indicated similar outcomes with home management (either in a day care unit or with home health care) as with in-patient hospital care (Crowther, Bouwmeester, and Ashurst, 1992; Tuffnell and others, 1992; Barton and others, 1994, 1995, 1997). Refer to home care guidelines for treatment of mild preeclampsia under the Nursing Management section of this chapter.

If the disease is severe—as indicated by worsening maternal symptoms, diagnostic tests showing evidence of end-organ dysfunction, or deterioration of the fetus—or if HELLP syndrome develops, the current treatment is to prevent convulsions with an anticonvulsant, control the blood pressure within a safe range with an antihypertensive agent, and evaluate maternal and fetal well-being frequently. Then expeditious delivery is initiated as the woman's condition indicates. If the patient manifests a bleeding tendency, fresh frozen plasma (FFP) and packed RBCs are usually transfused.

Activity Restriction

Resting in bed in the lateral recumbent position takes the pressure of the gravid uterus off the inferior vena cava. This facilitates venous return, thereby increasing the circulatory volume, which increases renal blood flow and promotes diuresis (Dekker, 2001). Blood pressure normally drops as a result, enhancing blood flow to the placenta and fetus. How much of the day should be spent in bed is currently controversial. According to the National High Blood Pressure Education Program Working Group (2000), there is lack of scientific support for the effectiveness of continuous bedrest when compared with maternal risks associated with bedrest (see Chapter 1).

Diet

A diet adequate in protein is therapeutic in promoting cellular growth, replacing the protein lost in the urine, and lowering the risk for hypertension. During pregnancy, the RDA for protein increases by 25 grams (Wardlaw and Smith, 2006). Protein also increases the plasma colloid osmotic pressure. As the plasma colloid osmotic pressure increases, it pulls fluid from the intracellular spaces back into the circulatory system. Adequate calcium, magnesium, and vitamins are also important. Vitamins C and E may be particularly important because of their antioxidant effect (Chappell and others, 1999).

Sodium intake should not exceed 6 g daily. According to the Cochrane Review (Duley, Henderson-Smart, and Meher, 2005), the patient should be instructed to salt foods to taste. An excessive salt intake can increase angiotensin II sensitivity and cause increased vasoconstriction. On the other hand, an inappropriate dietary sodium restriction below 2 g can further reduce the blood volume and decrease placental perfusion (Newman and Fullerton, 1990; IFIC, 2003). However, if the patient has salt-sensitive chronic hypertension or renal disease and was on a sodium-restricted diet before pregnancy, she should continue this diet during her pregnancy.

Fetal Surveillance

The most commonly used methods of fetal surveillance are serial ultrasounds to estimate fetal growth, amniotic fluid index (AFI) studies, biophysical profile (BPP) with nonstress test, and daily fetal movement counts to assess uteroplacental perfusion.

Pharmacologic Therapy

The following medications are commonly used in the treatment of preeclampsia.

Anticonvulsive Therapy

Magnesium sulfate is still the anticonvulsant drug of choice to prevent seizure activity with severe preeclampsia and to treat eclampsia (National High Blood Pressure Education Program Working Group, 2000; Duley and Henderson-Smart, 2002; Duley, Gulmezoglu, and Henderson-Smart, 2003). However, there is no evidence-based data concerning the use of prophylactic magnesium in mild preeclampsia. Phenytoin may be used as an alternative therapy when magnesium is contraindicated such as in renal failure and myasthenia gravis. It is not as effective as magnesium for prophylaxis or treatment of eclampsia seizures. For anticonvulsant therapy, refer to the section on critical case interventions for anticonvulsant therapy later in this chapter.

Antihypertensive Therapy

According to the Cochrane database of systematic reviews, the benefit of antihypertensive therapy for mild to moderate hypertension during pregnancy is unclear (Duley and Henderson-Smart, 2002). Antihypertensive therapy in preeclampsia does not appear to improve perinatal outcomes (Abalos and others, 2001). However, in situations in which the diastolic blood pressure goes above 110 or the systolic goes above 160 to 180, there are significant renal, hepatic, and neurologic risks, such as cerebrovascular accident, to the mother. Antihypertensive therapy is indicated. Treatment should be implemented to reduce the blood pressure to a level that provides a margin of maternal safety without compromising adequate uterine perfusion.

Hydralazine (Apresoline) has been the antihypertensive drug of choice in the United States because it is more effective in lowering MAP to safe levels than other drugs (National High Blood Pressure Education Program Working Group, 2000). However, it has been shown to be associated with more material side effects and low Apgar scores at 1 minute (von Dadelszen and Magee, 2005). Labetalol has extensively been be used during pregnancy. Another antihypertensive agent being tried is oral nifedipine (Procardia). However, it is not approved by the Food and Drug Administration for treating hypertensive emergencies (National High Blood Pressure Education Program Working Group, 2000). For antihypertensive therapy, refer to the section on critical case interventions for acute antihypertensive therapy later in this chapter.

Corticosteroid Therapy

The use of a single course of corticosteroids to facilitate fetal lung maturity is recommended if delivery is imminent before 34 weeks of gestation (NIH, 2000). In the presence of HELLP syndrome, glucocorticoids have been shown to decrease the severity of the disease, decreasing intraventricular hemorrhage and perinatal infection (Anumba and Robson, 1999) and normalizing platelet count and liver enzymes (O'Brien, Milligan, and Barton, 2000).

Blood Component Replacement

In the presence of severe persistent thrombocytopenia, FFP or packed RBCs are usually infused. Platelet transfusions are ineffective because platelet consumption occurs soon after administration (Mabie, 2001).

Intensive Hemodynamic Monitoring

Intensive hemodynamic monitoring is not considered a standard of practice for severe preeclampsia or eclampsia according to the National High Blood Pressure Education Program Working Group (2000). However, many clinicians find it helpful in determining appropriate therapy in the presence of pulmonary edema or oliguria or in situations in which blood pressure is unresponsive to therapy results.

Delivery

Vaginal delivery is preferred unless caesarean delivery is indicated for other obstetric reasons. Cervical ripening agents or oxytocin for induction or augmentation can be used to expedite labor within 24 hours. Regional anesthesia such as epidural, spinal, or combination spinal and epidural are safe. Laryngoscopy and tracheal intubation with a general anesthesia can increase hypertension. Pretreatment with an antihypertensive agent may decrease this risk.

NURSING MANAGEMENT

Prevention

Because the etiology of the disease is unknown, it is difficult to outline a protocol for prevention. Based on scientific studies, some general principles, however, appear to decrease the incidence of this disease.

Adequate Nutrition

All pregnant patients should receive instructions regarding the benefits of eating a nutritious, balanced diet containing at least 70 to 80 g of protein, 1200 mg of calcium, and an adequate amount of zinc, magnesium, sodium (salt), other minerals, and vitamins (especially folate, C, and E) every day (Chappell and others, 1999; Roberts and Hubel, 1999; Gunderson, 2003). According to the Cochrane Trials, supplementation of magnesium or zinc has not been shown to be beneficial (Madomed, 1997; Makrides and Crowther, 2001). With evidence that oxidative stress influences the disease process, a diet with adequate antioxidants such as lycopene, zinc, selenium, magnesium, and melatonin may decrease the incidence. (O'Scholl and others, 2005; Spinnato and Livingston, 2005). Drinking six to eight glasses of water or fluid per day should be included in the instructions. According to the Cochrane Database of Systematic Review, if the pregnant patient is not including adequate calcium in her diet, a calcium supplement reduces the risk for preeclampsia (Atallah, Hofmeyr, Duley, 2002).

Adequate Rest

Bedrest facilitates venous return, increasing the circulatory volume, enhancing renal and placental perfusion, and lowering blood pressure. Therefore high risk patients may benefit from 8 to 12 hours of sleep each night with a rest period in the middle of the day. Bedrest also mobilizes edematous fluid back into the intravascular space. However, according to the Cochrane Review, complete bedrest should not be considered unless the disease is severe (Meher, Abalos, and Carroli, 2005).

Water Therapy

In the presence of severe edema, research has demonstrated that shoulder-deep immersion in water can mobilize extravascular fluid, initiate diuresis, and decrease the renin, angiotensin, aldosterone, and vasopressin levels (Katz and others, 1990; Katz and others, 1992; Kent and others, 1999; Young and Jewell, 2001; DiPasquale and Lynett, 2003). Therefore water therapy may help prevent or slow the progression of preeclampsia. It has also been shown to help reverse oligohydramnios resulting from uteroplacental insufficiency (Strong, 1993).

Early and Appropriate Prenatal Care

Early, appropriate treatment is effective in preventing the severe form of preeclampsia or eclampsia. Therefore early detection of its development is effective in lowering the high maternal and fetal mortality associated with the disease (MacKay, Berg, and Atrash, 2001).

Detection begins on the first prenatal visit early in pregnancy. The nurse practitioner or nurse obtains an in-depth patient history that includes age and parity, a medical history of such things as diabetes and persistent hypertensive disorders, and a familial history of preeclampsia or eclampsia. On each prenatal visit, the patient is weighed, an accurate blood pressure reading is obtained, and an early-morning urine specimen is checked for protein. If protein is noted in the urine, it should be checked for bacteria and another specimen obtained by clean-catch midstream collection because bacteria, vaginal discharge, blood, and amniotic fluid can give a false-positive result. If urine protein is 11 or greater, follow up with a 24-hour urine test for protein and creatinine clearance.

Low-Dose Aspirin

The Cochrane Database of Systematic Review of the research on the effectiveness of low-dose aspirin therapy (60 to 75 mg/day) to reduce the incidence of preeclampsia in some women at risk for the disease concluded that there is a small to moderate benefit (Duley and others, 2003). Aspirin selectively inhibits thromboxane production with minimal effect on prostacyclin synthesis. Therefore it restores the prostacyclin/thromboxane balance. This low dose appears to have no harmful effects on the fetus or neonate and is safe for the mother, and epidural anesthesia is safe with the use of low-dose aspirin (CLASP Collaborative Group, 1995). Further studies are needed to assess which women would benefit and when treatment should be initiated (Duley and others, 2003).

Home Health Care for Mild Preeclampsia*

Criteria Selection

- Blood pressure lower than 150/100 mm Hg sitting and lower than 140/90 mm Hg in the left lateral position
- Proteinuria lower than 500 mg/day
- Platelet count more than 125,000/μl
- Normal liver enzymes: aspartate transaminase (AST) less than 50 units/L, alanine transaminase (ALT) less than 50 units/L, lactate dehydrogenase (LDH) less than 200 units/L
- Serum creatinine less than 1.32 mg/dl
- Reassuring fetal status with no intrauterine fetal growth restriction
- No worsening signs present
- A compliant, reliable patient

Home Care Protocols

- Limited home activity with 12 hours sleep each night and rest periods during the day to facilitate renal and placental perfusion by mobilizing the movement of extracellular fluid back into the intravascular space.
- Bed exercises to keep the muscles toned and increase blood flow; leg exercises, such as foot circles at least twice each day; the super Kegel and abdominal tightening exercises to keep the perineal and abdominal muscles in tone. If the patient complains of back pain, the pelvic rock can help relieve this discomfort (see Box 1-1).
- Balanced diet containing at least 60 to 70 g of protein, 400 mcg of folic acid, 1200 mg of calcium; adequate zinc and sodium (2 to 6 g); and six to eight glasses of water per day.
- Blood pressure monitored every 4 to 6 hours daily (while awake).
- Daily weighing at the same time.
- Urine tested for protein using first-voided specimen of the day.
- Understanding of the signs and symptoms that indicate the condition is worsening with instructions to report them immediately:
  - Headaches, severe and not relieved by acetaminophen
  - Vision changes, such as blurry vision or seeing spots
  - Epigastric pain or right upper quadrant (RUQ) pain

*Friedman and others, 2001.

- Increased edema indicated by a weight gain of more than 2 pounds in 1 day or 5 pounds in 1 week
- Vaginal bleeding or changes in vaginal discharge
- Severe abdominal pain
- Watery fluid leading from the vagina
- Uterine tightening
- Decreased fetal movements or fetal movements of fewer than four in 1 hour
- Tell her to expect home health nurse visits two times per week with daily telephone contact.
- Schedule weekly prenatal visits.
- Perform initial and frequent diagnostic laboratory assessments as follows:
  - 24-hour urine sample for protein and creatinine clearance
  - Serum creatinine and uric acid levels
  - Hematocrit
  - Serum albumin
  - Platelet count
  - Liver enzymes, such as AST, ALT, and LDH, if platelet count is low
- Instruct patient in fetal surveillance.
  - Daily fetal movement counts
  - Frequent evaluations with BPP, contraction stress test (CST), nonstress test (NST), and AFI
  - Fetal growth by ultrasound every 3 weeks
- Admit patient to hospital for worsening status.

Nursing Assessment for Severe Preeclampsia
General Criteria

The goal is *early* detection of indicators that the condition is deteriorating.

Instruct the patient to check her blood pressure every 4 hours while she is awake or more often if indicated. The blood pressure should be taken on the same arm with the patient in the same position each time. Preferably, the patient is lying on her left side with the cuff on the right arm.

Cardiovascular Alterations
- Measure pulse rate; assess quality and rhythm.
- Evaluate degree of edema every 8 hours and score as shown in Table 21-7.
- Obtain daily weight before breakfast.
- Check capillary refill and neck vein distention.
- Evaluate serum albumin to check for endothelial leakage.

Renal Alterations
- Evaluate urine for protein, specific gravity, pH, and glucose daily or every 8 hours with dipstick. The gram equivalent of protein, as indicated on the dipstick, is outlined in Table 21-8. A 24-hour urine collection for protein and creatinine clearance may be ordered if the dipstick protein is +1 or

Table 21-7   Degree of Edema

Physical Findings	Score
Minimal edema of lower extremities	1
Marked edema of lower extremities	2
Edema of lower extremities, face, hands	3
Generalized massive edema including abdomen and sacrum	4

Table 21-8   Proteinuria

Dipstick Reading	Protein
Trace	5–20 mg/L
1	30 mg/L
2	100 mg/L
3	300 mg/L
4	>1000 mg/L

Reference: Chernecky C, Berger B: *Laboratory tests and diagnostic procedures,* ed 4, Philadelphia, 2004, Saunders.

Table 21-9   Deep Tendon Reflex Grading

Physical Result	Grade
None elicited	0
Sluggish or dull	1
Active, normal	2
Brisk	3
Brisk with transient (few beats) or sustained (continuous) clonus	4

Reference: Hallett M: National Institute of Neurological Disorders and Stroke (NINDS) myotatic reflex scale. *Neurology* 43(12):2723, 1993.

greater. The loss of 5 g or more of protein in 24 hours indicates severe preeclampsia.
- Measure intake and output every 1 to 4 hours, and keep a record. If the urinary output is less than 30 ml/hour or 120 ml/4 hours, oliguria is present. This indicates that the condition is deteriorating. If output is increased, monitor electrolytes for indications of high output renal failure such as serum creatinine greater than 1.0.
- Measure serum creatinine and uric acid levels.

Central Nervous System Alterations
- Check deep tendon reflexes (DTRs) daily or more often if indicated. The easiest DTR to check is the patellar reflex (knee jerk). The response elicited should be graded as shown in Table 21-9.

- Determine whether clonus is present. In clonus, dorsiflexion of the foot causes spasms of the muscle. This is seen as a convulsive movement of the foot and indicates neuromuscular irritability.
- Assess for severe headaches not relieved by acetaminophen or visual changes that are indicative that the condition is worsening. Additionally, note changes in level of consciousness or changes in behavior.

Pulmonary Alterations

- Check respiration rate every 4 hours while the patient is awake or more often if indicated.
- Auscultate lung fields for wheezing or crackles, which can indicate pulmonary edema. Signs of dyspnea, tightness of the chest, shallow respiration, or a cough should be noted.
- Assess skin color and mucous membranes for cyanosis.
- Monitor oxygenation with pulse oximetry as indicated.

Hepatic Alterations

- Assess for epigastric pain, right upper quadrant pain, nausea, vomiting, and jaundice; these are all possible signs of liver injury.
- If platelet count is low, assess liver enzymes such as AST, ALT, and LDH to monitor for HELLP.
- Assess for hypoglycemia and coagulation defects in the presence of severe hepatic involvement.

Hematology Alterations

- Hematocrit for hemoconcentration
- Peripheral smear for hemolysis of RBCs
- Platelet counts to monitor for HELLP (If patient has been on low dose aspirin therapy, platelet function may be below normal even if platelet count is adequate.)
- Follow-up coagulation studies, such as fibrinogen, D-dimers, prothrombin, and partial thromboplastin time, if platelet count is lower than 100,000 mm^3
- Indications of possible DIC development include signs of bleeding, such as oozing from IV sites, nosebleeds, and petechiae

Reproductive System Status

- Assess for the presence of uterine contractions because decreased uteroplacental blood flow can initiate labor.
- Assess for signs of an abruptio placentae, including dark red vaginal bleeding, sustained abdominal pain, uterine tenderness, tetanic contractions, and increasing fundal height.

Fetal Surveillance Status

- Check fetal heart rate every 4 to 6 hours with a Doppler FHR device or a continuous electronic fetal monitor, if the condition indicates.

- Record fetal movements daily. Fetal movements have been shown to correlate with fetal well-being. Fewer fetal movements from the patient's previous pattern may indicate fetal hypoxia. Instruct the patient to report decreased fetal movements compared with the movements of the previous day or when there are fewer than 10 fetal movements in any 2-hour period (ACOG, 1999).
- Monitor for IUGR. Use serial ultrasounds and AFI for oligohydramnios.
- Severe uteroplacental insufficiency: Appropriate fetal surveillance tests, such as nonstress test (NST), contraction stress test (CST), or BPP with frequent AFI, are carried out at appropriate intervals after 28 to 30 weeks of gestation.

Nursing Interventions for Severe Preeclampsia

- *Manage patient in a tertiary care center* on a high risk obstetric unit that has a neonatal intensive care unit.
- *Follow systematic assessments* (as outlined under Nursing Assessment for Severe Preeclampsia) if critical to the ongoing management.
- *Limit activity to bathroom privileges.* Help the patient and her family problem-solve difficulties that implement limited activity.
- *Make appropriate referrals*, for example, to Sidelines or a social worker.
- *Encourage family participation* in patient's care and decision making as much as possible.
- *Encourage bed exercises* because they are important in keeping the muscles in tone and in increasing blood flow. The patient should be instructed to do leg exercises such as foot circles at least twice each day. She should also be instructed to do the super Kegel and abdominal tightening exercises to keep the perineal and abdominal muscles in tone. If the patient complains of back pain, the pelvic rock can help relieve this discomfort (see Box 1-1).
- *If IV fluids are indicated, administer isotonic crystalloid fluids or colloid-containing fluids* to increase colloid osmotic pressure. Avoid the use of hypotonic fluids in fluid replacement therapy because they may further decrease the serum osmolarity.
- *Base initial intake of fluid* on the need to combat dehydration. (Usual amount for first 24 hours is 1500 to 3000 ml of fluid. Therefore if patient is not dehydrated, fluid intake equals amount of urinary output of the previous 24 hours plus 1000 ml, except in acute renal failure, in which case intake should not exceed 500 ml.) If oliguria develops, fluid administration is best guided by pulmonary capillary wedge pressure.
- *Monitor maternal and fetal status* and for signs the condition is worsening (as outlined under Nursing Assessment for Severe Preeclampsia).
- *Baseline and frequent diagnostic laboratory assessments* (as outlined under Nursing Assessment for Severe Preeclampsia).
- *Monitor for HELLP* (see Table 21-6).
- *Prevent eclampsia* with anticonvulsant therapy (refer to Critical Care Intervention for Anticonvulsant Therapy, later in this chapter).

- *Treat hypertension* if blood pressure is higher than 160 to 180/110 mm Hg (refer to Critical Care Intervention for Antihypertensive Therapy, later in this chapter).
- *Initiate corticosteroid therapy* to improve premature fetal lung maturity and to decrease HELLP syndrome severity (Box 21-1).
- *Allay anxiety* by providing time for the patient and her family to express their concerns regarding the possible outcomes for the baby and the inconvenience to the mother and family during the treatment. Encourage them to vent any feelings, fears, and anger they may experience. Provide understandable information to the patient and her family regarding the disease process, plan of treatment, and implications for mother and fetus. Explain all treatment modalities and reasons for each. Keep patient informed of health status, results of tests, and fetal well-being.
- *Refer to a community support group* such as Sidelines *(http://www.sidelines. org)*.
- *Refer to a spiritual counselor or chaplain* on request.
- *Suggest diversional activities.* Assess patient's interest in various diversional activities within her activity limit. Provide crafts, reading, and puzzles that can be done in bed, or encourage patient to have these things brought in. Provide classes in preparation for childbirth by way of video, the hospital television, or group classes that can be attended while reclining. Refer to a diversional therapist or volunteer to provide reading materials, handicrafts, or other activities of interest.
- *Prepare for delivery* when indicated as outlined by Odendaal (2001):
  - Fetal lung maturity
  - Fetal stress
  - Abruptio placenta
  - Uncontrolled blood pressure
  - Oliguria
  - Pulmonary edema

Box 21-1   Corticosteroid Therapy

Betamethasone

Action

Betamethasone stimulates the production of a more mature surfactant in the fetal lung between 24 and 34 weeks of gestation. It has no effect in enhancing fetal lung maturity after 34 weeks of gestation (Odendaal, 2001). Optimal benefit begins 24 hours after initiation of therapy and lasts 7 days. This period of time is called the *steroid window.* Higher doses in the presence of the HELLP syndrome have been shown to improve platelet count and liver function enzymes (O'Brian, Milligan, and Barton, 2000). It has also been shown to shorten the recovery period during the postpartum period (O'Brien and Barton, 2005).

Dosage

For the treatment of immature surfactant, two doses of 12.5 mg are given intramuscularly 24 hours apart (NIH, 2000; Weiner and Buhimschi, 2004).

- • Persistent HELLP
- • Imminent eclampsia
- • *Postpartum considerations.* There is an increased risk for recurrence of preeclampsia of approximately 10% to 25% (Hayman, 2004). There is an increase risk for cardiovascular disease later in life. Van Pampus and Aarnoudse (2005) consider preeclampsia as a first manifestation of atherosclerosis. Lifestyle changes should be advised as indicated, as well as ongoing screening such as hyperlipidemia, hyperhomocystinemia, and thrombophilia. Overall, 35% develop chronic hypertension later in life (Witlin, 1999). This risk can be affected by or be related to lifestyle health habits, stress level, and current partner (Egerman and Sibai, 2001). Long-term follow-up is important because of the possible underlying medical problems such as coagulation disturbances, protein S and C deficiency, hyperhomocystinemia, and anticardiolipin antibodies (Odendaal, 2001).

Critical Care Interventions for Anticonvulsant Therapy: Magnesium

- • *Administer magnesium sulfate.* Normal dosing guidelines are provided in Box 21-2.
- • *Set the goal of therapy* to be decreased but not absent DTRs.
- • *Assess for magnesium toxicity* any patient receiving magnesium sulfate in the follow manner:
  - • The DTR should be checked every hour if the patient is on continuous IV drip and before administering each dose if the patient is on intermittent therapy (Table 21-10).
  - • Check the respiratory pattern and rate, pulse, blood pressure, oxygen saturation, and level of consciousness frequently if the patient is receiving a continuous IV drip or before administering each dose if the patient is receiving intermittent therapy.
  - • Monitor patient's intake and output closely and insert a Foley catheter because magnesium is excreted largely in the urine; the patient with kidney involvement can develop toxicity rapidly. If the patient is receiving a continuous IV drip, the urinary output should be at least 30 ml/hour. If the patient is receiving intermittent doses of magnesium, the urinary output should be obtained every 4 hours and should be at least 120 ml/4 hours.
- • To decrease the risk for pulmonary edema, limit the total fluid intake for 24 hours to not exceed 2000 ml.
- • Use serum magnesium levels to assess magnesium toxicity. Therapeutic levels are between 4 and 7 mEq/L and are effective in preventing convulsions, demonstrated by depressed DTRs. Plasma levels between 8 and 10 mEq/L cause a loss of DTRs, which is the first sign of toxicity. Other early signs are nausea, a feeling of warmth, flushing, somnolence, double vision, slurred speech, and weakness. Plasma levels above 13 to 15 mEq/L can cause respiratory paralysis, and levels greater than 20 to 25 mEq/L can cause cardiac arrest (see Table 21-10). Therefore assess serum magnesium levels

Box 21-2   Anticonvulsive Therapy in Preeclampsia

Magnesium Sulfate

The drug of choice to treat eclampsia.

Action

Decreases central nervous system irritability and blocks neuromuscular conduct by blocking the release of acetylcholine at neuromuscular junctions. Acetylcholine is the excitatory substance that transmits nerve messages across the synapse.

Other Beneficial Actions

Magnesium sulfate has been shown to cause peripheral vasodilation, increase uterine and renal blood flow, increase prostacyclin production by endothelial cells, reduce platelet aggregation, and decrease the action of plasma renin and angiotensin (Eclampsia Trial Collaborative Group, 1995). It is superior to phenytoin or diazepam (Duley, Gulmezoglu, and Henderson-Smart, 2003; Duley and Henderson-Smart, 2003a, 2003b).

Intravenous Dosage

Therapeutic administration of magnesium sulfate usually consists of an initial loading dose of 4 to 6 g by IV in 100 ml of fluid administered over 15 to 20 minutes, followed by a maintenance dose of 2 g/hr diluted in 5% dextrose and lactated Ringer's solution administered by an infusion pump to maintain serum magnesium levels in a therapeutic range of 4 to 8 mEq/L.

Intramuscular Dosage

The maintenance dose can also be administered intramuscularly. The normal dosage is 5 g every 4 hours in alternate buttocks. Intramuscular injections of magnesium sulfate are seldom used because the rate of absorption cannot be controlled, tissue necrosis can develop, and the injections are painful. If magnesium sulfate is administered intramuscularly, Z-track technique should be used with a 3-inch, 20-gauge dry needle to ensure that the medication is injected deep into the gluteal muscle, and the site should be gently massaged to facilitate absorption. A local anesthetic agent can be added to the magnesium sulfate solution to minimize the discomfort.

Side Effects

Frequently experienced side effects are lethargy, sensations of heat or burning, headache, nausea and vomiting, blurry vision, and constipation. The patient should be prepared for these normal side effects. Because magnesium sulfate decreases smooth muscle contractility by moving calcium out of the smooth muscle, it decreases uterine activity and can prolong labor. However, it is ineffective in suppressing uterine activity once labor becomes active. Because magnesium blocks neuromuscular and cardiac transmission of nerve impulses and depresses the central nervous system, respiratory paralysis and cardiac arrest can result if serum magnesium levels rise too high. Plasma levels of 4 to 7 mEq/L are very effective in preventing convulsions, demonstrated by depressed deep tendon reflexes (DTRs). Plasma levels between 8 and 10 mEq/L cause a loss of DTRs, which is the first sign of toxicity. Other early signs are nausea, a feeling of warmth, flushing, somnolence, double vision, slurred speech, and weakness.

Plasma levels above 13 to 15 mEq/L can cause respiratory paralysis, and levels greater than 20 to 25 mEq/L can cause cardiac arrest

Continued

Box 21-2 Anticonvulsive Therapy in Preeclampsia—cont'd

(see Table 20-8). Therefore serum magnesium levels should be assessed daily. Magnesium can have some detrimental effects on the fetus as well. Relatively less fetal heart rate variability at therapeutic levels and neonatal neuromuscular and respiratory depression have been seen.

Fetal Effect

Magnesium crosses the placenta, but there is no clear evidence of adverse effects (Weiner and Buhimschi, 2004).

Contraindications

Myasthenia gravis and myocardial ischemia or infarct (Aagaard-Tillery and Belfort, 2005)

Phenytoin

Can be used in situations when magnesium is associated with increased risk.

Action

Suppresses the influx of sodium ions across cell membranes during potential repetitive neuronal activity and blocks the changes in the concentrations of potassium and calcium ions that occur before seizure activity, thus lowering the neuronal excitation threshold.

Dosage

The therapeutic loading dose is usually 10 mg/kg of current weight, diluted in 250 ml of normal saline or lactated Ringer's solution. A dextrose solution should not be used since a precipitation will occur (Lucas and Jordan, 1997). The rate of infusion is between 25 and 40 mg/min. An additional dose of 5 mg/kg is given 2 hours later. Because the half-life of this drug is 12 hours, which is relatively long compared with that of magnesium sulfate, a maintenance dose may not be needed. It is given based on the serum phenytoin levels. The therapeutic range for phenytoin is 10 to 20 mg/ml.

Side Effects

Hypotension, the most common side effect, occurs if the IV infusion is given too rapidly (Lucas and Jordan, 1997). Other side effects seen are cardiac dysrhythmias, bradycardia, hypotension, and heart block; ataxia, slurred speech, mental confusion, and decreased coordination; nausea and vomiting; and double or blurred vision (Weiner and Buhimschi, 2004). Phenytoin has no effect on suppression of labor. Mothers are more alert, awake, and able to breastfeed compared with mothers who received magnesium (Lucas and Jordan, 1997).

daily. Magnesium can have some detrimental effects on the fetus as well. Relatively less FHR variability at therapeutic levels and neonatal neuromuscular and respiratory depression have been seen.

- *Signs of magnesium.* Discontinue or withhold magnesium sulfate and notify the attending physician if any of the following signs of magnesium toxicity develop:
  - No DTR or a sudden change in the DTR
  - Respirations fewer than 14/min or change in breath sounds

Table 21-10   Serum Magnesium Levels

Magnesium Levels (mEq/L)	Magnesium Levels (mg/dl)	Interpretation
1.5–2.5	1.7–2.4	Normal
4–7	5–8.4	Therapeutic
7–8	8.5–10	Depression of deep tendon reflexes
8–10	10–12	Loss of deep tendon reflexes
10–12	12–15	Respiration depression
12–15	15–18	Respiratory paralysis
15–20	18–25	Heart block
Above 20	Above 25	Cardiac arrest

Data from Nick J: Deep tendon reflexes, magnesium, and calcium: assessments and implications. *J Obstet Gynecol Neonatal Nurs* 33(2):221–230, 2004; Roberts J: Pregnancy-related hypertension. In Creasy R, Resnik R, and Iams, J, editors: *Maternal-fetal medicine: principles and practice*, ed 5, Philadelphia, 2004, Saunders; Sibai, B: Hypertension. In Gabbe S, Niebyl J, Simpson J, editors. *Obstetrics: normal and problem pregnancies*, ed 4, New York, 2002, Churchill Livingstone.

- Oxygen saturation below 95%
- Urinary output less than 30 ml/hour or 120 ml/4 hours
- Significant drop in pulse or blood pressure
- Double or blurred vision
- Signs of fetal distress
- Serum magnesium levels 8 mEq/L or greater

- *Use calcium gluconate as the antidote* for magnesium toxicity because calcium stimulates the release of acetylcholine at the nerve synapse. The normal dose is 10 ml of a 10% solution (1 g) given by IV push (Sibia, 2002). This is administered by the physician over 3 minutes to avoid undesirable reactions such as bradycardia, dysrhythmias, and ventricular fibrillation. It can also be administered IV at a rate of 1 g/hour if needed.
- *Prevent pulmonary edema* by closely monitoring the IV and oral fluids to avoid exceeding 125 ml/hour.
- *If magnesium sulfate* is contraindicated, use phenytoin. (Refer to Box 21-1 for dosage administration.)
- *Postpartum considerations*:
  - Continue magnesium sulfate or another anticonvulsant for 24 to 48 hours following delivery or longer if the HELLP syndrome coexisted (Friedman and others, 2001).
  - Monitor closely for pulmonary edema related to fluid replacement and mobilization of accumulated fluid back into the intravascular spaces.

Critical Care Interventions for Acute Antihypertensive Therapy

- *Initiate antihypertensive therapy* if the diastolic blood pressure is greater than 105 to 110 mm Hg or the systolic greater than 160 to 180 mm Hg.
- *Goal of therapy.* Maintain blood pressure below 160/100 mm Hg but above 140/90 mm Hg to reduce blood pressure for mother's benefit while maintaining uteroplacental perfusion for fetal oxygenation.

Box 21-3   Antihypertensive Medications for Acute Hypertensive Crisis
During Pregnancy

Hydralazine

Action

Directs peripheral vasodilation by relaxing smooth muscle; increases cardiac
output and heart rate.

Dosage

Administer 5 to 10 mg by intravenous (IV) push over 1 to 2 minutes. The dose can
be repeated every 20 minutes until the diastolic blood pressure is between 90
and 100 mm Hg or a maximum of 30 mg is reached. The diastolic blood
pressure should not be allowed to fall below 90 mm Hg to prevent further
reduction in blood flow to the placenta, cerebrum, and kidneys. Hydralazine is
administered whenever the diastolic blood pressure again reaches
110 mm Hg.

Side Effects

Possible side effects are tachycardia, dizziness, faintness, headache,
palpitations, numbness, tingling of the extremities, and disorientation. Fetal
effects such as adverse fetal heart rate and low Apgar score at **1 minute.**

Contraindication

Do not use in patients with hypertension and tachycardia because hydralazine
is ineffective in treating hypertension caused by elevated cardiac output.

Labetalol

Action

Labetalol is a combined alpha- and beta-blocker that decreases peripheral
vascular resistance without changing cardiac output or causing tachycardia.
Therefore it is the drug of choice for hypertensive patients with tachycardia
(Weiner and Buhimschi, 2004). It is less effective in black Americans.

Dosage

Administer 20 mg by a bolus IV injection. If effect is suboptimal, give 40 mg
10 minutes later and 80 mg 10 minutes after that, up to a maximum of
300 mg.

Side Effects

The patient can experience nausea, vomiting, orthostatic hypotension, sweating,
dizziness, headaches, bronchospasm, and dyspnea (Weiner and Buhimschi,
2004). Fetal effects such as respiratory depression and bradycardia can occur.

Contraindication

Labetalol is contraindicated in patients with asthma, congestive heart failure,
hypoglycemia, or with hepatotoxicity.

- *Two of the most commonly used drugs* are hydralazine and labetalol. Nifedipine and nitroprusside are used occasionally. Box 21-3 provides a listing of antihypertensive medications to use for acute hypertensive crisis during pregnancy.
- *Stabilize for transport* may be accomplished with hydralazine 5 mg intramuscularly or nifedipine 10 to 20 mg orally (Odendaal, 2001).

- *Check the blood pressure* every minute for the first 5 minutes following administration of antihypertensive medication and then every 5 minutes for the next 30 minutes, preferably with an automatic blood pressure cuff.
- *To prevent treatment-induced severe hypotension*, consider the need for 200 to 300 ml of IV fluid before drug administration unless contraindicated.

Critical Care Interventions for HELLP Syndrome

- *Transfer the patient to a tertiary care center*, if possible.
- *Assess and stabilize maternal condition.*
- *Implement the same monitoring protocol* as for the severe preeclamptic patient.
- *Provide oxygen*, 8 to 10 L via facemask to improve oxygen flow to vital organs and the placenta.
- *Prevent eclampsia* with anticonvulsant therapy. Infusion dose of magnesium sulfate is adjusted based on serum magnesium levels, patellar reflexes, and urinary output. The risk for magnesium toxicity is increased because of the possibility of renal dysfunction and hematoma in the presence of thrombocytopenia. Refer to Critical Care Interventions for Anticonvulsant Therapy.
- *Treat severe acute hypertension.* Refer to Critical Care Interventions for Antihypertensive Therapy.
- *When DIC is present, correct coagulopathy.*
- *Be aware that the patient is at increased risk for abruptio placenta*, pulmonary edema, acute renal failure, eclampsia, and subcapsular hematoma of the liver.
- *Consider the differential diagnosis of acute fatty liver of pregnancy (AFLP).* AFLP is a rare but potentially fatal third trimester complication that can manifest with symptoms similar to HELLP. A diagnostic laboratory finding that differs between AFLP and HELLP is that AFLP has prolonged prothrombin and partial thromboplastin, hypoglycemia, and increased ammonia.
- *Observe more closely for a subcapsular hematoma*, which is rare but life-threatening. Possible signs are a sudden exacerbation of severe epigastric or RUQ pain or unexplained hypotension (Williamson and Girling, 2006). If subcapsular hematoma is suspected, abdominal ultrasound is indicated for diagnosis. If subcapsular hematoma of the liver develops, perform the following:
  - Follow with serial abdominal ultrasounds.
  - Type and cross-match packed RBCs (30 units), FFP (20 units), and platelet concentration (30–50 units).
  - Monitor the hemodynamic state closely by assessing signs of shoulder pain, ascites, respiratory difficulty, and shock.
  - Be prepared for emergency surgery and aggressive management of coagulopathy if rupture occurs.
- *Provide continuous electronic monitoring of FHR*, and carry out ordered fetal surveillance studies such as an NST or BPP.

- *Be prepared to assist with fetal lung maturity studies* if less than 35 weeks of gestation.
- *Initiate corticosteroid therapy* if indicated to improve fetal lung maturity and a more rapid improvement of the condition (see Box 21-1).
- *Prepare for delivery.* If the fetus is immature, attempts may be made to stabilize the patient, undelivered, until corticosteroids can be administered. If the fetus is mature, vaginal delivery is preferred. Induction with oxytocin and or prostaglandins may be attempted if patient's condition is stable. If a cesarean delivery is indicated and the platelet count is below 40,000 mm^3, 10 units of platelets should be administered before the surgery.
- *Postpartum considerations*:
  - Continue intensive monitoring for 48 hours postpartum.
  - Consider corticosteroid therapy to shorten the disease process and improve recovery time (see Box 21-1).
  - Be aware that the onset of the HELLP syndrome develops 30% of the time during the postpartum period. Clinical manifestations of the syndrome usually occur within the first 48 hours postpartum.
  - There is a 19% to 27% risk for recurrence in subsequent pregnancies with the highest risk correlating with the severity of abnormal laboratory findings and a 15% risk for developing a non-HELLP preeclampsia (Witlin, 1999).

Critical Care Nursing Interventions for Eclampsia
Seizure Precautions

- *Assess for signs of impending eclampsia,* such as epigastric or right upper quadrant pain, nausea and vomiting, headache, jaundice, and hematuria.
- *Implement seizure precautions* by having oxygen, suction, a padded tongue blade, and supplies to pad side rails at bedside.
- *Provide a quiet, pleasant environment* with limited lighting so as not to activate further the already overstimulated central nervous system.
- *Limit visitors* except the patient's family.
- *Administer magnesium sulfate* or other anticonvulsant therapy as ordered. Refer to Critical Care Interventions for Anticonvulsant Therapy.
- *Assess for signs of magnesium toxicity,* such as absence of DTRs, respirations fewer than 12/min, or a significant drop in pulse or blood pressure. Monitor urinary output, since magnesium sulfate is excreted by way of the kidneys. Note serum magnesium levels.
- *Have antidote of calcium gluconate* at bedside.
- *Notify attending physician of any worsening signs,* including signs of magnesium sulfate toxicity.

During the Seizure

- *Remain with the patient.*
- *Reduce the risk for aspiration and establish airway patency* by lowering and turning the head to one side to keep the airway open and minimize aspiration. Suction any secretions from the mouth.

- *Observe seizure activity* for time of occurrence, length of seizure, and type of seizure activity.
- *Call for help* by turning on the patient's call light.
- *Notify attending physician* at the first sign of convulsive activity.
- *Prevent maternal injury.* If possible, a padded tongue blade should be inserted with care between the teeth to prevent tongue injury and to facilitate the insertion of an airway if needed. Make sure the side rails are up and padded if possible.

After the Seizure

- *Assess airway and suction* if needed. Maintain adequate oxygenation by administering oxygen via facemask at 10 L/min.
- *Start an IV line* as soon as possible. Monitor IV fluid closely with infusion pump.
- *Ensure maternal oxygenation after seizure.* Assess breathing pattern, and administer oxygen at 10 L/min by tight facemask as needed to increase the maternal oxygen concentration and improve the oxygen supply to the fetus, which is lessened during a convulsion. Assess blood pressure, pulse, and respirations every 5 minutes until stable. Auscultate lung sounds to rule out aspiration.
- *Ensure fetal oxygenation after seizure.* Assess the FHR continuously with a fetal monitor because the hypoxic and acidotic state of a seizure may cause fetal distress. Change the patient's position from left lateral to right lateral every 30 minutes to increase uterine and renal blood flow.
- *Provide a quiet environment.*
- *Establish seizure control with magnesium sulfate.* Magnesium sulfate therapy is usually initiated as soon as the seizure stops. Start an IV line with an 18-gauge intracatheter if it has not already been inserted. The normal dosage is a 4-g IV loading dose followed by a continuous infusion of 2 g/hour. Closely monitor delivery of IV fluid, and avoid exceeding 125 ml/hour to decrease risk for pulmonary edema. Insert a Foley catheter to measure hourly output, proteinuria, and specific gravity. Refer to Critical Care Interventions for Anticonvulsant Therapy.
- *Assess frequently for uterine contractions*; a seizure frequently stimulates labor. During the coma phase, restlessness may indicate uterine contractions.
- *Assess for abruptio placentae*, which occurs in 7% to 10% of eclamptic patients (Sibai, 2005a), by checking for fundal height changes, uterine hyperactivity, vaginal bleeding, or fetal bradycardia.
- *Assess for signs of the HELLP syndrome and DIC.* There is a high frequency of HELLP syndrome (8%) and DIC (7%–11%) in eclamptic patients (Sibai, 2005a).
- *The environment should be kept as quiet as possible* throughout the delivery of care, and bright lights should be avoided to decrease central nervous system stimulation.
- *Assess and treat severe hypertension if present.* Blood pressure is checked according to previously stated protocol as soon as possible to determine

whether a hypertensive agent will be needed. Be prepared to administer an antihypertensive agent, such as hydralazine, if the diastolic blood pressure is higher than 110 mm Hg. Refer to Critical Care Interventions for Antihypertensive Therapy.

- *Assess urine for protein.*
- *Keep hourly input and output measures.*
- *Correct maternal acidemia.* Obtain blood gas levels following a seizure, and administer sodium bicarbonate only if pH is lower than 7.10.
- *Initiate delivery.* Once the mother and fetus have been stabilized, delivery is usually initiated. If labor is not already underway, induction by a labor stimulant is usually attempted if there is no fetal malpresentation or distress and if the fetus is at least 33 weeks of gestation. If the fetus is less than 33 weeks of gestation but the cervix is ripe, labor induction may be attempted. Cesarean birth is the choice of delivery for all others.

Postpartum Considerations

- Remember that approximately 30% of eclampsia cases develop during the postpartum period (Sibai, 2005a).
- Monitor closely for pulmonary edema related to fluid replacement and mobilization of accumulated fluid back into the intravascular spaces.
- Remember that although the risk for recurrence of eclampsia in the next pregnancy is 2%, 22% to 35% do experience some form of preeclampsia; however, most is of the mild form (Sibai, 2005a). According to Witlin (1999), the risk for developing chronic hypertension later in life is 24%. Therefore the postpartum nurse should discuss lifestyle modifications for the prevention of hypertension after pregnancy as presented by the National Institutes of Health (JNC VII, 2003).

Critical Care Interventions for Invasive Hemodynamic Monitoring

- Recommended indications for use of invasive hemodynamic monitoring: Because it is impossible to differentiate clinically among the varying causative factors of severe preeclampsia or eclampsia, invasive hemodynamic monitoring is being recommended for severe preeclampsia or eclampsia complicated with pulmonary edema, oliguria unresponsive to fluid challenge, or severe hypertension unresponsive to hydralazine treatment (ACOG, 2002).
- A pulmonary artery catheter (Swan-Ganz catheter) that continuously evaluates central vein and pulmonary artery pressures and intermittent measurement of central venous pressure and pulmonary capillary wedge pressure should be used for hemodynamic monitoring. This allows precise assessment of the underlying pathophysiology, thus allowing the medical team to specifically tailor and evaluate the therapy.
- Table 21-11 lists manifestations of preeclampsia that should be evaluated with invasive hemodynamic monitoring and treatment protocols.
- *Oliguria,* defined as less than 25 ml of urine over 2 consecutive hours, requires fluid challenge of 500 to 1000 ml of normal saline or Ringer's lactate

Table 21-11   Manifestations of Preeclampsia That Should Be Evaluated with Invasive Hemodynamic Monitoring

Disease Manifestation	Causes	Hemodynamic Values	Possible Treatment
Hypertensive crisis	Increased cardiac output related to increased heart rate and stroke volume Increased systemic vascular resistance	Normal preload High cardiac output Increased PCWP ($\geq$18 mm Hg)	Reduce cardiac preload with beta-blocker agents and vasodilators Reduce systemic vascular resistance Bedrest in left lateral position Antihypertensive therapy such as hydralazine hydrochloride
Pulmonary edema	Noncardiogenic • Decreased colloid osmotic pressure • Increased pulmonary capillary permeability	Normal PCWP (<18 mm Hg) Normal PCWP	Administer colloid fluids Maintain filling pressures in lower-normal range
	Cardiogenic • Volume overload related to left ventricular failure resulting from high vascular resistance	Increased PCWP (>18 mm Hg)	Decrease afterload with bedrest and antihypertensive therapy
	• Volume overload related to iatrogenic fluid overload	Increased CVP	Attempt diuresis with diuretic such as furosemide, O$_2$, morphine
	• Volume overload related to normal postpartum mobilization of third-space fluid (diuresis)	Normal or increased PCWP	

Continued

Table 21-11   Manifestations of Preeclampsia That Should Be Evaluated with Invasive Hemodynamic Monitoring—cont'd

Disease Manifestation	Causes	Hemodynamic Values	Possible Treatment
Oliguria	*Hypovolemic:* Decreased renal blood flow related to intravascular volume depletion	Decreased PCWP Decreased cardiac output Increased SVR	Administer colloid or crystalloid fluid boluses
	Hypervolemic: Decreased renal blood flow related to severe vascular resistance causing left ventricular failure	Increased PCWP (>18 mm Hg) Increased SVR Decreased cardiac output Decreased vascular resistance	Decrease vascular resistance Bedrest in the left lateral position Aggressive afterload reduction and diuresis Antihypertensive drugs such as hydralazine hydrochloride
	Renal arteriospasms: Specific renal arteriospasms disproportionate to systemic vasospasms	Normal PCWP Normal cardiac output Normal SVR	Treat with low-dose dopamine infusion (1–5 mcg 1 kg/min)

CVP, Central venous pressure; *PCWP*, pulmonary capillary wedge pressure; *SVR*, systemic vascular resistance.

over 30 minutes. An unresponsive urine output in a patient not ready to deliver indicates the need for invasive hemodynamic monitoring.

- *Acute pulmonary edema* usually responds to the following treatment plan:
  - Have the patient sit upright.
  - Administer oxygen by facemask at 8 to 10 L to increase arterial oxygen saturation.
  - Reduce anxiety and dilate the pulmonary and systemic veins by administering morphine sulfate at 2 to 5 mg IV every 10 minutes unless near the time of delivery.
  - Improve diuresis with furosemide 40 mg IV.
  - Goal is 1800 to 2000 ml diuresis to improve pulmonary edema.
  - Use invasive hemodynamic monitoring.

Intrapartum Interventions for Preeclampsia

- *Delivery* is indicated in the preeclamptic patient for the following reasons: deterioration of fetal well-being, treatment ineffective in improving the disease as evidenced by worsening maternal symptoms or laboratory evidence of end-organ dysfunction, or eclampsia or warning signs of eclampsia.
- *Vaginal delivery* is usually attempted and achieved after induction with oxytocin.
- *Cesarean birth* is the method of delivery if the following conditions are present: labor does not begin promptly after attempted induction, vaginal delivery is contraindicated for other obstetric reasons, or the fetus weighs less than 1500 g.
- *Continue to assess and implement precise care* that was outlined for the antepartum period.
- *Continuous IV* of 5% D_5 and lactated Ringer's solution at 100 to 150 ml an hour or as assessment indicates is needed.
- *Hourly input and output* is evaluated.
- *Induce labor.* If oxytocin is used, the contractions must be assessed frequently for hypertonus because the uterus may be more sensitive to oxytocin than usual (Cunningham and others, 2005).
- *Monitor labor progress* closely because the patient may not be aware of the strength and frequency of her contractions.
- *Continuous electronic fetal monitoring* is required because the uteroplacental blood flow is already compromised, and the added stress of labor may be too much for the fetus. Magnesium sulfate crosses the placenta readily. It can cause decreased beat-to-beat variability as seen on the fetal monitor strip. However, there is no indication that it adversely affects the fetus as long as the mother's serum magnesium level does not reach toxic levels.
- *Allay anxiety.* The patient is usually very anxious about the well-being of the fetus and her own condition. Most women with preeclampsia or eclampsia are transferred to a high risk center. This can mean that they are a long way from home without any family members available. This adds to the anxiety and stress of the condition. Therefore it is important for nurses who are providing skilled care to attempt to allay anxiety.

- *Analgesia during labor* is limited to small doses and is withheld during the 2 hours before delivery. If the fetus is premature, analgesics should be avoided; they further depress an already compromised fetus. Administering anesthesia to a patient with preeclampsia has added risks. Regional anesthesia such as intrathecal or epidural block is the preferred method except in the presence of coagulopathy. Because of the hemorrhagic risk, regional anesthesia should not be used in the presence of coagulopathy (ACOG, 2002). A general anesthesia may further elevate the blood pressure, especially during induction and awakening.

Postpartum Interventions for Preeclampsia
Nursing Interventions

If the patient has been receiving magnesium sulfate or another anticonvulsant, it is usually continued for 24 to 48 hours following delivery or longer if the HELLP syndrome coexisted (Friedman and others, 2001). During this time, the patient's condition is monitored as closely as before; her condition can still deteriorate. This risk may be enhanced by normal postpartum diuresis. As diuresis takes place, an increased loss of magnesium leads to a drop in serum magnesium below therapeutic levels, and a convulsion could result. Blood loss is not tolerated as well as in the healthy postpartum patient because of the reduced blood volume caused by the disease process. Therefore the nurse should monitor the blood loss closely. If the HELLP syndrome coexists, platelets, AST, ALT, and LDH levels are appropriate indicators of severity and progress toward recovery. There is a direct correlation between severity of the disease and the length of time for recovery.

Psychologic needs are great during the postpartum period. If the mother was not fully alert for all or part of the labor and delivery, it is important to fill in the gaps of the event for her. Most parents are also very concerned about their neonate's well-being. If the neonate was born prematurely or has IUGR and is in the intensive care nursery (ICN), the mother should be shown pictures of the infant and kept informed about the infant's condition. The father should be encouraged to visit the ICN. Then, when the mother's condition becomes stable, arrangements should be made for her to visit the ICN. Even if the neonate is healthy, the mother will need extra support because she will be separated from her infant for a large portion of the first day or two following delivery. The mother needs limited neuromuscular stimulation and therefore is kept in a dark, quiet environment with limited visitors.

The parents might be concerned about the effects of magnesium on their neonate. It is a relatively safe drug in relationship to the disease process (Weiner and Buhimschi, 2004). The neonate may appear hypotonic at first. The parents should be informed that this is a temporary condition and it does not indicate neurologic damage. The mother may also be concerned about breastfeeding and the effects of magnesium. She should be reassured that no negative effect has been implicated and that the levels of magnesium in breast milk are usually less than even in some formulas (Weiner and Buhimschi, 2004).

On the other hand, the patient who has chronic hypertension and must continue on hypertensive therapy should understand that antihypertensives are excreted in breast milk. The effect on the infant is unknown. If the patient has mild hypertension, the health care provider may withhold the medication during breastfeeding and closely observe the patient's blood pressure. For the patient with severe hypertension, the same antihypertensive drugs that are recommended during pregnancy seem to be the safest during breastfeeding, as long as they are taken at the lowest dose possible for hypertensive management (National High Blood Pressure Education Program Working Group, 2000).

Long-term effects are listed under the respective nursing intervention sections. However, the increased risk for preeclampsia and hypertension and cardiovascular disease later in life direct the nurse to encourage lifestyle modifications for the prevention of hypertension as outlined by the National Institutes of Health (Irgens and others, 2001; JNC VII, 2003; Kestenbaum and others, 2003; Freeman and others, 2004; Van Pampus and Aarnoudse, 2005).

All types of contraception are available to hypertensive women, provided that compliance and close follow-up can be guaranteed, according to Repke (2001). However, the risks of oral contraceptives must be discussed completely if that method is considered. Estrogen has a negative effect on various clotting factors, total cholesterol, triglycerides, and angiotensinogen. Progesterone has a negative effect on high-density lipoprotein, low-density lipoprotein, and insulin resistance. In contrast, the benefits of these methods should also be presented.

CONCLUSION

The ultimate goal of the nurse is to prevent hypertensive disorders of pregnancy or to assist in early diagnosis and appropriate treatment of these disorders to maximize outcome. Preeclampsia is a much studied disease of pregnancy, but the triggering factor remains unknown. This makes prevention difficult; however, because research indicates that several factors, such as early appropriate prenatal care, adequate fluid intake, and optimal nutrition, play important roles, the nurse should include these in the prenatal instructions. When a patient develops preeclampsia during pregnancy, the goal becomes the prevention of eclampsia and uteroplacental insufficiency while attempting to facilitate fetal maturity. Therefore, preeclampsia is treated in hopes of stabilizing the condition until fetal maturity is reached. If treatment is effective, diuresis should occur within 18 to 36 hours. Positive signs of stabilization are increased output and a decrease in weight, blood pressure, edema, and proteinuria. If preeclampsia does not respond to treatment, delivery is the treatment of choice to prevent eclampsia and uteroplacental insufficiency.

Other hypertensive disorders of pregnancy are treated to keep the diastolic blood pressure below 100 mm Hg to prevent maternal cardiovascular complications and uterine insufficiency.

BIBLIOGRAPHY

Aagaard-Tillery K, Belfort M: Eclampsia: morbidity, mortality, and management, *Clin Obstet Gynecol* 48(1):12–23, 2005.

Abalos E and others: Antihypertensive drug therapy for mild to moderate hypertension during pregnancy, *Cochrane Database Syst Rev* Issue 2, 2001.

Al-Mulhim A and others: Pre-eclampsia: maternal risk factors and perinatal outcome, *Fetal Diagn Ther* 18(4):275–280, 2003.

American College of Obstetricians Gynecologists: Antepartum fetal surveillance, *ACOG Technical Bulletin,* No. 9, Washington DC, 1999, ACOG.

American College of Obstetricians Gynecologists: Chronic hypertension in pregnancy, *ACOG Practice Bulletin,* No. 29, Washington DC, 2001, ACOG.

American College of Obstetricians Gynecologists: Diagnosis and management of preeclampsia and eclampsia, *ACOG Practice Bulletin,* No. 33, Washington DC, 2002, ACOG.

Anumba D, Robson S: Management of pre-eclampsia and haemolysis, elevated liver enzymes, and low platelets syndrome, *Curr Opin Obstet Gynecol* 11(2):149–156, 1999.

Atallah A, Hofmeyr G, and Duley L: Calcium supplementation during pregnancy for preventing hypertensive disorders and related problems, *Cochrane Database Syst Rev* Issue 1, 2002.

Barton J, Sibai B: HELLP syndrome. In Sibai B: *Hypertensive disorders in women,* Philadelphia, 2001, Saunders.

Barton J and others: Does advanced maternal age affect pregnancy outcomes in women with mild hypertension remote from term? *Am J Obstet Gynecol* 176(6):1236–1240, 1997.

Barton J and others: Monitored outpatient management of mild gestational hypertension remote from term in teenage pregnancies, *Am J Obstet Gynecol* 173(6):1865–1868, 1995.

Barton J, Stanziano G, and Sibai B: Monitored outpatient management of mild gestational hypertension remote from term, *Am J Obstet Gynecol* 17(3):765–769, 1994.

Baylis C and others: Recent insights into the roles of nitric oxide and renin-angiotensin in the pathophysiology of preeclamptic pregnancy, *Semin Nephrol* 18(2):208–230, 1998.

Boggess K and others: Maternal periodontal disease is associated with an increased risk for preeclampsia, *Obstet Gynecol* 101(2):227–231, 2003.

Branch D, Dudley D, and Michell M: Preliminary evidence for homeostatic mechanism regulating endothelin production in preeclampsia, *Lancet* 337(8747):943–945, 1991.

Branch D and others: Outcome of treated pregnancies in women with antiphospholipid syndrome: an update of the Utah experience, *Obstet Gynecol* 80(4):614–620, 1992.

Brown M and others: Randomised trial of management of hypertensive pregnancies by Korotkoff phase IV or phase V, *Lancet* 352(9130):777–781, 1998.

Cox S, Kilpatrick S, and Geller S: Preventing maternal deaths, *Contemporary OB/GYN* Sept 1, 2004.

Chappell L and others: Effect of antioxidants on the occurrence of pre-eclampsia in women at increased risk: a randomised trial, *Lancet* 354(9181):810–816, 1999.

Chesley L, Cooper D: Genetics of hypertension in pregnancy: possible single gene control of pre-eclampsia and eclampsia in the descendants of eclamptic women, *Br J Obstet Gynaecol* 93(9):898–908, 1986.

Churchill D, Duley L: Intraventionist versus expectant care for severe pre-eclampsia before term, *Cochrane Database Syst Rev* Issue 3, 2002.

Clark B and others: Plasma endothelin levels in preeclampsia: elevation and correlation with uric acid levels and renal impairment, *Am J Obstet Gynecol* 166(3):962–968, 1992.

CLASP Collaborative Group: Low dose aspirin in pregnancy and early childhood development: follow up of collaborative low dose aspirin study in pregnancy, *Br J Obstet Gynaecol* 102(11):861–868, 1995.

Conde-Agudelo A, Villar J, and Lindheimer M: World Health Organization systematic review of screening tests for preeclampsia, *Obstet Gynecol* 104(6):1367–1391, 2004.

Cotter A and others: Elevated plasma homocysteine in early pregnancy: A risk factor for the development of nonsevere preeclampsia, *Am J Obstet Gynecol* 189(2):391–394, 2003.

Crowther C, Bouwmeester A, and Ashurst H: Does admission to hospital for bedrest prevent disease progression or improve fetal outcome in pregnancy complicated by nonproteinuric hypertension? *Br J Obstet Gynaecol* 99(1):13–17, 1992.

Cunningham F and others: *Williams' obstetrics,* ed 22, New York, 2005, McGraw-Hill.

Davey D, MacGillivray I: The classification and definition of the hypertensive disorders of pregnancy, *Am J Obstet Gynecol* 158(4):892–898, 1988.

Dekker G: Prevention of preeclampsia. In Sibai B: *Hypertensive disorders in women*, Philadelphia, 2001, Saunders.

Dekker G, Sibai B: The immunology of preeclampsia, *Semin Perinatol* 23(1):24–33, 1999.

DiPasquale L, Lynett K: The use of water immersion for treatment of massive labial edema during pregnancy, *MCN Am J Matern Child Nurs* 28(4):242–245, 2003.

Duley L and others: Antiplatelet agents for preventing pre-eclampsia and its complications, *Cochrane Database Syst Rev* Issue 4, 2003.

Duley L, Henderson-Smart D: Drugs for treatment of very high blood pressure during pregnancy, *Cochrane Database Syst Rev* Issue 4, 2002.

Duley L, Henderson-Smart D, and Meher S: Altered dietary salt for preventing pre-eclampsia, and its complications, *Cochrane Database Syst Rev* Issue 4, 2005.

Duley L, Gulmezoglu A, and Henderson-Smart D: Magnesium sulfate and other anticonvulsants for women with pre-eclampsia, *Cochrane Database Syst Rev* Issue 2, 2003.

Duley L, Henderson-Smart D: Magnesium sulphate versus diazepam for eclampsia, *Cochrane Database Syst Rev* Issue 3, 2003a.

Duley L, Henderson-Smart D: Magnesium sulphate versus phenytoin for eclampsia, *Cochrane Database Syst Rev* Issue 3, 2003b.

Eclampsia Trial Collaborative Group: Which anticonvulsant for women with eclampsia? Evidence from the collaborative eclampsia trial, *Lancet* 345(8963):1455–1463, 1995.

Egerman R, Sibai B: Preconception counseling for women with a history of hypertensive disorders. In Sibai B: *Hypertensive disorders in women*, Philadelphia, 2001, Saunders.

Foley M: *Hypertensive emergencies during pregnancy: a general overview.* Presented at Obstetrical Challenges of the New Millennium, Phoenix, Ariz, April 7, 2001.

Flack J and others: Hypertension in special populations, *Cardiol Clin* 20(2):303–319, 2002.

Freeman D and others: Short- and long- term changes in plasma inflammatory markers associated with preeclampsia, *Hypertension* 44(5):708–714, 2004.

Friedman S and others: Mild gestational hypertension and preeclampsia. In Sibai B: *Hypertensive disorders in women*, Philadelphia, 2001, Saunders.

Ghabour M and others: Immunohistochemical characterization of placental nitric oxide synthase expression in preeclampsia, *Am J Obstet Gynecol* 173(3 Pt 1):687–694, 1995.

Green L, Froman R: Blood pressure measurement during pregnancy: auscultatory versus oscillatory methods, *J Obstet Gynecol Neonatal Nurs* 25(2):155–159, 1996.

Gregg A: Hypertension in pregnancy, *Obstet Gynecol Clin North Am* 31(2):223–241, 2004.

Gudnasson H, Dubiel M, and Gudmundsson S: Preeclampsia: Abnormal uterine artery Doppler is related to recurrence of symptoms during the next pregnancy, *J Perinat Med* 32(5):400–403, 2004.

Gunderson E: Nutrition during pregnancy for the physically active woman, *Clin Obstet Gynecol* 46(2):390–402, 2003.

Haddad B, Sibai S: Expectant management of severe preeclampsia: proper candidates and pregnancy outcome, *Clin Obstet Gynecol* 48(2):430–440, 2005.

Hayman R: Hypertension in pregnancy, *Curr Obstet Gynecol* 14(1):1–10, 2004.

International Food Information Council Foundation (IFIC): Healthy eating during pregnancy, Washington, DC, 2003, Author. Retrieved *http://www.ific.org/publications/brochures/pregnancy-broch.cfm*

Irgens H and others: Long term mortality of mothers and fathers after pre-eclampsia: Population based cohort study, *BMJ* 323(7323):1213–1217, 2001.

Joint National Committee (JNC) VII: *Prevention, detection, evaluation, treatment of high blood pressure,* NIH Publication No. 03-5233, Bethesda, Maryland, 2003, U.S. Dept of Health and Human Services. Retrieved from *http://www.nhlbi.nih.gov/guidelines/hypertension/jncintro.htm*

Katz V and others: A comparison of bed rest and immersion for treating the edema of pregnancy, *Obstet Gynecol* 75(2):147–151, 1990.

Katz V and others: Effect of daily immersion on the edema of pregnancy, *Am J Perinatol* 9(4):225–227, 1992.

Kent T and others: Edema of pregnancy: a comparison of water aerobics and static immersion, *Obstet Gynecol* 94(5 Pt 1):726–729, 1999.

Kestenbaum B and others: Cardiovascular and thromboembolic events following hypertensive pregnancy, *Am J Kidney Dis* 42(5):982–989, 2003.

Levine R, Karumanchi S: Circulating angiogenic factors in preeclampsia, *Clin Obstet Gynecol* 48(2):372–386, 2005.

Levine R and others: Two-stage elevation of cell-free fetal DNA in maternal sera before onset of preeclampsia, *Am J Obstet Gynecol* 190(3):707–713, 2004.

Levine R and others: Urinary placental growth factor and risk of preeclampsia, *JAMA* 293(1):77–85, 2005.

Lowenstein C, Dinerman J, and Snyder S: Nitric oxide: a physiologic messenger, *Ann Intern Med* 120(3):227–237, 1994.

Lucas L, Jordan E: Phenytoin as an alternative treatment for preeclampsia, *J Obstet Gynecol Neonatal Nurs* 26(3):263–269, 1997.

Mabie W: Life-threatening complications of hypertension in pregnancy. In Sibai B: *Hypertensive disorders in women*, Philadelphia, 2001, Saunders.

MacKay A, Berg C, and Atrash H: Pregnancy-related mortality from preeclampsia and eclampsia, *Obstet Gynecol* 9(4):533–538, 2001.

Madomed K: Zinc supplementation in pregnancy, *Cochrane Database Syst Rev* Issue 3, 1997.

Magee L, Duley L: Oral beta-blockers for mild to moderate hypertension during pregnancy, *Cochrane Database Syst Rev* Issue 3, 2003.

Magee I, Sadeghi S: Prevention and treatment of postpartum hypertension, *Cochrane Database Syst Rev* Issue 1, 2005.

Makrides M, Crowther C: Magnesium supplementation in pregnancy, *Cochrane Database Syst Rev* Issue 2, 2001.

Manten G and others: The role of lipoprotein (a) in pregnancies complicated by pre-eclampsia, *Med Hypotheses* 64(1):162–169, 2005.

Martin J and others: The natural history of HELLP syndrome: patterns of disease progression and regression, *Am J Obstet Gynecol* 164(6 Pt 1):1500–1509, 1991.

Matthys L and others: Delayed postpartum preeclampsia: An experience of 151 cases, *Am J Obstet Gynecol* 190(5):1464–1466, 2004.

Meher S, Abalos E, and Carroli G: Bed rest with or without hospitalization for hypertension during pregnancy, *Cochrane Database Syst Rev* Issue 4, 2005.

Mignini L and others: Mapping the theories of preeclampsia: the role of homocysteine, *Obstet Gynecol* 105(2):411–425, 2005.

Mills J and others: Prostacyclin and thromboxane changes predating clinical onset of preeclampsia: a multicenter prospective study, *JAMA* 282(4):356–362, 1999.

Myatt L, Miodovnik M: Prediction of preeclampsia, *Semin Perinatol* 23(1):45–57, 1999.

National High Blood Pressure Education Program Working Group: Report on high blood pressure in pregnancy, *Am J Obstet Gynecol* 183(1):S1–S22, 2000.

National Institutes of Health (NIH): Antenatal corticosteroids revisited. Consensus development conference statement, Maryland, 2000, NIH. Retrieved from *http://consensus.nih.gov*

Newman V, Fullerton J: Role of nutrition in the prevention of preeclampsia: review of the literature, *J Nurse Midwifery* 35(5):282–291, 1990.

Nick J: Deep tendon reflexes, magnesium, and calcium: assessments and implications, *J Obstet Gynecol Neonatal Nurs* 33(2):221–230, 2004.

Nick J: Deep tendon reflexes: The what, why, where, and how of tapping, *J Obstet Gynecol Neonatal Nurs* 32(3):297–306, 2003.

Nova A and others: Maternal plasma level of endothelin is increased in preeclampsia, *Am J Obstet Gynecol* 165(3):724–727, 1991.

O'Brien J, Barton J: Controversies with the diagnosis and management of HELLP syndrome, *Clin Obstet Gynecol* 48(2):460–477, 2005.

O'Brien J, Milligan D, and Barton J: Impact of high-dose corticosteroid therapy for patients with HELLP (hemolysis, elevated liver enzymes, and low platelet count) syndrome, *Am J Obstet Gynecol* 183(4):921–924, 2000.

Odendaal H: Severe preeclampsia eclampsia. In Sibai B: *Hypertensive disorders in women*, Philadelphia, 2001, Saunders.

Paruk F, Moodley J: Antihypertensive therapy for the management of mild-to moderate hypertension? In Studd J, editor: *Progress in obstetrics and gynaecology*, Edinburgh, 2005, Churchill Livingstone.

Patrick T, Roberts J: Current concepts in preeclampsia, *MCN Am J Matern Child Nurs* 24(4):193–200, 1999.

Peters R, Flack J: Hypertensive disorders of pregnancy, *J Obstet Gynecol Neonatal Nurs* 33(2):209–220, 2004.

Phelan J, Easter T: HELLP syndrome: the great masquerader, *Female Patient* 15(2):79, 1990.

Reif M: Managing hypertension during pregnancy, *Womens Health Primary Care* 6(4):194, 2003.

Repke J: Contraception on the woman with hypertension. In Sibai B: *Hypertensive disorders in women*, Philadelphia, 2001, Saunders.

Roberts J: Endothelial dysfunction in preeclampsia, *Semin Reprod Endocrinol* 16(1):5–15, 1998.

Roberts J: Pregnancy-related hypertension. In Creasy R, Resnik R, and Iams J editors: *Maternal-fetal medicine: principles and practice*, ed 5, Philadelphia, 2004, Saunders.

Roberts J and others: Summary of the NHLBI Working Group on research on hypertension during pregnancy, *Hypertension* 41(3):437–445, 2003.

Roberts J, Hubel C: Is oxidative stress the link in the two-stage model of pre-eclampsia? *Lancet* 354(9181):788–789, 1999.

Sandruck J, Grobman W, and Gerber S: The effect of short-term indomethacin therapy on amniotic fluid volume, *Am J Obstet Gynecol* 192(5):1443–1445, 2005.

Scholl T and others: Oxidative stress, diet, and the etiology of preeclampsia, *Am J Clin Nutr* 81(6):1390–1396, 2005.

Sibai B: Diagnosis prevention, management of eclampsia, *Obstet Gynecol* 105(2):402–410, 2005a.

Sibai B: Magnesium sulfate prophylaxis in preeclampsia: Evidence from randomized trials, *Clin Obstet Gynecol* 48(2):478–488, 2005b.

Sibai B: Hypertension. In Gabbe S, Niebyl J, and Simpson J editors: *Obstetrics: Normal and problem pregnancies*, New York, 2002, Churchill Livingstone.

Sibai B, Mabie W: Hemodynamics of preeclampsia, *Clin Perinatol* 18(4):727–747, 1991.

Sibai B and others: Maternal morbidity and mortality in 442 pregnancies with hemolysis, elevated liver enzymes, and low platelets (HELLP syndrome), *Am J Obstet Gynecol* 169(4):1000–1006, 1993.

Simpson K, Knox G: Obstetrical accidents involving intravenous magnesium sulfate: recommendations to promote patient safety, *MCN Am J Matern Child Nurs* 29(3):161–169, 2004.

Spinnato J, Livingston J: Prevention of preeclampsia with antioxidants: evidence from randomized trials, *Clin Obstet Gynecol* 48(2):416–429, 2005.

Strong T: Reversal of oligohydramnios with subtotal immersion: a report of five cases, *Am J Obstet Gynecol* 169(6):1595–1597, 1993.

Taylor R: Review: immunobiology of preeclampsia, *Am J Reprod Immunol* 37(1):79–86, 1997.

Tuffnell D and others: Randomised controlled trial of day care for hypertension in pregnancy, *Lancet* 339(8787):224–227, 1992.

U.S. Department of Health and Human Services: *Healthy People 2010: understanding and improving health*. Washington, DC, 2000, USDHHS.

van Beck E, Peeters L: Pathogenesis of preeclampsia: a comprehensive model, *Obstet Gynecol Surv* 53(4):233–239, 1998.

Van Pampus M, Aarnoudse J: Long-term outcomes after preeclampsia, *Clin Obstet Gynecol* 48(2):489–494, 2005.

Vedernikov Y, Saade G, and Garfield R: Vascular reactivity in preeclampsia, *Semin Perinatol* 23(1):34–44, 1999.

Var A and others: Endothelial dysfunction in preeclampsia: increased homocysteine and decreased nitric oxide levels, *Gynecol Obstet Invest* 56(4):221–224, 2003.

von Dadelszen P, Magee L: Antihypertensive medications in management of gestational hypertension-preeclampsia, *Clin Obstet Gynecol* 48(2):441–459, 2005.

Walfisch A, Hallak M: Hypertension. In James D and others, editors: *High risk pregnancy: management options*, ed 3, Philadelphia, 2006, Saunders.

Walker J: Hypertensive drugs in pregnancy. In Sibai B: *Hypertensive disorders in women*, Philadelphia, 2001, Saunders.

Walsh S: Physiology of low dose aspirin therapy for the prevention of preeclampsia, *Semin Perinatol* 14(2):152–170, 1990.

Wang Y and others: Evidence of endothelial dysfunction in preeclampsia: decreased endothelial nitric oxide synthase expression is associated with increased cell permeability in endothelial cells from preeclampsia, *Am J Obstet Gynecol* 190(3):817–824, 2004.

Wang Y and others: Maternal levels of prostacyclin, thromboxane, vitamin E, and lipid peroxides throughout normal pregnancy, *Am J Obstet Gynecol* 165(6 Pt 1):1690–1694, 1991a.

Wang Y and others: The imbalance between thromboxane and prostacyclin in preeclampsia is associated with an imbalance between lipid peroxides and vitamin E in maternal blood, *Am J Obstet Gynecol* 165(6 Pt 1):1695–1700, 1991b.

Wardlaw G, Smith A: *Contemporary nutrition,* ed 6, Boston, 2006, McGraw-Hill.

Weinstein L: Preeclampsia/eclampsia with hemolysis, elevated liver enzymes, and thrombocytopenia, *Obstet Gynecol* 66(5):657–660, 1985.

Weiner C, Buhimschi C: *Drugs for pregnant and lactating women,* Philadelphia, 2004, Churchill Livingstone.

Williamson C: Molecular biology related to pre-eclampsia, *Institute Reprod Dev Biol* 1279:282, 2005.

Williamson C, Girling J: Hepatic gastrointestinal disease. In James D and others, editors: *High risk pregnancy: management options,* ed 3, Philadelphia, 2006, Saunders.

Witlin A: Counseling for women with preeclampsia and eclampsia, *Semin Perinatol* 23(1):91–98, 1999.

Witlin A, Sibai B: Epidemiology classification of hypertension in women. In Sibai B: *Hypertensive disorders in women,* Philadelphia, 2001, Saunders.

Young G, Jewell D: Interventions for varicosities leg edema in pregnancy (Cochrane Review). In *The Cochrane Library,* Issue 3, Oxford, 2001, Update Software.

Zhou Y, Damsky C, and Fisher S: Preeclampsia is associated with failure of human cytotrophoblasts to mimic avascular adhesion phenotype: one cause of defective endovascular invasion in this syndrome? *J Clin Invest* 99(9):2152–2164, 1997.

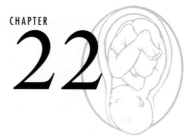

22

Preterm Labor and Multiple Gestation

PRETERM LABOR

Preterm labor (PTL) can be defined as regular uterine contractions that cause progressive dilation of the cervix after 20 weeks of gestation and before 36 completed weeks.

MULTIPLE GESTATION

A multiple gestation can result from fertilization of one egg by one sperm that splits, which is called *monozygotic multiple fetus*. Multiple gestations can also result from fertilization of two or more eggs called *dizygotic*. Or multiple gestations can result from a combination of these two processes.

Because of the increased likelihood for infertile couples who become pregnant with any fertility method to have twins or more, we now see many more successful pregnancy outcomes. However, with this success comes an increased incidence of preterm births of the multiples. Currently, some perinatal programs are reporting equally successful outcomes with quadruplet and triplet births as with twin births (Elliott, 2000). Although quadruplets and triplets are more likely to deliver by 32 to 34 weeks than are twins, ultimately their outcome successes rival twins (Elliott, 2000). Multiple gestations with more than four fetuses have an extremely high loss rate of all fetuses and probably fall more in the "miraculous" survival rather than a statistical prediction model (Elliott, 2000).

PTL with multiple gestation is more difficult for the pregnant woman to identify. It can be confused with the extra aches and pains from rapid stretching and pressure, and it can be confused with kicks and movements of multiple babies. In addition, the overdistention of the uterus contributes to increased irritability of the uterus.

INCIDENCE

Approximately 12% of all pregnancies end in PTL. The rate is increasing despite innovative perinatal technology. Prematurity in the newborn continues to account for 75% to 80% of neonatal morbidity and mortality (Iams, 2003).

491

The rate of multiple gestations is rapidly rising (19% increase), secondary to new technologies in infertility treatment. Twins have a 50% preterm birth rate, and triplets and higher-order multiples have a 90% preterm birth rate (Russell and others, 2002). In addition, there are significant racial differences in preterm birth rates: whites, 9.9%; blacks, 17.6%; Native Americans, 12.2%; Hispanics, 11.2%; and Asians, 7.4% (NCHS, 2000). Sociodemographics affect preterm birth as well, with rates of preterm birth being highest among the socially disadvantaged (Freda and Patterson, 2001).

ETIOLOGY

The cause of PTL cannot be identified in 50% of patients who experience it (Moos, 2004). It is currently thought to be a chronic, long-term, multifactorial process (Iams and Creasy, 2004). The primary cause for multiparas is a history of previous preterm delivery (McParland, Jones, and Taylor, 2004). Factors frequently related to PTL can be classified as altered lifestyle practices, stress, altered uterine factors, and infections. Another factor that predisposes a woman to PTL is a disadvantaged socioeconomic status. The deterrent factor is unknown, but altered nutrition and bacterial or viral flora of the reproductive tract caused by inadequate hygiene, lack of education, higher incidence of teenage pregnancies, higher frequency of grand multiparity, and psychologic and physical stress have all been suggested.

Modifiable risk factors include the following:

- Tobacco, alcohol, and illegal substance use (e.g., cocaine) (ICSI, 2004)
- Low prepregnancy weight or low weight gain (USDHHS, 2000)
- Vaginal infections especially bacterial vaginosis, gonorrhea, chlamydia, and trichomonas vaginalis
- Asymptomatic group B streptococcal bacteriuria
- Domestic violence (USDHHS, 2000; ICSI, 2004)
- Periodontal disease (Wener and Lavigne, 2004)
- Maternal stress (Hobel, 2004)
- Long working hours or strenuous work (Hobel, 2004)

Nonmodifiable factors that may contribute to the risk for PTL include the following (Pschirrer and Monga, 2000):

- Socially disadvantaged status
- Less than high school education
- Extremes of maternal age
- Multiple gestation
- African-American descent
- Pregnancy complication such as preeclampsia, hyperthyroidism, anemia, hepatitis, cholestasis, heart disease

Box 22-1 provides a summary of predisposing factors of PTL.

NORMAL ANATOMY OF THE CERVIX

Normal cervical lengths, according to gestation, are as follows:

- 14–22 weeks of gestation: 35 to 40 mm cervical length

| **Box 22-1** | Predisposing Factors of Preterm Labor |

Behavior and Environmental Risk Factors
- Unhealthy lifestyle practices such as use of tobacco, alcohol, or illicit drugs, especially cocaine
- Altered nutrition that leads to low maternal weight gain
- High stress, physical and emotional
- Domestic violence
- Long, tiring commutes
- Physically demanding work, prolonged standing, night work

Demographic Risk Factors
- Asian or non-white race, especially black race
- Extreme maternal age
- Low socioeconomic status
- Unmarried

Medical Risk Factors
- Autoimmune problems
- Hereditary thromboembolic disorders
- Diabetes
- Renal disease
- Cardiovascular disease
- Hypertension
- Anemia
- Infections such as sexually transmitted infections especially bacterial vaginosis, trichomosis, gonorrhea, and chlamydia
- **Reproductive Risk Factors**
- History of preterm labor—single most important factor
- Preterm rupture of membranes—a significant factor in one third of these patients (NICH, 2001)
- Multiple gestation
- No or inadequate prenatal care
- Cervical abnormality such as surgery, cone biopsy, loop electrical excision procedure (LEEP), diethylstilbestrol (DES) exposure, incompetent cervix
- In vitro fertilization
- Polydramnios
- Uterine anomalies
- Abruptio placenta or placenta previa
- Trauma, motor vehicle accident

Modified from Maloni J: Preventing preterm birth: evidence-based interventions shift toward prevention, *AWHONN Lifelines* 4(4):26–33, 2000; Institute for Clinical Systems Improvement (ICSI): *Preterm birth prevention*, Bloomington (MN), 2004, Institute for Clinical Systems Improvement.

- 24–28 weeks of gestation: 35 mm cervical length
- 32 weeks or more of gestation: 30 mm cervical length

NORMAL PHYSIOLOGY OF LABOR CONTRACTIONS

Muscle contraction and relaxation occur in response to the movement of the thick (myosin) and the thin (actin) filaments. The flow of calcium regulates the movement of the filaments. Multiple mechanisms regulate the flow of calcium affecting the balance between muscle relaxation and contraction. Hormones are one importance regulator of myometrial contraction.

To have a physiologic understanding of possible causes and current medical treatments for preterm labor, one must understand the physiology of labor contractions. A fetal signal (surfactant protein A [SP-A]) from the maturing lungs probably initiates normal labor (Condon and others, 2004). Following initiation, there is strong scientific evidence that various hormones interplay to influence uterine activity.

PROSTAGLANDINS

The fetal adrenal glands' production of dehydroepiandrosterone (DHEA), related to certain fetal maturational milestones, may interrupt the support of systems that serve to promote uterine quiescence and maintain pregnancy (Lockwood, 1999). This unknown fetal signal appears to stimulate macrophage-like decidua, the endometrium of pregnancy, to release interleukin-1-beta (IL-1β). IL-1β, an immune hormone, causes hydrolysis of glycerophospholipids found in the decidua, fetal membranes, and myometrium. Esterified arachidonic acid, which is stored in the glycerophospholipids, is released to free arachidonic acid (Challis and Lye, 2004). The release of arachidonic acid is accomplished either directly by phospholipase A2 or indirectly by phospholipase C. Both of these agents hydrolyze the membrane to release arachidonic acid.

Free arachidonic acid is then converted into prostaglandins (PGs) and thus stimulates the platelet-activating factor. Each tissue synthesizes a type of PG. For example, the decidua produces primarily PGF2α and a small amount of PGE2. The amniotic and chorionic fetal membranes produce PGE2, and the myometrium produces prostacyclin (PGI2) and a small amount of PGF2α.

During labor, prostaglandins PGF2α and PGE2 and platelet-activating factor accumulate in the amniotic fluid. Along with arachidonic acid and IL-1β, PGF2α, PGE2, and platelet-activating factor remain active for 4 to 6 hours.

Thromboxane, PGF2α, and PGE2 prepare the myometrial muscle for labor by promoting the development of gap junctions, which are cell-to-cell contact areas, and coordinate smooth muscle contractions. These three substances stimulate myometrial contractions by facilitating the movement of calcium into the smooth muscle so that the muscle can contract and promote cervical ripening.

During pregnancy, PGI2 quiets the uterus by inhibiting the function of gap junctions, by inhibiting release of phospholipases A2 and C, and by blocking movement of calcium into cells. Production of PGI2 is suppressed during labor secondary to high levels of maternal and fetal cortisol (Lockwood, 2000).

Estrogen

Estrogen is produced by the corpus luteum for the first 2 to 4 weeks of gestation. Then the placenta takes over the production. Low-density lipoprotein (LDL) cholesterol is used by the fetal and maternal adrenal glands to secrete a precursor for placental estrogen. Near term, the adrenal gland, the largest fetal organ, is the primary source for placental estrogen precursor.

Estriol, one form of placental estrogen, stimulates the fetal membranes and decidua to deposit glycerophospholipids.

Estrogen influences the increased number of cells and size of the myometrium, stimulates Braxton-Hicks contractions, facilitates the development of gap junctions (Castracane, 2000), and promotes oxytocin receptors. It is for this reason that oxytocin is an ineffective stimulator of myometrial contractions until late in pregnancy when estrogen levels are high. Estrogen also stimulates prostaglandin biosynthesis and inhibits progesterone synthesis in fetal membranes, thus effecting a local change in the progesterone-estrogen ratio in amniotic fluid at term.

Progesterone

Progesterone is produced by the corpus luteum for the first 4 to 6 weeks of gestation. Then it is produced by the fetal syncytiotrophoblasts at an increasing rate until 32 to 34 weeks of gestation by converting maternal plasma LDL cholesterol into progesterone. Then progesterone is maintained at a constant level, approximately 250 mg/day, until birth. Progesterone withdrawal does not cause the initiation of true labor but may stimulate the synthesis of the precursor for IL-1β. At the same time, progesterone prevents the release of IL-1β and of phospholipase A2 and blocks the effect of estrogen on the induction of oxytocin receptors. Therefore progesterone appears to influence preparation for labor while maintaining quiescence of the myometrial muscle.

Oxytocin

It was once thought that oxytocin initiated normal labor, but it is now known to maximize uterine contraction of second-stage labor and, after delivery, to stimulate decidual prostaglandin release. Oxytocin is ineffective at stimulating uterine contractions during early pregnancy because high estrogen levels are necessary first for the formation of oxytocin receptors in the uterus. Oxytocin is also ineffective at promoting gap junctions and cervical ripening.

NORMAL PHYSIOLOGIC ADAPTATION OF MULTIPLE GESTATION

In a multiple gestation, cardiac output is increased 20% to 40% greater than in a singleton pregnancy. Renal plasma flow increases and the systemic vascular resistance decreases more than in a singleton pregnancy. Placentation may differ as well. In monozygotic multiples, the fetal membranes may surround one or more fetuses and their placentas may be separate or fused. When splitting of the zygotic occurs, dichorionic diamniotic placentation results. When the splitting occurs during the morula phase, the placentation is usually monochorionic and diamniotic. If the splitting occurs after the eighth day, the placentation is monochorionic and monoamniotic.

PATHOPHYSIOLOGY

PTL is usually caused by a breakdown in the mechanism that maintains uterine quiescence (Norwitz and others, 1999).

Infection

Inflammatory cytokines or bacterial endotoxins can stimulate prostaglandin release directly or indirectly by stimulating the release of corticotropin-releasing hormone (CRH) or IL. In this manner, a urinary tract, vaginal, uterine, or fetal infection may stimulate PTL. Infection may be predictive as a marker in preterm birth at least 50% of the time (Lockwood, 2000).

Altered Uterine Factors

Uterine factors such as myometrial stretch, hyperosmolarity, rupture of fetal membrane, or uterine trauma cause lysosomes to release phospholipase A2. Prostaglandins are then produced, stimulating the myometrium to contract. In this way, premature rupture of membranes (PROM), abdominal trauma, multiple gestations, uterine anomalies causing overdistention of the uterus, and polyhydramnios can stimulate PTL.

Stress

Emotional stress increases the release of epinephrine, and physical stress increases the release of norepinephrine. Epinephrine and norepinephrine increase the release of catecholamines, leading to uterine irritability and decreased placental function. They can also can stimulate the release of corticotropin-releasing hormone (CRH), which stimulates the fetal adrenal to produce early the signal to interrupt the support of systems serving to promote uterine quiescence, thus resulting in PTL (Lockwood, 1999; Majzoub and others, 1999; Hobel, 2004).

Factors that decrease blood flow to the uterus may also cause the release of CRH. Therefore conditions during pregnancy that interfere with uterine or placental blood flow can trigger PTL. Some of these conditions are preeclampsia, poorly controlled diabetes, heart disease, renal disease, abruptio placentae, or placenta previa. Altered nutrition, smoking, or illicit drug use may stimulate PTL in this manner as well.

Table 22-1 summarizes the interrelationships among the different endocrine factors that contribute to the control of labor or the development of PTL. Fig. 22-1 shows the pathophysiologic effects of the causative factors of PTL.

MATERNAL EFFECTS

Preterm Labor

The most common direct effect on the mother is psychologic stress from the threat of a preterm delivery on the health and well-being of the expected baby. Other maternal consequences are related to the side effects of the medical treatment, such as prolonged bedrest and the use of labor suppressant drugs, on the mother's health.

Multiple Gestation

Complications such as pregnancy-induced hypertension, abruptio placenta, and anemia are more likely in the multiple gestation pregnancy. Labor suppressant

Table 22-1   Factors Influencing Uterine Activity

Factor	Role	Maintain Pregnancy	Promote Labor
Cervix	Collagen and fibrous connective tissue (ground substance) resist gravity force	Closure of cervix maintained by progesterone	Cervix ripened by: • Breakdown of collagen by collagenase • Breakdown of connective tissue • Addition of more water Estrogen increases collagenase activity Prostaglandin E$_2$ increases cervical extensibility Cervical trauma can cause early cervical dilation
Gap junctions	Cell-to-cell contact areas that coordinate smooth muscle contraction	Kept inactive by prostacyclin	Formed by: • Estrogen • Thromboxane
Calcium	Free calcium in the cytoplasm of the cell essential for smooth muscle contractions	Decreases in intracellular calcium favor myometrial relaxation • Prostacyclin Calcium channel blockers: nifedipine • Magnesium calcium substitution	Increases intracellular calcium • Oxytocin • Prostaglandin F$_{2\alpha}$ • Thromboxane
Autonomic nervous system	Innervate uterus • Beta receptors—inhibit uterine contractility • Alpha receptors—stimulate uterine contractility	Medications that stimulate beta receptors: • Ritodrine • Terbutaline	Hormone that stimulates alpha receptors: • Norepinephrine Stress stimulates norepinephrine release

Continued

Table 22-1 Factors Influencing Uterine Activity—cont'd

Factor	Role	Maintain Pregnancy	Promote Labor
Progesterone	Placenta hormone of pregnancy	Normally promotes uterine relaxation Keeps cervical collagen together	As estrogen-to-progesterone ratio increases, collagenase is released, breaking down cervical collagen; cervical softening results When combined with oxytocin and prostaglandins, relaxation effect may be lost
Relaxin	Protein hormone produced by the corpus luteum	Suppresses myometrial contraction with progesterone	Promotes cervical ripening Increased levels increase preterm labor
Oxytocin	Promotes uterine contractility if oxytocin receptors are present Oxytocin receptors are myometrial cell components that allow oxytocin to attach	Normally held in check by: • Progesterone Oxytocin antagonist may be beneficial in stopping preterm labor Oxytocin sensitivity decreased in postterm patients	Estrogen promotes formation of oxytocin receptors in the myometrial muscle Levels normally do not rise before labor but during active labor enhance contraction strength Uterine oxytocin release is stimulated by: • DHEA • Fetal hormone • Estrogen

		Production stimulated by:	Production suppressed by:
Prostaglandins	Prostaglandins E2, F2α thromboxane cause uterine contractions and cervical ripening	• Estrogen • Uterine hypoxia caused by maternal smoking, drug use (e.g., cocaine), or hypertension	• Progesterone • Prostaglandin synthetase inhibitors help arrest: • PTL • Indomethacin
Vasopressin	Antidiuretic hormone related structurally to oxytocin Primary action is to conserve body water	Dehydration can cause increased release and uterine contractile activity	Hydration can reduce secretion of and decrease uterine contractile
Endothelin and cytokines	Potent uterine contractility substances that are released during an infectious process	Infection releases endothelin and cytokines, which stimulate increased release of oxytocin and prostaglandins	Early diagnosis and treatment of genitourinary infections, especially bacterial vaginosis and UTIs

DHEA, Dehydroepiandrosterone sulfate; *PTL,* preterm labor; *UTIs,* Urinary track infections.
Reference: Castracane V: Endocrinology of preterm labor, *Clin Obstet Gyn* 43(4):717–726, 2000; Ruiz R: Mechanism of full-term and preterm labor: factors influencing uterine activity, *J Obstet Gynecol Neonatal Nurs* 27(6):652–660, 1998.

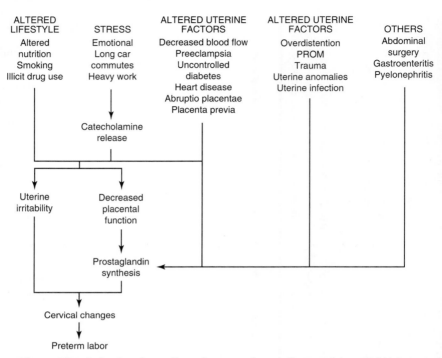

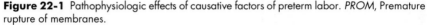

Figure 22-1 Pathophysiologic effects of causative factors of preterm labor. *PROM,* Premature rupture of membranes.

drugs place the multifetal gestation at higher risk than a singleton pregnancy, especially to pulmonary edema. When one fetus dies, disseminated intravascular coagulation result.

FETAL AND NEONATAL EFFECTS

Preterm Labor

PTL leads to the birth of an infant whose body processes are immature. These infants have an increased risk for birth trauma and an increased difficulty adjusting to extrauterine life. Special problems seen in the preterm infant are as follows:

- Respiratory distress syndrome
- Intraventricular or pulmonary hemorrhage
- Patent ductus anteriosis
- Necrotizing enterocolitis
- Retinopathy
- Hyperbilirubinemia
- Increased susceptibility to infections
- Anemia
- Ineffective temperature regulatory mechanism

- Development delay
- Chronic lung disease
- Later in life, increased risk for type 2 diabetes mellitus (Hofman and others, 2004)

The severity of each of these problems depends greatly on the gestational age of the infant. The greatest potential problem the preterm infant has is respiratory distress. If it is severe, hypoxia can ensue and cerebral hemorrhage, seizure disorders, and neonatal death can result. In fact, PTL accounts for 75% to 85% of all neonatal mortality and morbidity (Bernhardt and Dorman, 2004).

Multiple Gestation

Prematurity is the greatest risk that occurs in multiple gestations. Monoamniotic and monochorionic placentation is associated with high fetal uncertainty because of the risk for twin-to-twin transfusion syndrome (Malone and D'Alton, 2000). This type of placentation usually results in vascular communication between placentas. One fetus tends to receive a volume overload, leading to polyuria and polyhydramnios at the expense of another fetus who becomes hypovolemic, resulting in oligohydramnios. Both fetuses are at extreme risk if untreated.

NATIONAL EFFECTS

Despite technologic and pharmacologic advances in the treatment of PTL, the preterm birth rate is higher in the United States than in 18 other industrialized nations. At the same time, the economic importance of preterm births has direct and indirect effects on us as a nation. Neonatal intensive care, primarily because of premature births, is the most expensive care service in our health care system, with estimated costs of $5 billion annually (Elliott, 2000).

DIAGNOSTIC TESTING

Risk Assessment

No routine screening tool has been effective in predicting those at high risk for PTL. Current biochemical markers being used to assist in the diagnosis of PTL in symptomatic high risk patients are listed next.

Fetal Fibronectin

Fibronectins are a family of proteins found in extracellular matrix. Fetal fibronectins (fFns) are found in fetal membranes and decidua throughout pregnancy. As the gestational sac implants and attaches to the interior of the uterus in the first half of pregnancy, fFn is normally found in cervicovaginal fluid. After 22 weeks, the presence of fFns can no longer be detected in normal vaginal secretions. It is present again in the vaginal secretions within 2 weeks of the onset of delivery, term or preterm. It is suggested that fFns be released into the cervix and the vagina when mechanical- or inflammatory-mediated damage occurs to the membranes (McParland, Jones, and Taylor, 2004).

The test is done during a speculum examination by taking a sterile Dacron polyester swab and collecting the vaginal and cervical secretions near the external os of the cervix. The swab should remain in place approximately 10 seconds and then be transferred to a tube of sample buffer for transport. This test is for women who have PTL signs and symptoms and who are at 24 to 35 weeks of gestation to assist in avoiding unnecessary interventions (ACOG, 2001). A positive fFn (50 ng/ml or greater) in a singleton pregnancy is a moderate predictor that more significant preterm cervical changes are likely within 1 to 2 weeks (Andersen, 2000; Iams, 2003; Ruiz, Fullerton, and Brown, 2004). A negative fFn is a strong predictor that preterm delivery in the next 1 to 2 weeks is unlikely. False positives may result from recent sexual intercourse, vaginal bleeding, amniotic fluid, or recent cervical examination.

Cervical Length

Transvaginal ultrasound to measure cervical length is also being used to assess risk for PTL. Women with short cervical length have an increased risk for PTL. According to Iams (2003), a cervical length less than 25 mm between 22 and 24 weeks of gestation indicates an increased risk for PLT. Cervical funneling is also a predictive sign. The role of cervical length in assessing risk for PTL in multiple gestations is less defined (Welch and Nicolaides, 2002).

Criteria for Diagnosis of Preterm Labor

When a patient comes in experiencing regular, rhythmic uterine contractions, the medical team must first determine whether the patient is in true labor. The diagnosis is usually made in the presence of (1) four contractions in a 20-minute period, (2) a cervix that is beginning to dilate more than 2 cm, and (3) 80% or greater cervical effacement (ISCI, 2004). Therefore the diagnosis of PTL requires both uterine contractions and cervical change. Cervical length and fetal fibronectin are used to facilitate diagnosis. Fibronectin swab must be obtained at the initial speculum exam to prevent a false positive. If the patient is experiencing uterine contractions but the cervix is less than 80% effaced and 3 cm dilated, cervical length is usually determined with transvaginal ultrasound. A cervical length of more than 30 mm indicates that preterm labor is unlikely (Iams, 2003).

USUAL MEDICAL MANAGEMENT AND PROTOCOLS FOR NURSE PRACTITIONERS

When the diagnosis of PTL is made, the medical team attempts to determine the cause and whether further continuation of the pregnancy will be beneficial or harmful to the fetus or harmful to the mother. The choice of treatment depends on the answers to these questions and the age and maturity of the fetus.

Diagnostic Data to Direct Preterm Management

Diagnostic data in PTL to direct management include the following:
- Blood studies: a complete blood cell count with differential and platelets
- Urinalysis for culture and sensitivity to rule out a urinary tract infection, especially for group B streptococcus

- Cervical cultures for bacterial vaginosis, gonorrhea, chlamydia, and trichomonas vaginalis to rule out an infection
- Drug screen if indicated
- Fetal surveillance studies to determine signs of fetal compromise
- Fetal lung maturity if gestational age is between 32 and 36 weeks
- fFn evaluation
- Transvaginal ultrasound to determine cervical length

Contraindications to Halting Preterm Labor

In 20% of the cases that present in PTL, delivery is indicated because of a medical or obstetric reason (ACOG, 2003), such as the following:
- Mature fetus as demonstrated by a lecithin/sphingomyelin (L/S) ratio of 2:1 or greater or the presence of phosphatidyl glycerol in the amniotic fluid
- Fetal death
- Fetal anomaly incompatible with life
- Intrauterine growth restriction related to an unfavorable intrauterine environment
- Fetal compromise
- Active hemorrhage
- Intraamniotic infection
- Severe preeclampsia, heart disease, or significant bleeding from placenta previa or abruptio placentae

Preterm Labor Management Options

Despite all our advances in technology and treatments, it must be understood that preterm birth rates have increased, rather than declined. No treatment has been shown to reduce the rate of preterm delivery with clinical significance (McParland, Jones, and Taylor, 2004). There is some clinical evidence that some tocolytic agents used to initially suppress uterine contractions for an acute episode of PTL may have limited benefit by delaying delivery for a few days, thus allowing time for steroid administration and maternal transport to a tertiary care center (King and others, 2003; Anotayanonth and others, 2004). However, all these drugs have risks. Tocolytic drugs being used include magnesium sulfate, beta-mimetic agonists, calcium channel blockers, oxytocin antagonists, and nonsteroidal antiinflammatory drugs (NSAIDs). According to the Cochrane Database of Systematic Review, data are too inadequate to identify one specific tocolytic agent over another (Anotayanonth and others, 2004). However, the use of calcium channel blockers (such as nifedipine) and oxytocin antagonists (such as atosiban) is increasing because these drugs have fewer adverse side effects than beta-mimetic agonists and magnesium with equal effectiveness (King and others, 2003; Svigos, Robinson, and Vigneswaran, 2006). Atosiban has recently been approved as a tocolytic agent in Europe and United Kingdom (Chandraharan and Arulkumaran, 2005).

According to several systematic reviews of relevant published random-control clinical trials by Gyetvai and others (1999), Nanda and others, (2002), Sanchez-Ramos and Kaunitz (1999), and Thornton (2005), maintenance tocolytic therapy with the subcutaneous infusion pump or oral tocolytic therapy, after parenteral tocolytic therapy, does not significantly reduce the rates of recurrent PTL. Therefore because of the risk and consequences of the medication, routine use of maintenance tocolytic therapy is not currently recommended (Svigos, Robinson, and Vigneswaran, 2006).

Devoe and Ware (2000), after reviewing the six published meta-analyses of the major home uterine activity monitoring (HUAM) clinical trials, concluded that the only benefit of HUAM results from the nursing contact—and not the device. Self-palpation and weekly nursing contact, according to Dyson and others (1998), appear to be the most effective. Therefore HUAM devices offer only limited benefit to a very select group of women at high risk for PTL who live a long distance from their health care providers (Devoe and Ware, 2000).

Current management options of PTL include the following:

- Evaluate the symptomatic patient by assessing her contraction pattern, obtaining a vaginal swab for fibronectin, ruling out rupture of membranes and vaginal bleeding, and assessing the cervical status of effacement and dilation. If cervix is less than 80% effaced, perform a transvaginal ultrasound, assessing length of cervix.
- Determine whether possible contributing causes, such as infection or PROM, are present.
- Treat any sexually transmitted infections or any other infection other than group B streptococcus. Treat for group B streptococcus when the patient goes into active labor (as outlined in Chapter 25).
- Restrict activity.
- Hydrate with 500 ml of isotonic crystalloid solution if the patient is dehydrated (Stan and others, 2002); if the patient is not dehydrated, this may lead to pulmonary edema if tocolytic drugs are used.
- Initially monitor fetal heart rate (FHR) and uterine activity continuously, then periodically.
- Transfer to a tertiary care center if possible.
- Initially use tocolytic agents to suppress uterine contractions for an acute episode of PTL until the patient can be transported to tertiary care or complete corticosteroid therapy initiated (Anotayanonth and others, 2004). These tocolytic agents include magnesium sulfate, beta-sympathomimetics, calcium channel blockers, prostaglandin inhibitors, and oxytocin antagonists.
- Use a single course of corticosteroids to facilitate fetal lung maturity if delivery is imminent before 34 weeks of gestation (NIH, 2000; Crowther and Harding, 2003; Dudley, Thaddeus, Peter, 2003).
- Do not use prophylactic antibiotics. They are not proven beneficial and are not recommended except to treat B streptococcus during active labor (King and Flenady, 2006; ACOG, 2003).
- Instruct the patient to use self-palpation uterine activity at home or to use HUAM with a device. If a home uterine contraction monitor is ordered, it can be rented from a privately owned perinatal home care company. The equipment consists of a monitoring device and a battery-operated

recording unit. The monitoring device is a large disk with a curved surface and serves as a tocodynamometer. It is designed so that the entire surface, unlike a conventional electronic fetal monitor tocodynamometer, is capable of sensing a low-intensity contraction and making a printout. Daily follow-up is provided by the nursing services of the uterine contraction monitoring company, guided by the orders of the attending physician.

Experimental Treatment

One treatment modality still in experimental protocols is the use of progesterone for patients with a history of preterm labor. Progesterone (17P) injections, administered weekly between 16 and 20 weeks of gestation, have been shown to decrease the chance of preterm labor in the current pregnancy by 33% (Petrini and others, 2005).

Abdominal Surgery Management

If a surgical emergency presents itself before 36 weeks of gestation, regardless of previous risk, the pregnant patient is at high risk for PTL and delivery. It is postulated that the higher production of prostaglandins for the healing process increases the likelihood of preterm contractions. The pregnant woman may find it difficult or impossible to distinguish preterm contractions from abdominal pain at the surgical site. Add pain medication, which masks contraction discomfort as well, and it becomes even more unlikely that contractions will be the identified complaint. After abdominal surgery, it is a good idea to monitor with an electronic monitor the contraction pattern of the uterus. Some providers treat with subcutaneous terbutaline every 2 to 4 hours or with IV magnesium sulfate as a preventative for 24 to 48 hours after abdominal surgery, if the woman is more than 20 weeks pregnant.

Multiple Gestation Management

The most common components of multiple gestation management are increased nutritional requirement (see Chapter 1), increased rest, PTL prevention, and antepartum testing every 3 to 4 weeks after 25 weeks.

Bedrest, except for being allowed up to the bathroom and for meals, is still the preferred treatment once signs of preterm cervical changes are identified. Usually, larger doses of magnesium sulfate or other tocolytics are needed than with a singleton preterm pregnancy. Tocolytic home therapy with the terbutaline pump is more successful than any of the other home tocolytic therapies. Ultimately, the most effective tocolytic is IV magnesium sulfate. There is no evidence to support hospitalization for bedrest in the absence of significant cervical changes. Prolonged hospitalized bedrest does not reduce the risk for preterm birth or perinatal death. There is some suggestion that hospitalization may increase fetal growth in the higher order multiples (e.g., more than twins) (Crowther, 2001).

Other complications are also more likely with a multiple gestation pregnancy, including pregnancy-induced hypertension, which may be modified by hydrotherapy beginning at 24 to 26 weeks, thus allowing the fetuses more time in utero. Hydrotherapy has a number of beneficial effects:

- Forces fluid from tissue back into the circulating volume
- Improves blood flow to the uterus and thus to the babies, thereby improving growth potential in multiple gestation
- Buoyancy with water relieves weight from the skeletal structures and muscles and therefore improves comfort

There is no doubt that multiple gestation presents management problems to the provider, as well as self-management challenges for the patient and her family. Bedrest is the ultimate treatment of choice. This places an additional strain on the family unit. It requires additional support financially, physically, and emotionally. The emotional strain can be a prenatal precursor to postpartum depression even when the infant outcomes are optimal. The deconditioning from prolonged inactivity makes recovery more difficult and the fatigue factor more pronounced. Counseling prenatally and postpartum can help to shorten the term of depression or avoid most or all of the more serious sequelae.

NURSING MANAGEMENT

Prevention

The most prescient and compelling shift in PTL and birth care since the 1990s has been toward prevention of PTL and birth. This is the most important area on which we must focus if we are to change preterm birth outcomes, which is a national health priority in the United States and Canada (Maloni, 2000). Preventive measures must center on counteracting or improving the modifiable risk factors for PTL while keeping in mind that 50% of patients who experience PTL have no identifiable risk factors. Thus any prevention program must consider the inclusion of all pregnant women (Freda and Patterson, 2001; ICSI, 2004). It is the single most important aspect of obstetric management of multiple gestation.

Prevention consists of first screening all pregnancies for risk. If a patient is found to be at moderate to high risk, extra evaluation and more frequent evaluation can help identify signs and symptoms before advanced changes occur. If the patient is not at risk, she should be made aware of early signs of PTL and be made to feel comfortable reporting these for evaluation by her health care provider. PTL cannot be diagnosed over the phone and must be evaluated by seeing the patient, talking with her, and physically examining her for early signs of cervical change. This antepartum preterm prevention program should include the following assessments:

- Assess smoking habits and intervene.
- Assess for substance use, if substance abuse is determined (see Chapter 26 for interventions).
- Screen for medical risks.
- Screen for bacterial vaginosis, as well as other urogenital infections, and treat appropriately.

- Assess for domestic violence and provide appropriate intervention and referrals if identified (see Chapter 24).
- Evaluate the patient's employment and home responsibilities to determine the amount of stress, level of heavy work, duration of prolonged standing, and length of commute. Instruct her to modify or stop activities that cause fatigue and plan daily rest periods to increase blood flow to the uterus, which decreases the risk for prostaglandin release. If work responsibilities involve strenuous activities, problem-solve with the patient and her family about ways to avoid or lessen these activities (ICSI, 2004).
- Assess for exposure to toxic substances.
- Assess the patient's level of anxiety, as well as for the presence of economic or family stressors. Teach relaxation techniques to decrease the effects of stress (Hobel, 2004). Encourage problem solving to reduce stress by avoiding or altering stressful situations. Make appropriate referrals as needed.
- Assess for symptoms of PTL at each prenatal visit after 20 weeks.

The antepartum preterm prevention program should include the following general education components to be taught to all pregnant women to facilitate lifestyle modification and risk reduction:

- Plan pregnancies with at least an interval of 16 months between births.
- Encourage early and regular prenatal care.
- Provide nutritional counseling to achieve appropriate weight for height and avoid fasting, which can cause accelerated ketosis and release stress hormones (Hobel, 2004).
- Provide oral health education to decrease periodontal disease that can increase risk for PTL (Wener and Lavigne, 2004).
- Encourage patients to drink 8 ounces of water or fruit juice every waking hour except for the last couple of hours before sleep to decrease release of ADH and oxytocin from the posterior pituitary gland and increase uterine blood flow, thereby stabilizing decidual lysosomes. Drinks containing caffeine should be avoided.
- Instruct the patient to empty bladder every 2 hours while awake. A full bladder can stimulate the uterus to contract and increase the risk for urinary tract infections.
- Help the patient avoid infection. Because of the stimulating effect of cytokines and bacterial endotoxins in prostaglandin production, infection prevention should be taught. Prevention of urinary tract and vaginal infections is most important. Adequate fluid, perineal hygiene, the wearing of cotton-lined underwear, the avoidance of scented bath salts, and the limiting of sexual contacts to only one person are beneficial in lowering the risk for these infections. The patient should understand the signs of an infection and the need to report any signs immediately.
- Encourage rest periods during the day to prevent fatigue, to decrease pressure of the fetus on the cervix, and to increase blood flow to the uterus. However, remember that bedrest, hydration, and pelvic rest are not effective in decreasing the risk for preterm birth (ACOG, 2003).

- Emphasize that appropriate exercise such as walking or swimming can be beneficial in decreasing fatigue and stress.

The antepartum preterm prevention program includes the following specific education components. It is to be taught to all pregnant women and their significant others between 20 and 36 weeks of gestation to enhance early recognition:

- PTL is subtle.
- Contractions may feel like a tightening sensation; they are not necessarily painful (avoid use of the term *Braxton-Hicks contractions*).
- Uterine contractions should be felt for twice a day for 1 hour.
- Symptoms of PTL that should be reported to the health care provider include menstrual-like cramps, low dull backache, pelvic pressure, changes in vaginal discharge, and intestinal cramping with or without diarrhea.
- If any PTL symptoms occur, the patient should empty her bladder, lie down on her side, drink two to three glasses of fluid, and palpate for uterine contractions. She should come in for a vaginal examination if the symptoms continue or if she experiences four or more contractions in 1 hour. If symptoms stop, she may resume light activity. If the symptoms resume, she should call the health care provider or go directly to the hospital.
- The nurse should provide sensitive care when women report symptoms of PTL, making a through evaluation and reinforcing the importance to continue to report any symptoms experienced.

Hospitalization Management of Preterm Labor

- Determine estimated age of delivery through history and an ultrasound for fetal growth and gestational age assessment.
- Place the electronic fetal monitor to continually assess FHR, fetal well-being, and uterine contraction pattern.
- Initiate orders for treatment of PTL contractions within 30 minutes of initial hospital evaluation if the patient reports symptoms.
- Treat preterm contractions by having the patient void and placing her in a lateral recumbent position.
- Use IV hydration only if patient manifests signs of dehydration (Freda and Patterson, 2001; Stan and others, 2002).
- If tocolytic drugs are to be used, start an IV infusion and administer the tocolytic drug as outlined in this chapter under the respective IV tocolytic drug therapy (Box 22-2). Tocolytic agents are currently divided into five classes: (1) beta-sympathomimetics, (2) magnesium sulfate, (3) calcium antagonists, (4) prostaglandin inhibitors, and (5) oxytocin antagonists.
- Assess for signs of infection by palpating for abdominal tenderness unassociated with contractions; assess for changes in vaginal discharge (either watery, bloody, with increased mucus, or foul- smelling); assess laboratory data for rapid rise in white blood cells; evaluate FHR for tachycardia, late decelerations, and absence of variability; assess maternal vital signs for temperature rise or drop in blood pressure.

Box 22-2   Tocolytic Therapy for Preterm Labor

Beta Sympathomimetics
Action

Sympathomimetic drugs supplement or mimic the effects of norepinephrine and
epinephrine on the body's organs innervated by the adrenergic nerve fibers.
There are two types of adrenergic receptors: alpha and beta. Alpha receptors
primarily cause contractions of smooth muscle; beta receptors primarily cause
relaxation of smooth muscle by preventing the release of calcium from the
sarcoplasmic reticulum, except in the heart, where they cause cardiac
stimulation.

There are two types of beta receptors: $beta_1$ and $beta_2$. $Beta_1$ receptors are
more predominant in the heart, and their stimulation results in tachycardia and
increased myocardial contractility. $Beta_2$ receptors are more predominant in
the uterus, blood vessels, bronchioles, and diaphragm. The contractility of the
smooth muscle is decreased, which results in uterine and bronchial relaxation
and peripheral vasodilation. Contractility of smooth muscle is decreased by
binding calcium to the sarcoplasmic reticulum and therefore blunting the
movement of the myosin and actin filaments (Pryde and others, 2001).

Contraindications

Contraindications for beta sympathomimetics are cardiovascular disease, cardiac
dysrhythmias, hypertension, uncontrolled maternal hyperthyroidism, and
migraine headaches. Because beta sympathomimetics antagonize the body's
normal compensatory mechanism for blood loss by their effects on heart rate
and systolic and diastolic pressure, these drugs should not be
used if there are any indications that bleeding is present.

Acute Dosage for Intravenous Terbutaline

When intravenous (IV) terbutaline is ordered, a diluent is used of 500 ml of
lactated Ringer's solution or normal saline. Begin at a rate of 0.01 mg/min and
increased 0.01 mg/min every 10 to 30 minutes until one of the
following occurs (Iams and Creasy, 2004).
- Uterine contractions cease.
- Intolerable side effects develop.
- A maximum rate of 0.08 mg/min is reached.
   The patient is usually maintained on a dose that is effective for her for
   12 to 24 hours after uterine contractions cease. The medication is then tapered
   off.
   Subcutaneous injections of 0.25 mg every 30 to 60 minutes up to 3 doses
   are also used to treat acute preterm labor. A dose should be held if the maternal
   pulse is greater than 120 beats a minute.

Maternal Side Effects

Side effects that frequently occur with terbutaline include the following:
- Slight hypotension or a widening of maternal pulse pressure related to
   a slight increase in systolic and a slight decrease in diastolic pressure,
   thereby decreasing coronary perfusion

Continued

Box 22-2   Tocolytic Therapy for Preterm Labor—cont'd

- Lightheadedness, tremors, and a flushed feeling related to relaxation of vascular smooth muscle
- Restlessness, emotional upset, and anxiety related to epinephrine release
- Maternal and fetal tachycardia, heart palpitations, and frequent skipping of a heartbeat related to cardiac stimulation
- Transient maternal hyperglycemia related to drug stimulation of the liver and muscle, causing glycogenolysis, gluconeogenesis, and decreased uptake of glucose by peripheral tissue
- Elevated lactate and free fatty acids, related to hyperglycemia, cause drug stimulation of the pancreas
- Decreased serum potassium caused by intracellular shift from the extracellular space
- Decreased hematocrit or vomiting by 20% to 25% related to plasma volume expansion
- Nausea
- Increased insulin and glucagon secretion related to decreased intestinal motility
- Bronchial relaxation
  Intolerable side effects are maternal tachycardia greater than 120 beats/min, drop in blood pressure to less than 90/60, chest pain or tightness, and cardiac dysrhythmias.
  Life-threatening complications are pulmonary edema, which may result from myocardial failure and fluid overload; subendocardial myocardial ischemia; cardiac dysrhythmias, such as premature ventricular contractions, premature nodal contractions, and atrial fibrillation; or cerebral vasospasm in patients who have a history of migraine headaches.

Long-Term Fetal Effects of Terbutaline

The major side effect to the fetus is tachycardia, but other side effects are hyperinsulinemia, hyperglycemia, hypocalcemia, myocardial hypertrophy, and ischemia (Hearne and Nagey, 2000).

Magnesium Sulfate

Action

Magnesium relaxes the smooth muscle of the uterus by substituting itself for calcium. It may also decrease the amount of cellular calcium by hyperpolarizing the cell membrane (Jeyabalan and Caritis, 2002).

Contraindications

A contraindication for magnesium sulfate is myasthenia gravis (ACOG, 2003).

IV Dosage

A loading IV dose of 4 to 6 g, given over 20 to 30 minutes, is usually recommended in the treatment of preterm labor, followed by a maintenance dose of 2 to 4 g/hour until uterine contractions cease or signs of toxicity develop (ACOG, 2003; ICSI, 2004; Rident, 2005). The patient being treated for preterm labor can tolerate a much higher dose of magnesium than the preeclamptic patient. Kidney function is usually not compromised in the preterm labor patient as it can be in the preeclamptic patient.

Box 22-2   Tocolytic Therapy for Preterm Labor—cont'd

Signs of Toxicity

Signs of toxicity are fewer than 12 respirations/min, absence of deep tendon reflexes, severe hypotension, or extreme muscle relaxation.

Maintenance Oral Magnesium Dosing

Oral magnesium oxide or magnesium gluconate may be used for maintenance tocolysis. The normal dose for magnesium gluconate is 500 mg to 2 g every 2 to 4 hours. Research has indicated that certain oral forms of magnesium may be as effective as an oral beta sympathomimetic in suppressing preterm labor with fewer side effects. Research in this area of oral tocolysis is again evolving after about a 15-year hiatus (Iams and Creasy, 2004).

Side Effects

During the loading dose, the patient frequently complains of hot flashes, nausea, vomiting, drowsiness, headaches, muscle weakness, and blurred vision. These side effects usually subside when the loading dose is completed. Less common but more problematic side effects are bone demineralization, paralytic ileus, shortness of breath, and pulmonary edema.

Signs of magnesium toxicity include the following:

- Respirations fewer than 12/min
- Absence of deep tendon reflexes
- Severe hypotension
- Extreme muscle relaxation
  Antidote for magnesium toxicity
- Calcium gluconate 1 gm (10 ml of a 10% solution) IV over 3 minutes

Long-Term Effects on Neonate

There are no reliable data as to the long-term effect on the neonate (Duley, Gulmesoglu, and Henderson-Smart, 2003).

Calcium Channel Blockers

Action

Calcium channel blockers, such as nifedipine, do not allow the movement of calcium into the smooth muscle of the uterus. Contraction of smooth muscle depends on the availability of calcium.

Dosage

Initial dosage is 10 mg po every 20 minutes for up to three doses. Maintenance dosage is 10 to 20 mg every 4–6 hours orally (Iams and Creasy, 2004).

Maternal Side Effects

Uncommon side effects related to peripheral vasodilation are flushing, headache, fatigue, mild hypotension, dizziness, and peripheral edema (Weiner and Buhimschi, 2004). Another side effect is tachycardia. The dose should be held if the maternal heart rate is higher than 120 or blood pressure is lower than 90/50 (Freda and Patterson, 2001).

Fetal Side Effects

Negative effects to the fetus appear to be minimal. In the presence of severe maternal hypertension, decreased uteroplacental blood flow can result (Weiner, and Buhimschi, 2004).

Continued

Box 22-2   Tocolytic Therapy for Preterm Labor—cont'd

Prostaglandin Inhibitors
Action

Prostaglandin inhibitors, such as indomethacin or ibuprofen (Motrin), act by inhibiting prostaglandin synthesis.

Contraindications

Prostaglandin inhibitors are contraindicated in patients who have an active peptic ulcer, renal disease, hypertension, nonsteroidal antiinflammatory drug sensitive asthma, or a coagulation disorder.

Dosage

The initial loading dose of indomethacin is 50 to 100 mg orally or by rectal suppository followed by a maintenance oral dose of 25 to 50 mg every 4 hours for 24 to 48 hours (Freda and Patterson, 2001). If contractions recur, a second course of indomethacin may be given. Patients have been treated for 1 month or more with the drug. Ibuprofen, 600 mg every 6 hours, may be used instead (Elliott, 2001).

Maternal Side Effects

Maternal side effects are uncommon but can include nausea and heartburn. They can mask the symptoms of a fever.

Fetal and Neonatal Side Effects

Side effects are premature closure of the ductus arteriosus that can cause oligohydramnios, neonatal pulmonary hypertension, intraventricular hemorrhage, hyperbilirubinemia, and necrotizing enterocolitis. The risk for transient obstruction of the ductus arteriosus increases with increasing gestational age and long duration of treatment. It rarely occurs if the drug is not used after 32 weeks of gestation (Hearne and Nagey, 2000).

Oxytocin Antagonists
Actions

Oxytocin antagonists, such as atosiban, inhibit oxytocin release.

Dosage

If used, IV infusion of 300 mg/min is given for a maximum of 12 hours (Hearne and Nagey, 2000).

Maternal Side Effects

This research drug has been well tolerated with few side effects. The side effects are nausea and vomiting, headache, chest pain, palpitations, tachycardia, and hypertension (Svigos, Robinson, and Vigneswaran, 2006).

- Educate as to the importance of promotion of fetal lung maturity with corticosteroids between gestational weeks 24 and 34 to decrease respiratory distress syndrome, intraventricular hemorrhage, and necrotizing enterocolitis (ACOG, 2003). See Box 21-3 for information about corticosteroid therapy.
- Include supportive family members in all instructions.
- Make needed referrals—for example, to the social worker—if problems are identified.

- Encourage the patient's participation in her own care and decision making as much as possible.
- Provide time for the patient and her family to express their concerns regarding the possible outcome for the baby and inconvenience to the mother and family during treatment. Encourage them to vent any feelings, fears, and anger they may experience.
- Assess family's support system and coping mechanisms.
- Provide patient and her family with honest appraisal of the situation and plan of treatment.
- Give adequate information for decisions about alternatives of care.
- Refer to a high risk pregnancy support group such as Sidelines, a national support group for women experiencing a high risk pregnancy (*www.sidelines.org*).
- Refer to a spiritual counselor or chaplain on request or based on your assessment of need and patient acceptance.

Nursing Interventions for Acute Tocolytic Therapy

- Talk with the patient and her family to assess their understanding of the prescribe management plan.
- Obtain a patient history to assess contraindications to the prescribed tocolytic agent or to suppression of labor.
- Obtain such baseline data as FHR, uterine activity, maternal vital signs, weight, electrocardiogram, and laboratory studies that include a complete blood cell count with differential, blood glucose, colloid osmotic pressure, urea nitrogen, and serum electrolytes to determine maternal response to the drug therapy.
- Follow the 2003 National Patient Safety Goals from the Joint Commission on Accreditation of Healthcare Organization (JCAHO, 2003) when administering a tocolytic agent.
- If the IV route is to be used, start an IV infusion of normal saline with an 18-gauge needle to piggyback the IV administration of the drug. Because incremental titration is essential, an infusion pump should be used. Refer to Box 22-2 tocolytic therapy for PTL for normal dosing.
- Encourage the patient to maintain a left lateral position to minimize the risk for hypotension.
- Provide psychosocial support.
- Use an external monitor to record FHR and uterine activity continuously.
- Monitor blood pressure, pulse rate and rhythm, and temperature closely. Notify health care provider if systolic blood pressure is higher than 140 or lower than 90 mm Hg, diastolic blood pressure is higher than 90 or lower than 50 mm Hg, maternal pulse is higher than 120 beats per minute, or hyperthermia is present.
- Keep total fluid intake below 2500 ml/24 hours to avoid fluid overload and pulmonary edema.
- Accurately measure and record intake and output and a daily weight. Notify the health care provider if output is less than 30 ml per hour.

- Auscultate lung sounds for evidence of pulmonary edema.
- Assess for intolerable side effects and potential life-threatening complications to the drug.
- Have available cardiopulmonary resuscitation equipment and appropriate antidote such as propranolol (Inderal) 0.25 mg or verapamil for beta-sympathomimetics or calcium gluconate 1 gm (10 ml of a 10% solution) for magnesium sulfate.
- If pulmonary edema develops, be prepared to treat as outlined under Critical Care Interventions for Pulmonary Edema, later in this chapter.
- If beta-sympathomimetics are used, be prepared to obtain diagnostic data, such as serum potassium, hemoglobin, hematocrit, and renal function studies, periodically during the IV treatment. Although hypokalemia can develop as the result of potassium moving from the extracellular space to the intracellular space, there is no change in the total body potassium level. Therefore supplemental potassium is usually not necessary. The potassium level will return to normal within 24 hours after the IV therapy is discontinued.
- If beta-sympathomimetics are used, measure blood glucose twice daily with B-G Chemstrips or the Dextrometer. Patients with diabetes can become hyperglycemic if treated with terbutaline. Therefore they require careful monitoring of plasma glucose and usually require IV insulin administration.
- If magnesium sulfate is being used, check deep tendon reflex every hour and refer to serum magnesium levels daily. Therapeutic serum levels of 4.0 to 7.5 mEq/L are effective in reducing uterine contractions. Toxicity can develop with levels of 10 mEq/L or greater.
- If prostaglandin inhibitors are being used, be prepared to assist with fetal surveillance studies such as an echocardiogram and amniotic fluid index. These drugs should not be used after 35 weeks of gestation because of the potential seriousness of the fetal side effects after this gestational age.

Critical Care Interventions for Pulmonary Edema*

- Position in upright tilted position.
- Start strict I&O
- Administer oxygen at a rate indicted by pulse oximetry and arterial blood gases to maintain maternal SaO_2 greater than 95%.
- Be prepared to use continuous positive airway pressure by facemask if oxygen levels are difficult to maintain.
- Administer diuretics as ordered using the lowest effective dose. Usual dose is furosemide 10 to 80 mg IV.
- Monitor blood pressure and be prepared to administer IV hydralazine or labetalol as indicated.
- Use invasive hemodynamic monitoring if conservative methods are not effective, if indicated.

---

*Powrie, 2006

Home Management of Preterm Labor

- Conduct a physical and functional health pattern assessment as outlined in Boxes 22-3 and 22-4.

Box 22-3   Home Visit Physical Assessment

- Vital signs, including blood pressure, respiratory rate, and temperature
- Breath sounds
- Fetal heart rate
- Fetal activity
- Cervical status
- Fasting blood glucose because of possible drug-induced alteration in glucose metabolism
- Weight
- Fundal height
- Urine for ketones, protein, leukocyte esterase
- Signs of pathologic edema

Box 22-4   Functional Health Pattern Assessment for Home Visit

Health-Perception/Health-Management Assessment
- Which prenatal health care resources have you used or do you plan to use, such as childbirth education classes, support groups, social service, and community agencies?

Nutritional Assessment
- What is a typical daily food and fluid intake?
- Appetite?
- Is weight increase appropriate (usual problem is a deficient gain)?

Elimination Assessment
- Urinary elimination pattern: changes or problems perceived, such as odor or burning pain on urination?
- Bowel elimination pattern: changes or problems perceived, such as flatulence or constipation?

Activity/Exercise Assessment
- What activity level are you maintaining? What kinds of limited activity exercises are you doing?

Sleep/Rest Assessment
- How do you feel after a night's sleep?
- Can you sleep comfortably for at least 4 hours at night?
- Is a sleep aid needed for periodic relief of expected insomnia from discomforts and lack of regular exercise and activities of daily living?

Cognitive/Perceptual Assessment
- Describe your uterine activity pattern. How many contractions do you palpate during the assessment hour? What activities seem to stimulate contractions?
- What kind of management problems have you experienced with the pump, home bedrest, or other recommendations?

Continued

Box 22-4   Functional Health Pattern Assessment for Home Visit—cont'd

Self-Perception/Self-Concept Assessment
- Describe how you and your family feel everything is going.

Role-Relationship Assessment
- How are all of your role responsibilities being managed while you are maintaining limited activity?
- How are you dealing with boredom?

Sexuality/Reproductive Assessment
- Have you experienced any warning signs of preterm labor?
- How are you and your partner dealing with the restricted sexual activity?

Coping/Stress-Tolerance Assessment
- What are you most concerned or worried about at this time?
- How are other family members dealing with their concerns, anxieties, or fears?

Spiritual Distress/Distress of the Human Spirit
- How are individuals and family dealing with loss of spiritual guidance?
- Is this a necessary part of daily life and are there creative ways to incorporate this with bedrest modification?

- Provide nursing support because research suggests that this has the most beneficial effect in preventing recurring PTL.
- Educate as to the importance of limited activity. Empower the patient and her family to implement this prescribed intervention by providing her with helpful hints (Boxes 22-5 and 22-6). Refer her to a high risk support group such as Sidelines (*www.sidelines.org*) or *http://www.parentsplace.com/pregnancy/complications.*
- Reinforce the primary prevention strategies again to decrease the risk for PTL recurrence.
- The effectiveness of home uterine activity monitoring is controversial. If HUAM is ordered, see Box 22-7 for components of uterine activity monitoring program.
- If maintenance therapy with a subcutaneous terbutaline pump or oral terbutaline therapy is ordered, obtain a 24-hour uterine contraction pattern to be used by the physician in ordering the basal rate and setting the bolus schedule.

Box 22-5   Entertaining Children While Mother is on Bedrest

- Keep supplies in a laundry basket near your bed.
- Keep a roll of paper towels near your bed for spills.
- Use an old sheet or blanket as a playtime cover to spare your bedspread.
- Keep activities brief.
- Have a remote-control television.
- Do not feel guilty about "neglecting your children." They live through it, and it is a small portion out of their lives in comparison with the rest of your unborn baby's life.
- Let your child play under the covers.
- Play "bed bowling" with paper cups and a small ball.
- Play "bed basketball" with rolled-up socks and an empty laundry basket.
- Direct bedspread traffic using small cars to follow the design on the bedspread.
- Use a mirror to make faces. This would be a good time to express feelings and show them on your face in the mirror.
- Make hand shadows on the wall with a flashlight.
- Build with blocks.
- Play board games.
- Go "bed fishing" using magnets and paper fish.
- Play "red light, green light" with mom as the traffic cop.
- Cut up magazines and paste them on cardboard.
- Make an alphabet book by cutting up magazines and pasting the pieces in a photograph album using a separate page for each letter.
- Get children's books from the library, and read to your child.
- Color in coloring books.
- Play with Colorforms sets.
- Play "I see something"—find something in the room, say its color, and then ask your child to guess what you are "seeing."
- Play with Play-doh.
- Trace letters or numbers on your child's back and have him or her guess what you wrote.
- Use this time constructively. Once the baby gets here, you will have few opportunities to spend this "special" time with this child again!

Modified from Maurer L: *Confinement connection: a home support program*, Phoenix, 1992, Author.

Box 22-6   Helpful Hints for Preterm Labor Patients on Bedrest

- Wear clothes (not pajamas) during the day if possible.
- Be neat and clean; keep up personal hygiene.
- Have as much contact and involvement with children as possible.
- Set goals, and keep them in mind.
- Shop by phone using the Yellow Pages and catalogs.
- Plan your menus, and organize the grocery list.
- Do projects you have long put off, such as putting pictures in albums, writing letters, sewing or stitchery, or writing holiday cards.
- Keep a journal of your pregnancy.
- Do fun things with your children: watch television, read books, play games, play video games, have special "just talking" time, do puzzles, make a paper chain of the days you have left on bedrest and let your child take one piece of the chain off every day
- When you feel up to it, allow visitors, but keep this under control.
- If you do not have child care, make your bedroom into a giant playpen. Put everything out of reach, and shut the door so that you do not have to worry about where your child is.
- Have a small ice chest next to your bed packed with the day's supplies of drinks and snacks.
- Do something special to pick you up when you are down, such as doing a manicure or facial or watching favorite show.
- Keep a calendar close by to chart your progress. Focus on how far you have come, not how far you have to go!
- Listen to books on tape if you tire of reading.
- Make a list of things that people can do for you, so that when they ask, you can easily come up with something and you can even give them a choice. And do take them up on their offers; people mean it, or they would not offer in the first place.
- Attend a childbirth class in your home, if this is available in your area.
- Have "dates" with your partner: have him pick up take-out food and bring in candles.
- Do craft projects such as cross-stitch, needlepoint, or knitting. Make something special for the baby or maybe someone else!
- Do passive bedrest exercises with prior approval from your physician.
- Read available books on high risk pregnancy and premature babies. Be informed, and become involved as a partner with your physician in your care.
- Focus on *why* you are doing this, not on *what* you are doing.
- Use a local support group for empathy and understanding when you need to talk to someone who can understand your feelings and fears.
- Pay the bills.
- Compile tax data.
- Reorganize files.
- Update your address book.
- Do mending.
- Learn a new language with tapes from the library.

Box 22-6   Helpful Hints for Preterm Labor Patients on Bedrest—cont'd

- Order and address birth announcements.
- Call a friend, relative, or support person each day.
- Do crossword, word search, or jigsaw puzzles.

Modified from Maloni J: Home care of the high-risk pregnant woman requiring bed rest, *J Obstet Gynecol Neonatal Nurs* 23(8):696–706, 1994; Maurer L: *Confinement connection: a home support program*, Phoenix, 2001; McCann M: *Days in waiting: a guide to surviving pregnancy bedrest*, St Paul, Minn, 2003, deRuyter-Nelson Publications. Retrieved from Sidelines High Risk Pregnancy Support, Laguna Beach, Calif, 2004, Sidelines National Support Network.

Box 22-7   Home Uterine Activity Monitoring

Program Initiation

The provider may order home uterine contraction monitoring when a woman who is at risk for preterm labor reports or is treated for signs of preterm labor. In the event home uterine contraction monitoring is ordered, the patient monitors for uterine contractions either by self-palpation or with a home uterine contraction monitor. Self-palpation is done by teaching the woman
to spread her fingers across all four quadrants of her abdomen, pressing in just enough to feel the uterine wall through the abdominal muscle (Fig. 22-2). If a home uterine contraction monitor is to be used, the patient must be referred to one of the uterine contraction monitoring companies to rent the monitor. She is taught how to place the ambulatory tocodynamometer,
which is connected to a battery-operated recording unit, just below the umbilicus and comfortably secure it with a belt. When the device for home uterine activity monitoring is used, self-palpation must also be taught to the patient.

Uterine Monitoring

Whether using the device for monitoring or self-palpation alone, the woman should record uterine activity for 1 full hour twice each day. With the monitoring equipment, contraction data are stored for later transmission via the telephone. With self-palpation alone, the woman is instructed to record the period of cramping or the numbers of contractions and whether they were palpated only or also perceived as a specific sensation, such as backache, tightening, tingling, or discomfort.

Daily to Weekly Nursing Contact

Once a day or less frequently, depending on assessed need, a preterm birth prevention nurse contacts the patient at home, discusses with her any home management problems, and encourages her to share her perceptions of how the past 24 hours have been.

Transmission of Data

After the nurse contact, the patient, using the monitoring equipment, is instructed to transmit both of the stored hours of contraction information. This is done by connecting the home telephone receiver into the recorder and pressing a button on the recorder to send. Within a matter of minutes, the 2 hours worth of contraction monitoring is received on the receiving center's equipment.

Continued

Box 22-7   Home Uterine Activity Monitoring—cont'd

If self-palpation is used, the woman describes times and type of uterine activity noted to the nurse.

Analysis of Data

The received data are analyzed by the nurse and are relayed verbally to the patient, and instructions for further monitoring, continuing care, or reporting to the hospital for treatment are given. The instructions are based on a tolerable baseline of no more than four contractions (or other number determined by the attending physician) per hour or patient's report of symptoms. Standing physician orders or immediate referral to the attending physician guides the nurse's instructions to the patient.

Expense

The patient's third-party reimbursement is charged a separate daily fee for rental of the equipment and for the nursing care follow-up. The cost/benefit ratio for indiscriminate use of the uterine contraction monitor has not been firmly established by research.

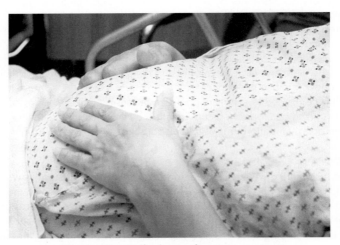

Figure 22-2 Self-palpation for uterine contractions.

CONCLUSION

The ultimate goal of prevention and treatment of PTL is delivery of a healthy term infant. It is a fact that neonatal outcomes are greatly improved when intrauterine life can be extended until fetal lungs mature. It is therefore suggested that delaying labor for even days can be beneficial. Early and ongoing risk assessment, education of all pregnant women in preterm prevention, and psychosocial intervention regarding smoking, alcohol use, illegal substance use, and domestic violence are important components of primary prevention. Early diagnosis and frequent health care contact can have a positive effect on early treatment of PTL before advanced cervical changes take place. Perinatal nurses can have a positive impact on neonatal morbidity by doing what nurses do so uniquely well. Screening, motivating, providing health care education, and frequent caring and sensitive contact with at-risk pregnant women can make a significant contribution to lowering neonatal morbidity and mortality from preterm delivery.

BIBLIOGRAPHY

Abramov Y and others: Indomethacin for preterm labor: a randomized comparison of vaginal and rectal-oral routes, *Obstet Gynecol* 95(4):482–486, 2000.

Adams M and others: Rates of and factors associated with recurrence of preterm delivery, *JAMA* 283(12):1591–1596, 2000.

American College of Obstetricians and Gynecologists: Management of preterm labor, *ACOG Practice Bulletin* number 43, Washington, DC, 2003, ACOG.

American College of Obstetricians Gynecologists: Clinical management guidelines for obstetrician-gynecologists. *Assessment of risk factors for preterm birth, ACOG Practice Bulletin Number 31.* Washington DC, 2001, Author. Retrieved from *http://www.fedstats.gov/qf/states/12/12097.html*

Andersen H: Use of fetal fibronectin in women at risk for preterm delivery, *Clin Obstet Gynecol* 43(4):746–758, 2000.

Anotayanonth S and others: Betamimetics for inhibiting preterm labour, *Cochrane Database Syst Rev* Issue 4, 2004.

Bernhardt J, Dorman K: Exploring fetal fibronectin and cervical length for validating risk, *AWHONN Lifelines* 8(1):39–44, 2004.

Castracane V: Endocrinology of preterm labor, *Clin Obstet Gynecol* 43(4):717–726, 2000.

Challis J, Lye S: Characteristics of parturition. In Creasy R, Resnik R, and Iams J, editors: *Maternal-fetal medicine: principles and practice,* ed 5, Philadelphia, 2004, Saunders.

Chandraharan E, Arulkumaran S: Acute tocolysis, *Curr Opin Obstet Gynecol* 17(2):151–156, 2005.

Cockey C: Prematurity Hits record high: More babies born at risk for lifetime disabilities, *AWHONN Lifelines* 9(5):365–367, 2004.

Colombo D, Iams J: Cervical length and preterm labor, *Clin Obstet Gynecol* 43(4):735–745, 2000.

Condon J and others: Surfactant protein secreted by the maturing mouse fetal lung acts as a hormone that signals the initiation of parturition, *Proc Natl Acad Sci USA* 101(14): 4978–4983, 2004.

Crowley P: Prophylactic Corticosteroids for Preterm Birth (Cochrane Review), *The Cochrane Library,* Issue 1, Chichester, UK, 2004, Wiley.

Crowther C: Hospitalization and bedrest for multiple pregnancy. In *The Cochrane Library,* Issue 2, Oxford, 2001, Update Software.

Crowther CA, Harding J: Repeat doses of prenatal corticosteroids for women at risk of preterm birth for preventing neonatal respiratory disease, *Cochrane Database Syst Rev* Issue 2, 2003.

Crowther CA: Hospitalisation and bed rest for multiple pregnancy, *Cochrane Database Syst Rev* Issue 1, 2001.

Devoe L, Ware D: Home uterine activity monitoring: a critical review, *Clin Obstet Gynecol* 43(4):778–786, 2000.

Dudley D, Thaddeus W, and Peter N: Current status of single-course antenatal steroid therapy, *Clin Obstet Gynecol* 46(1):132–149, 2003.

Duley L, Gülmezoglu AM, and Henderson-Smart DJ: Magnesium sulphate and other anti-convulsants for women with pre-eclampsia, *Cochrane Database Syst Rev* Issue 2, 2003.

Dyson D and others: Monitoring women at risk for preterm labor, *N Engl J Med* 338(1): 15–19, 1998.

Elliott J: Overview of the problem and higher order multiples, what have we learned. Presented at Preterm Delivery: A National Disgrace, Phoenix, AZ, November 2000.

Elliott J: Preterm labor: OB challenges of the millennium. Presented in Phoenix, AZ, April 2001.

Freda M, Patterson E: *Preterm labor: prevention and nursing management,* ed 2, White Plains, NY, 2001, March of Dimes.

Freda M: Nursing's contribution to the literature on pre-term labor and birth, *J Obstet Gynecol Neonatal Nurs* 32(5):659–667, 2003.

Gaunekar NN, Crowther CA: Maintenance therapy with calcium channel blockers for preventing preterm birth after threatened preterm labour, *Cochrane Database Syst Rev* Issue 3, 2004.

Gyetvai K and others: Tocolytics for preterm labor: a systematic review, *Obstet Gynecol* 94(5 Pt 2): 869–877, 1999.

Haas J and others: Prepregnancy health status and the risk of preterm delivery, *Arch Pediatr Adolesc Med* 159(1):58–63, 2005.

Hearne A, Nagey D: Therapeutic agents in preterm labor: tocolytic agents, *Clin Obstet Gynecol* 43(4):787–801, 2000.

Hendler I and others: The preterm prediction study: Association between maternal body mass index and spontaneous and indicated preterm birth, *Am J Obstet Gynecol* 192(3):882–886, 2005.

Hobel C: Stress and preterm birth, *Clin Obstet Gynecol* 47(4):856–880, 2004.

Hofman P and others: Premature birth and later insulin resistance, *N Engl J Med* 351(21):2179–2186, 2004.

Iams J, Creasy R: Preterm labor and delivery. In Creasy R, Resnik R, and Iams J, editors: *Maternal-fetal medicine: principles and practice,* ed 5, Philadelphia, 2004, Saunders.

Iams J: Prediction and early detection of pre-term labor, *Obstet Gynecol* 101(2):402–412, 2003.

Institute for Clinical Systems Improvement (ICSI): *Preterm birth prevention,* Bloomington, MN, 2004, Institute for Clinical Systems Improvement.

Jeavons W: Sterile speculum exams and fFN collection, *AWOHNN Lifelines* 9(3):237–240, 2005.

Jeyabalan A, Caritis S: Pharmacologic inhabitation of pre-term labor, *Clin Obstet Gynecol* 45(1): 99–113, 2002.

Joint Commission on Accreditation of Healthcare Organizations: *National patient safety goals,* Oakbrook, IL, 2003, Author.

Kenyon S, Boulvain M, and Neilson J: Antibiotics for preterm rupture of membranes, *Cochrane Database Syst Rev* Issue 2, 2003.

King J and others: Calcium channel blockers for inhibiting preterm labour, *Cochrane Database Syst Rev* Issue 1, 2003.

King J, Flenady V: Prophylactic antibiotics for inhibiting preterm labour with intact membranes, *Cochrane Database Syst Rev,* Issue 3, 2006.

Leitich H and others: Cervical length and dilation of the internal os detected by vaginal ultrasonography as markers for preterm delivery: a systematic review, *Am J Obstet Gynecol* 181(6):1465–1472, 1999.

Lockwood C: Biochemical predictors of preterm delivery. Presented at Preterm Delivery: a National Disgrace, Phoenix, AZ, November 2000.

Lockwood C: Stress-associated preterm delivery: the role of corticotropin releasing hormone, *Am J Obstet Gynecol* 180(1 Pt 3):S264–S266, 1999.

Majzoub J and others: A central theory of preterm and term labor: putative role for corticotropin-releasing hormone, *Am J Obstet Gynecol* 180(1 Pt 3):S232–S241, 1999.

Malone F and D'Alton M: Anomalies peculiar to multiple gestations, *Clin Perinatol* 27(4):1033–1046, 2000.

Maloni J: Preventing preterm birth: evidenced based interventions shift toward prevention, *AWHONN Lifelines* 4(4):26–33, 2000.

Maurer L: Confinement connection: a home support program, Phoenix, AZ, 1992, Sidelines Newsletter.

Maxwell C, Amankwah K: Alternative approaches to preterm labor, *Semin Perinatol* 25(5):310–315, 2001.

McParland P, Jones G, and Taylor D: Preterm labour and prematurity, *Curr Obstet Gynaecol* 14:309–319, 2004.

Mercer B and others: The preterm prediction study: effect of gestational age and cause of preterm birth on subsequent obstetric outcome, *Am J Obstet Gynecol* 181(5 Pt 1): 1216–1221, 1999.

Moore M: Preterm labor and birth: What have we learned in the past two decades? *JOGNN Clin Issues* 32(5):638–649, 2003.

Moos, M: Understanding prematurity: Sorting fact from fiction, *AWHONN Lifelines* 8(1): 32–37, 2004.

Mozurkewich E and others: Working conditions and adverse pregnancy outcomes: a meta-analysis, *Obstet Gynecol* 95(4):623–635, 2000.

Nanda K and others: Terbutaline pump maintenance therapy after threatened preterm labor for preventing preterm birth, *Cochrane Database Syst Rev* Issue 4, 2002.

National Center for Health Statistics (NCHS): Births, marriages, divorces, and deaths: provisional data for July 1999, *Natl Vital Stat Rep* 48, 2000.

National Center for Health Statistics: *Health, United States 2001*, Hyattsville, MD, 2002, U.S. Department of Health and Human Services.

National Institute of Child Health and Human Development: *Perinatology research branch annual report excerpt on pathophysiology of premature labor and complications of prematurity*, Washington, DC, 2001, NICHHD. Retrieved from *http://dir2.nichd.nih.gov*

National Institutes of Health (NIH): Antenatal corticosteroids revisited, Consensus development conference statement, Maryland, 2000, NIH. Retrieved from *http://consensusnih.gov*

Norwitz E, Robinson J, and Challis J: The control of labor, *N Engl J Med* 341(9):660–666, 1999.

Olsen S: Is supplementation with marine omega-3 fatty acids during pregnancy a useful tool in the prevention of preterm birth? *Clin Obstet Gynecol* 47(4):768–774, 2004.

Petrini J and others: Estimated effect of 17 alpha-hydroxyprogesterone caproate on preterm birth in the United States, *Am College Obstet Gynecol* 105(2):267–272, 2005.

Powrie R: Respiratory disease. In James D and others, editors: *High risk pregnancy: management options*, ed 3, Philadelphia, 2006, Saunders.

Pryde P and others: Adverse and beneficial effects of tocolytic therapy, *Semin Perinatol* 25(5):316–340, 2001.

Pschirrer E, Monga M: Risk factors for preterm labor, *Clin Obstet Gynecol* 43(4):727–734, 2000.

Raynes-Greenow CH and others: Antibiotics for ureaplasma in the vagina in pregnancy, *Cochrane Database Syst Rev* Issue 1, 2004.

Rideout S: Tocolytics for pre-term labor, *AWHONN Lifelines*, 9(1):56–61, 2005.

Ruiz R, Fullerton J, and Brown C: The utility of fFN for the prediction of preterm birth in twin gestations, *J Obstet Gynecol Neonatal Nurs* 33(4):446–454, 2004.

Ruiz R: Mechanism of full-term and preterm labor: factors influencing uterine activity, *J Obstet Gynecol Neonatal Nurs* 27(6):652–660, 1998.

Russell R and others: The changing epidemiology of multiple births in the United States, *Obstet Gynecol* 101(1):129–135, 2002.

Sanchez-Ramos L and others: Efficacy of maintenance therapy after acute tocolysis: a meta-analysis, *Am J Obstet Gynecol* 181(2):484–490, 1999.

Sanchez-Ramos L, Kaunitz A: Reassessing the value of maintenance tocolysis in preterm labor, *Contemp OB/GYN* 46(7):45, 2001.

Simpson K, Knox G: Obstetrical accidents involving intravenous magnesium sulfate, *MCN Am J Matern Child Nurs* 29(3):161–169, 2004.

Sosa C and others: Bed rest in singleton pregnancies for preventing preterm birth, *Cochrane Database Syst Rev* Issue 1, 2004.

Stan C and others: Hydration for treatment of preterm labour, *Cochrane Database Syst Rev* Issue 2, 2002.

Svigos J, Robinson J, and Vigneswaran R: Threatened and actual preterm labor including mode of delivery. In James D and others, editors: *High risk pregnancy: management options*, ed 3, Philadelphia, 2006, Saunders.

U.S. Department of Health and Human Services: *Healthy People 2010: understanding and improving health*, Washington, DC, 2000, USDHHS.

Varma R, James D: Antenatal care of women with previous preterm delivery, *Curr Obstet Gynecol*, 4(3):207–215, 2004.

Weiner C, Buhimschi C: *Drugs for pregnant and lactating women*, Philadelphia, 2004, Churchill Livingstone.

Welsh A, Nicolaides K: Cervical screening for preterm delivery, *Curr Opin Obstet Gynecol* 14(2):195–202, 2002.

Wener M, Lavigne S: Can periodontal disease lead to premature death: How the mouth affects the body, *AWOHNN Lifelines* 8(5):424–431, 2004.

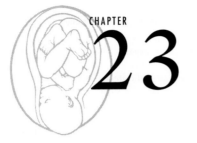

Premature Rupture of Membranes

*P*remature or *prelabor rupture of membranes* (PROM) is defined as rupture of the amniotic sac surrounding the fetus before the onset of labor. *Preterm PROM* is commonly used to refer to the rupture of the membranes when it occurs before term. The period between preterm rupture of membranes and the onset of labor is called the *latency period*. It is called *prolonged rupture of membranes* when the latency period is extended beyond 24 hours.

INCIDENCE

PROM occurs in 6% to 10% of all pregnancies, and approximately 20% of these cases occur before 36 weeks of gestation (Weitz, 2001; Mercer, 2003).

ETIOLOGY

The cause of PROM is unknown in most cases. Increased intrauterine pressure with multiple gestation and polyhydramnios, inflammatory processes such as cervicitis and amnionitis, placenta previa, abruptio placentae, abnormalities of the internal cervical os, multiple amniocenteses, and therapeutic abortions are factors sometimes associated with PROM.

It was once believed that an inherently weak fetal membrane might be a cause of PROM. However, when fetal membranes were tested after premature rupture, they were found to be just as strong as membranes from normal term deliveries (Garite, 2004). Current information reveals that a bacterial invasion often precedes and may possibly be the cause of PROM in 30% to 40% of the cases. However, this is usually related to an ascending vaginal infection and does not mean the patient has an intraamniotic infection.

Another etiologic factor for PROM is a positive history in a prior pregnancy (Garite, 2004). The risk for PROM is increased in socioeconomically disadvantaged patients; sexually promiscuous teenagers; patients who have nutritional deficiencies, especially in zinc, vitamins C and E, and copper (Perry and Strauss, 1998; Woods, Plessinger, and Miller, 2001); patients who smoke (Woods, Plessinger, and Miller, 2001); and patients with decreased immunity.

NORMAL PHYSIOLOGY

The developing fetus is protected from the outside world by two fetal membranes—the amnion, composed of five distinct layers, and the chorion, composed of three layers—which form a sac around the fetus. These membranes are thin but tough. They contain no blood vessels or nerve endings. However, they are rich in collagen, which gives them their strength and elasticity. Regulatory inhibitors control collagenolytic enzymes such as trypsin and collagenase from breaking down the collagen throughout pregnancy.

As the pregnancy nears term, a normal decrease in regulatory inhibitors and an increase in collagenolytic enzyme activity occur. Among these enzymes are relaxin and cytokines. At the same time, phospholipase enzymes are activated, which convert phospholipids to arachidonic acid, the precursor of prostaglandins. These prostaglandins initiate labor. The decrease in phospholipids creates a rubbing force between the chorion and amnion. During labor this increase in collagenolytic enzymes and the decrease in phospholipids are what normally cause the membranes to rupture.

Amniotic fluid is produced within the amniotic sac, allowing the developing fetus to float freely. The fluid is slightly alkaline (pH 7.0 to 7.5). In early pregnancy, the primary source of the fluid appears to be the amnion, which produces the amniotic fluid by actively transporting solute and passively transporting water from maternal serum to the amniotic fluid space throughout pregnancy. As pregnancy advances, fetal urine significantly contributes. By way of fetal swallowing and breathing, amniotic fluid is reabsorbed. Thus the fluid is constantly being formed and reabsorbed with replacement about every 3 hours. At 12 weeks of gestation, the average volume is 50 ml; at 20 weeks, the average volume is 400 ml. The maximum volume of 1000 ml is reached between 36 and 38 weeks.

Amniotic fluid serves many functions. It provides a medium in which the fetus can move, grow, and develop symmetrically without pressure on its delicate tissue. Blood flow is also unrestricted as blood is transported through the umbilical cord. The fluid also helps to maintain an even environmental temperature for the fetus.

Normal amniotic fluid contains an antibacterial substance, which gradually increases with gestational age until term and then decreases. The level of this antibacterial substance varies among individuals. A diet deficient in protein, zinc, and antioxidants such as vitamin C may decrease the antibacterial and antiviral activity of the amniotic fluid (Sikorski, Juszkiewicz, and Paszkowski, 1990; Brace, 1997; Connors and Merrill, 2004).

PATHOPHYSIOLOGY

Premature rupture of the fetal membranes occurs when there is focal weakening as the result of extensive changes in collagen metabolism or when the intraamniotic pressure is increased (Parry and Strauss, 1998; Woods, Plessinger, and

Miller, 2001). In the presence of many bacteria, bacterial proteases and collagenases are produced. These enzymes and the inflammatory response of neutrophils act together to decrease the collagen content of the membranes, thus focally weakening the strength and elasticity of the membranes (Garite, 2004). Bacterial proteases also activate the prostaglandin cascade.

After prolonged rupture of membranes, an intraamniotic infection often develops as the result of ascending vaginal organisms such as *Ureaplasma urealyticum, Mycoplasma hominis, Bacteroides bivius,* group B streptococci, and *Gardnerella vaginalis. Neisseria gonorrhoeae,* herpes simplex virus, cytomegalovirus, and *Candida albicans* have been implicated as well.

There are two possible mechanisms that cause an intraamniotic infection. Some patients have normal inhibitory activity of the amniotic fluid, but when large volumes of bacteria enter the amniotic cavity, they are unable to overpower the inhibitors. In other patients, inhibitory activity in the amniotic fluid may be lacking. These patients are susceptible to an intraamniotic infection if any bacteria enter the amniotic fluid.

It is also hypothesized that tissue-damaging molecules called *reactive oxygen species* (ROS) damage the integrity of the collagen, causing membrane weakening (Connors and Merrill, 2004). Overproduction of relaxin increases collagenase activity and has been linked with preterm PROM.

MATERNAL EFFECTS
Infection
If an intraamniotic infection develops as a result of rupture of membranes, it can quickly cause a serious maternal infection. This can lead to septicemia and death if not treated promptly. If maternal infection occurs, it usually develops during the postpartum period (Svigos, Robinson, and Vigneswaran, 2006).

Abruptio Placenta
Abruptio placenta also occurs more frequently in the woman with preterm PROM.

Postpartum Hemorrhage
Postpartum hemorrhage occurs more frequently related to increased retained placenta and intrauterine infection.

FETAL AND NEONATAL EFFECTS
Prematurity
Preterm PROM causes one third of all preterm births (Weitz, 2001). Before 36 weeks of gestation, respiratory distress syndrome is the main cause of morbidity and mortality of the neonate resulting from a preterm PROM (Garite, 2004; Svigos, Robinson, and Vigneswaran, 2006).

Fetal and Neonatal Infection

The incidence of fetal/neonatal sepsis is small, 2% to 4%, with the rate correlating directly with the length of time the membranes are ruptured and the gestational age. The earlier the gestation, the greater the risk for an infection (Svigos, Robinson, and Vigneswaran, 2006). If an intraamniotic infection develops, the fetus has a 15% to 20% risk for developing septicemia, pneumonia, or a urinary tract infection (Garite, 2004).

Fetal Compromise

PROM can cause fetal compromise as a result of a prolapsed cord or oligohydramnios. The cord can prolapse if the presenting part is not well engaged. If the amniotic fluid volume is affected to a large degree, pressure can be applied on the cord as the fetus moves, thereby causing fetal compromise. Seventy-five percent of patients with PROM will experience variable decelerations related to cord compression (Garite, 2004). If fetal compromise is allowed to persist for any length of time, fetal hypoxia can result, causing the anal sphincter to relax and release meconium into the amniotic fluid. Deep, gasping respiratory movements are triggered, which moves the meconium-stained amniotic fluid deep into the alveoli. Then the neonate is at risk for developing aspiration pneumonia.

Developmental Anomalies

If the membranes rupture before 23 to 26 weeks of gestation and marked oligohydramnios results, the fetus is at an increased risk (20% to 50%) for skeletal compression deformities, amniotic band syndrome, and pulmonary hypoplasia (Garite, 2004). Pulmonary hypoplasia is more common with PROM because lung development depends more on extrinsic factors such as amniotic fluid than other fetal organs. Amniotic band syndrome occurs when the fetal membranes adhere to and constrict fetal parts causing deformities (Weitz, 2001). Other developmental abnormalities associated with an early rupture are intestinal obstruction, diaphragmatic hernia, clubfoot, scoliosis, and hip dislocation (Weitz, 2001; Mercer, 2003).

DIAGNOSTIC TESTING

Sterile Speculum Examination

When PROM is suspected, a sterile speculum examination is done. If amniotic fluid is observed leaking from the cervix and collecting in the posterior fornix of the vagina, an accurate diagnosis of PROM can be made. A digital vaginal examination should *never* be done if any attempt is to be made in delaying the labor. Vaginal bacteria could be transported into the cervical canal from the vaginal examination, thereby increasing the risk for an intraamniotic infection and thus precipitating early delivery.

Nitrazine Test

If there is no visual sign of loss of amniotic fluid from the cervix, the secretions of the posterior fornix of the vagina should be tested with Nitrazine paper for pH determination. Because amniotic fluid is alkaline and vaginal secretions are acidic, the Nitrazine paper turns blue in the presence of amniotic fluid. Blood, cervical mucus, and povidone-iodine (Betadine) should not be allowed to contaminate the specimen; they are also alkaline.

Microscopic Examination

A small amount of the fluid should then be spread on a slide and allowed to dry. Microscopic examination of dried amniotic fluid shows a fernlike pattern because of the fluid's concentration of salt.

USUAL MEDICAL MANAGEMENT AND PROTOCOLS FOR NURSE PRACTITIONERS

The treatment of PROM is one of the most controversial subjects in obstetrics today because of conflicting scientific research. Management generally depends on variables such as gestational age, presence of fetal stress, presence of maternal or fetal infection, and presence of labor.

Documentation of Fetal Age

Gestational age is usually verified with review of prenatal records and ultrasounds. If this information is unavailable because of late prenatal care, the biparietal diameter may not be accurately determined because the head is low in the pelvis. In this case, femur length, abdominal circumference, or both are used.

Fetal Maturity Assessment

Fetal lung maturity can be determined in one of two ways. First, the amniotic fluid from the vaginal pool can be tested for phosphatidyl glycerol (PG); if PG is present, fetal lung maturity is probable (Garite, 2004; Svigos, Robinson, and Vigneswaran, 2006). Second, fetal lung maturity can be determined by collecting amniotic fluid through amniocentesis and evaluating for lecithin/sphingomyelin (L/S) ratio. An L/S ratio of 1:8 to 2:1 indicates probable lung maturity.

It may be difficult to collect fluid by amniocentesis if the leak is large. Amniocentesis may be facilitated by having the patient drink large amounts of fluids and having her remain in the Trendelenburg position for a period of time before the procedure. Fluid collected by amniocentesis is less likely than that collected from vaginal pooling to be contaminated by blood, which can create false-positive results. It may then be determined solely by the presence of PG. If lung maturity is positive, delivery is the management decision of choice.

Assessment of Fetal Stressors

Fetal heart rate (FHR) monitoring, fetal movement monitoring, nonstress tests (NSTs), biophysical profiles (BBPs), and amniotic fluid index (AFI) are used to determine fetal compromise in the presence of PROM. Fetal compromise may result from cord compression caused by oligohydramnios. This would manifest itself as variable decelerations of the FHR. Decreased fetal movements may indicate an infected fetus because an infected fetus is usually lethargic. A reactive NST indicates an uninfected fetus.

In the presence of a nonreactive NST, further testing should be done because of the high false-positive rate of this test (Garite, 2004). The fetal BBP and AFI have been used to detect early signs of an intraamniotic infection after PROM. Late decelerations accompanying variable decelerations may indicate a coexistent abruption.

Assessment of Intraamniotic Infection

Maternal fever, maternal and fetal tachycardia, uterine tenderness, and an elevated maternal white blood cell count are earlier clinical indicators of an intraamniotic infection. Fetal heart rate reactivity can be used as a screening assessment. Nonreactive fetal heart rate is associated with an intraamniotic infection. Laboratory tests such as serial white blood cell differential and C-reactive protein estimates coupled with weekly vaginal cultures can facilitate diagnosis of an intraamniotic infection. Daily BBPs to assess for a subclinical infection are used. Some obstetricians take a culture of the amniotic fluid by way of an amniocentesis. The amniotic fluid is then tested for bacteria by doing a Gram stain and glucose level (Garite, 2004).

Assessment of Signs of Labor

If the fetal membranes rupture before the onset of labor at term, 70% will begin labor within 24 hours (Parry and Strauss, 1998). The latency period after preterm PROM decreases inversely with gestational age; therefore the earlier the gestation, the longer the latency period.

Expectant Management Before 34 Weeks of Gestation

When the fetus is not mature, there are no signs of infection, and when no fetal compromise is identified, expectant management consisting of bedrest with bathroom privileges and observation for signs of infection and fetal compromise is the preferred treatment. This is done in the hope that, by lengthening the pregnancy, fetal lungs may mature and the risk for respiratory distress will decrease in the neonate. It is currently recommended that prophylactic antibiotics and corticosteroids be implemented during expectant management of preterm ROM. The use of tocolytics is very controversial.

Before 23 weeks of gestation, care must be individualized because of the very early gestation, as well as the risk for maternal infection and fetal developmental abnormalities. Most providers inform and involve parents in the decision-making process (Mercer, 2003; Garite, 2004; ICSI, 2005).

Expectant Management After 34 Weeks of Gestation

The preferred treatment of term PROM is delivery. According to *The Cochrane Review* (Dare and others, 2006), the woman with gestational rupture of membranes at 34 to 36 weeks should be allowed to choose between labor induction and expectant management after presentation of the risks and benefits of both options. The benefits of induction with oxytocin or prosta-glandin have been demonstrated, through research results, to lower the risk for chorioamnionitis and neonatal infection as well as decrease the length of stay in the neonatal intensive care setting without increased risk for cesarean birth or operative vaginal birth. The risks associated with induction were increased use of epidural analgesia at an early stage of labor dilation, use of anesthesia or analgesia, and use of internal FHR monitoring in the presence of prolonged rupture of membranes (Wilkes and Galan, 2004).

Variations in Management

Prophylactic Antibiotic Therapy

According to *The Cochrane Review* (Kenyon, Boulvain, and Neilson, 2003, 2004), the use of antibiotic therapy to prevent an ascending infection in patients with preterm PROM has been shown to lengthen the latency period, decrease the incidence of chorioamnionitis, decrease postpartum maternal endometritis, and decrease neonatal morbidity related to sepsis, pneumonia, RDS, and necrotizing enterocolitis. One protocol is ampicillin and erythromycin intrave-nously for 48 hours, followed by oral amoxicillin (250 mg orally every 8 hours) and erythromycin (333 mg orally every 8 hours) for 5 days (Kenyon, Boulvain, and Neilson, 2003; Mercer, 2003). This regimen does not always treat group B strep. The intrapartum prophylaxis therapy for prevention of neonatal GBS infection should still be followed as outlined by the Centers for Disease Control and Prevention (see below and Chapter 25).

Corticosteroids

Antenatal corticosteroids in women with preterm PROM at less than 34 weeks of gestation, in the absence of chorioamnionitis, is recommended according to the National Institutes of Health (NIH, 2000). Antenatal corticosteroids have been shown to significantly reduce respiratory distress syndrome and intraven-tricular hemorrhage in the neonate. The treatment consists of a single course of betamethasone or dexamethasone. For betamethasone dosing, give two doses of 12 mg intramuscularly 24 hours apart. For dexamethasone dosing give four doses of 6 mg intramuscularly 12 hours apart (NIH, 2000). There are insuffi-cient scientific data from randomized clinical control trials to recommend repeat courses of corticosteroids routinely (NIH, 2000).

Tocolysis

The use of tocolysis in the presence of PROM is controversial. Tocolytic agents are less effective when membranes are ruptured, and they may increase the risk for or mask the signs of an intrauterine infection (Garite, 2004). According to ICSI (2005), if tocolytics are used, they should be used to facilitate transfer, only long enough to allow sufficient time for gestational age and other assess-ments to be completed, for antibiotics to take effect, or if corticosteroids are used, for there to be sufficient time to have any benefit. (See Chapter 22 for further discussion of drug therapies.)

Intrapartum Prophylaxis for Group B Streptococcus (GBS)

The benefit of narrow-spectrum intrapartum prophylaxis with either intravenous penicillin or ampicillin to prevent transmission of GBS to the neonate is well documented. In the presence of rupture of membranes for 18 hours or more, with unknown GBS status, intrapartum antibiotic prophylaxis is indicated (CDC, 2002).

NURSING MANAGEMENT

Prevention

Because the actual cause of PROM is unknown, prevention is difficult. However, it may be helpful to look at the risk factors and guard against these during pregnancy. Statistics indicate that socioeconomically disadvantaged patients and teenagers have an increased risk for PROM. The reason for this is unknown, but nutrition probably plays an important role. Therefore these patients should be instructed early in pregnancy regarding a healthful diet for pregnancy and should be provided with reasons to follow this diet. They may also need referral to sources of financial assistance and food supplement programs, as well as instruction in how to prepare nutritious foods.

Cleanliness can also be a factor in decreasing the risk for PROM; vaginal bacterial flora should be kept to a minimum. Daily bathing and wiping the perineum from front to back are important prenatal instructions. Multiple sexual relationships also increase the vaginal bacterial count and should be avoided.

Any attempt to facilitate increased immunity against infection is beneficial. Therefore maintaining cleanliness, drinking 6 to 8 ounces of fluid per waking hour, exercising daily, resting adequately to avoid fatigue, and eating an adequate diet that is high in protein, zinc, and antioxidants are all beneficial in guarding against PROM.

A relationship between smoking and PROM has been demonstrated in numerous studies. Therefore patients who smoke while pregnant should be instructed regarding its effect on pregnancy and should be supported in their attempts to stop smoking.

All pregnant women should be instructed regarding the danger signs in pregnancy, and PROM should be pointed out as one of these signs. The signs of membrane rupture and the necessity of prompt notification if these signs occur should be explained early in prenatal care.

Nursing Interventions to Decrease the Risk for Infection After PROM

- Assess and prove membrane rupture by a sterile speculum examination (two out of three positive tests proving positive); by positive pooling; by positive ferning on collected slide specimen when viewed under a microscope; or by Nitrazine-positive result (turns from yellow to blue).
- Assess temperature every 4 hours or as indicated. (Maternal fever is one of the earlier signs of an intraamniotic infection.)

- Assess maternal pulse and blood pressure as indicated. (Tachycardia is one of the earlier signs of an intraamniotic infection.)
- Assess FHR as indicated. (Fetal tachycardia is one of the earlier signs of an intraamniotic infection.)
- Assess vaginal discharge for odor or color change.
- Assess for uterine tenderness.
- Assess for signs of a urinary tract infection.
- Determine nutritional habits.
- Determine activities since PROM.
- Refer to such diagnostic data as white blood cell count and C-reactive protein. A white blood cell count above $18,000/mm^3$ is a significant sign of an infection during pregnancy. A normal C-reactive protein level is a valuable predictor of no intraamniotic infection.
- Assist in obtaining vaginal and urethral cultures for group B streptococci, chlamydia, and gonococcus. If any of these organisms is present, be prepared to start antibiotic therapy to decrease neonatal infection risk. (Group B streptococcus is the most common cause of neonatal sepsis.)
- Assist with an amniocentesis to measure for gram-positive bacteria.
- Teach the benefits of bedrest with bathroom privileges only.
- Teach the importance of perineal care after each voiding and stool.
- Perform no vaginal examinations until the patient is in active labor.
- If patient is discharged home, instruct regarding having no intercourse, doing no douching, taking temperature twice daily, taking showers only, notifying the physician if temperature is more than 38° C or if amniotic fluid loss increases or becomes foul-smelling, and returning to the clinical laboratory for a white blood cell count twice weekly.
- Notify the provider if temperature is greater than 38° C, fetal or maternal tachycardia develops, foul-smelling amniotic fluid develops, or amniotic fluid changes from straw color.
- If signs of an intraamniotic infection are manifested, be prepared to begin broad-spectrum antibiotic therapy, such as penicillin G and gentamicin, ampicillin and gentamicin, or cephalosporin. If the patient has a cesarean delivery, clindamycin may also be administered.

Nursing Interventions to Decrease Impaired Fetal Gas Exchange

- Continuously monitor FHR initially for about 48 to 72 hours after membrane rupture, to rule out fetal stressors.
- Assess maternal temperature, palpable abdominal tenderness unassociated with contractions, purulent vaginal discharge.
- During expectant management, periodically monitor FHR for variable decelerations and fetal activity.
- Observe amount of amniotic fluid that is being lost.
- Reposition mother, and administer oxygen by mask if variable decelerations occur.
- Instruct patient to report any decrease in fetal activity.

- Prepare the patient for ordered fetal well-being and maturity studies. BBPs, ultrasound, NSTs, AFI, and amniocentesis are usually ordered on a frequent basis in an attempt to determine the optimal time for delivery.
- Notify physician if a baseline or periodic FHR change occurs, an NST is nonreactive, or a BBP of 6 or less is noted.

Nursing Interventions to Decrease Fear and Stress

- Assess family's anxiety over maternal, fetal, and neonatal well-being.
- Assess family's coping strategies and resources.
- Encourage expectant parents to communicate openly about their feelings and concerns.
- Clarify any misconceptions.
- Provide information to the patient and her family regarding the pregnancy complication, treatment plan, and implications for mother and fetus in understandable terms.
- Arrange a tour of the intensive care nursery in the event of a possible preterm delivery.
- Refer to the social worker if inadequate coping is noted.
- Refer to pastor, priest, or chaplain per parents' request.

Nursing Interventions to Promote Prescribed Bedrest

- Assess the patient's responsibilities to determine difficulties she will have in implementing prescribed bedrest.
- Teach the patient and her family about the importance of bedrest in the lateral position.
- Facilitate the family in problem solving if difficulties arise in implementing bedrest.
- Make needed referrals (for example, to the social worker) if problems are identified.
- Encourage patient's participation in her own care and decision making as much as possible.
- Assess for side effects of prolonged bedrest and implement therapeutic interventions as outlined in Chapter 22.

Nursing Interventions to Decrease Other Antepartum Complications

- Assess for signs of preterm labor.
- Administer tocolytics if ordered.
- Provide routine prenatal education and care, as well as education for special care needs of a premature infant.

Intrapartum Nursing Interventions

- Use continuous fetal monitoring for early detection of nonreassuring FHR changes.
- Be prepared to administer intrapartum prophylaxis for group B streptococcus if vaginal and rectum culture is positive or unknown.

- Assess amniotic fluid for meconium.
- Reposition patient, administer oxygen by mask at 8 to 10 L, and increase the intravenous fluid rate if variable decelerations occur.
- Be prepared to manage a saline amnioinfusion if multiple variable decelerations occur related to decreased amniotic fluid. Refer to Chapter 29 for the nursing interventions.
- Notify the physician at the first signs of a nonreassuring FHR change.
- Once delivery is imminent, notify the intensive care nursery of a possible high risk infant.

CONCLUSION

Because infections and lower amniotic fluid immunity play a significant role in PROM, the ultimate goal of the nurse should be to educate the patient. Prenatal education should cover the need for adequate fluids and nutrition, appropriate hygiene, and the significance of reporting any signs of an infection immediately. This decreases the risk for PROM. Once the membranes rupture, the goal of treatment is to allow for fetal maturity by maintaining the pregnancy as long as the uterine environment is healthy. If the uterine environment becomes infected or causes fetal compromise, the fetal outcome may be improved by premature delivery.

BIBLIOGRAPHY

Brace R: Physiology of amniotic fluid volume regulation, *Clin Obstet Gynecol* 40(2):280–289, 1997.

Centers for Disease Control and Prevention: Prevention of perinatal group B streptococcal disease: revised guidelines from CDC, *MMWR Morb Mortal Wkly Rep* 51:RR–11, 2002.

Connors N, Merrill D: Antioxidants for prevention of preterm delivery, *Clin Obstet Gynecol* 47(4):822–832, 2004.

Dare MR and others: Planned early birth versus expectant management (waiting) for prelabour rupture of membranes at term (37 weeks or more), *Cochrane Database Syst Rev* Issue 1, 2006.

Garite T: Premature rupture of membranes. In Creasy R, Resnik R, and Iams J, editors: *Maternal-fetal medicine: principles and practice*, ed 5, Philadelphia, 2004, Saunders.

Institute for Clinical Systems Improvement (ICSI): *Management of labor.* Bloomington, Minn, 2005, ICSI, 73 p. Retrieved from *http://www.guideline.gov*

Kenyon S, Boulvain M, and Neilson J: Antibiotics for preterm rupture of membranes: a systematic review, *Obstet Gynecol* 104(5 Pt 1):1051–1057, 2004.

Kenyon S, Boulvain M, and Neilson J: Antibiotics for preterm rupture of membranes, *Cochrane Database Syst Rev* Issue 2, 2003.

Mercer B: Preterm premature rupture of the membranes, *Obstet Gynecol* 101(1):178–193, 2003.

National Institutes of Health (NIH): *Antenatal corticosteroids revisited.* Consensus development conference statement, Maryland, 2000, NIH. Retrieved from *http://www.consensus.nih.gov*

Parry S, Strauss J: Premature rupture of fetal membranes, *N Engl J Med* 338(10):663–670, 1998.

Svigos J, Robinson J, and Vigneswaran R: Prelabor rupture of membranes. In James D and others, editors: *High risk pregnancy: management options*, ed 3, Philadelphia, 2006, Saunders.

Sikorski R, Juszkiewicz T, and Paszkowski T: Zinc status in women with premature rupture of membranes at term, *Obstet Gynecol* 76(4):675–677, 1990.

Stringer M and others: Nursing care of the patient with preterm premature rupture of membranes, *MCN Am J Matern Child Nurs* 29(3):142–150, 2004.

Weitz B: Premature rupture of membranes: an update for advanced practice nurse, *MCN Am J Matern Child Nurs* 26(2):86–92, 2001.

Wilkes P, Galan H: Premature rupture of membranes, *Emedicine.com, Inc*, 2004.

Woods J, Plessinger M, and Miller R: Vitamins C and E: missing links in preventing preterm premature rupture of membranes? *Am J Obstet Gynecol* 185(1):5–10, 2001.

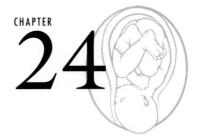

CHAPTER

24

Trauma

T
rauma during pregnancy varies in degree and causation. It is caused by motor vehicle accidents (MVAs), accidental injury, and domestic violence. An estimated 7% of all pregnant women suffer some type of trauma during their pregnancy, and trauma is the leading cause of nonobstetric maternal death (Grossman, 2004a). The frequency of injury increases with each trimester; therefore, the highest risk for injury is in the third trimester. Trauma causes death of the fetus more often than death of the mother (Bobrowski, 2006).

When pregnancy is complicated by trauma, providers who are not routinely accustomed to problems associated with trauma may provide emergency care in a variety of settings outside trauma units, including obstetric units and outpatient settings. In addition, trauma teams in emergency centers are often unfamiliar with some of the physiologic considerations specific to pregnancy and with caring for a second, invisible patient (the fetus).

INCIDENCE

Statistics support recognition of trauma as a significant complication in pregnancy:
- Seven percent of pregnant women seek medical care for trauma-related injury (Grossman, 2004a).
- It is more common for trauma to occur during the third trimester.
- Of all injuries during pregnancy, 54% are from MVAs; 70% of the major, life-threatening injuries are from MVAs (Divekar and Keith, 2004).
- Approximately 25% to 30% of pregnant women are physically or sexually abused (Guth and Pachter, 2000; Hedin and Janson, 2000) but only 3% to 8% of these abuses are detected (Cox, Kilpatrick, and Geller, 2004; FVPF, 2004).

ETIOLOGY

MVA and domestic violence are the leading causes of maternal trauma during pregnancy, and MVAs lead to the most deaths (FVPF, 2004; Grossman, 2004a; Chang and others, 2005). Falls, burns, and penetrating injuries, such

535

as stabbing and gunshot wounds (Pearlman and others, 2000), are also significant causes of maternal and fetal trauma.

Battering is reported as a source of serious injury during pregnancy, but it is difficult to acquire specific statistics because these crimes are generally underreported. Abuse can be physical, emotional, or sexual; it can also be in the form of economic abuse or isolation. The cause of domestic violence and abuse involves the need for the partner in a domestic relationship to exert power and control over the pregnant woman.

Violent assaults and suicide are other causes of maternal death from trauma. Most of the maternal deaths from trauma of this type are the result of head trauma or intraabdominal hemorrhage.

Normal Physiology

A thorough review of maternal physiologic adaptations is provided in Chapter 1.

Pathophysiology

The pathophysiology to be considered obviously depends on the type of injury, the source of injury, and the system or part of the body affected. Because head injury and abdominal hemorrhage are the most common lethal maternal effects, discussion of pathophysiology focuses on both. The adverse fetal effects of preterm labor, delivery, abruption, preterm rupture of membranes (PROM), and intrauterine death are conditions reviewed in Chapters 15 to 18, 22, and 23.

Hemorrhage

Because of the total blood volume increase during pregnancy, trauma involving abdominal hemorrhage has profound hemodynamic consequences that place the pregnant woman at much greater risk than a nonpregnant counterpart. These consequences include the following (Grossman, 2004a; Bobowski, 2005):

- By 32 to 34 weeks of gestation, there is an average of 50% blood volume increase. Because clinical signs of shock usually present as a function of percentage of total blood loss, the pregnant patient has a greater absolute amount of blood loss than a nonpregnant person in a similar state. Thus a larger amount of blood replacement is needed in resuscitative efforts.
- Because of the increased blood volume available to her, the pregnant woman may be able to more readily, although temporarily, maintain hemodynamic stability at the expense of the fetus. Reflex, compensatory, vasoconstrictive responses can significantly decrease uteroplacental perfusion, compromising the fetal compartment.
- Although cardiac output is increased by 30% to 40% near term, supine positioning is likely to confuse the general picture of potential shock by enhancing hypotension. Supine positioning decreases cardiac output secondary to decreased cardiac return from mechanical obstruction of the inferior vena cava by the gravid uterus.
- Because the pregnant woman's heart rate is already increased by approximately 10 to 15 beats/min and blood pressure falls in the second trimester, these two parameters may confuse the clinical picture for the provider

who is unfamiliar with normal, physiologic, hemodynamic alterations in pregnancy.

- When the gravid abdomen sustains trauma, both the uterus, with its increased circulating volume, and the bladder are more anatomically prone to injury. Abdominal injury adds an additional risk for significant maternal hemorrhage secondary to placental abruption.

- The kidneys and ureters are relatively protected from injury by the uterus. However, normal dilation of the ureters may be misinterpreted on radiologic examination of the abdomen following injury.

- Anatomically, the bowel is pushed upward and is more prominent during pregnancy. As a result, the small and large intestines are at greater risk for injury from blunt or penetrating trauma.

- Because pregnancy is a hypercoagulable state, risks for thrombosis after injury are increased.

- Disseminated intravascular coagulopathy (DIC), a frequent complication of severe abdominal trauma, may also present atypically. Normal fibrinogen level in pregnancy is four to five times the nonpregnant level. As a result, the lower nonpregnant levels, when applied to pregnant women, may signify early DIC. (See Chapters 18 and 19 for signs and symptoms of shock, DIC, and placental abruption.)

Neurologic Injury

Head injury is often severe enough to result in maternal death. No significant neurophysiologic adaptations in pregnancy alter presentation of the clinical picture. However, if maternal brain death occurs, the fetus may remain viable. Therefore, maternal brain death needs to be considered from an ethical perspective because of the presence of the fetus.

Brain death is the unequivocal and irreversible loss of total brain function. It is a concept used to determine when death has occurred even though cardiopulmonary resuscitation (CPR) and life support technology obscure the conventional criteria for diagnosis of life or death. Once the diagnosis of brain death is made, cardiopulmonary collapse may be expected within 72 hours. In any situation in which brain death has occurred, it is generally considered unethical to squander costly medical resources to continue to support life with artificial means. However, even if the woman has given an advance directive for removal of life support in such a situation, maternal brain death presents a case for continued artificial support for the sake of the fetus. The new, advance directive law (see Chapter 8) does not change this.

Spinal cord injury is another type of neurologic injury that can have pathophysiologic consequences in the pregnant woman. When spinal cord injury occurs during the course of an established pregnancy, the following complications may occur (Carbuapoma, Tomlinson, and Levine, 2006).

With lesions above the tenth thoracic segment, the woman will not note onset of abdominal pain or discomfort. Because of the caudal entrance of the afferent uterine nerves, the nerve supply to the uterus is interrupted. Thus the uterus can contract normally, but there is an absence of associated pain sensation with onset of labor contractions.

Complete cord lesions above the fifth or sixth thoracic segment, above the splanchnic outflow, may cause the development of the syndrome of hyperreflexia with the onset of contractions.

Signs and symptoms of hyperreflexia are caused by the sudden release of catecholamines. These include throbbing headache, hypertension, reflex brady-cardia, sweating, nasal congestion, and vasodilation.

Chest Injury

Physiologic adaptations in respiratory functions may confuse the understanding of the pathophysiology of chest injury and confound resuscitative efforts. During pregnancy there is increased oxygen (O_2) consumption, increased tidal volume, decreased arterial carbon dioxide partial pressure (PCO_2), and decreased serum bicarbonate. Chronic, compensatory respiratory alkalosis may mislead the resuscitation team in evaluation of blood gases. Blood buffering capabilities decrease during pregnancy; therefore reestablishing acid-base homeostasis is more difficult.

Pelvic Fractures

The major complications of pelvic fractures include retroperitoneal bleeding and placental abruption in the pregnant woman. The pelvis usually fractures in two places in the bony ring. If the fetal head is engaged, fetal skull fracture may occur.

Thermal (Burn) Trauma

Classification of thermal injury is according to the percentage of the body burned, the depth involved, and gestational age. If more than 60% of the body is affected, there is significant risk for maternal death. Because of the normally hypervolemic state in pregnancy, fluid resuscitation must be vigorous, with prompt evaluation and correction of electrolyte imbalance. Maternal sepsis secondary to burns can lead to intrauterine death or fetal compromise.

SIGNS AND SYMPTOMS

Signs and symptoms of complications of trauma are given in Chapters 12, 13, 15, 18, 19, 22, and 23. Signs of domestic violence or abuse include the following:

- Delayed prenatal care
- Frequent visits to emergency units
- Recurrent or unexplained chronic pain or vague complaints of fatigue, depression, or difficulty swallowing without apparent etiology
- Unexplained injuries or injuries at different stages of healing
- Very low self-esteem or flattened affect
- Jealous or possessive partner
- Partner speaking for the patient, acting overprotective, or refusing to leave the room for any part of examination or interview

MATERNAL EFFECTS

Trauma is the leading cause of nonobstetric maternal death from head injury, hemorrhage, shock, DIC, respiratory compromise, cardiopulmonary arrest, or syndrome of hyperreflexia with spinal cord injury. With blunt abdominal trauma, injury to the liver or spleen can occur, causing severe hemorrhage. Indirect injury due to abuse during pregnancy can have indirect adverse effects as well, including causing chronic health problems such as depression, substance abuse, delayed prenatal care, and inadequate nutrition (ANA, 2000).

FETAL EFFECTS

The fetus is extremely vulnerable to the effects of maternal trauma, especially blunt or penetrating trauma to the abdomen (Bobowski, 2006). Once trauma has occurred, maternal shock is the leading cause of fetal death; the second most common cause is abruptio placenta, which can occur without a direct blow to the abdomen (Bryan and Bledsoe, 2002; Grossman, 2004a). Abruptio placenta is the most common cause of fetal death when the mother survives (Divekar and Keith, 2004). There is a 40% to 50% risk for an abruption following severe trauma or blunt abdominal trauma. There is also a 5% risk following a minor injury. Other common fetal effects include the following:

- PROM
- Premature labor and delivery
- Spontaneous abortion or stillbirth
- Fetal maternal transfusion
- Fetal skull injuries, especially when the fetal head is engaged and there is a maternal pelvic fracture
- Hypoxic compromise secondary to maternal respiratory embarrassment, shock, DIC, thermal injury, or maternal cardiopulmonary arrest

MEDICAL DIAGNOSIS AND USUAL TRAUMA MANAGEMENT

Minor Injury Management

A minor injury may be described as losing one's balance and falling, with or without a blow to the abdomen. It may also be described as a minor MVA with no obvious injuries or marks, but in which some degree of jarring occurred. After a minor injury, the initial assessment usually takes place in the trauma unit, emergency department, or obstetric triage unit. The following areas should be covered in the initial assessment:

- History of the circumstances surrounding the incident
- Diagnostic tests and procedures as dictated by the initial injury
- Monitoring of mother and fetus for contractions and fetal heart rate (FHR) if 20 weeks of gestation or more
- Follow-up evaluation for occult abruption with continuous fetal monitoring usually for a minimum of 6 to 8 hours and a Kleihauer-Betke test for fetal to maternal hemorrhage

Major Injury Management

Immediately after major trauma, diagnosis and treatment occur almost simultaneously in three phases.

Initial Care Phase

The initial response to a major trauma usually involves two teams, each with members assigned to very specific and limited components of care. The A team, or first team, focuses on the mother and responds immediately, begins an assessment, and sets priorities for stabilization management. Their focus is on identification of immediate life-threatening injuries and is directed at assessment of airway, breathing, and circulation for the mother. Neurologic injuries, especially head injuries, should next be evaluated as appropriate depending on the type of injury.

As soon as the initial assessment is done, the A team moves out of the way and the B team moves in to focus on the fetus and pregnancy-related issues. Next, the A team reevaluates the effects of resuscitation efforts for the mother. Finally, the B team reevaluates resuscitation of the mother as it affects the fetus. The specific efforts of each team are directed toward immediate stabilization and basic life support resuscitation. (See Table 24-1 for a summary of management of the pregnant patient after major trauma. The acronym *TRAUMA* is used to summarize priorities for immediate management and stabilization.)

Resuscitation

The standard CPR procedure should be followed with a pregnant woman. There is increased likelihood that artificial ventilation will be needed because of the anatomic shift of the diaphragm. The patient should be tilted or positioned laterally to prevent supine hypotension. Certain modifications to the conventional CPR procedures should be considered:

- *Vasopressor drugs.* Avoid use of vasopressor drugs such as epinephrine, dopamine, or norepinephrine bitartrate; these cause vasoconstriction of the placental bed. Epinephrine is a better choice when fetal outcome is also a high priority because it enhances placental blood flow.
- *Antidysrhythmics.* Lidocaine hydrochloride does not appear to cross the placenta and may be helpful in treating some dysrhythmias. Other antidysrhythmics may be toxic to the fetus.
- *Open heart massage.* If circulatory function is not restored after 5 to 10 minutes, open heart massage may be needed with an emergency cesarean performed once fetal viability is established by ultrasound.
- *Defibrillation.* If defibrillation is necessary and a fetal spiral electrode is being used to monitor the FHR, the wires should be disconnected from the leg plate to reduce the risk for conducting through the fetal spiral electrode to the fetus.
- *Fluid replacement.* Give vigorous and aggressive fluid replacement.
- *Perimortem.* If maternal resuscitation efforts are not successful after 15 minutes, a perimortem (agonal or postmortem) cesarean delivery should be done unless the fetus is no longer viable or less than 23 weeks of gestation.

Table 24-1   Priorities for Perinatal TRAUMA Management

Activity	Team A (Mother)	Team B (Fetus)

T = Triage*	Assess ABCs
	  Airway
	  Breathing
	  Circulation
		Assess fetus
		  Cardiac activity
		  Gestational age
		Assess placenta for
		  abruption

R = Resuscitation	Perform CPR
	Infuse crystalloid fluids
	Administer oxygen at 8–10 L/
	  min by mask
	Administer blood as indicated
	  (in emergency situation,
	  O-negative blood can be
	  used)
		Position mother in left lateral
		  tilt
		Kleihauer-Betke test may be
		  done to rule out fetal
		  hemorrhage

A = Assessment	Assess for maternal injuries
	  (similar to nonpregnant
	  patients)
	Assess vital signs; level of
	  consciousness; respiratory
	  status as to depth,
	  irregularity, and breath
	  sounds
		Assess FHR and uterine
		  contractions with EFM
		
		Assess for vaginal bleeding
		  and rupture of membranes

U = Ultrasound
and uterine
evaluation
	Evaluate uterine cavity for
	  hemorrhage
		Evaluate fundal height
		Palpate for uterine
		  tenderness, contractions,
		  or irritability
		Ultrasound may be done to
		  determine placental or
		  fetal injury and placental
		  location
		Amniocentesis may be done
		  to assess fetal lung
		  maturity or intrauterine
		  bleeding

M = Management
and monitor
	Decide initial management
	  and needed continual
	  monitoring
		Decide to monitor or deliver
		  depending on status of
		  mother and fetus and risk
		  for prematurity

A = Activate
transport/
transfer
	After stabilization, transport/
	  transfer to critical care,
	  operating suite, or level III
	  perinatal unit
		Activate neonatal team for
		  consultation, transfer, or
		  transport as necessary

CPR, Cardiopulmonary resuscitation; *EFM*, electronic fetal monitor; *FHR*, fetal heart rate.
*Mother is first priority, then fetus.

Continued Care Phase

Although initial emergency assessment and stabilization may be carried out in any level trauma center, emergency department, or surgical service, continued maternal care for serious trauma commonly is delivered in critical care units.

If the mother is pronounced dead and the fetus is older than 24 weeks of gestation and alive, a cesarean delivery is performed. If the mother is brain-dead, she may be kept on life support until the fetus has an opportunity to grow to maturity.

Recovery and Rehabilitation Phase

During the recovery and rehabilitation phase, assessments are directed at identification of potential long-term complications and sequelae. Interventions during this phase are focused on restoration of optimal functional capabilities.

NURSING MANAGEMENT

Prevention

All pregnant women should be made aware of their potential for injuries and trauma and ways to prevent them, especially those related to MVAs and domestic violence and abuse. Prevention of violence against women is one of the top priority health issues for the United States as identified in the *Healthy People 2010* report (USDHHS, 2000). Association between domestic violence and 8 of the 10 leading health indicators of the federal Healthy People 2010 initiative have been recognized (FVPF, 2003) These indicators are obesity, tobacco use, substance abuse, responsible sexual behavior, mental health, injury, immunization, and access to health care.

Motor Vehicle Accident Prevention

Efforts to teach and demonstrate safe and consistent use of car safety belts can have a major impact on the degree of injury, especially blunt trauma to the abdomen. Every pregnant patient should be taught that the seat belt harness should be used, no matter how short the trip. The current recommendation for seat belt use during pregnancy is for the shoulder strap to cross between the breasts and over the upper abdomen above the uterus. The lap belt should cross over the pelvis below the uterus (McGwin and others, 2004; Grossman, 2004b). A discussion of the pregnant woman's vulnerability should include encouragement to avoid fatigue, avoid late departures, and avoid distractions such as loud music, cell phones, and arguing children.

The major risk in an MVA is from the impact and resultant momentum causing gross traumatic separation of the placenta from the wall of the uterus. If a small amount separates at the beginning, the signs may occur slowly and insidiously (an occult abruption) or quickly (an overt massive separation), usually accompanied by obvious signs of shock and hemorrhage (Harris, 2001).

Other Accidental Injuries

Pregnant women should be made aware of sources of injury, such as falls resulting from the displaced center of gravity or increased joint flexibility.

Domestic Violence Prevention

Routine prenatal care should include an assessment for physical or sexual abuse (ICSI, 2003). Families that are known to be at risk should be observed and provided preventive intervention as needed, such as referral for stress reduction, emotional support, improving communication, and improving interpersonal relationships. Battering during pregnancy is a significant health risk and hazard. Therefore an environment friendly and conducive to disclosure should be established in every obstetric care setting. Ways to accomplish this include the following:

- Place posters and brochures in accessible areas in the health care setting such as in the waiting room, in the bathrooms, and near the scales.
- Ensure privacy during the screening assessment.
- Have referral information available.

According to Dunn and Oths (2004), prenatal predictors of domestic violence are:

- Stressful life
- Depression
- Lack of spiritual values
- Lack of contraceptive use

An abuse assessment screen that can be reproduced was developed by the Nursing Research Consortium on Violence and Abuse (Parker, McFarlane, and Soeken, 1994; Christian, 1995; Norton and others, 1995). The assessment screen includes four basic questions and a scoring system for the degree of threat pertaining to specific types of abuse. It is important to construct the questions in a comfortable manner and in a setting likely to encourage disclosure from the patient. You may formulate the questions below into a less formalized questionnaire or use a preprinted form with an explanation that makes the patient feel comfortable, cared about, and not singled out—for example, "This is a questionnaire we have found helpful in assessing all our patients so that we are better able to help keep you and your baby healthy." Most assessment tools include the following questions:

- Has your partner or someone important to you ever emotionally or physically abused you?
- Within the last year, have you been hit, slapped, kicked, or otherwise physically hurt by someone?
- Since you have been pregnant, have you been hit, slapped, or otherwise physically hurt by someone?
- Are you afraid of your partner or anyone else listed above?

Perinatal nurses should screen all pregnant women at the earliest opportunity and again at intervals during the pregnancy. Box 24-1 presents an abuse assessment screening tool. Pregnant women who are battered need education,

Box 24-1 Abuse Assessment Screen

Assessment Questionnaire

Have you ever been emotionally or physically abused by your partner or someone important to you?
- Yes or ▪ No

Within the last year, have you been hit, slapped, kicked, or otherwise physically hurt by someone?
- Yes or ▪ No

If yes, by whom? _____

Total number of times? _____

Since you have become pregnant, have you been hit, slapped, kicked, or otherwise physically hurt by someone?
- Yes or ▪ No

If yes, by whom? _____

Total number of times? _____

Are you afraid of your partner or anyone you have already mentioned?
- Yes or ▪ No

Reference: Christian A: Home care of the battered pregnant woman: one woman's battered pregnancy, *J Obstet Gynecol Neonatal Nurs* 24(9):836–842, 1995; Norton L and others: Battering in pregnancy: an assessment of tool screening methods, *Obstet Gynecol* 85(3):321–325, 1995; Parker B, McFarlane J, Soeken K: Abuse during pregnancy: effects on maternal complications and birth weight in adult and teenage women, *Obstet Gynecol* 84(3):323–328, 1994.

support, and intervention to break the cycle of abuse that includes an immediate risk assessment and safety plan. A new Danger Assessment instrument by Campbell (2004) is available online *(http://www.dangerassessment.org/webapplication)*. Other excellent resource material regarding documentation, intervention, and referral are available from Family Violence Prevention Fund (FVPF, 2004) entitled *National Consensus Guidelines*. This material can also be accessed online *(endabuse.org/programs/healthcare/files/Consensus.pdf)*.

General Nursing Interventions for Psychosocial and Physical Diagnoses Related to Domestic Violence

- Provide education about battering.
- Provide information about community resources and how to use them.
- Assist in planning strategies for safety crisis intervention.
- Support and advocate for the pregnant woman when she is unable to advocate for herself.
- Encourage a problem-solving approach with the woman so that she is able to look at and evaluate various options. Support her choices whenever possible.
- Be aware of the local laws regarding reporting procedures and assist the woman if she wishes to file a report.
- Be prepared to make appropriate referrals to available resources for the family. If the woman or children are in danger of harm, refer immediately to a battered women's shelter.

- Refer the woman's partner to a resource for abusers if the opportunity presents and it does not violate issues of trust for the woman.

Specific Nursing Interventions for Domestic Violence

If the woman reveals that she has been abused, respond using the ABCDs for universal screening:

A: Acknowledge to the woman that she is not alone—"Many women are in abusive relationships."

B: Believe the woman and acknowledge her grief and pain—"No one deserves to be hurt" and "It is not your fault."

C: Confidentiality is vitally important. Reassure the woman that health care providers will keep all the information she provides confidential. Know the state laws about mandatory reporting. A few states such as California, Kentucky, New Mexico, New Hampshire, and Rhode Island currently mandate reporting. If child abuse is reported or suspected, all states require that the local child protection agency be informed. Child abuse occurs in 50% of domestic violence situations (U.S. Advisory Board on Child Abuse and Neglect, 1995).

D: Document specific details and place the patient's statements in quotation marks. Document any visual injury by using a body map or photograph with size referencing such as a coin or ruler next to the injury if the woman signs a consent. If injuries are in various stages of healing, record this as well. Documentation can be helpful to the woman later during any legal encounters. Document referrals and information provided as well. If prenatal records are sent to the labor and delivery area, an undefined coding system might be used and the documentation written in a form separate from the chart. A documentation form is available for use from the Family Violence Prevention Fund.

E: Educate the woman regarding the cyclic nature of abuse, safety measures, importance of a safety plan, legal issues such as restraining and protection orders, and referrals. National resources are listed in Table 24-2. If social services are available, provide referral.

S: Safety is the key. Communicate concern for the woman's safety and assure her that help is available when she is ready. Assist the woman if she wishes to file a report and obtain a restraining/protective order. If the woman or children are in danger of harm, refer immediately to a battered women's shelter. Refer the woman's partner to a resource for abusers if the opportunity presents and it does not violate issues of trust for the woman. If she is not ready to report or leave the situation, support her by providing her with information about how to develop a safety plan. Many community agencies provide written materials to help the woman develop a plan. Provide her with resources as well.

For resource material and guidelines, refer to the National Consensus Guidelines on Identifying and Responding to Domestic Violence Victimization in Health Care Settings (FVPF, 2004). For information on mandatory reporting of domestic violence by health care providers, contact the local

Table 24-2   Domestic Violence Resources

Agency	Phone Number or Web Address
National Domestic Violence Hotline	(800) 799-SAFE (7233)
Family Violence Prevention Fund	(888) RX-ABUSE
Online resources	http://www.endabuse.org/health
National guidelines and health care protocols	
Health screening for domestic violence	
Coding and documentation of domestic violence	
Rape Abuse & Incest National Network (RAINN)	(800) 656-HOPE (4673)
Prevent Domestic Violence	http://www.domesticviolence.org/ plan.html
Assists in developing a personalized safety plan	
Shelter Hotline	(800) 799-7739
Legal Advocacy Hotline	(800) 782-6400
Community Information and Referral	(800) 352-3792
List of state domestic violence or sexual assault coalitions	http://www.ojp.usdoj.gov/vawo/ state.htm

District Attorney's office or health facility counsel. This information can also be accessed online *(http://www.endabuse.org/health/mandatoryreporting)*.

Nursing Interventions for Minor Trauma

- Treat any area of abrasion with antibiotic ointment or oral antibiotics.
- Treat ecchymotic areas with ice applications.
- Provide mild pain relief medications such as Tylenol 3 or nonsteroidal antiinflammatory agents. Monitor FHR and uterine contractions for 4 hours after administration of these agents.
- Provide a Kleihauer-Betke screen to detect fetomaternal hemorrhage and quantitated fetal blood loss and to determine the dosage of RhoGAM for the Rh-negative woman.
- Administer RhoGAM to Rh-negative woman.
- If FHR decelerations or uterine contractions are noted in the initial 4-hour monitoring period or if there is a positive Kleihauer-Betke screen, admit for 24 hours of continuous observation, FHR and uterine contraction monitoring, evaluation for PROM, and evaluation for signs of abruptio placenta.
- Repeat nonstress test and Kleihauer-Betke in 24 hours.
- Toxicity screen for illicit drug or alcohol use may be indicated.
- Manage expectantly.

Critical Care Interventions for Acute Severe Trauma Maternal Focus ("A Team")

Stabilization

- Stabilize mother first; then be concerned about the fetus.
- Keep airway patent.
- Maintain breathing and circulation.
- Control bleeding.
- Position patient in a left lateral tilt or lateral displacement hip, if no spinal cord injury below thoracic region is suspected, to prevent spine hypotension and vena cava syndrome. If spinal immobilization is indicated, the backboard can be tilted slightly to the left.
- Administer oxygen at 8 to 10 L/min as indicated because of increased maternal oxygen consumption and high fetal sensitivity to material hypoxia.
- Assess level of consciousness.
- Assess and document respiratory status for rate, depth, regularity, and breath sounds.
- Assess and document peripheral pulses, skin color, and capillary bed refill.
- Monitor blood pressure frequently.
- Start an intravenous infusion with a 14- to 16-gauge needle.
- Infuse crystalloid fluids such as lactated Ringer's and blood as indicated.
- If the patient remains hypotensive, a suit of medical antishock trousers (MAST) can be applied without using the abdominal flap.
- Auscultate more laterally for bowel sounds.
- Intermittent nasogastric suctioning may be ordered because of the increased risk for regurgitation and aspiration related to trauma, further decreasing gastrointestinal motility.
- Monitor urinary output. A Foley catheter may be ordered to monitor urine output and evaluate urologic injuries after some types of trauma.
- Refer to diagnostic data, such as complete blood cell count, blood type, antibody screen, and Kleihauer-Betke test to determine a fetomaternal hemorrhage, platelet count, arterial blood gases, or coagulation studies, in case signs of DIC develop; refer to a toxicity screen for illicit drug or alcohol use if indicated.
- If a computed tomography scan of the abdomen is ordered, shield the fetus if at all possible. Magnetic resonance imaging and computed tomography scans are good choices for evaluation.
- In the event of a maternal cardiopulmonary arrest, be prepared to assist with a cesarean delivery within 4 hours to enhance maternal and fetal survival.
- If placental abruption, maternal injury resulting in persistent fetal compromise, intrauterine infection, or maternal death occurs and the fetus is more than 24 weeks of gestation and alive, prepare for a cesarean birth (Divekar and Keith, 2004; Grossman, 2004a).

Continued Care

- Work together. Perinatal nurse works with the critical care nurse unless the patient is in a tertiary care center with a critical care obstetrics unit.
- Provide consultation, such as physiologic changes related to pregnancy, fetal monitoring, and signs and treatment of pregnancy complications, such as abruptio placentae, preterm labor, and PROM.
- Assist physician with a quick abdominal ultrasound to evaluate fetal status and general gestational age.
- After stabilization, assess FHR and uterine contractions with electronic fetal monitor (EFM) for 4 to 24 hours after an MVA or abdominal injury for early detection of abruptio placentae and preterm labor (Bobrowski, 2006).
- Assess for signs of abruptio placentae, such as dark vaginal bleeding, sustained abdominal pain, uterine tenderness, or increasing fundal height.
- Assess for uterine contractions, warning signs of preterm labor, and PROM.
- If placental abruption, maternal injury resulting in persistent fetal compromise, intrauterine infection, or maternal death occurs and the fetus is more than 24 weeks of gestation and alive, prepare for a cesarean birth.
- Explain any ordered test such as biophysical profile or nonstress test for fetal surveillance and amniocentesis for fetal lung maturity or intrauterine bleeding.
- Check injury areas for redness, swelling, and drainage every shift.
- Administer prophylactic tetanus shot if there is no recent reliable history of administration.
- If the patient is D(Rh)-negative, administer D immune globulin as ordered for fetomaternal hemorrhage, which occurs in approximately 8% to 30% of patients who experience trauma.

Critical Care Interventions for Acute Severe Trauma with Fetal Focus ("B Team")

- Initially determine FHR.
- Assist physician with a quick abdominal ultrasound to evaluate fetal status and general gestational age.
- After stabilization, assess FHR and uterine contractions with EFM for 4 to 24 hours after an MVA or abdominal injury for early detection of abruptio placentae and preterm labor (Harris, 2001; Bobrowski, 2006).
- If signs of fetal compromise develop, prepare for emergent or postmortem cesarean birth.
- Prepare for transfer of premature or injured infant to an intensive care nursery.
- If not delivered in the initial phase or in early gestation, assess for spontaneous abortion, preterm labor, PROM, or intrauterine fetal compromise.
- If the mother needs to be positioned supine, place a small wedge under right hip if no spinal cord injury.

- Assist physician with a quick abdominal ultrasound to evaluate fetal status and general gestational age.
- Assess for signs of abruptio placentae, such as dark vaginal bleeding, sustained abdominal pain, uterine tenderness, or increasing fundal height.
- Assess for uterine contractions, warning signs of preterm labor, and PROM.

Recovery and Rehabilitation Nursing Interventions

- Educate patient in self-care and self-assessment after discharge.
- Teach patient to keep a daily fetal movement chart.
- Explain any ordered test such as biophysical profile or nonstress test for fetal surveillance and amniocentesis for fetal lung maturity or intrauterine bleeding.
- Instruct patient about the importance of immediately reporting the development of signs of an infection, abruption, or preterm labor.
- If the mother is left physically disabled because of the trauma, physical and occupational therapy may be needed to teach skills for caring for other children and a new baby.

CONCLUSION

As the leading cause of maternal death, maternal trauma is a serious consequence of the increase in societal violence, lack of protection of pregnant women, and a general apathy to the need for maternal protection from injury. Many life-threatening injuries to mother and fetus resulting from MVAs could be prevented by safe and consistent use of car seat belts. Other injuries related to falls, burns, and acts of individual violence might be prevented by education. Pregnant women, family members, employers, and society in general need to be made more aware of the incidence of, risks for, and potential dangers of exposure of pregnant women to possible physical injury and trauma.

BIBLIOGRAPHY

American College of Obstetricians and Gynecologists: Domestic Violence, *ACOG Technical Bulletin*, No. 257, Washington, DC, 1999, ACOG.

American Nurses Association (ANA): Position Statement on violence against women, Washington, DC, 2000, Author.

Bobrowski R: Trauma in pregnancy. In James D and others, editors: *High risk pregnancy: management options*, ed 3, Philadelphia, 2006, Saunders.

Bryan E, Bledsoe M: Trauma during pregnancy, *Merginet* 7(4): 2002.

Campbell J: Danger Assessment, Baltimore, Md, 2004, John Hopkins University. Retrieved from *http://endabuse.org/programs/display.php3?DocID=350*

Carbuapoma J, Tomlinson M, and Levine S: Neurologic disorders. In James D and others, editors: *High risk pregnancy: management options*, ed 3, Philadelphia, 2006, Saunders.

Chang J and others: Homicide: a leading cause of injury deaths among pregnant postpartum women in the United States, 1991–1999, *Am J Public Health* 95(3):471–477, 2005.

Christian A: Home care of the battered pregnant woman: one woman's battered pregnancy, *J Obstet Gynecol Neonatal Nurs* 2(9):836–842, 1995.

Cox S, Kilpatrick S, and Geller S: Preventing maternal deaths in America, *Contemporary OB/GYN*, Sept 1, 2004.

Divekar P, Keith L: Pregnancy outcome in motor vehicle accidents, *Female Patient* 29:3135, 2004.

Dunn L, Oths K: Prenatal predictors of intimate partner abuse, *J Obstet Gynecol Neonatal Nurs* 33(1):54–63, 2004.

Family Violence Prevention Fund (FVPF): *Fact sheet: Intimate partner violence and healthy people 2010 fact sheet,* San Francisco, Calif, 2003, FVPF. Retrieved from *http://endabuse.org/hcadvd/2003/tier4.pdf*

Family Violence Prevention Fund (FVPF): *National consensus guidelines on identifying and responding to domestic violence victimization in health care settings,* ed 2, San Francisco, Calif, 2004, FVPF. Retrieved from *http://endabuse.org/programs/healthcare/files/screpol.pdf*

Grossman N: Blunt trauma in pregnancy, *Am Fam Physician* 70(7):1303–1310, 2004a.

Grossman N: Seat belt use during pregnancy, *Am Fam Physician* 70(7):1313, 2004b.

Guth A, Pachter L: Domestic violence and the trauma surgeon, *Am J Surg* 179(2):134–40, 2000.

Harris C: Trauma in pregnancy, Presented at OB Challenges of the Millennium, Phoenix, Ariz, April 2001, 2001.

Hedin L, Janson P: Domestic violence during pregnancy: the prevalence of physical injuries, substance use, abortions, and miscarriages, *Acta Obstet Gynecol Scand* 79(8):625–630, 2000.

Institute for Clinical Systems Improvement (ICSI): *Domestic violence,* Bloomington, Minn, 2003, Institute for Clinical Systems Improvement.

McGwin G and others: A focused educational intervention can promote the proper application of seat belts during pregnancy, *J Trauma* 56(5):1016–1021, 2004.

Norton L and others: Battering in pregnancy: an assessment of tool screening methods, *Obstet Gynecol* 8(3):321–325, 1995.

Parker B, McFarlane J, and Soeken K: Abuse during pregnancy: effects on maternal complications and birth weight in adult and teenage women, *Obstet Gynecol* 84(3):323–328, 1994.

Pearlman M and others: A comprehensive program to improve safety for pregnant women and fetuses in motor vehicle crashes: a preliminary report, *Am J Obstet Gynecol* 182(6): 1554–1564, 2000.

Plichta S, Falik M: Prevalence of violence and its implications for women's health, *Womens Health Issues* 11(3):244–258, 2001.

U.S. Advisory Board on Child Abuse and Neglect: *A nation's shame: fatal child abuse and neglect in the United States,* 5th report, Washington, DC, 1995, Department of Health and Human Services, Administration for Children and Families.

U.S. Department of Health and Human Services: *Healthy people 2010: understanding and improving health,* Washington, DC, 2000, USDHHS. Retrieved from *http://health.gov/healthypeople/Document/tableofcontents.htm*

VI

Teratogens and Social Issues Complicating Pregnancy

T he rise in the incidence of sexually and nonsexually transmitted infections and substance abuse during pregnancy poses increased threats to fetal and maternal well-being. Chapter 25 describes the implications of the most common sexually and nonsexually transmitted infections on pregnancy and discusses nursing care responsibilities. Knowledgeable and involved perinatal nurses and nurse practitioners can significantly decrease the risk to the pregnant woman and her fetus.

Abuse of substances known to be teratogenic during pregnancy has increased dramatically since the early 1990s. Any pattern of habitual use and some isolated uses of substances such as alcohol, cocaine, heroin, marijuana, and tobacco can have adverse teratogenic effects on the development and growth of the fetus. Nurse practitioners and nurses have a unique opportunity during preconceptual and early prenatal care to educate and empower patients to abstain from contact with all substances that might potentially threaten the well-being of the fetus. Chapter 26 focuses on the six most commonly abused substances (alcohol, amphetamines, cocaine, heroin, marijuana, and tobacco) and describes nursing assessment techniques and interventions.

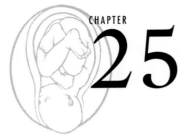

25

Sexually and Nonsexually Transmitted Genitourinary Infections

C urrently, more than 20 sexually transmitted diseases (STDs) and numerous other genitourinary infections are recognized that affect the outcome of pregnancy (NIH, 2005). Because of the continuing rise in the incidence of sexually and nonsexually transmitted infections, the development of microbial resistance to antibiotics, the emergence of incurable and fatal disease types, and the risk that they pose to the fetus and expectant mother, it is imperative that nurse practitioners and nurses caring for families who are in their childbearing years have an in-depth understanding of these diseases. This chapter focuses on the seven most common STDs and the six most common nonsexually transmitted diseases and how each can affect pregnancy.

BACTERIAL VAGINOSIS
Organism

The organisms responsible for bacterial vaginosis (BV) are anaerobic bacteria, such as *Gardnerella vaginalis*; *Mobiluncus, Mycoplasmas hominis, and Prevotella.* (CDC, 2006; Nyirjesy, Boserge, and Taylor, 2003).

Transmission

BV is not considered an STD. It usually results from a disturbance in normal vaginal flora initiated by sexual intercourse, hormonal changes, pregnancy, antibiotic administration, or use of nonoxynol-9 spermicidal products, which have a bactericidal effect on lactobacilli (Andrist, 2001). Douching may wash out the normal bacteria flora and increase the risk for BV (Hillier, 2004).

Signs and Symptoms

Up to 50% of women with BV may be asymptomatic (Gibbs, Sweet, and Duff, 2004). Signs and symptoms of BV follow:

*   Thin, gray or white homogeneous vaginal discharge
*   Increased vaginal discharge odor (fishy) after intercourse
*   Alkaline pH (>4.5)
    BV does not cause vaginal itching or dysuria.

Screening

Patients should be screened for BV if they are symptomatic. According to ACOG's meta-analysis, there is no evidence to support the benefit of screening asymptomatic patients with a positive history for preterm labor (Okun, Gronau, and Hannah, 2005). Clinical diagnosis is made if three of the following four characteristics (Mayeaux, 2001) are present:

1   Saline wet mount showing clue cells that are characterized by 1:5 epithelial cell margins obscured by bacteria; no white blood cells
2   Whiff test (fishy odor prevalent when vaginal fluid is mixed with 10% potassium hydroxide [KOH])
3   Anterior fornix or lateral vaginal wall pH greater than 4.5
4   Homogeneous white to gray discharge that adheres to the vaginal wall

No cervical or vaginal inflammation is usually present. Smoking and douching increase the risk for developing BV.

Treatment in Pregnancy

Symptomatic

According to the Centers for Disease Control and Prevention (CDC, 2006), the recommended treatment regimen during pregnancy is metronidazole (Flagyl), 500 mg orally twice a day for 7 days or 250 mg orally three times daily for 7 days. Alternative regimen is clindamycin, 300 mg orally twice daily for 7 days. Clindamycin vaginal cream is not recommended during the second half of pregnancy because of the increased risk low birth weight and neonatal infections (CDC, 2006). During breastfeeding, the woman should be treated with one dose of metronidazole, 2 g orally, and instructed to pump and discard breast milk for 24 hours (Lawrence, 2005).

Current treatment of the woman's sexual partner or partners is not necessary and does not improve outcome.

Asymptomatic

According to ACOG's meta-analysis, there is no benefit to treating asymptomatic pregnant patients with antibiotics for BV to prevent preterm labor (Okun, Gronau, and Hannah, 2005).

Effect on Pregnancy Outcome

BV is the most common vaginal infection (CDC, 2004) and has the following effects on pregnancy:

- Increases the risk for spontaneous abortion, premature rupture of membranes (PROM), and preterm labor (Leitich and others, 2003; Macones and others, 2004)
- Increases the risk for vaginosis and postpartum endometritis (Gibbs, Sweet, and Duff, 2004)
- May cause neonatal septicemia

Pregnancy Considerations

BV affects up to 16% of all pregnancies (CDC, 2004). It changes the normal vaginal flora to (1) a small amount of lactobacilli, which normally produce lactic acid and protect against vaginal pathogens by maintaining an acid pH, and (2) a high concentration of anaerobes. Instruct all women regarding the risks and nonbenefits of douching, which can increase the risk for BV, chlamydia, pelvic inflammatory disease, HIV transmission, and cervical cancer (Cottrell, 2006).

CANDIDIASIS

Organism

Candida albicans is the most common cause (90% of cases) of candidiasis. *Candida tropicalis* and *Candida glabrata* are two other possible causes of candidiasis, a fungal (yeast) infection.

Transmission

Candidiasis is not considered an STD. It usually results from a disturbance in normal vaginal flora, conditions that cause vaginal pH to be more alkaline, and high estrogen levels causing increased production of vaginal glycogen (Gibbs, Sweet, and Duff, 2004).

Signs and Symptoms

Signs and symptoms of candidiasis follow:
- Vaginal and vulvar irritation (erythematous and edematous)
- Pruritic, white, curdlike vaginal discharge
- Yeasty odor
- Dysuria
- Dyspareunia

Screening

Screening for candidiasis is as follows:
- Saline or KOH wet mount microscopically examined: shows hyphae, pseudohyphae, and budding yeast
- Usually pH lower than 4.7
- Whiff test absent amine (fishy) odor

Treatment in Pregnancy

Only symptomatic women should be treated for candidiasis. Use an antifungal, intravaginal agent, such as butoconazole (e.g., Femstat 3), clotrimazole (e.g.,

Gyne-Lotrimin and Mycelex), miconazole (e.g., Monistat), or terconazole (e.g., Terazol). These drugs come in a vaginal suppository or cream form. Duration of treatment is 7 days during pregnancy (CDC, 2006).

Sitz baths twice daily may decrease the external irritation. Instruct the patient to abstain from intercourse, avoid bubble baths, wear cotton undergarments, and practice good perineal hygiene. To treat recurrent yeast infections or to prevent yeast infections when taking antibiotics, eating yogurt or inserting a tampon dipped in plain (unsweetened) yogurt can help restore *Lactobacillus acidophilus* in the vagina (Sierpina, 2001). Echinacea has been demonstrated by research to decrease the recurrence rate of *Candida* infections as well (Freeman and Lawlis, 2001).

Pregnancy Considerations

Candidiasis is the second most common vaginal infection (Andrist, 2001). The risk for acquiring candidiasis during pregnancy is increased; the highest risk is in patients with diabetes and patients receiving antibiotic therapy because they have decreased levels of lactobacilli.

Candidiasis may be more resistant to treatment during pregnancy. Treat all symptomatic pregnant patients vigorously to avoid neonatal thrush.

CHLAMYDIA
Organism

Chlamydia trachomatis, an obligate-intracellular, bacteria-like parasite, is the organism responsible for chlamydia.

Transmission

Chlamydia is transmitted by close sexual contact.

Signs and Symptoms

The pregnant woman with chlamydia is asymptomatic approximately 75% of the time. However, she may exhibit some or all of the following symptoms (CDC, 2004):
- Increased, clear, white to yellowish mucous vaginal discharge
- Painful, frequent urination
- Dyspareunia
- Rectal pain, discharge, or bleeding from chlamydial infection in the rectum from anal sex
- Posterior pharyngitis from chlamydial infection in the throat from oral sex

Objective Findings
- Bartholin, urethral, and Skene glands: swelling and abnormal discharge
- External genitalia: erythema, edema, and excoriation
- Vagina: abnormal discharge
- Cervix: mucopurulent cervicitis; edematous, erythematous, and friable; cervical motion tenderness

Screening

To reduce pelvic inflammatory infections, screening for chlamydia should be offered to all women who are 25 years of age or younger who come for gynecologic care and to women over 25 who have new or multiple sex partners (AHRQ, 2001; CDC, 2006). All pregnant women should be screened on the first prenatal visit, and high risk patients should be screened again during the third trimester because the disease is asymptomatic in 70% to 85% of cases (CDC, 2006; NGC, 2005). Screening methods (Ward, 2003) follow:

- **Gene amplification molecular diagnostics,** such as polymerase chain reaction (PCR) or ligase chain reaction (LCR), are the newest screening methods that identify chlamydia and gonorrhea organisms via hybridization or nucleic acid amplification. These tests are popular because of their sensitivity, specificity, and ease of sampling (endourethral, endocervix, or noninvasive sampling of a fresh voided urine).
- **Tissue culture,** which was previously considered the screening method of choice, is only 70% to 90% sensitive related to decrease survival during transportation (Tiller, 2002).
- Two other classic diagnostics are **antigen detection enzyme immunoassay (EIA) and direct fluorescent antibody detection (DFA).**

Treatment in Pregnancy

Treatment of choice for the pregnant woman with chlamydia is one dose of azithromycin 1 g. An alternative treatment is erythromycin base, 500 mg orally four times daily for 7 days (NGC, 2005). If gastrointestinal side effects occur, erythromycin base, 250 mg four times daily for 14 days (NGC, 2005), is given. Erythromycin should be taken with 8 ounces of water 1 to 2 hours after a meal. For patients who cannot tolerate erythromycin, amoxicillin, 500 mg orally three times daily for 7 days, is an acceptable alternative (Brocklehurst and Rooney, 1998; NGC, 2005). Because of the decrease effectiveness and compliance of these drugs, the National Guidelines Clearinghouse (2005) recommends follow-up testing with cultures 3 weeks after completion of therapy.

Avoid tetracycline, doxycycline, and ofloxacin during pregnancy because they have harmful effects on fetal teeth and cartilage. All sexual partners within 60 days before onset and diagnosis should be tested and treated as well.

Effect on Pregnancy Outcome

Chlamydia is an ascending infection and, if left untreated, can lead to pelvic inflammatory diseases (PIDs) up to 40% of the time (Parratt and Hay, 2003), which can later cause infertility, ectopic pregnancies, and chronic pelvic pain (Rawlins, 2001). However, PID is unlikely during pregnancy. Women infected with chlamydia have an increased risk for acquiring human immunodeficiency virus (HIV), if exposed.

Pregnancy Considerations

Chlamydia is the most frequently reported STD in the United States and in most developed countries (CDC, 2006). If the infection is present at the time of vaginal birth, the neonate is at a 15% to 25% risk for conjunctivitis, which can lead to blindness and a 5% to 15% risk for pneumonitis (Brocklehurst and Rooney, 2001); therefore all neonates' eyes should be treated with either 0.5% erythromycin or 1.0% tetracycline ophthalmic ointment on delivery. This does not prevent pneumonitis caused by chlamydia infection. Any neonate who develops conjunctivitis should be screened for chlamydia.

Postpartum endometritis is associated with chlamydia as well (Brocklehurst and Rooney, 1998).

GONORRHEA

Organism

The organism responsible for gonorrhea is *Neisseria gonorrhoeae*, a gram-negative intracellular diplococcus bacterium.

Transmission

Gonorrhea is transmitted by close sexual contact. The risk for transmission from an infected man to an uninfected woman is 50% to 90%, and there is a 20% risk from an infected woman to an uninfected man (Gibbs, Sweet, and Duff, 2004).

Signs and Symptoms

Gonorrhea is commonly asymptomatic (Gibbs, Sweet, and Duff, 2004). Signs and symptoms of gonorrhea if present are as follows:
- Vaginal discharge: may be profuse, purulent, yellow-green
- Anal discharge
- Itching or swelling of vulva
- Dysuria
- Dyspareunia
- Joint and tendon pain
- Anal discharge, discomfort, and pain with a rectal infection

Objective Findings
- Inguinal or cervical adenopathy
- Bartholin, urethral, and Skene glands tender to palpation
- External genitalia: erythematous, edematous; excoriation may be present
- Vagina: abnormal discharge; blood or pus may be seen
- Cervix: mucopurulent cervicitis indicated by erythema; friable, cervical os with cervical motion tenderness
- Rectal examination: assess for discharge, bleeding, or tenderness

Screening

Routine screening for gonorrhea is standard practice. All pregnant women should be screened on the first prenatal visit, and high risk patients should be screened again during the third trimester (Miller and others, 2003) because the disease is commonly asymptomatic. Screening should also be done before procedures such as dilation and curettage and chorionic villus sampling. Screening methods follow:

- **Molecular diagnostics** are the newest screening methods that identify chlamydia and gonorrhea organisms via hybridization or nucleic acid amplification. Because of their sensitivity, specificity, and easy of sampling (endourethral, endocervix, or noninvasive sampling of a fresh voided urine sample), these tests are popular.
- **Endocervical culture** was previously considered the gold standard. To collect a culture, insert a cotton, polyester, or calcium alginate swab moistened with warm water 2 to 3 cm into the cervical canal and move it in and out with a rotary motion for 10 seconds to allow absorption of exudate. If a Pap smear is to be taken during the same examination, it should be obtained first. There is a new DNA amplification test of urine that is used for screenings (CDC, 2006).

Treatment in Pregnancy

For the pregnant woman with gonorrhea, the drug of choice is one dose of cefixime, 400 mg orally, or one dose of ceftriaxone, 125 mg intramuscularly (IM). If chlamydia is suspected, follow up with either azithromycin or amoxicillin (CDC, 2006). If the patient is allergic to cephalosporins, one dose of spectinomycin, 2 g IM, can be given, followed by erythromycin base, 500 mg four times daily for 7 days if cotreating for chlamydia (Brocklehurst, 2002).

Avoid tetracyclines and quinolones during pregnancy because of their injurious effect on fetal teeth and cartilage (CDC, 2006).

Sexual partners within the preceding 60 days should be identified, examined, cultured, and treated.

Effect on Pregnancy Outcome

Gonorrhea can affect pregnancy outcome in any trimester, causing spontaneous abortion, preterm delivery, or PROM (Brocklehurst, 2002). If the organism is present at the time of delivery, the greatest neonatal risk (30%–47% risk) is an eye infection called *gonococcal ophthalmia*, which can cause blindness (Brocklehurst, 2002). This is one of the reasons all newborns' eyes should be treated with either 0.5% erythromycin or 1% tetracycline ophthalmic ointment as soon as possible after birth (CDC, 2006). If the organism is known to be present in the birth canal at delivery, the infant is treated with a single 1 gram IM injection of ceftriaxone (CDC, 2006).

Pregnancy Considerations

Gonorrhea is an ascending infection. If it is left untreated, it can cause a PID (CDC, 2006). PID can in turn cause infertility. Untreated gonorrhea is a significant cause of postpartum endometritis. The risk for coexisting chlamydia infection is 20% to 40% (Parratt and Hay, 2003).

GROUP B STREPTOCOCCUS INFECTION

Organism

Streptococcus agalactiae is a gram-positive encapsulated coccus, a two-cell wall polysaccharide.

Pregnancy Considerations

Streptococcus agalactiae is present in the lower genital tract or rectum of 10% to 30% of all healthy pregnant women. These women are asymptomatic carriers of group B streptococcal (GBS) infection, which causes a 1% to 2% risk for GBS disease in the newborn (CDC, 2002). Approximately 80% of these neonates develop early-onset invasive GBS disease in the first 7 days of their life. If a newborn contracts early-onset invasive GBS, mortality is 4% (Schrag and others, 2000).

GBS has maternal morbidity implications as well. During pregnancy, there is an increased risk for urinary tract infection (UTI), chorioamnionitis, sepsis, postpartum endometritis, and rarely meningitis (CDC, 2002).

Risk Factors

The following risk factors increase the likelihood of early onset neonatal GBS infection:
- Positive prenatal culture for GBS this pregnancy
- Preterm birth of less than 37 weeks of gestation
- PROM for longer than 18 hours
- Intrapartum maternal fever greater than 38°C
- Positive history for early onset neonatal GBS

Screening

The CDC (2002), American College of Obstetricians and Gynecologists (ACOG, 20020), and The Society of Obstetricians and Gynecologists of Canada (Money and Dobson, 2004) recommend prenatal lower vaginal and ano-rectal GBS screening (IDI-Strep B) between 35 and 37 weeks of gestation for all pregnant women. The only exceptions are cases of GBS bacteriuria during current pregnancy or a planned cesarean prior to labor or amniotic membrane rupture. The culture should be obtained without use of a speculum. The swabs should be placed in transport broth immediately (CDC, 2002).

Recommendations for Intrapartum Prophylaxis and Appropriate Therapy

The CDC (2002) recommends intrapartum antimicrobial prophylaxis for positive GBS screening culture, GBS bacteriuria during this pregnancy, and an unknown GBS status and any of the following:
- Preterm labor before 37 weeks of gestation
- Duration of ruptured membranes longer than 18 hours
- Intrapartum temperature greater than 100.4°F (38°C)

The antibiotic of choice is penicillin G, 5 million units by IV load and then 2.5 million units IV every 4 hours during labor. Ampicillin, 2-g loading dose

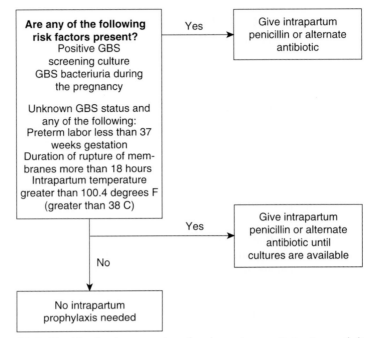

Figure 25-1 Algorithm for the prevention of early-onset group B streptococcal disease in neonates, using prenatal screening at 35–37 weeks of gestation.

and then 1 g IV every 4 hours during labor, is an alternative therapy. If the patient is allergic to penicillin, the alternative is cefazolin, 2 g IV loading dose and then 1 g IV q 8 hours. If the patient is at high risk for anaphylaxis, then clindamycin, 900 mg IV every 8 hours, or erythromycin, 500 mg IV every 6 hours, can be administered during labor (CDC, 2002). Fig. 25-1 shows the algorithm for prevention of early onset GBS disease according to the 2002 CDC recommendations.

Other Considerations

Treat all symptomatic or asymptomatic pregnant patients who have a positive urine culture for group B streptococcus with a 10-day course of antibiotics. Notify the pediatrician of any group B streptococcal infection during pregnancy.

HEPATITIS B

Organism

Hepatitis B virus (HBV), a hepadnavirus, is a partially double-stranded DNA virus consisting of a core antigen (HBcAg) carried in a lipoprotein envelope that contains the surface antigen (HBsAg). It carries a third antigen, the e antigen (HBeAg), which is highly infectious (Landon, 2004).

Transmission

Hepatitis B is transmitted by blood and body fluids, such as semen, vaginal secretions, and saliva. The organism is extremely hardy and can survive outside the body in dried blood or body secretions for 1 week or more. Therefore the two major modes of HBV transmission are contact with contaminated blood or blood products and participation in sexual intercourse.

Signs and Symptoms

Acute HBV infection usually resolves as the body develops protective antibodies, but a chronic infection (the carrier state) may result. The risk for becoming a carrier is inversely associated with the age at which the infection is acquired. Young children have the greatest risk (Landon, 2004). The pregnant woman with acute hepatitis B may be asymptomatic, or she may exhibit some or all of the following signs and symptoms:
- Chronic low-grade fever
- Anorexia
- Nausea and vomiting
- Fatigue
- Skin rashes
- Arthralgia

Screening

The Centers for Disease Control and Prevention (CDC), American College of Obstetricians and Gynecologists (ACOG), American Academy of Pediatrics (AAP), and Advisory Committee for Immunization Practice (ACIP) recommend routine prenatal HBV screening of all pregnant women at the initial visit and rescreening of all high risk women during the third trimester. Women who were not screened prenatally should be screened on admission to labor and delivery (CDC, 2005). Individuals at high risk for contracting HBV infection are the following (Corrarino, 1998):
- People of Central African, Southeast Asian, Middle Eastern, Pacific Island, and Alaskan descent
- IV drug users
- People with multiple sexual partners
- Health care workers with blood and needlestick exposure
- Recipients of multiple blood transfusions

Screening for the presence of HBV is easily done by drawing blood and testing it for HBsAg. If HBsAg is positive, order HBeAg, anti-HBe, anti-HBc, aspartate transaminase (AST), alkaline phosphatase, and liver profile studies per consult. In the presence of an acute HBV infection, HBsAg, HBeAg, and immunoglobulin M (IgM) anti-HBc are all elevated. In chronic HBV infection (the carrier state), HBsAg remains elevated, as does the IgG anti-HBc, but IgM anti-HBc is absent (IAC, 2004). If HBsAg is positive but HBeAg is negative, this indicates a carrier state without active liver disease.

If HBsAg and HBeAg are positive, it indicates a carrier state with most likely active liver disease (IAC, 2004).

Treatment in Pregnancy

If exposure occurs during pregnancy and the patient is HbsAg-negative, hepatitis B immunoglobulin (HBIG), 0.06 mL/kg IM, should be given; the HBIG dose is repeated 1 month later, followed by the hepatitis B vaccination series (CDC, 2005). If an expectant mother contracts the disease during pregnancy, symptomatic treatment only is given. This usually includes increased bedrest, a diet high in protein and low in fat, adequate hydration, and avoidance of medications that are metabolized in the liver.

Pregnancy Considerations

Acute HBV infection does not usually affect the course of pregnancy, except when the severe acute phase occurs during the third trimester, it can increase the risk for preterm delivery. The risk for transmission to the fetus during an acute HBV infection in the first and second trimester is low (3%). However, risk for transmission to the fetus during an acute HBV infection in the third trimester is 70% (Corrarino, Walsh, and Anselmo, 1999).

If the mother is a carrier, she is infectious and can transmit the disease to her child as well. If the mother is positive for both HbsAg and HbeAg, the child has a 70% to 90% risk for becoming infected. If she is HbsAg-positive only, the risk is less than 10% from perinatal transmission and approximately 40% from horizontal transmission (CDC, 2005). The infant rarely develops signs and symptoms, but 90% become chronic carriers if not treated (CDC, 2005). Chronic carriers have a 25% risk for developing liver cancer or cirrhosis by 50 years of age (CDC, 2005; Landon, 2004). To prevent perinatal HBV infection and development of a chronic carrier state, the following care of the newborn is important.

Newborn Care if the Mother is HbsAg-Negative

The CDC recommends routine HBV vaccination of all newborns to prevent HBV infection later in life. Vaccine for these infants is Recombivax HB 5 mcg or Engerix-B 10 mcg IM in the anterolateral thigh. The three-injection schedule recommended currently by the CDC is as follows: the first dose is given between 0 and 2 months, the second dose between 1 and 4 months, and the third between 6 and 18 months.

Newborn Care if the Mother is HbsAg-Positive

To prevent the chronic carrier state if the mother has a positive HBsAg test, the newborn is treated with HBIG 0.5 ml by 12 hours postdelivery and an initial dose of Recombivax HB 5 mcg or Engerix-B 10 mcg IM. Follow-up care includes a subsequent hepatitis B vaccination at 1 and 6 months of age and diagnostic studies between 12 and 15 months to determine the infant's carrier status. If anti-HB antibodies are present (greater than 10 mIU/ml), the prophylactic program was effective. Revaccinate nonresponders. However, if HBsAg is detected, the prophylactic program was ineffective and the infant is a carrier of HBV (CDC, 2005).

The prophylactic program just described is 85% to 95% effective in preventing exposed infants from becoming chronic carriers (CDC, 2002). It is ineffective in 5% to 15% of all infants and may be related to a transplacental exposure.

Breastfeeding is not contraindicated if the infant has been immunized.

HEPATITIS C

Organism

Hepatitis C virus (HCV) is an RNA virus of the *Flaviviridae* family. It is currently the most common chronic bloodborne infection (CDC, 2006).

Transmission

The primary route of transmission of hepatitis C is parenteral, including illicit IV drug use, accidental needlesticks, and blood transfusions. Transmission by sexual contact occurs, but it is rare, the rate varying from 0% to 4.4% (Strader and others, 2004). The body's immunologic defenses have difficulty clearing the virus. Therefore HCV becomes chronic in 60% to 85% of acute infected people (CDC, 2006).

Signs and Symptoms

The majority of people with HCV are asymptomatic; therefore the infection often goes undetected until significant liver damage results.

Screening

The CDC (2002) recommends screening women at risk for HCV, but they do not recommend routine prenatal screening of all pregnant women. Individuals at high risk for HCV infection are follows (CDC, 2006; NGC, 2004):

- IV drug users or women who ever injected an illegal drug
- Women who received clotting factor products before 1987
- Recipients of blood transfusions or organ transplants before July 1992
- Health care workers with blood and needlestick exposure

The EIA test for anti-HCV is the preferred screening test; if this test is positive, it is confirmed by a recombinant immunoblot assay (RIBA) (NGC, 2002). In an HCV-positive patient, a polymerase chain reaction RNA for hepatitis C may be drawn to estimate viral load, and an HIV screen is encouraged because of the increased association with this infection. In the presence of a coinfection, the maternal to fetal transmission is increased.

Treatment in Pregnancy

Routine prenatal care is recommended with baseline liver function studies including alanine transaminase (ALT). Currently, no method has been found to lower vertical transmission. Cesarean delivery, unless otherwise indicated, has not proved beneficial in lowering the rate of transmission (CDC, 2006; NGC, 2004). For patients with a high viral load, avoiding artificial rupture of membranes and fetal scalp electrode may be beneficial. Interferon alpha and ribavirin treatment of HCV is not currently recommended during pregnancy but is reserved for the postpartum period as indicated by a liver biopsy.

Pregnancy Considerations

There does not appear to be an increased risk to the pregnancy if the woman is HCV-positive unless other behavioral influences coexist. The risk for vertical transmission can occur antepartally, intrapartally, or postpartally. According to the NIH (2002), the risk for transmission to the fetus is approximately 4% to 7%. If the patient is also HIV-positive, the risk increases to 20% (NIH, 2002). There also appears to be an increased transmission rate as the viral load increases (Thomas and others, 1998). However, there are no current data to indicate whether antiviral therapy reduces perinatal transmission. The current antiviral drugs used in the treatment of chronic hepatitis C—ribavirin and interferons—are contraindicated during pregnancy (NIH, 2002). Breastfeeding does not seem to be contraindicated because there has been no increase transmission risk shown (NGC, 2002) unless the nipples are cracked or bleeding (CDC, 2006).

After 12 months of age, the infant born to an HCV-positive mother should be screened for HCV. Passively acquired maternal antibodies persist up to 1 year of life (AAP, 1998).

HERPES SIMPLEX VIRUS TYPE 2

Organism

The organism responsible for genital herpes is herpes simplex virus (HSV-2), a double-stranded DNA virus.

Transmission

Transmission occurs through direct, intimate, oral-genital, or genital-genital contact (Steben and Sacks, 1997).

Signs and Symptoms

HSV-2 is a chronic infection characterized by periods of remissions and exacerbations. There are three different infectious states: primary, first episode nonprimary, and recurrent infections. Signs and symptoms of primary infection are as follows:
- Prodrome: lasts 2 to 10 days
- Neuralgia
- Paresthesia
- Hypesthesias
- Vesicle pustule: lasts approximately 6 days
- Painful vesicular lesions
- Dysuria
- Fever
- Malaise
- Cervicitis
- Wet ulcer: lasts approximately 6 days

- Dry crust: lasts approximately 8 days
Recurrent infections are usually less severe and of shorter duration.

Objective Findings with Lesions

- Papules, vesicles, ulcerations, pustules, or crusts on the vulva, vagina, or perianal area
- Cervical lesions resembling mucus patches, with central necrosis and elevated borders
- General cervicitis

Screening

The first prenatal assessment should include questions regarding a history of HSV infection of both the father and mother. If the history is positive, screen for other STDs, such as gonorrhea, chlamydia, syphilis, hepatitis B, and HIV. Status-unknown pregnant women who have atypical symptoms suggestive of atypical HSV, an HSV-positive partner, or history of another sexual transmitted disease or HIV should be screened with an FDA-approved serologic test such as a viral culture, which has previously been considered the most accurate screening method.

New polymerase chain reaction (PCR) HSV type-specific glycoprotein gG-based type serology such as HerpeSelect ELISA or HerpeSelect immunoblot IgG for HSV-1 and HSV-2 are more cost-effective and 10 times more sensitive than viral culture (Wald, and others, 2003). Also, HSV IgG type-specific serology is effective in predicting nonspecific or asymptomatic shedding, whereas viral cultures are not (Morrow, 2004).

Treatment in Pregnancy

No therapy can eradicate HSV, and this chronic infection is noted for its frequent asymptomatic viral shedding (Leone, 2004). Oral Acyclovir is highly selective of infected cells, and the international acyclovir pregnancy registry has concluded that observed rates and types of birth defects are not significantly different for pregnancies exposed to Acyclovir and the general population (Stone and others, 2004). Therefore suppressive therapy with acyclovir is the current treatment of choice during pregnancy. Acyclovir antiviral suppressant therapy is started at 36 weeks and continued until delivery (Baker, 2004). Sheffield and others' (2003) meta-analysis of five studies indicated a five-fold decrease in genital HSV recurrence at delivery with the used of antiviral suppressant therapy during pregnancy.

At the time of delivery, if primary or recurrent active HSV lesions or prodromal symptoms are present, a cesarean delivery should be performed. All maneuvers that might cause a break in the infant's skin should be avoided, such as following:

- Artificial rupture of membranes
- Fetal scalp electrode
- Fetal scalp pH
- Forceps and vacuum

Discordant couples (female seronegative, male seropositive) should be counseled to avoid oral and genital sex and to use condoms during pregnancy. The male should also be encouraged to consider suppressive antiviral therapy once daily. Valacycovir significantly reduces the risk for transmission among heterosexual HSV–2 discordant couples (Corey and others, 2004).

Pregnancy Considerations

Intrauterine infection is rare and is caused a primary maternal infection during pregnancy. If infection occurs, it may cause spontaneous abortion, birth anomalies, intrauterine growth restriction, or preterm labor (ACOG, 1999). Contact at the time of delivery is the most common mode of transmission to the baby. Primary HSV infections during pregnancy have the greatest risk for transmission to the baby (USPSTF, 2005). Exposure may lead to serious neonatal complications such as learning disabilities, psychomotor retardation, seizures, spasticity, blindness, and even death (Wald and Link, 2002).

Infected parents should be counseled regarding the importance of good handwashing and hygiene in preventing transmission to their infant. Any skin lesions present at birth should be cultured for HSV-2. The currently accepted antiviral therapy for the neonate is acyclovir IV 20 mg/kg/8 hours for 14 to 21 days (CDC, 2006).

HUMAN IMMUNODEFICIENCY VIRUS

Organism

The HIV organism is a retrovirus of the lentivirus family that has an affinity for the T-lymphocytes (or "T helper cells"), macrophages, and monocytes.

Transmission

Transmission occurs from exposure to infected blood or body secretions of semen or vaginal fluid. The most common means is unprotected sexual activity or the sharing of contaminated needles. Pediatric HIV primarily results from perinatal or breastfeeding transmission (NIAID, 2004).

Normal Physiology of Immune System of Pregnancy

In HIV, the helper T cells (T4) are suppressed, which is important in cell-mediated immunity. The suppressor T cells (T8) are not affected. The polymorphonuclear leukocyte function is decreased. Antibody formation is not affected. The net result is the pregnant woman is not more susceptible to an infection, but once she contracts an infection, it is harder to eradicate.

Pathophysiology

HIV is an envelope virus consisting of a p24 protein capsule (p24 antigen) containing two short strands of genetic material (RNA) and a unique reverse transcriptase enzyme encapsulated in a lipid envelope.

A virus can reproduce only inside a cell. To enter the cell, there must be an attachment molecule on the cell wall for the virus to attach to and then enter the cell. HIV attaches to the glycoprotein antigen (CD4) receptors on the T4 cells, B-lymphocytes, macrophages, and monocytes, as well as other cells in the immune system and CNS, and then enters these cells.

The virus reproduces inside the CD4 cells, such as the T4 cells, and eventually destroys them. The T4 cells are the master immune cells. They send out alerting messages, by way of hormones, to the rest of the immune system. This activates the killer T-lymphocytes that hunt down and destroy microbes, monocytes that engulf microbes, and B cells that produce antibodies. Therefore HIV weakens the immune system, causing the patient to be susceptible to opportunistic infections that can lead to death.

HIV Disease Continuum

Initial infection with HIV may manifest with mononucleosis-like symptoms, such as fever, fatigue, sore throat, lymphadenopathy, and occasionally spleno-megaly. In the asymptomatic phase the patient is infectious without any signs or symptoms for months to 10 or more years. Next is persistent generalized lymphadenopathy that lasts at least 3 months.

Acquired immunodeficiency syndrome (AIDS) is the final phase. In this phase, the immune system is suppressed, making the person susceptible to opportunistic infections.

Screening

Preconception Screening for Known HIV-Positive Women

Preconception screening is being emphasized for the HIV-positive woman to discuss maternal infection status, viral load, immune status, and therapeutic regimen, perinatal transmission risks, and prevention strategies (PHSTF, 2004, 2005). Additional screening for maternal psychological and substance abuse disorders may be in order. Ideal nutritional status is important in optimizing the woman's health and preparing her body for a pregnancy.

Screening if HIV Status is Unknown

The U.S. Preventive Services Task Force (USPSTF, 2005) recommends that all pregnant women be screened for HIV antibodies. The current recommendation for health care providers is the "opt out" screening policy, which informs all pregnant women that HIV screening is a standard prenatal test unless they decline. This recommendation is based on the evidence that early identification of HIV:

- Allows for early antiretroviral treatment that has been shown to signifi-cantly reduce mother-to-fetus transmission.
- Alerts provider so that invasive procedures are minimized to avoid the increased risk for transmission.
- Allows time for teaching regarding the increase risk for transmission with breastfeeding.

Screening Methods Currently Used

Currently, there are two categories of screening methods: rapid HIV tests and confirmatory tests. The new rapid HIV tests allow for screening at the point of care, as well as the traditional laboratory, increasing compliance with the "opt out" HIV screening policy. Three currently available rapid HIV tests are FDA-approved:

- OraQuick Advance HIV-1Antibody Test (whole blood can be used and test is CLIA-waived)
- Uni-Gold Recombigen HIV Test (whole blood can be used)
- Reveal Rapid HIV-1 Antibody Test (serum or plasma is required)

For information about the rapid testing waiver for the OraQuick test, go to the CDC's website *(http://www.cdc.gov/hiv/rapid-testing)*. These test have a high sensitivity and specificity (Lampe and others, 2004). A positive result is to be followed up with one of the two confirmatory tests:

- Western blot
- Immunofluorescence assay (IFA).

A false-negative can result if the tests are done sooner than 3 months after exposure to HIV.

Risk Factors

Risk factors for HIV are as follows:

- Has multiple sex partners or has practiced serial monogamy
- Is infected with another STD
- Personally has used or sexual partner has used illicit IV drugs
- Is an emigrant from an HIV-endemic area, such as Haiti or Africa
- Has been or is employed in the sex trades (prostitution)
- Received a blood transfusion between 1977 and 1985

Pregnancy Outcome

The risk for transmission to the fetus or neonate is approximately 25% without the use of antiretroviral therapy (ACOG, 2000; Lampe and others, 2004). Transmission appears to occur transplacentally, during delivery, and through breast milk (Penn and Ahmed, 2003). In areas where breastfeeding is not the norm for HIV-positive patients, the greatest risk is during delivery; more than 60% of transmissions occur during exposure to birth canal secretions and blood (Penn and Ahmed, 2003).

With the use of antiretroviral (ARV) therapy as a regimen used to treat HIV infection or as prophylaxis to prevent HIV transmission to the fetus/neonate, the risk for perinatal transmission can be significantly lowered. Research has indicated that zidovudine (ZDV) administered during pregnancy can reduce the transmission rate to 8% (PHSTF, 2005a). With the use of combination ARV therapy, which can lower the viral loads more effectively, a number of retrospective studies have reported reduction of HIV transmission rates to below 2% (McGowan and others, 1999; Clarke and others, 2000; Cooper and others, 2000; PHSTF, 2005). Therefore mother-to-child transmission of HIV is virtually eliminated (Moodley and Wennberg, 2005). The risk was similarly reduced in women with viral loads greater than 1000 copies/ml if delivered by cesarean (ACOG, 2000; PHSTF, 2005).

Pregnancy may mask the symptoms of HIV infection because clinical manifestations of HIV such as fatigue, nausea, and weight loss can be common discomforts of pregnancy. However, pregnancy does not appear to accentuate the course of HIV infection (Minkoff and others, 2003).

Treatment in Pregnancy, During Intrapartum, and of the Newborn

The treatment goals are to treat the woman's HIV infection and reduce the risk for perinatal HIV transmission by reducing and maintaining the viral load at or as close to an undetectable level as possible. Initial assessment includes the CD4+ count and HIV-1 RNA copy number, history of medication use, and gestational age. This is followed by serial monitoring of the CD4+ counts and HIV-1 RNA copy number. Liver function should be followed monthly when the woman is taking nevirapine during pregnancy (PHSTF, 2005).

ARV regimens take on two forms: antiretroviral prophylaxis or antiretroviral treatment. Prophylaxis is used to prevent transmission from mother to child when the mother herself has no indication for ARV therapy. The current ART prophylaxis, according to the PHSTF (2004, 2005) and World Health Organization (2004), is as follows:

- Antepartum: Give oral ZDV, 100 mg five times daily, or 200 mg tid or 300 mg bid, initiated at 28 weeks of gestation and continued throughout pregnancy.
- Intrapartum: Continue ZDV plus a single-dose nevirapine (NVA) at onset of labor.
- Neonate: Dose the neonate with ZDV for 1 week.

Alternative regimens include ZDV in combination with lamivudine (3TC) or single-dose nevirapine (NVP).

For women who are on antiretroviral (ARV) treatment before pregnancy, the current recommendation is to stay on the medications and to avoid known teratogenic drugs such as ribonucleotide reductase hydroxyurea and nonnucleoside reverse transcriptase inhibitor efavirenz. ZDV may be added or substituted to the current regimen, avoiding incompatible drug combinations. Screen for therapy-associated side effects such as hyperglycemia, anemia, and hepatic toxicity (PHSTF, 2005). ARV treatment can be started during pregnancy if the viral load indicates. These women should be given the option of starting their medications after the first trimester to decrease the risk for teratogenicity, while also weighing the risk for delayed therapy (PHSTF, 2004, 2005). For a complete evidence-based resource on nucleoside analogue inhibitors, refer to the CDC's *Safety and Toxicity of Individual Antiretroviral Agents in Pregnancy (http://www.aidsinfo.nih.gov/guidelines)* or the World Health Organization's Guidelines *(http://www.who.int/hiv/pub/mtct/guidelines/en)*.

Women with HIV infection who are in labor and who have had no prior ART therapy are currently being treated using several regimens. One regimen is a single dose of nevirapine given to mother, 200 mg orally, at the onset of labor and to the newborn, 2 mg/kg orally, between 48 and 72 hours of life. Other regimens involve oral or IV ZDV to the mother during labor and then to the infant in combination with lamivudine (3TC) (PHSTF, 2004, 2005; WHO, 2004).

Counseling regarding scheduled cesarean at 38 weeks should take into consideration the viral load and gestational age confirmation, as well as the risk to the mother. If the viral load is less than 1000 copies/ml, given the low risk for transmission, it is unlikely that the cesarean would further reduce transmission. However, if the viral load is greater than 1000 copies/ml or if the viral load is unknown and the mother has been receiving only ZDV monotherapy, or not receiving antiretroviral therapy, a cesarean further reduces the risk for transmission (Lampe and others, 2004; PHSTF, 2004, 2005). Refer to the antiretroviral clinical scenarios for varying situations to obtain specific guidelines for individualized treatment found in the Public Health Service Task Force (2005) recommendations for use of antiretroviral drugs in pregnant women with HIV-1 infection.

To enhance the treatment of HIV during pregnancy, an Antiviral Pregnancy Registry (800-258-4262; fax: 800-800-1052) is being maintained to collect data to follow the long-term safety of exposure of the fetus to antiretroviral agents. Patient handouts are available at AIDSinfo, a service of the U.S. Department of Health and Human Services (USDHHS), http://www.aidsinfo.nih.gov

Pregnancy Considerations

Antepartum

If HIV infection is diagnosed during pregnancy, the woman needs initial and ongoing counseling for the social, emotional, and economic ramifications. She also needs education as to potential consequences of pregnancy on HIV disease progression as well as risk for transmission and consequences to her child. To facilitate health promotion, the woman needs adequate instructions in ways to enhance the immune system, such as (1) adequate sleep; (2) decreased stress; (3) adequate protein because a deficiency can cause depression of cell-mediated immunity, complement, and phagocytes; (4) balanced intake of polyunsaturated fatty acids and vitamin E because a high intake can depress the humoral- and cell-mediated immunity; (5) adequate zinc and vitamin A for overall growth and development of immune cells; (6) adequate pyridoxine, pantothenic acid, and folic acid for general cell synthesis (a deficiency in any of these nutrients can impair both humoral- and cell-mediated immunity); (7) avoidance of infections; and (8) cessation of cigarette smoking because smoking further alters immunity. Screen for other STDs. Assist in the notification plan of all sexual partners.

Intrapartum

Another current recommendation is that all women presenting in labor without documentation of HIV status be screened for HIV using one of the rapid HIV tests unless the woman declines through the "opt out" approach. Measures must be taken to protect confidentiality.

Elective cesarean delivery before rupture of membranes has been shown to further decrease the risk for mother-to-child transmission of HIV infection in women whose viral loads are greater than 1000 copies/ml (PHSTF, 2005). However, cesarean delivery increases the HIV-positive mother's risk for post-partum complications. Therefore the woman should be allowed to make the decision after receiving current information about the known and potential benefits and risks to her and her infant (CDC, 2004). If cesarean delivery is chosen, schedule the procedure for 38 weeks of gestation. A ZDV infusion should be started 3 hours prior to surgery (PHSTF, 2005).

If vaginal delivery is chosen, care should be taken to decrease risk for inoculation of the virus into the neonate during labor by not using a scalp electrode for fetal monitoring or doing a scalp blood sampling for fetal pH (Penn and Ahmed, 2003). Delay amniotomy to possibly decrease the transmission rate of HIV because of the evidence that increasing duration of membrane rupture is associated with an increasing transmission risk. Avoid such invasive procedures as forceps- or vacuum-assisted delivery and episiotomy if clinically appropriate (Lampe and others, 2004).

Postpartum

According to the Perinatal HIV Guidelines Working Group (PHSTF, 2005), comprehensive care and support services are important for the HIV-positive postpartum woman and should include the following:
- Case management coordination of care by the primary care provider, obstetrician, pediatrician, and HIV clinical specialist
- Observation for signs of clinical depression with appropriate referrals made as indicated
- Reemphasis on safe-sex practices and referral for family planning
- Counseling regarding importance of adherence to use of antiretroviral agents and prophylactic drugs against opportunistic infections, if indicated
- Review of immunization status, updating vaccines, and reviewing prevention of opportunistic infections
- Reference for substance abuse treatment, if appropriate

A recent Kenyan study added to the plethora of existing research that shows a significant transmission during breastfeeding (Nduati and others, 2000). If formula is readily available, as it is in all industrialized countries, the mother should not breastfeed her baby.

Neonate

Because the length of exposure appears to be important, bathe the infant as soon as possible after delivery (Lampe and others, 2004). Percutaneous needlesticks should be done only after the initial bath and with thorough cleansing of the skin just before the injections. Refer parents to a pediatric HIV specialist for follow-up care.

Because of the risk for anemia, a baseline complete blood count with differential should be obtained prior to starting antiretroviral therapy. After the 6-week antiviral prophylaxis regimen, prophylaxis antibiotic treatment for *Pneumocystis carinii* pneumonia should be initiated (PHSTF, 2005).

Antibody screening is not reliable during infancy because maternally produced immunoglobulin G (IgG) antibodies to HIV are present in the body up to 18 months of age. However, an HIV DNA PCR virologic test is used to determine whether the neonate received the virus from the mother. The test is usually performed within 48 hours after birth, at 14 days of life, at age 1 to 2 months, and at age 4 to 6 months. HIV is diagnosed by two positive test results at two different times. Two negative test results, one of which must be after 4 months, means HIV can be reasonably ruled out (Pediatric HIV Working Group, 2005).

Health Care Workers

Use standard precautions when caring for all pregnant women during labor, during delivery, and during the postpartum period and for infants until they have had their first bath. This includes wearing gloves, protective eyewear, and water-repellent gowns.

HUMAN PAPILLOMAVIRUS

Organism

The organisms responsible for human papillomaviruses (HPVs) are human wart viruses of the papillomaviridae family of DNA viruses. Currently, more than 100 HPV types are identified, 40 of which infect the genital area (ACOG, 2005). Ninety-five percent of cervical cancer cases are associated with HPV. HPV types 16, 18, 45, and 56 are found to be strongly associated with genital dysplasia and invasive cancer. HPV types 31, 33, and 35 are more commonly associated with squamous intraepithelial neoplasia (Canavan and Doshi, 2000; Thomas, 2001). HPV types 6 and 11, the most common types, have a lower but increased risk for dysplasia (CDC, 2002).

Transmission

Sexual contact is the most common form of transmission, with a higher transmission rate in young adolescents and multiple sex partners (Gerberding, 2004). Other risk factors associated with HPV infection are smoking and poor nutrition, which affect the immune response, and lack of male circumcision (Gerberding, 2004).

Signs and Symptoms

Most women with HPV are asymptomatic. The virus requires magnification or acetic acid for visualization and can be transmitted before visual lesions appear. Visible warty growths are single or multiple growths called *condylomata acuminata* (genital warts); these warts may be fleshy-colored, pale pink or red, raised or flat, and small or large. If clustered together, they may have a cauliflower-shaped appearance (CDC, 2002). Mucosal warts located on non-hairy areas of the genital tract are softer. Hyperkeratotic warts located in outer hairy skin of the vulva are firm (Thomas, 2001).

Screening

Screening for HPV includes the following:
- Hybrid capture HPV DNA test with liquid-based cytology (Thin-Prep)
- Visualization
- Application of acetic acid to wart to magnify its presence

Treatment in Pregnancy

Most HPV infections are controlled by the body's immune system. Research studies indicate that 70% of HIV infections clear within 1 year and 90% clear within 2 years (Ho and others, 1998; Moscicki and others, 1998; Syrjanen, 2002; Molano and others, 2003). However, reactivation or reinfection occurs (CDC, 2002). No treatment has been shown to eradicate HPV. Therefore the goal is to remove the visible lesions and ameliorate the signs and symptoms only, not to eliminate the virus (Thomas, 2001). After removal of visible lesions, wait for the immune response to control replication of the virus. Various treatments are used to do this. A safe treatment regimen during pregnancy is the use of trichloroacetic acid (TCA), bichloroacetic acid (BcA), or cryotherapy with liquid nitrogen.

Electrocautery effectively removes small lesions throughout pregnancy. Surgical removal during pregnancy has an increased risk for hemorrhage related to the increased vascularity. Podophyllum resins and interferon are not safe treatment modalities during pregnancy because of their teratogenic potential. Safety of the patient-applied medications podofilox, imiquimod, and podophyllin is unknown and should not be used during pregnancy (CDC, 2006).

If the patient smokes, instruct her regarding the effect that smoking has on the immune system, which can decrease the effectiveness of any HPV treatment.

All sexual partners should be examined for any evidence of warts and instructed to use condoms to decrease transmission.

Effect on Pregnancy Outcome

Condylomata acuminata, genital warts, have an insignificant adverse effect on pregnancy.

Pregnancy Considerations

HPV is currently the most common viral STD in North America (Thomas, 2001) and, according to the CDC, HPV is the most common STD in young, sexually active women 25 years and under (CDC, 2006). Warts tend to proliferate and become friable during pregnancy (CDC, 2006). During delivery, condylomata can cause pelvic outlet obstruction and severe hemorrhage related to lacerations of the friable condylomatous tissue.

There is a 2% to 5% risk for HPV, especially types 6 and 11, causing laryngeal papillomas in infants and children exposed during delivery through an infected birth canal (McCance and Huether, 2006). These laryngeal papillomas usually appear between 2 and 5 years of age, causing such symptoms as an abnormal cry, voice changes, stridor, or evidence of airway obstruction.

Cesarean delivery is indicated only when warts are so large at the time of delivery that the risk for dystocia and hemorrhage is great (CDC, 2006).

There is a 25% to 33% risk for coexisting STDs such as trichomoniasis, BV, and chlamydia. Coinfection with chlamydia and herpes simplex type 2 may increase the risk for cervical cancer (Smith and others, 2002; Castle and Giuliano, 2003).

There is strong research evidence regarding the association between HPV and the development of cervical cancer (Gerberding, 2004). Therefore all patients with HPV should be instructed regarding the risk and reminded of the importance of a yearly Pap smear. Thin-Prep Pap test is the preferred test for any patient with a history of HPV or with a prior positive Pap. If the report comes back as positive for atypical squamous cells of undetermined significance (ASCUS), ask for a hybrid capture HPV DNA assay, a diagnostic test for HPV, on the Thin Prep (ACOG, 2003). If the HC_2 is positive, colposcopy is appropriate follow-up.

A healthy lifestyle with exercise, with a healthy diet low in fat and high in vegetables and fruits, and without cigarette smoking enhances the immune system and is important in decreasing the cervical cancer risk. Smoking and deficiencies in vitamin A, vitamin C, and folic acid can increase the risk for progressive development of invasive carcinoma in the presence of HPV (Carson, 1997; Thomas, 2001).

SYPHILIS

Organism

The organism responsible for syphilis is *Treponema pallidum,* an anaerobic spirochete bacterium.

Transmission

Syphilis is transmitted by way of sexual contact during the primary, secondary, and early latent stages.

Signs and Symptoms

After exposure to syphilis, there is an incubation period before the first stage of the disease. This time period can last 10 to 90 days, during which the patient is serononreactive. After this incubation phase, syphilis has four distinct stages:

- **Primary syphilis.** Stage one is evidenced by a chancre, which is a highly infectious, painless, round, ulcerated sore that does not get better fast. It may last 3 to 6 weeks.
- **Secondary syphilis.** Stage two is evidenced by a maculopapular rash that typically occurs on the face, palms of the hands, or soles of the feet and is characterized by brown sores about the size of a penny. This rash is usually exhibited between 1 week and 3 months after the primary chancre. It

typically clears in 2 to 6 weeks but can last up to a year. Other manifestations include wartlike genital "growth," lymphadenopathy, fever, sore throat, patchy hair loss, headaches, weight loss, muscle aches, and tiredness.

- **Latent syphilis.** Stage three is usually asymptomatic. The spirochete goes into hiding for 5 to 20 years. The patient is seroreactive during this stage. However, in about one third of patients, the infection may develop into the tertiary stage of syphilis. The other two thirds will experience no further consequences of the disease. During the first year of this stage (early latent), the patient is infectious.

- **Tertiary syphilis.** The fourth stage is a remanifestation of the disease; it slowly destroys the heart, eyes, brain, central nervous system, and occasionally, the liver, bones, and skin.

Screening

Routine screening is considered a standard of practice to be performed on the first prenatal visit and repeated at 28 weeks of gestation and at delivery if the patient is at high risk (CDC, 2006). Some states mandate syphilis screening at delivery for all pregnant women. All cord blood should be tested as well. Increased cord blood sample error occurs if the cord is milked to obtain the sample. Common screening tests for syphilis are the nontreponemal tests, that is, either the Venereal Disease Research Laboratory (VDRL) test or the rapid plasma reagin (RPR) test. Common tests used to confirm the diagnosis are the treponemal antibody titer tests, either the microhemagglutination assay for antibodies to *T. pallidum* (MHA-TP) or the fluorescent treponemal antibody absorption test (FTA-ABS).

Treatment in Pregnancy

If the patient has had the disease for less than 1 year, she is given benzathine penicillin G, 2.4 million units IM for one dose. If the patient has had the disease for more than 1 year, she is given Bicillin L-A (penicillin G benzathine), 2.4 million units IM for three doses 1 week apart for 3 consecutive weeks, for a total of 7.2 million units (CDC, 2006).

This therapy cures a maternal infection and prevents congenital syphilis (CDC, 2006). Sixty percent of women who receive this treatment experience a Jarisch-Herxheimer reaction, that is, a fever, myalgia, headache, mild hypotension, tachycardia, decreased fetal activity, and uterine contractions (CDC, 2006).

If the patient is allergic to penicillin, the CDC (2006) guidelines suggest skin testing and referral for penicillin desensitization. This is indicated because tetracycline and doxycycline are contraindicated during pregnancy and nonpenicillin drugs such as erythromycin fail to prevent congenital syphilis (CDC, 2006).

Monthly quantitative nontreponemal serologic tests for the remainder of the pregnancy should be drawn. If the titers show a four-fold rise, the pregnant woman is retreated.

All sexual partners are managed according to the CDC latest guidelines.

Effect on Pregnancy Outcome

The syphilis spirochete can cross the placenta at any time. However, treatment is very effective if given before 16 weeks of gestation; this is related to fetal immune competence before that gestational age (Gibbs, Sweet, and Duff, 2004).

Untreated syphilis can profoundly affect the fetus, depending on the stage of maternal infection and the length of exposure to the organism. During the active phases of the disease, the organism load is the highest and has the gravest effect on the fetus. If the mother has untreated early latent syphilis, infection of the fetus is possible but there is significantly lower risk (Gibbs, Sweet, and Duff, 2004).

Consequences of congenital syphilis are the following:
- Spontaneous abortion
- Prematurity
- Stillbirth
- Multisystem failure of the heart, lungs, spleen, liver, and pancreas, as well as structural bone damage and nervous system involvement and mental retardation.

TRICHOMONIASIS

Organism

The organism responsible for trichomoniasis is *Trichomonas vaginalis*, a flagellated protozoan that is sexually transmitted.

Transmission

Trichomoniasis generally is caused by sexual activity. However, it may be contracted by swimming in contaminated water, using contaminated towels, or sitting in contaminated hot tubs.

Signs and Symptoms

The pregnant woman with trichomoniasis may be asymptomatic, or she may exhibit some or all of the following signs and symptoms:
- Frothy, yellow-green or gray, foul-smelling discharge
- Constant perineal itching
- Erythema (strawberry spots)
- Vaginal pH alkaline (>4.5)
- Vaginal mucosa erythematous
- Cervix with punctate hemorrhages

Screening

If the pregnant woman is symptomatic for trichomoniasis, a saline wet mount shows motile trichomonads with an increased number of white blood cells. The amine odor (Whiff test) may or may not be positive for a fishy odor, and the vaginal pH is greater than 4.5 and often greater than 6.0. The routine Pap smear may detect trichomonads.

Treatment in Pregnancy

Symptomatic

Treatment of choice for trichomoniasis during pregnancy is metronidazole (Flagyl), a single oral dose of 2 g (CDC, 2006). Some health care providers prefer to avoid treatment until after the first trimester; however, according to the CDC (2006), there is no indication of teratogenicity. According to the *Cochrane Review*, it is unknown whether this treatment has any adverse effect on the pregnancy (Gulmezoglu, 2002). The U.S. National Institute of Child Health and Human Development trial has shown an increased risk for preterm labor when trichomoniasis is treated with metronidazole (Kigozi and others, 2003).

No alcoholic beverages or vinegar products are allowed for 48 hours after therapy to avoid nausea, vomiting, cramping, and headaches. No intercourse is allowed for 2 weeks to allow pelvic and cervical rest.

During breastfeeding the woman could be treated with metronidazole, 2 g orally for one dose, and instructed to pump and discard breast milk for 24 hours (Lawrence, 2005). All sexual partners should be treated also.

Asymptomatic

According to ACOG's meta-analysis, there is an increase risk for preterm labor when asymptomatic trichomoniasis is treated with metronidazole (Okun, Gronau, and Hannah, 2005). It is speculated that the dying organisms elicits an inflammatory response that stimulates preterm contractions.

Effect on Pregnancy Outcome

Trichomonas vaginalis is diagnosed in 20% of all pregnancies and has been implicated in PROM and preterm delivery (CDC, 2006).

URINARY TRACT INFECTION

UTI is manifested by the following three clinical types:

1   Asymptomatic bacteriuria
2   Cystitis
3   Pyelonephritis

Organism

The common causative organisms of UTIs are coliforms, particularly *Escherichia coli* gram-negative pathogenic bacteria. They account for approximately 85% of all UTIs. Other gram-negative pathogenic bacteria (*Klebsiella pneumoniae*, *Proteus* species) are important pathogens, especially in recurrent UTIs. Less frequent causative organisms involved in UTIs are gram-positive organisms: group B streptococci, enterococci, and staphylococci. They account for approximately 3% to 7% of the infections (Delzell, 2000). Two other causative organisms are *N. gonorrhoeae* and *C. trachomatis* (sexually transmitted pathogens).

Transmission

Coliform organisms are a normal part of the perineal flora and may be introduced into the urethra during intercourse or improper wiping after defecation. *N. gonorrhoeae* and *C. trachomatis* are transmitted by sexual contact.

Signs and Symptoms

Signs and symptoms of a UTI depend on the location of the infection. In 5% to 10% of cases, they are asymptomatic. In cystitis or lower UTI, the following symptoms are common:
- Urinary frequency
- Urinary urgency
- Dysuria
- Hesitancy or dribbling
- Suprapubic tenderness
- Gross hematuria

Accompanying symptoms with pyelonephritis (upper UTI) are usually chills, fever, and back pain with costovertebral angle (CVA) tenderness. Signs of a lower UTI may be present as well.

Screening

Routine screening for UTI is standard practice at the first prenatal visit and is repeated at 32 to 34 weeks of gestation. It should also be performed if there are complaints of any signs or symptoms:
- Microscopic examination shows white blood cells; bacteria may or may not be present
- Dip urine may be positive for nitrites and leukocyte esterase
- Clean-catch midstream specimen for culture and sensitivity

Treatment in Pregnancy for Asymptomatic or Acute Cystitis

According to the *Cochrane Review*, antibiotic therapy for asymptomatic bacteriuria is effective in lowering the risk for pyelonephritis and preterm labor (Smaill, 2001). Table 25-1 lists the most common antibiotics used in treatment of asymptomatic or acute cystitis. In the initial infection, a 7- to 10-day course of treatment is usually preferred (Delzell, 2000). However, with a recurrent infection, a 7- to 10-day course of treatment is necessary. To facilitate antibacterial action, acidify urine by having the woman take ascorbic acid (vitamin C) or cranberry tablets (Fontaine, 2000; Sierpina, 2001). Griffiths (2003) review of the literature did not support treating UTI with cranberry juice. Instruct the patient to drink at least one glass of water or low sugar juice per waking hour and to void before and after intercourse to decrease the risk for recurrent UTIs. At all remaining prenatal visits, screen the urine for nitrites and leukocyte esterase. If either of these tests is positive, repeat urine culture and retreat as culture indicates.

Table 25-1   Antibiotics for Asymptomatic Bacteriuria or Cystitis

Antibiotics	Organism Sensitivity	Oral Dose	Administration Considerations
Penicillin (Amoxicillin)	70%–80% of *Escherichia coli,* most *Proteus* species, group B streptococci, enterococci, some staphylococci	500 mg three times daily	Do not use this drug unless sensitivity test indicates sensitivity Side effects: diarrhea and candidiasis
Penicillin (Augmentin)	Most gram-negative aerobic bacilli Most gram-positive cocci	500–875 mg bid	Best to use if drug-resistant *E. coli is* suspected Side effects: diarrhea and candidiasis
Cephalosporin (Keflex)	Most *E. coli* *Klebsiella* *Proteus* species Group B streptococci Staphylococci	250–500 mg four time daily	
Nitrofurantoin (Macrobid)	Most gram-negative aerobic bacilli	100 mg four time daily	Best to use if drug-resistant *E. coli is* suspected
Sulfonamides (Bactrim)	Most gram-negative aerobic bacilli	160/800 mg twice daily	Pregnancy category C drug Avoid first trimester use and do not use near delivery date because it has possible effect on protein binding of bilirubin causing hemolytic anemia

Data from Gibbs R, Sweet R, Duff W: Maternal and fetal infectious disorders. In Creasy R, Resnik R, Iams J: *Maternal-fetal medicine: principles and practice,* ed 5, Philadelphia, 2004, Saunders; Weiner C, Buhimschi C: *Drugs for pregnant and lactating women,* Philadelphia, 2004, Churchill Livingstone.

Treatment in Pregnancy for Pyelonephritis

The patient may be treated on an outpatient basis if the disease manifestations are mild and the patient is hemodynamically stable and without evidence of preterm labor. The usual treatment is amoxicillin clavulanate (Augmentin), 875 mg bid for 7 to 10 days, trimethoprim and sulfamethoxazole (Bactrim DS), twice daily for 7 to 10 days, or ceftriaxone (Rocephin) IM plus oral cephalexin (Keflex). If the patient is hemodynamically unstable, disease manifestations are severe, including high fever, chills, and tachycardia. If the patient is experiencing uterine contractions, she must be hospitalized for treatment. Obtain a catheterized urine sample and send immediately for culture and sensitivity. Initiate antibiotic therapy immediately.

If the patient is hemodynamically stable, common IV antibiotic therapy is a first-generation cephalosporin, such as cefazolin (Ancef), 1–2 g IV piggyback every 8 hours, or a third-generation penicillin, such as ampicillin, 1–2 g IV piggyback every 6 hours (Gibbs, Sweet, and Duff, 2004). If the patient has a high fever, chills, and tachycardia, alternate ampicillin and gentamicin. The usual dose of gentamicin is 1 mg/kg every 8 hours. Consider changing the IV antibiotic therapy if the culture and sensitivity indicate or if the patient has not responded to therapy within 48 hours (Gibbs, Sweet, and Duff, 2004). Obtain blood cultures if the patient has an unexplained heart murmur or signs of subacute bacterial endocarditis.

Discontinue the IV antibiotics when the patient is afebrile for 48 hours, and continue on oral antibiotics to complete a 10-day course of therapy. Commonly used oral antibiotics are listed in Table 25-1. Repeat a urine culture and sensitivity before discharge from hospital.

Effect on Pregnancy Outcome

The endotoxins released from gram-negative bacteria may stimulate the production of prostaglandins and thus cause preterm labor (AAP and ACOG, 2002; Cram and others, 2002). If the causative organism was GBS, the woman should be treated with antibiotics during labor to decrease the risk for GBS infection in the newborn. Refer to the Group B Streptococcus section earlier in this chapter.

Pregnancy Considerations

Approximately 10% of all pregnancies are complicated with a UTI. Approximately 2% of these cases are pyelonephritis, usually as a consequence of undiagnosed asymptomatic bacteruria or inadequately treated cystitis. The risk to preterm labor is increased (ACOG, 2002).

GENERAL NURSING MANAGEMENT FOR GENITOURINARY INFECTIONS

Prevention

Prevention is the cornerstone of nursing practice and includes three steps: primary, secondary, and tertiary prevention. Primary prevention of genitourinary infections, including sexually transmitted infections (STIs), involves health promotion and prevention activities. When primary prevention fails, secondary prevention, involving activities for early detection, is the next important step in the prevention of serious consequences. Tertiary prevention involves appropriate treatment to prevent or reduce disability once the infection is contracted.

Primary Prevention of Sexually Transmitted Infections

- Nurses should be actively involved in accurate, timely education programs that teach about the method of transmission and risk reduction behaviors.

- The only absolutely safe sexual practice is abstinence until one establishes a mutually monogamous relationship. Health care providers should not avoid mentioning this option, especially with teens (Tumolo, 2000).
- Safe sexual practice, if one chooses to have sex outside a mutually monogamous relationship, is use of condoms. Use of condoms decreases the risk but is not 100% effective. The health care provider must inform the patient that she can contract an infection, especially viral herpes or HPV, from viral shedding in the genital area not covered by the condom (Waldrop, 2001).
- Abstinence from illegal drug use, especially the sharing of needles and syringes with anyone, is important.
- Conduct a sexual history. A guide to taking a sexual history is an excellent resource provided by the CDC in the Syphilis Elimination Effort (SEE) Tool Kit. This resource can be retrieved online *(http://www.cdc.gov/std/see/ description.htm)*.
- Periodic examinations for STDs in the at-risk woman are beneficial.
- Expression of values and beliefs that might not following this type of suggested lifestyle are allowed.
- Motivation seminars can increase one's reasons to delay sex, including the following examples:
  - Job training
  - Staying in school
  - Building self-esteem
  - Life planning and counseling
  - Recreational activities

Secondary Prevention of Sexually Transmitted Infections

- When women of childbearing age seek health care, a thorough history should be taken and should include the following:
  - Cultural background
  - Sexual practices
  - Drug use
- Periodic examinations for STDs in the at-risk group are beneficial.
- Further investigation of the following manifested signs should be conducted:
  - Perineal, vaginal, or cervical lesions or sores
  - Increased, abnormal, or malodorous vaginal discharge
  - Dysuria
- Teach the significant signs and symptoms to at-risk patients, and instruct them to report to health care workers to enable effective treatment to be initiated early.

Tertiary Prevention of Sexually Transmitted Infections

- Implement treatment according to the CDC guidelines.
- Inform of the requirement to report specific STDs, such as syphilis, gonorrhea, and HIV, to community health officials, and explain local follow-up procedures in this event.

- Educate as to the importance of notifying all sexual partners who could have been infected when an STD is diagnosed.
- Encourage abstinence from sex until follow-up cultures are negative.
- Educate as to the importance of using condoms lubricated with a spermicide containing nonoxynol-9 to prevent reinfection.
- Educate as to the importance of seeking immediate medical treatment if any symptoms reappear or if a sexual partner is diagnosed with an STD.
- Inform that cigarette smoking may accelerate the pathogenic course of many STIs, especially HPV.

Affect Self-Esteem When Diagnosed with an Incurable Sexually Transmitted Infection

- Provide opportunities to discuss feelings in a nonjudgmental environment.
- Provide referrals to support groups if indicated.
- Assist in planning for future with regard to sexual activity.
- Provide assistance with notification of sexual partners if applicable.
- Provide opportunities for family members to discuss feelings in a nonjudgmental environment.
- Provide appropriate referrals as needed.
- Suggest alternative methods of sexual gratification for couples who have an active STD.
- Educate regarding the importance of ongoing screening protocols and treatment regimens.
- Empower in self-care strategies.

Primary Prevention of Vaginal Infections Related to Nonsexually Transmitted Infections

- Teach behaviors to promote normal vaginal flora:
  - Wear cotton undergarments and avoid tight fitting clothing.
  - Maintain good perineal hygiene.
  - Reduce simple sugars in the diet.
  - Refrain from douching for hygienic reasons.
  - Eat yogurt or drink milk containing active acidophilus cultures when taking an antibiotic.

CONCLUSION

Most STDs pose a risk not only to the pregnant woman but also to the fetus she carries. It is particularly important that childbearing women be free of STDs. Nurses who provide health care to childbearing families can participate in primary prevention by conducting education programs and consistently providing ongoing education about the risk and prevention of these diseases. Nurses should also be involved in secondary and tertiary prevention, which includes early diagnosis and appropriate intervention if the problem arises. Only by addressing these diseases at every level will progress be made in diminishing their prevalence and devastating effects.

BIBLIOGRAPHY
Bacterial Vaginosis

Andrist L: Vaginal health and infections, *J Obstet Gynecol Neonatal Nurs* 30(3):306–315, 2001.

Centers for Disease Control and Prevention: *Bacterial vaginosis,* Factsheet, Rockville, MD, 2004. Author. Retrieved from *http://www.cdc.gov/std/healthcomm/fact_sheets.htm*

Centers for Disease Control and Prevention (CDC): Sexually transmitted diseases treatment guidelines, 2006, *MMWR Morb Mortal Wkly Rep* 55(RR11):1–94, 2006.

Cottrell B: Vaginal douching practices of women in eight Florida panhandle counties, *J Obstet Gynecol Neonatal Nurs* 35(1):24–33, 2006.

Gibbs R, Sweet R, and Duff W: Maternal fetal infectious disorders. In Creasy R, Resnik R, and Iams J, editors: *Maternal-fetal medicine: principles and practice,* ed 5, Philadelphia, 2004, Saunders.

Hillier S: Treatment of recurrent bacteria vaginosis, *Clinician Rev* 14:98–101, 106, 2004.

Lawrence R, Lawrence M: *Breastfeeding: a guide for the medical profession,* ed 6, Philadelphia, 2005, Mosby.

Leitich H and others: Bacterial vaginosis as a risk factor for preterm delivery: a meta-analysis, *Am J Obstet Gynecol* 189(1):139–147, 2003.

Mayeaux E: Work-up of bacterial vaginosis, *Female Patient* 26(5):21, 2001.

Macones G and others: A polymorphism in the promoter region of TNF and bacterial vaginosis: preliminary evidence of gene-environment interaction in the etiology of spontaneous preterm birth, *Am J Obstet Gynecol* 190(6):1504–1508, 2004.

Nyirjesy P, Bosarge P, and Taylor P: Diagnosis of bacterial vaginosis: pathways to effective treatment, *Clinical Reviews: A Self-Study Supplement* March 2003.

Okun N, Gronau K, and Hannah M: Antibiotics for bacterial vaginosis or trichomonas vaginalis in pregnancy: a systematic review, *Obstet Gynecol* 105(4):857–868, 2005.

Candidiasis

Andrist L: Vaginal health and infections, *J Obstet Gynecol Neonatal Nurs* 30(3):306–315, 2001.

Centers for Disease Control and Prevention (CDC): Sexually transmitted diseases treatment guidelines, 2006, *MMWR Morb Mortal Wkly Rep* 55(RR11):1–94, 2006.

Freeman L, Lawlis G: *Mosby's complementary and alternative medicine: a research-based approach,* St Louis, 2001, Mosby.

Gibbs R, Sweet R, and Duff W: Maternal fetal infectious disorders. In Creasy R, Resnik R, and Iams J, editors: *Maternal-fetal medicine: principles and practice,* ed 5, Philadelphia, 2004, Saunders.

Sierpina V: *Integrative health care: complementary and alternative therapies for the whole person,* Philadelphia, 2001, FA Davis.

Chlamydia

Agency for Healthcare Research and Quality: *U.S. Preventive Services Task Force calls for chlamydia, lipid screening among first four recommendations,* Rockville, Md, 2001, U.S. Department of Health and Human Services.

Brocklehurst P, Rooney G: Interventions for treating genital chlamydia trachomatic infection in pregnancy, *Cochrane Database Syst Rev* Issue 4, 1998.

Centers for Disease Control and Prevention: *Chlamydia,* Factsheet, Rockville, MD, 2004. Author. Retrieved from *http://www.cdc.gov/std/healthcomm/fact_sheets.htm*

Centers for Disease Control and Prevention (CDC): Sexually transmitted diseases treatment guidelines, 2006, *MMWR Morb Mortal Wkly Rep* 55(RR11):1-94, 2006.

National Guideline Clearinghouse: *Guideline synthesis: screening for and management of chlamydial infection.* Rockville, Md, 2005, NGC. Retrieved from *http://www.guideline.gov*

Rawlins S: Nonviral sexually transmitted infections, *J Obstet Gynecol Neonatal Nurs* 30(3):324–331, 2001.

Parratt J, Hay D: Sexually transmitted infections, *Curr Obstet Gynaecol* 13(4):224, 2003.

Schachter J, Barnes R: Chlamydia. In Morse S, Moreland A, and Holmes K, editors: *Atlas of sexually transmitted diseases and AIDS,* ed 2, Baltimore, 1996, Mosby-Wolfe.

Tiller C: Chlamydia during pregnancy: implications and impact on perinatal and neonatal outcome, *J Obstet Gynecol Neonatal Nurs* 31(1):93–98, 2002.

Ward M, webmaster: *A portal to the Chlamydia literature and news,* England, 2003, University of Southampton. Retrieved from *http://www.Chlamydiae.com*

Gonorrhea

Brocklehurst P: Interventions for treating gonorrhoeae in pregnancy, *Cochrane Database Syst Rev* Issue 2, 2002.

Centers for Disease Control and Prevention (CDC): Sexually transmitted diseases treatment guidelines, 2006, *MMWR Morb Mortal Wkly Rep* 55(RR11):1–94, 2006.

Centers for Disease Control and Prevention: National Center for Chronic Disease Prevention and Health Promotion: *2001 performance plan,* 2001 [online]. Retrieved from *http://www.cdc.gov/od/pertplan/2001perfplan.pdf*

Gibbs R, Sweet R, and Duff W: Maternal fetal infectious disorders. In Creasy R, Resnik R, and Iams J, editors: *Maternal-fetal medicine: principles and practice,* ed 5, Philadelphia, 2004, Saunders.

Koumans E and others: Laboratory testing for *Neisseria gonorrhoeae* by recently introduced non-culture tests: a performance review with clinical and public health considerations, *Clin Infect Dis* 27(5):1171–1180, 1998.

Miller J and others: Initial and repeated screening for gonorrhea during pregnancy, *Sex Transm Dis* 30(9):728–730, 2003.

Parratt J, Hay D: Sexually transmitted infections, *Curr Obstet Gynaecol* 13(4):224, 2003.

Group B Streptococcus

American College of Obstetricians and Gynecologists: Prevention of early-onset group B Strepto-coccal disease in newborns, *ACOG Committee Opinion* No 279, Washington, DC, 2002, Author.

Centers for Disease Control and Prevention: Prevention of perinatal group B streptococcal disease: revised guidelines from CDC, *MMWR Morb Mortal Wkly Rep* 51:RR-11, 2002.

Money D, Dobson S: The prevention of early-onset neonatal group B streptococcal disease, *J Obstet Gynaecol Can* 26(9):826–840, 2004.

Parratt J, Hay D: Sexually transmitted infections, *Curr Obstet Gynaecol* 13(4):224, 2003.

Schrag S and others: Group B streptococcal disease in the era of intrapartum antibiotic prophylaxis, *N End J Med* 342(1):15–20, 2000.

Hepatitis B

Centers for Disease Control and Prevention (CDC): A Comprehensive immunization strategy to eliminate transmission of Hepatitis B virus infection in the United States, *MMWR Morb Mortal Wkly Rep* 54(RR16):1–33, 2005.

Corrarino J: Perinatal hepatitis B: update and recommendations, *MCN Am J Matern Child Nurs* 23(5):246–252, 1998.

Corrarino J, Walsh P, and Anselmo D: A program to educate women who test positive for the hepatitis B virus during the perinatal period, *MCN Am J Matern Child Nurs* 24(3):151–155, 1999.

Immunization Action Coalition: *Hepatitis B facts: testing and vaccination,* St Paul, 2004, IAC. Retrieved from *http://www.immunize.org/catg.d/p2110.htm*

Landon M: Diseases of the liver, biliary system, pancreas. In Creasy R, Resnik R, and Iams J, editors: *Maternal-fetal medicine: principles and practice,* ed 5, Philadelphia, 2004, Saunders.

Hepatitis C

Centers for Disease Control and Prevention (CDC): Sexually transmitted diseases treatment guidelines, 2006, *MMWR Morb Mortal Wkly Rep* 55(RR11):1–94, 2006.

Landon M: Diseases of the liver, biliary system, pancreas. In Creasy R, Resnik R, and Iams J, editors: *Maternal-fetal medicine: principles and practice,* ed 5, Philadelphia, 2004, Saunders.

National Guideline Clearinghouse: *National guideline for the management of the viral hepatitides A, B, and C, 2002,* 2002. Retrieved from *http://guideline.gov*

National Guideline Clearinghouse: Screening for hepatitis C virus infection in adults: re-commendation statement, *Ann Intern Med* 140(6):462, 2004. Retrieved from *http://guideline.gov*

National Institutes of Health: Management of hepatitis C. *NIH Consensus and State-of-the-Science Statements* 19(3), 2002. Retrieved from *http://consensus.nih.gov/cons/cons.htm*

Thomas S and others: A review of hepatitis C virus (HCV) vertical transmission: risks of transmission to infants born to mothers with and without HCV viraemia or human immunodeficiency virus infection, *Int J Epidemiol* 2(1):108–117, 1998.

Herpes Simplex Virus-2

American College of Obstetricians and Gynecologists: Management of herpes in pregnancy, *ACOG Practice Bulletin*, No. 8, Washington, DC, 1999, ACOG.

Baker D and others: Cost-effectiveness of HSV-2 Serologic testing and antiviral therapy in pregnancy, *Am J Obstet Gynecol* 191(6):2074–2084, 2004.

Centers for Disease Control and Prevention (CDC): Sexually transmitted diseases treatment guidelines, *MMWR Morb Mortal Wkly Rep* 55(RR11):1–94, 2006.

Corey L and others: Once daily valacyclovir to reduce the risk of transmission of genital herpes, *N Engl J Med* 350(1):11–20, 2004.

Leone P: Asymptomatic shedding in the transmission, prevention, and treatment of genital herpes, *Medscape Infectious Diseases* 6(1): 2004. Retrieved from *http://www.medscape.com/viewarticle/478550*

Morrow R: Importance of testing and diagnosis in genital herpes, *Medscape Infectious Diseases* 6(2), 2004. Retrieved from *http://www.medscape.com/viewarticle/483440*

Parker L, Montrowi S: Neonatal herpes infection: a review. *NBIN* 4(1):62, 2004. Retrieved from *http://www.medscape.com/viewarticle/472408*

Sandhaus S: Genital herpes in pregnant and nonpregnant women, *Nurs Pract* 26(4):15, 2001.

Sheffield J and others: Acyclovir prophylaxis to prevent herpes simplex virus recurrence at delivery: a systematic review, *Obstet Gynecol* 102(6):1396–1403, 2003.

Steben M, Sacks S: Genital herpes: the epidemiology and control of a common sexually transmitted disease, *Can J Human Sex* 6:127, 1997.

Stone K and others: Pregnancy outcomes following systemic prenatal acyclovir exposure: conclusions from the international acyclovir pregnancy registry, 1984–1999, *Birth Defects Res A Clin Mol Teratol* 70(4):201–207, 2004.

Thomas D: Sexually transmitted viral infections: epidemiology and treatment, *J Obstet Gynecol Neonatal Nurs* 30(3):316–323, 2001.

U.S. Preventive Services Task Force (USPSTF): Screening for genital herpes: Recommendation statement. Rockville, Md, 2005, Agency for Healthcare Research and Quality.

Wald A and others: Polymerase chain reaction for detection of herpes simplex virus (HSV) DNA on mucosal surfaces: comparison with HSV isolation in cell culture, *J Infect Dis* 188(9):1345–1351, 2003.

Wald A, Link K: Risk of human immunodeficiency virus infection in herpes simplex virus infection type 2-seropositve persons: a meta-analysis, *J Infet Dis* 185(1):45–52, 2002.

Wyckoff M: Neonatal herpes simplex virus type II, *MCN Am J Matern Child Nurs* 25(2):100–103, 2000.

HIV

American College of Obstetricians and Gynecologists: *Committee opinion: scheduled cesarean delivery and the prevention of vertical transmission of HIV infection*, No. 234, Washington, DC, 2000, ACOG.

Bardeguez A and others: Effect of cessation of zidovudine prophylaxis to reduce vertical transmission on maternal HIV disease progression and survival, *J Acquir Immune Defic Syndr* 31(2):170–181, 2003.

Brocklehurst P, Volmink J: Antiretrovirals for reducing the risk of mother-to-child transmission of HIV infection, *Cochrane Database Syst Rev* Issue 2, 2002.

Centers for Disease Control and Prevention: Successful implementation of perinatal HIV prevention guidelines, *MMWR Morb Mortal Wkly Rep* 50:15, 2001.

Centers for Disease Control and Prevention: Introduction of routine HIV testing in prenatal care, *MMWR Morb Mortal Wkly Rep* 53(46), 2004.

Clarke S and others: The efficacy and tolerability of combination antiretroviral therapy in pregnancy: infant and maternal outcome, *Int J STD AIDS* 11(4):220–223, 2000.

Cooper E and others: Trends in antiretroviral therapy and mother-infant transmission of HIV, *J Acquire Immune Defic Syndr* 24(1):45–47, 2000.

Department of Health and Human Services: HIV during pregnancy, labor and delivery, and after birth: health information for HIV positive pregnant women, Rockville, Md, 2005a, Author. Retrieved from *http://aids.info.nih.gov/guidelines*

Department of Health and Human Services: Safety and toxicity of individual antiretroviral agents in pregnancy, Rockville, Md, 2005b, Author. Retrieved from *http://aids.info.nih.gov/guidelines*

Lampe M and others: Rapid HIV-1 antibody testing during labor and delivery for women of unknown HIV status. A Practical Guide and Model Protocol, Washington, DC, 2004, Centers for Disease Control and Prevention (CDC). Retrieved from *http://www.cdc.gov/hiv/projects/perinatal*

McGowan J and others: Combination antiretroviral therapy in human immunodeficiency virus-infected pregnant women, *Obstet Gynecol* 94(5 Pt 1):641–646, 1999.

Minkoff H and others: The relationship of pregnancy to human immunodeficiency virus disease progression, *Am J Obstet Gynecol* 189(2):552–559, 2003.

Moodley J, Wennberg J: HIV in pregnancy, *Curr Obstet Gynecol* 17(2):117–121, 2005.

National Institute of Allergy and Infectious Disease (NIAID). HIV infection in infants and children, Bethesda, Md, 2004, NIH. Retrieved from *http://www.niaid.nih.gov/factsheets/hivchildren.htm*

Nduati R and others: Effect of breastfeeding and formula feeding on transmission of HIV-1: a randomized clinical trial, *JAMA* 283(9):1167–1174, 2000.

Pediatric HIV Working Group on Antiretroviral Therapy and Medical Management of HIV-Infected Children: Guidelines for the use of antiretroviral agents in pediatric HIV infection, 2005b. Retrieved from *http://aidsinfo.nih.gov*

Penn Z, Ahmed S: Human immunodeficiency virus in pregnancy, *Curr Obstet Gynaecol* 13(6):321–328, 2003.

Public Health Service Task Force (PHSTF): *Recommendations for use of antiretroviral drugs in pregnant HIV-1 infected women for maternal health and interventions to reduce perinatal HIV-1 transmission in the United States,* Rockville, Md, 2005, Public Health Service Task Force.

Public Health Service Task Force (PHSTF): *Recommendations for use of antiretroviral drugs in pregnant HIV-1 infected women for maternal health and interventions to reduce perinatal HIV-1 transmission in the United States,* Rockville, Md, 2004, Public Health Service Task Force.

Santhanam H, Goins M: Antiretroviral update: recent advances expand options for patients with HIV, Adv Nurse Pract, Retrieved from *http://www.advanceweb.com*

U.S. Preventive Services Task Force (USPSTF): Screening for HIV: recommendation statement. Rockville, Md, 2005, Agency for Healthcare Research and Quality (AHRQ). Retrieved from *http://guidelines.gov*

World Health Organization: *Antiretroviral drugs for treating pregnant women and preventing HIV infection in infants,* Geneva, Switzerland, 2004, Department of HIV/AIDS, Department of Reproduction Health and Research.

Human Papillomavirus

American College of Obstetricians and Gynecologists: Cervical cytology screening: clinical management guidelines for obstetrician-gynecologists, *ACOG Practice Bulletin,* 45, 2003.

American College of Obstetricians and Gynecologists: Human papillomavirus, *ACOG Practice Bulletin,* 61, 2005.

Burk R: Pernicious papillomavirus infection, *N Engl J Med* 341(22):1687–1688, 1999.

Canavan R, Doshi N: Cervical cancer, *Am Fam Physician* 61(5):1369–1376, 2000.

Carson S: Human papillomatous virus infection update: impact on women's health, *Nurse Pract* 22(4):24–25, 1997.

Castle P, Giuliano A: Genital tract infections, cervical inflammation, and antioxidant nutrients assessing their roles as human papillomavirus cofactors, *J Natl Cancer Inst Monogr* 31:29–34, 2003.

Centers for Disease Control and Prevention: Genital HPV infection, *Factsheet* 2004 [online]. Retrieved from *http://www.cdc.gov/std/healthcomm/fact_sheets.htm*

Centers for Disease Control and Prevention: 2002 guidelines for treatment of sexually transmitted diseases, *MMWR Morb Mortal Wkly Rep* 51:No.RR-6, 2002.

Centers for Disease Control and Prevention: Prevention of genital HPV infection and sequelae: report of an external consultants' meeting., *Executive summary*, 2000 [online]. Retrieved from *http://cdc.gov/nchstp/dstd/ReportsPubliciations/99HPVReport.htm*

Gerberding J: Report to congress: Prevention of genital human papillomavirus infection, 2004, CDC. Retrieved from *http://www.cdc.gov/std/hpv/default.htm*.

Ho G and others: Natural history of cervicovaginal papillomavirus infection in young women, *N Engl J Med* 338(7):423–428, 1998.

McCance K, Huether S: *Pathophysiology: the biologic basis for disease in adults and children*, ed 5, St Louis, 2006, Mosby.

Molano M and others: Determinants of clearance of human papillomavirus infections in Colombian women with normal cytology: a population-based, 5 year follow-up study, *Am J Epidemiol* 158(5):486–494, 2003.

Moscicki A and others: The natural history of human papillomavirus infection as measured by repeated DNA testing in adolescent and young women, *J Pediatr* 132(2):277–284, 1998.

Smith J and others: Evidence for Chlamydia trachomatis as a human papillomavirus cofactor in the etiology of invasive cervical cancer in Brazil and the Philippines, *J Infect Dis* 185(3):324–331, 2002.

Syrjanen K: HPV infections and oesophageal cancer, *J Clin Pathol* 55(10):721–728, 2002.

Thomas D: Sexually transmitted viral infections: epidemiology and treatment, *J Obstet Gynecol Neonatal Nurs* 30(3):316–323, 2001.

Syphilis

Centers for Disease Control and Prevention: 2002 guidelines for treatment of sexually transmitted diseases, *MMWR Morb Mortal Wkly Rep* 51:No.RR-6, 2002.

Gibbs R, Sweet R, and Duff W: Maternal fetal infectious disorders. In Creasy R, Resnik R, and Iams J, editors: *Maternal-fetal medicine: principles and practice*, ed 5, Philadelphia, 2004, Saunders.

Trichomoniasis

Centers for Disease Control and Prevention: 2002 guidelines for treatment of sexually transmitted diseases, *MMWR Morb Mortal Wkly Rep* 51:No.RR-6, 2002.

Gulmezoglu A: Interventions for trichomoniasis in pregnancy, *Cochrane Database Syst Rev* 2002.

Kigozi G and others: Treatment of Trichomonas in pregnancy and adverse outcomes of pregnancy, *Am J Obstet Gynecol* 189(5):1398–1400, 2003.

Lawrence R, Lawrence M: *Breastfeeding: a guide for the medical profession*, ed 6, Philadelphia, 2005, Mosby.

Okuh N, Gronau K, and Hannah M: Antibiotics for bacterial vaginosis or trichomonas vaginalis in pregnancy: a systematic review, *Obstet Gynecol* 105(4):857–868, 2005.

Urinary Tract Infection

American Academy of Pediatrics and American College of Obstetricians and Gynecologists: *Guidelines for perinatal care*, ed 5, Washington, DC, 2002, Author.

American College of Obstetricians and Gynecologists: Prevention of early-onset group B streptococcal disease in newborns, *ACOG Committee Opinion* No 279, Washington, DC, 2002, Author.

Cram L and others: Genitourinary infections and their association with preterm labor, *Am Fam Physician* 65(2):241–248, 2002.

Delzell J, Lefevre M: Urinary tract infections in pregnancy, *Am Fam Physician* 61(3):713–721, 2000.

Fontaine K: *Healing practices: alternative therapies for nursing*, Upper Saddle River, NJ, 2000, Prentice Hall.

Gibbs R, Sweet R, and Duff W: Maternal fetal infectious disorders. In Creasy R, Resnik R, and Iams J, editors: *Maternal-fetal medicine: principles and practice*, ed 5, Philadelphia, 2004, Saunders.

Morgan K: Management of UTIs during pregnancy, *MCH* 29(4):54–258, 2004.

Sierpina V: *Integrative health care: complementary and alternative therapies for the whole person,* Philadelphia, 2001, FA Davis.

Smaill F: Antibiotics for asymptomatic bacteriuria in pregnancy (Cochrane Review), In *The Cochrane Library* Issue 3, Oxford, 2001, Update Software.

General Nursing Management

National Institute of Health: Sexually transmitted diseases and infections and HIV/AIDS research, Bethesda, Md, 2005, Author. Retrieved from *http://www.nichd.nih.gov/womenshealth/STDHIV. cfm*

Tumolo J: Sweet 16 and infected: sexually transmitted diseases in adolescents, *Adv Nurse Pract* 8(9):49–52, 2000.

Waldrop J: Tough lessons in STD prevention, *Clin Advis NPs* 92, June, 2001.

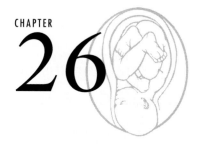

Substance Abuse

T he rate of substance abuse among childbearing women continues to increase dramatically. Approximately 15% of all pregnant women have a substance abuse problem (USDHHS, 2000). Four percent use illicit drugs (SAMHSA, 2005; USDHHS, 2005). Abusing any kind of substance increases the risk for pregnancy complications and the risk for adverse physical and mental outcomes in the fetus. It is imperative that nurse practitioners and nurses caring for families during their childbearing years understand substance abuse and implement care in a collaborative effort to support the *Healthy People 2010* goal of increased abstinence from alcohol, cigarettes, and illicit drug use among pregnant women. This chapter focuses on six of the most commonly abused substances and provides insight into the management of care for pregnant women who are using any of these six substances.

ALCOHOL
Incidence
Currently, alcohol is the most common teratogen. According to the National Survey on Drug Use and Health (USDHHS, 2005), 10% of childbearing women drink alcohol, 1% are heavy drinkers, consuming at least 7 drinks per week, and 4% binge-drink, consuming five or six drinks on occasion (USDHHS, 2005). The highest incidence is in the Native American population (Gardner, 2000).

Pathophysiologic Effects
Alcohol use during pregnancy can have varied pathophysiologic effects, including the following:
- Interferes with the absorption of such nutrients as thiamin (vitamin B_1), vitamin B_{12}, folic acid, and zinc related to its irritation effect on the GI tract
- Interferes with nerve cell growth and development in various ways (USDHHS, 2000)
- Impairs neuronal differentiation and facilitates free radical damage (USDHHS, 2000)

- Induces premature death of cells that develop into facial bones and cartilage (USDHHS, 2000)

Maternal Complications

Maternal complications with alcohol use during pregnancy include increased risk for the following problems:
- Infertility
- Spontaneous abortion
- Abruptio placentae
- Preterm labor

Fetal Complications

Alcohol is the leading preventable cause of birth defects and mental retardation (ACOG, 2004). Alcohol can have varying adverse effects on the fetus, depending on factors such as genetic sensitivity, time of exposure, and dose (Goodlett and Johnson, 1999). The continuum for adverse fetal outcome can range from no effect to fetal alcohol syndrome (FAS).

FAS is a pattern of defects that are the result of prenatal exposure to alcohol; it is characterized by three clinical features. To make the diagnosis of FAS, two of the three facial abnormalities and one manifestation from each of the other deficits must be present (Table 26-1) (NCBDDD, CDC, and DHHS, 2004). Prenatal alcohol exposure can cause other alcohol-related problems referred to as fetal alcohol spectrum disorders (FASD). The Institute of Medicine (IOM) of the National Academy of Science classifies prenatal alcohol exposure into four diagnostic categories (Stratton, Howe, and Battaglia, 1996; USDHHS, 2000; Avner and Nulman, 2005). In 2005, diagnostic clarification was been published (Table 26-2) (Hoyme and others, 2005).

Childhood Effects

Current research indicates that newborns are at increased risk for an infection if exposed to alcohol during fetal life (Gauthier and others, 2005).

Children with FAS continue to demonstrate growth deficiency, facial dysmorphic characteristics, performance deficits, and varying degrees of learning difficulties. FAS is the most common cause of mental retardation (Gardner, 2000; ACOG, 2004). The social and emotional development of these children can be affected by their lack of understanding of consequences, aggressiveness, and destructive behavior. They also have a high pain tolerance (Gardner, 2000).

Screening

The American Medical Association (AMA) has endorsed universal screening in a nonjudgmental and supportive manner (ACOG, 2004; NCBDDD, CDC, and DHHS, 2004). The best screening method for alcohol abuse is a self-administered questionnaire given to all pregnant women on their first prenatal visit. The questions should be worded in a manner that assumes alcohol use in order to lessen defensive responses and increase honesty. Two different ways of wording

Table 26-1   Possible Characteristics in Each of the Three Categories for Diagnosis of Fetal Alcohol Syndrome

Categories	Characteristics
Facial anomalies	*Exhibit two of the following three:*
	Flattened philtrum (the groove between the nose and upper lip)
	Thin vermilion border (flat upper lip)
	Short palpebral fissures (eye openings)
Prenatal and/or postnatal growth deficits	*Exhibit one of the following:*
	Low birth weight for gestational age
	Failure to thrive
Neurodevelopmental abnormalities	*Exhibit one of the following:*
	Microcephaly at or below 10th percentile
	Impaired fine motor skills
	Neurosensory hearing loss
	Poor tandem gait
	Poor eye-hand coordination
	Attention deficit disorder
	Aggressiveness
	Mental retardation
	Poor short-term memory
	Difficulty in problem solving

Data taken from National Center on Birth Defects and Developmental Disabilities (NCBDDD), Centers for Disease Control and Prevention (CDC), Department of Health and Human Services (DHHS): *Fetal alcohol syndrome: guidelines for referral and diagnosis,* Atlanta, Ga, 2004, NCBDDD, CDC.

the questions have been found to facilitate disclosure. The first way is a simple question such as "How many times per week do you drink beer, wine, or liquor?" (Mason and Lee, 1995). A second way is to use Ewing's 4 Ps (yes and no questions) to assess use of alcohol or other drugs (Taylor, Zaichkin, and Bailey, 2002). The four questions are as follows (see Box 26-3):

- Have you ever used drugs or alcohol during this **P**regnancy?
- Have you had a problem with drugs or alcohol in the **P**ast?
- Does your **P**artner have a problem with drugs or alcohol?
- Do you consider one of your **P**arents to be an addict or alcoholic?

If it is determined that the pregnant woman drinks, administer a questionnaire to determine at-risk levels of drinking. The T-ACE (Table 26-3), CAGE (Table 26-4), and TWEAK (Table 26-5) questionnaires are three such instruments. According to research done by Bradley and others (1998), these questionnaires provide the most reliable screening survey for women, especially during pregnancy.

Very carefully screen women who are particularly at risk, including the following groups:

- Single pregnant women
- Women of Native American descent

Table 26-2   Diagnostic Criteria for Fetal Alcohol Spectrum Disorders

Diagnosis	Criteria for Diagnosis
Fetal alcohol syndrome (FAS)	Facial anomalies
With confirmed maternal alcohol exposure	Exhibits two of the three
	Evidence of prenatal and/or postnatal growth deficits
	Neurodevelopmental abnormalities
Without confirmed maternal alcohol exposure	Evidence of one or more
Partial fetal alcohol syndrome (PFAS)	Facial anomalies
With confirmed maternal alcohol exposure	Exhibits two of the three
	Prenatal and/or postnatal growth deficits or neurodevelopmental abnormalities
Without confirmed maternal alcohol exposure	Exhibits one
Alcohol-related birth defects (ARBD)	Facial anomalies
Confirmed maternal alcohol exposure	Exhibits two of the three
	One or more congenital structural defects associated with alcohol such as congenital heart defect, skeletal anomaly, kidney defect, hearing impairment, or other characteristic anomalies
Alcohol-related neurodevelopmental disorders (ARND)	Evidence of one deficient brain growth or abnormal prenatal or postnatal growth deficit
Confirmed maternal alcohol exposure	Evidence of complex pattern of behavioral or cognitive abnormalities such as impairment of performance of complex tasks
	Higher-level receptive and expressive language deficits
	Disordered behavior

Reference: Hoyme H and others: A practical clinical approach to diagnosis of fetal alcohol spectrum disorders: clarification of the 1996 institute of medicine criteria, *Pediatrics* 115(1):39–47, 2005.

- Smokers
- Women with alcoholic husbands

Pregnancy Considerations

No level of alcohol has been proved to be safe for the fetus, and alcohol should be completely avoided when planning for conception and during pregnancy (U.S. Surgeon General, 2005). Because alcohol readily passes to the infant through breast milk and research has shown that when it contains alcohol,

Table 26-3   T-ACE Questionnaire for At-Risk Drinking Patterns

Questions	Score
T How many drinks does it take to make you feel high (**T**olerance)?	≥6 drinks = 2 <6 drinks = 1
A Have people **A**nnoyed you by criticizing your drinking?	No = 1 Yes = 2
C Have you felt you ought to **C**ut down on your drinking?	No = 1 Yes = 2
E Have you ever had a drink first thing in the morning to steady your nerves or get rid of a hangover (**E**ye opener)?	No = 1 Yes = 2

A score of 2 on any question indicates a high probability of being a risk drinker.
Modified from Sokol R, Martier S, Ager J: The T-ACE questions: practical prenatal detection of risk drinking, *Am J Obstet Gynecol* 160(4):863–868, 1989; American College of Obstetricians and Gynecologists: *ACOG Technical Bulletin*, No. 195, 1994.

Table 26-4   CAGE Questionnaire for At-Risk Drinking Patterns

Questions	
C	Have you ever felt you ought to **C**ut down on drinking?
A	Have people **A**nnoyed you by criticizing your drinking?
G	Have you ever felt bad or **G**uilty about your drinking?
E	Have you ever had a drink first thing in the morning to steady your nerves or get rid of a hangover (**E**ye opener)?

More than one positive response suggests an alcohol at-risk problem.
Reference: American Society of Addiction Medicine: *Questions to ask,* patient pocket card, 2001. Retrieved from http://www.asam.org/publ/CAGE.htm

Table 26-5   TWEAK Questionnaire for At-Risk Drinking Patterns

T	**T**olerance. How many drinks can you hold?
W	**W**orry. Does your spouse or do your other family members ever worry or complain about your drinking?
E	**E**ye opener. Have you ever had a drink first thing in the morning to steady your nerves or get rid of a hangover?
A	**A**mnesia. Have you ever awakened the morning after drinking the night before and found that you could not remember a part of the evening before?
K	**K**ut. Have you ever felt you ought to cut down on your drinking?

Positive answers to the first two questions score 2 points each; the other three questions score 1 point each for a positive answer.
Modified from Chan A and others: Use of the TWEAK test in screening on alcoholism/heavy drinking in three populations, *Alcohol Clin Exp Res* 17(16):1188–1192, 1993.

infants consume significantly less breast milk, sleep less, and show developmental delays (Lawrence and Lawrence, 2005), drinking is not recommended during breastfeeding either. Health care providers should avoid prescribing alcohol to help with letdown.

The teratogenic effect of alcohol is dose-related, and *risk drinking* is of greatest concern. This is defined as maternal drinking that produces blood alcohol levels high enough and for long enough to produce fetal damage (Hankin and Sokol, 1995). However, the precise level of alcohol varies with each individual. Therefore no safe drinking level has been established.

Maternal nutrition is usually affected if the pregnant woman drinks. Ethanol is a source of energy; therefore a person with alcoholism usually has a low intake of nutrients. Ethanol can also interfere with intestinal absorption of certain vitamins and nutrients, such as calcium, amino acids, thiamin, vitamin B_6, vitamin B_{12}, folate, and zinc.

Women are frequently more receptive to making lifestyle changes during pregnancy than at any other time during their lives. Offering advice that can be easily remembered versus mass media education is more effective in motivating a woman to choose to stop drinking (Hankin and Sokol, 1995). Examples follow:

- You have a whole life to drink but only 9 months to grow a healthy baby.
- Although only 1 in 10 heavy drinkers has a baby with FAS, you cannot predict that you will not be the one.
- The most important thing you can do to influence the health of your baby is to cut your drinking or quit altogether.

Treatment During Pregnancy

The risk for FAS decreases if an alcohol-abusing pregnant woman stops her alcohol use during the third trimester. Therefore when a pregnant woman identifies that she does use alcohol to some degree, classify her drinking pattern according to (1) social drinking, (2) symptom-relief drinking (drinking to relieve depression or to elevate mood), or (3) syndrome drinking (physiologic and psychologic dependence on alcohol). Then implement nursing interventions based on the woman's drinking pattern to facilitate her quitting or at least decreasing her drinking.

The social drinker just needs complete information as to the effects of alcohol on her unborn child, and she will most likely quit. Yet in a qualitative study, Barbour (1990) found that 60% of pregnant women received information that occasional drinking was not likely to be harmful. However, as stated previously, no safe drinking level during pregnancy has been established. On the other hand, to decrease undue anxiety, a woman who has had a few social drinks before the pregnancy was recognized should be reassured of a relatively low risk for fetal damage but instructed as to the importance of avoiding alcohol for the remainder of the pregnancy.

The symptom-relief drinker should receive the same education as to the effects of alcohol but needs supportive counseling as well. This can be provided effectively in the prenatal office setting by trained health care workers. The woman with alcoholism requires referral to an appropriate detoxification program, as well as support programs. However, the nurse practitioner and the prenatal nurse need to remain actively involved after making the appropriate referrals.

One technique shown to be effective in reducing excessive alcohol consumption is defined by the acronym FRAMES (Fleming and others, 1997):

F   *Feedback* about the adverse effects of alcohol
R   *Responsibility* for change
A   *Advice* about appropriate drinking amounts
M   *Menu* of available options
E   *Empathy* for the patient
S   *Self-efficacy*

METHAMPHETAMINES

Methamphetamines, stimulants known as *meth, chalk, glass, ice,* or *blue ice,* have vasoconstrictive properties like cocaine and are used in a similar manner. Methamphetamine is snorted, swallowed, injected, or smoked.

Maternal Complications

The following complications are known to occur with amphetamine use:
- Abruptio placentae
- Preterm labor
- Insomnia
- Loss of appetite
- Cardiac dysrhythmias
- "Meth mouth" (gum erosion and infection)

Perinatal Effects

- Strongest correlations are intrauterine growth restriction (IUGR) and reduced brain growth (Smith and others, 2003).
- Congenital anomalies and fetal stress have been reported, but there is not one consistent associated anomaly (Andres, 2004).
- May cause neonatal withdrawal.
- Developmental effects occur related to prenatal exposure and postnatal environment (Medical Study News, 2004).
- Risk for SIDS is increased (DEA, 2006).

Treatment During Pregnancy

Ideal treatment is as follows:
- Cessation of use
- Optimal nutrition
- Ongoing prenatal care

COCAINE

Cocaine can be snorted, injected, or smoked as *freebase* or *crack.* Cocaine comes in two forms: powder and crystals. Cocaine hydrochloride, cocaine sulfate, and cocaine base come in the form of a powder and are inhaled (snorted or sniffed);

therefore they are readily absorbed through the mucous membranes or dissolved and taken intravenously (IV). Cocaine powders are only 15% to 25% pure and have many street names, such as *lady, snow, coke, white girl, nose candy, Cadillac,* and *gold dust.* Crack, which is 90% pure cocaine, comes in the form of crystals called *rocks* and is smoked (freebased); therefore it is absorbed through the lung tissue.

Sniffing cocaine produces a high after several minutes, and the effect lasts for more than 1 hour. Cocaine that is smoked or taken IV produces a high in seconds that causes rapid euphoria that lasts only about 30 minutes. Thus the latter two methods are usually repeated more often and are therefore more highly addicting. Many people are hooked after their first experience with it.

Incidence

The use of cocaine during pregnancy has continued to dramatically increase in the past few years. It is estimated that 11% of pregnant women use cocaine (Beers and Berkow, 2005).

Pathophysiologic Effects

Cocaine interferes with the reuptake of dopamine and norepinephrine at the nerve synapses, resulting in increased circulating levels of these two neurotransmitters. Cocaine also alters the metabolism of serotonin and acetylcholine. The resulting neurotransmitter imbalance overactivates certain receptors that regulate (1) mood, causing euphoria (a feeling of confidence and sexual arousal); (2) sleep, causing a hyperaroused state; (3) motor function, causing excitation and restlessness; and (4) sympathetic nervous system stimulation, causing tachycardia, tachypnea, hyperthermia (38.8° C to 46° C [102° F to 106° F]), hypertension (increased mean arterial pressure approximately 50%), and intense, generalized vasoconstriction (Schiller and Allen, 2005). After depletion of the neurotransmitters, depression, malaise, and an extreme craving for the drug ensue.

Resulting complications that can occur from cocaine use are as follows (Wagner and others, 1998; Kuczkowski, 2003; Vidaeff and Mastrobattista, 2003):

- Decreased blood flow to the heart muscle, which predisposes to dysrhythmias, a myocardial infarction, and platelet aggregation
- Decreased blood flow to the brain, which predisposes to seizures, stroke, and cerebral infarction
- Decreased blood flow to the intestines, which can cause peristaltic stimulation but can also lead to tissue death
- Decreased uterine blood flow by 50% and increased uterine vascular resistance
- Increased levels of fetal neurotransmitters (The resulting consequences are the same as for the adult, such as increased fetal mean arterial pressure by 24%, increased FHR by 50%, and decreased fetal oxygen partial pressure [PO_2] by 30%, which may cause various teratogenic effects [Dolkart, Plessinger, and Woods, 1990; Buehler, Conover, and Andres, 1996].)

Cocaine is metabolized by plasma and liver cholinesterase to water-soluble substances called *metabolites* that are excreted in the urine. Because the plasma cholinesterase is decreased during pregnancy and is much less in the fetus and neonate, cocaine is more toxic during pregnancy and to the fetus (Wagner and others, 1998).

Maternal Complications

Cocaine can stimulate uterine contractions. Therefore its use in the first trimester of pregnancy increases the risk for a spontaneous abortion. Its use in the second and third trimesters can increase the risk for preterm labor and premature rupture of membranes (Bateman and Chiriboga, 2000; Bandstra and others, 2001; Fajemirokun-Odudeyi and Lindow, 2004). It is not known whether these risks are directly related to cocaine use or to the frequent associated use of tobacco and inadequate prenatal care.

Cocaine decreases blood flow to the heart, brain, and uterus to a greater extent during pregnancy. Because of this vasoconstrictor effect of the drug, cardiovascular failure, intracerebral hemorrhage, respiratory failure, seizures, and hypertensive crises that may mimic pregnancy-induced hypertension (PIH) occur significantly more frequently (Plessinger and Woods, 1998).

Abruptio placentae and stillbirth occur more frequently in cocaine users and may be related to the effect on blood pressure (Singer and others, 2002; Fajemirokun-Odudeyi and Lindow, 2004; MOD, 2004).

Fetal and Neonatal Complications

Because of the dramatic decrease in uterine blood flow with resultant fetal hypoxia and the blocking reuptake of the neurotransmitters that occur with maternal cocaine use, complications are prevalent. Prematurity caused by a preterm delivery is related to cocaine-induced uterine contractions (Bandstra and others, 2001; Bada and others, 2002). Cocaine-exposed infants have been observed to be small for gestational age, including small head circumference (Bateman and Chiriboga, 2000; Bandstra and others, 2001; Singer and others, 2002). Congenital malformations have been reported in the literature and include cardiac anomalies, urinary tract defects, segmental intestinal atresia, and central nervous system (CNS) abnormalities (Potter and others, 2000; Hepburn, 2004). However, available research data do not provide unequivocal proof.

Infants exposed to cocaine during pregnancy do not exhibit physiologic withdrawal symptoms as seen when other types of substances are abused but frequently manifest neurobehavioral abnormalities (AAP, 1998), such as the following:

- Hyperreflexia, which can be seen as an exaggerated startle response and tremulousness
- Abnormal state patterns such as difficulty sleeping and maintaining an alert, inactive state, thus spending prolonged time in the crying and alert active state

- Inappropriate interactive behaviors and inability to respond appropriately to parents, affecting parent-infant attachment
- Difficulty in habituating and therefore extreme sensitivity to environmental stimuli
- Extremely short attention to a stimulus before showing signs of agitation, such as color changes, rapid respirations, and agitated motor activity
- Deficient self-consoling abilities and poor response to comforting by care providers
- Difficulty eating because of an ineffective suck

The preceding neurobehavioral abnormalities may partially correct but frequently lead to learning difficulties caused by attention deficits and behavioral problems, such as a flat, apathetic mood later in life. In their longitudinal prospective study, Singer and associates (2002) found that prenatal cocaine exposure has a significant effect on later cognitive development. According to Frank and others (2001), systematic review of studies assessing the possible relationship between maternal prenatal cocaine use and childhood effects concluded that the data are not persuasive that in utero exposure to cocaine alone causes these developmental problems. Co-factors such as prenatal exposure to tobacco, marijuana, or alcohol and the later quality of the child's environment may be contributing factors, along with cocaine exposure.

Effect of Paternal Cocaine Use

If the man is exposed to cocaine just prior to the intercourse that results in conception, the offspring has an increased risk for abnormalities. Research has demonstrated that cocaine binds to the human spermatozoa (Yazigi, Odem, and Polakoski, 1991).

Screening

During the initial prenatal assessment, all pregnant women should be asked about cocaine use. Health care providers may screen prenatally for cocaine use with various biologic specimens if the history is positive, as shown by one of the following:

- No or inadequate prenatal care
- Inadequate prenatal weight gain
- Previous induced abortion
- Preterm labor
- Abruptio placentae
- History of substance abuse, such as cigarettes, alcohol, or cocaine
- Presence of a sexually transmitted disease
- Inconsistent support system
- Chronic nasal congestion

The American Medical Association recommend urine toxicology screening be performed on all pregnant women because the chances of missing drug use are significant if one screens only those with an indicating history (ACOG, 2004).

Various biologic specimens such as blood, urine, hair, meconium, saliva, amniotic fluid, and perspiration are used. Toxicology urine screen can detect cocaine use by the pregnant woman during the previous week because of its slow metabolism during pregnancy. Newborn meconium (stool of the first 3 days of life) can be analyzed by radioimmunoassay (RIA) for drug metabolites, and analysis of hair is being used as well because the drug remains embedded for the life of the hair shaft (Ursitti, Klein, and Koren, 2001; Drug Facts and Comparisons, 2004).

Treatment During Pregnancy

Be able to recognize the signs of possible cocaine use, such as sweatiness, tachycardia, flushed skin, tremulousness, irritability, difficulty sitting still, and being "high" or sleepy. Dispel myths, such as the misconception that recreational use is not harmful or that cocaine use will bring about a shorter, easier labor. Education as to the harmful effects of cocaine is essential because many feel it is harmless.

When it is determined that the pregnant woman is taking cocaine, she should be told that the best thing to do is to stop immediately. Then provide supportive services so that she can stop, such as referrals to drug rehabilitation programs that address women's needs, individual and family counseling, support groups such as Narcotics Anonymous, financial assistance, and home nurse visitation. A cocaine addict usually resists treatment. Therefore the health care provider must persist in all avenues appropriate for the patient, such as patient support systems and multidisciplinary resources, in attempting to help her understand and admit that cocaine is harmful to her and her fetus and that she should stop using the drug.

Compose a list of available community and state resources. A helpful national treatment referral and information service resource is 800-COCAINE. This resource can give health care providers names of local perinatal cocaine treatment centers. This same number serves as a cocaine hotline that is available for cocaine addicts and family members.

Assess for multiple risk factors, such as cigarette smoking, alcohol use, use of other drugs, and inadequate prenatal care.

Become familiar with the legislative issues related to drug testing, reporting drug use, and fetal rights for your state. Become involved, in cooperation with the risk management department of your institution, in policy development to legally manage the care of pregnant women who use cocaine.

Care of the laboring patient who has recently used cocaine should include close observations for signs of complications, oxygen by mask at 7 to 10 L/min to enhance fetal oxygenation, and notification of the intensive care nursery of a potential high risk neonate. Cocaine may induce fetal tachycardia and affect variability (Lynch and McKeon, 1990). These patients experience labor pains as much as any other patient, and withholding pain medication is not beneficial. If epidural anesthesia is necessary, the nurse should monitor closely for hypotension because it seems to occur more frequently in the cocaine-positive laboring woman (Kain and others, 1996; FIRST Consult, 2006).

If there is a chance that the mother will use cocaine after the birth of her infant, she should be counseled not to breastfeed because cocaine readily passes to the infant by way of breast milk (Lawrence and Lawrence, 2005).

HEROIN

Heroin is most common drug injected intravenously, referred to as *mainlining*. Smoking or inhaling the drug is becoming more popular because of the fear of contracting HIV from needles. Taken by any route, heroin is extremely addicting. Street names for this drug are *snow, stuff, junk, smack, horse,* and *joy powder.*

Maternal Complications

Infertility is common because heroin frequently inhibits ovulation. A woman usually becomes pregnant when heroin levels drop.

It is difficult to ascribe specific maternal effects to heroin because 75% of women who use heroin report using more than one drug (Little and others, 1990). A pregnant heroin addict has a three-fold to seven-fold increased risk for preterm labor, preeclampsia, and postpartum hemorrhage (Archie, 1998). Infections such as syphilis, hepatitis, tuberculosis, cellulitis, thrombophlebitis, and HIV are common complications of heroin because the route of administration is likely IV (NIDA, 2005).

Fetal and Neonatal Complications

Fetal and neonatal complications of heroin use include the following:
- Preterm birth and prematurity (Lee, 1995)
- IUGR, which is compounded by maternal abuse of other substances and malnutrition (Archie, 1998)
- Appears to accelerate fetal lung maturity but increases the risk for meconium-stained amniotic fluid and the risk for SIDS (Kendig, 1996)
- Signs of withdrawal (Box 26-1) manifested by 60% to 80% of the infants exposed to prenatal heroin; withdrawal usually occurring within the first 24 to 72 hours but may be delayed up to 10 days of life (Archie, 1998)
- Postnatal growth deficiency, mild developmental delays, and behavior problems observed in follow-up studies of children exposed to perinatal heroin; however, these problems are reported to be more related to poor maternal nutrition and inappropriate postnatal environment than to the direct effect of the perinatal heroin (Robins and Mills, 1993)

Treatment During Pregnancy

Screening for other STDs is essential. Sudden withdrawal from heroin can be harmful and is not recommended during pregnancy because of heroin's significant physical and psychological addictive properties. Methadone treatment is frequently used to help the pregnant mother stop using heroin. Because heroin can cause detrimental fetal effects and neonatal withdrawal, a pregnant woman

Box 26-1	Signs of Drug Withdrawal
W	**W**akefulness
I	**I**rritability
T	**T**remulousness, **T**emperature variation, and **T**achypnea
H	**H**yperactivity and **H**igh-pitched or continuous cry
D	**D**iarrhea, **D**iaphoresis, and **D**isorganized suck
R	**R**ub marks, **R**estless sleeping, and **R**espiratory difficulty
A	**A**pneic attacks
W	**W**eight loss or failure to gain weight
A	**A**lkalosis (respiratory)
L	**L**acrimation (runny eye syndrome)

Modified from American Academy of Pediatrics Committee on Drugs: Neonatal drug withdrawal, *Pediatrics* 72:895, 1983; Torrence C, Horns K: Appraisal and caregiving for the drug addicted infant, *Neonatal Netw* 8(3):49–59, 1989.

should be withdrawn from heroin with a small dose (1–20 mg) of methadone to control symptoms of withdrawal (Andres, 2004). This also decreases the exposure to infectious diseases and to repeated intoxication and withdrawal cycles.

During labor, methadone may be continued and narcotics can be used to manage pain. Avoid narcotics with mixed agonist-antagonist properties because they may precipitate acute withdrawal. The newborn needs withdrawal treatment. Breastfeeding is not contraindicated during methadone maintenance therapy if the mother is not abusing other drugs.

Marijuana

Street names for marijuana are *grass, pot, joint, reefer,* and *weed.*

Incidence

It is estimated that approximately 14% of pregnant women use marijuana (Beers and Berkow, 2005). It is the most commonly used illicit drug among childbearing women (DPNA, 2004).

Pathophysiologic Effects

One of the active ingredients of marijuana is delta–9-tetrahydrocannabinol, which crosses the placenta and is fat-soluble. Therefore, it may take 30 days for the drug to be excreted from the fetal body (Hubbard, Franco, and Onaivi, 1999).

Marijuana interferes with the production of follicle-stimulating hormone, luteinizing hormone, and prolactin, thereby inhibiting ovulation.

Marijuana increases the carbon monoxide levels in blood five times more than tobacco smoke and therefore decreases fetal oxygenation.

Maternal Complications

- Marijuana can cause infertility problems, especially in the male.
- Marijuana does not cause physical addiction, but it can cause psychologic addiction.
- Marijuana smoke contains more cancer-causing properties than tobacco smoke. One joint affects the lungs as much as smoking 16 cigarettes (Wu and others, 1988).

Fetal Complications

Research results are equivocal as to the teratogenic effects of marijuana on fetal growth, neurobehavioral activities, and length of gestation (Lee, 1998). Marijuana has been linked to low birth weight, preterm birth, and such neurobehavioral effects as attention deficit and impulsiveness (Faden and Graubard, 2000; Fried and Smith, 2001; Fergusson, Horwood, and Northstone, 2002). Significantly, executive function deficiency, causing lower scores in childhood verbal and memory abilities, poor focused attention, and self-directed responses have been associated with maternal marijuana use (Fried and Smith, 2001).

Screening

Many marijuana users, as well as substance users of most illegal drugs, go undetected if a drug toxicity screen is not done on all pregnant patients. A commonly used toxicity urine screen is the enzyme-multiplied immunoassay. It is effective in detecting marijuana use for the past 3 to 30 days (Hubbard, Franco, and Onaivi, 1999).

Meconium is a useful sample for drug screening in newborns (Maynard, Amoruso, and Oh, 1991).

Treatment During Pregnancy

Because no drug has proved safe for the unborn child, marijuana is not safe. Therefore a woman is encouraged to stop using it. She should be closely evaluated for the use of other substances as well.

TOBACCO

Incidence

According to the National Survey on Drug Use and Health, 18% of all pregnant women smoke (USDHHS, 2005). The *Healthy People 2010* goal is that no more than 1% of pregnant women will smoke.

Pathophysiologic Effects

A cigarette contains more than 2500 chemicals and 200 poisonous compounds (Cleveland Clinic, 2004; MOD, 2004). One of them, carbon monoxide, readily crosses the placenta and decreases the oxygen-carrying capacity of the hemoglobin. Nicotine, another substance in cigarettes, stimulates adrenergic release, which causes generalized vasoconstriction, leading to decreased uterine perfusion and narrowing of the umbilical arteries. Compensatory signs are manifested, such as increased maternal and FHR and decreased fetal movement.

Research indicates that cigarette smokers eat a poorer diet than nonsmokers (Haste and others, 1990). Cigarette smoking also interferes with the assimilation of various essential vitamins and minerals, resulting in an increased loss of calcium caused by mobilization from bones, decreased intestinal synthesis of vitamin B_{12}, and increased usage of vitamin C (Wardlaw and Smith, 2006).

Maternal Complications

The risk for the following complications is increased in the pregnant woman who smokes (Maloni, 2000; USDHHS, 2004):
- Infertility related to ovulatory dysfunction and alteration in sperm
- Spontaneous abortion or ectopic pregnancy
- Placenta previa
- Abruptio placentae
- Premature rupture of membranes
- Preterm delivery

Fetal and Neonatal Complications

The risk for the following complications is increased in the fetus, neonate, and infant when exposed to cigarette smoke:

According to *Healthy People 2010* (2002), 20% to 30% of low birth weight and very low birth weight may be attributed to smoking. The severity of low birth weight is in direct proportion to the number of cigarettes smoked per day or the amount of exposure to passive ("side stream") smoke (MOD, 2004). Perinatal and neonatal mortality is increased 10% when the fetus is exposed to cigarette smoke (ACOG, 2000).
- IUGR and stillbirth are increased.
- Teratogenic effects of cleft palate and lip are seen.
- Increased risk for childhood cancer related to prenatal exposure to cigarette smoking exists.
- Lower IQ and behavioral abnormalities, such as attention deficit hyperactivity disorder (ADHD), resulting in later learning difficulties have been observed in follow-up studies (Dobson, 2005; Li and others, 2005).
- Smoking can reduce breast milk and expose the infant to harmful compounds that pass freely into breast milk (Lawrence and Lawrence, 2005).
- Children exposed in utero or through second-hand smoke have an increased risk for developing asthma (Li and others, 2005).
- Postnatal exposure to passive smoke can increase the infant's risk for developing SIDS (USDHHS, 2004) and childhood respiratory illnesses such as respiratory syncytial virus (RSV), pneumonia, bronchitis, and inner ear infections (Bradley and others, 2005).

Treatment During Pregnancy

The goal of treatment for smokers during pregnancy is to convince all pregnant women and those around them to stop smoking. Quitting before conception is most beneficial. However, even quitting before 16 weeks of gestation significantly decreases the adverse risks (Maloni, 2001). According to the *Cochrane Review*, smoking cessation programs during pregnancy are effective, and it is recommended that all health care providers provide smoking cessation programs to all pregnant women in all maternity care settings (Lumley and others, 2004).

Based on recommendations of the U.S. Department of Health and Human Services (USDHHS) (Melvin and others, 2000), the American College of Obstetrics and Gynecology (2000) offers guidelines to help health care practitioners implement an effective smoking cessation program (Box 26-2). The outlined steps to this smoking cessation program are available from the Publications Clearinghouse (800-358-9295).

Implementing a smoking cessation program is challenging, and the counseling must be individualized. Health professionals must motivate their patients to choose to stop smoking and empower them to be successful. Some additional general guidelines follow:

- Set the right example as a health care provider by not smoking—or at least not smoking in the presence of patients. Make the health care facility a smoke-free environment.
- If the woman is reluctant to quit, assess her reasons. For example, she may be afraid of gaining too much weight or going through withdrawal symptoms. She may feel that she needs smoking as a psychologic support or may have tried and failed to quit in the past. Keep in mind that a woman may believe that smoking will not hurt her baby because it did not hurt someone else's baby or because she discovers that her health care provider smokes.
- If the woman chooses to keep smoking, encourage her to reduce the amount she smokes but remind her that quitting entirely is the best for her and her fetus. Counsel her to increase her intake of calcium, vitamins B_{12} and C, and folic acid to compensate for the smoking-induced loss of these vitamins and minerals.
- Also, give family members a clear, brief message on the need to quit or at least never smoke in the presence of the expectant mother or young child because passive smoke is harmful prenatally, as well as postnatally.
- Take an active part in legislative and legal strategies to reduce cigarette smoking, such as increasing cigarette taxes, banning cigarette advertisements, or enforcing provisions to make public places smoke-free.
- If necessary, encourage short-term use of nicotine gum, nasal spray, or the patch because they deliver less nicotine than usual cigarette smoking and can be considered during pregnancy if nonpharmacologic treatment fails and if potential benefits outweighs the unknown risk (CDC, 2000). Pharmacotherapy such as bupropion SR (Zyban) should be considered only when a pregnant woman is otherwise unable to quit through other forms of treatment.

Box 26-2   Smoking Cessation Plan for Expectant Mothers

Ask every woman about her smoking habits. Improve disclosure by using multiple-choice questions rather than "yes" or "no" type questions.

Choose the answer that best describes your pattern of cigarette smoking:

_ I smoke regularly now, about the same amount as before I was pregnant.

_ I smoke regularly now, but I have cut down since finding out I was pregnant.

_ I smoke every once in a while.

_ I quit after finding out I was pregnant.

_ I do not currently smoke and was not smoking at the time I got pregnant.

_ I have NEVER smoked.

Advise
Advise every smoking woman to stop smoking now. Present a clear, strong message on the need to quit. Personalize the advice to her health and to the health of her fetus. Compliment and affirm the patient who has stopped smoking.

Assess
Assess the woman's willingness to set a stop date now. You could say, "Quitting smoking is the most important thing you can do for your health and the health of your baby. If we provide you with help, are you willing to try to quit?"

_ If the woman is willing to make a quit attempt, provide assistance by moving to the next step.

_ If the woman is not willing at this time to make a quit attempt, provide a motivation intervention

Assist
Assist the woman by helping her with a plan to quit smoking using the acronym **STAR**:

- **S**et a quit date within 2 weeks
- **T**ell your family, friends, and coworkers—and request their support.
- **A**nticipate challenges such as withdrawal symptoms and triggers.
- **R**emove tobacco products from the environment.

Provide self-help materials that are pregnancy-specific (see Table 26-6).

Provide encouragement and help patient obtain social support.

Arrange
Arrange for immediate follow-up, within 1 week after the quit date, and provide ongoing follow-up to congratulate, support, and reinforce success—or to encourage her to try again if a relapse occurs. During the postpartum period, use relapse prevention strategies because of the high relapse rate during this time.

If patient continues to smoke, assess smoking status at all prenatal visits and keep encouraging cessation.

NURSING MANAGEMENT

Prevention and Early Detection

Nurse practitioners and nurses should be actively involved in accurate, timely education programs that teach about the effects of practicing substance abuse on one's personal health and the potential teratogenic effects on the growing fetus.

These programs should be available in grade school, in high school, during contraceptive counseling, and on gynecologic visits.

- Develop and consistently use a matter-of-fact, nonjudgmental question-naire to obtain a substance abuse assessment because a screening tool is the most effective method for detecting substance abuse (Morse, Gehshan, and Hutchins, 1997). Laboratory tests and urine toxicologies have been found to be ineffective in determining substance abuse (Morse, Gehshan, and Hutchins, 1997).
- Prepare the patient by introducing the screening with a statement such as "I ask all my patients these questions because it is important to their health and the health of their baby" (Morse, Gehshan, and Hutchins, 1997).
- The four Ps is one screening device often used as a way of beginning the discussion about substance abuse (Box 26-3).

Intervention for a Positive Screen*

- Assess for barriers such as peer pressure, socioeconomic status, psychologic stress, or other environmental factors.
- In a positive, nonjudgmental manner, motivate the woman who is consid-ering childbearing or who is pregnant to want to make lifestyle changes to improve health-related behavior by providing her with information about health risks and the effects of substance abuse on her fetus.
- Assess the family's need for detoxification; if they need it, determine whether outpatient, inpatient, or family treatment would be most effective. The CAGE questionnaire for at-risk drinking patterns has been adapted for general drug use as well by substituting drug use or a specific abused substance in place of drinking (Archie, 1998).
- State the need to stop and verbalize assistance.
- Discuss possible options such as individual counseling, a 12-step program, or addition treatment programs.
- Provide supportive counseling to help the patient make changes, build self-esteem, and overcome feelings of inadequacy. Avoid using threatening statements that make her feel like a bad mother for abusing a substance.

---

*(Morse, Gehshan, and Hutchins, 1997).

Box 26-3   General Screening for Substance Abuse Using the Four Ps

Have you ever used drugs or alcohol during this **P**regnancy?
Have you had a problem with drugs or alcohol in the **P**ast?
Does your **P**artner have a problem with drugs or alcohol?
Do you consider one of your **P**arents to be an addict or alcoholic?
    If the pregnant woman answers "yes" to one or more of these questions, it is considered a positive screen for substance abuse.

Reference: Ewing H, Medical Director, Born Free Project. Contra Costa County, 111 Allen Street, Martinez, Calif, (510) 646–1165; Morse B, Gehshan S, Hutchins E: *Screening for substance abuse during pregnancy: improving care, improving health,* Arlington, Va, 1997, National Center for Education in Maternal and Child Health.

- Make appropriate referrals to self-help groups: 12-step programs such as Alcoholics, Cocaine, or Narcotics Anonymous.
- Provide smoking cessation materials (Table 26-6).
- Refer to the cocaine hotline: 800-COCAINE
- Refer to local clinics dealing specifically with pregnant substance abusers.
- If use is related to defined problems in the woman's life, such as depression, marital discord, domestic violence, or history of abuse, make appropriate community referrals to resources that address these issues.

Table 26-6   Resources for Smoking Cessation Materials

Title/Type	Resource	Website
Tobacco and Pregnancy (general reference for tobacco and pregnancy material)	Addressing Tobacco in Managed Care (313) 874-6815	www.aahp.org/atmc.htm
You Can Quit Smoking (consumer guide)	Agency for Healthcare Research and Quality	www.ahrq.gov/ consumer/tobacco/ quits.htm
Make Yours a Fresh Start Family (comprehensive program package for health care professionals to help counsel pregnant women to stop smoking)	American Cancer Society 1599 Clifton Road NE Atlanta, GA 30329 (800) 277-2345 or call local chapter	www.cancer.org
Freedom From Smoking for You and Your Baby (a 10-day quit smoking program for pregnant women)	American Lung Association 1703 Broadway New York, NY 10017 (800) LUNG-USA	www.lungusa.org/ tobacco/smosmpreg. html
Clinical Practice Guidelines: Treating Tobacco Use and Dependence *You Can Quit Smoking Consumer Guide* *You Can Quit Smoking Tear Sheet*	Centers for Disease Control and Prevention Office on Smoking and Health Publications Clearinghouse (800) 358-9295	www.cdc.gov/tobacco/ how2quit.htm
Nurses Help Your Patients Stop Smoking Publication No. 92-2962	National Heart, Lung, and Blood Institute 4733 Bethesda Avenue, Suite 350 Bethesda, MD 20814 (301) 951-3260	www.nhlbi.nih.gov/ health/prof/lung/ other/nurssmok.txt
Smoke-Free Families	Robert Wood Johnson Foundation	www.smokefreefamilies. org

- Provide ongoing encouragement and support.
- If efforts to encourage total abstinence fail, provide a message of the potential benefits from reduction of use.
- Become active in legislative issues to block punitive legislation dealing with childbearing women who are substance abusers because if these women are punished legally, they will be driven away and perhaps not seek help when they need it the most.

CONCLUSION

Health care providers have a unique opportunity to help prevent birth defects by providing education about the effects of substance abuse on the fetus and by early identification of childbearing women who are abusing substances such as alcohol, cigarettes, and illicit drugs. Women who abuse substances are at greater risk for spontaneous abortion, preterm labor, low-birth-weight infants, and abruptio placentae (USDHHS, 2000).

Nurses who provide health care to childbearing families can participate in primary prevention by conducting education programs and consistently providing ongoing education about the risks of practicing substance abuse. Nurses should also be involved in secondary prevention, which includes early diagnosis and appropriate intervention if the problem exists. Obtaining an accurate assessment can be exceptionally complex because of the varying symptoms manifested and the need of the patient to conceal her habit. Planning appropriate nursing care for these patients is challenging.

BIBLIOGRAPHY
General

Substance Abuse and Mental Health Services Administration: *Over four percent of pregnant women used illicit drugs in past month,* Rockville, MD, 2005, USDHHS.

U.S. Department of Health and Human Services (USDHHS): *Healthy People 2010: understanding and improving health:* Maternal, Infant, and Child Health. Rockville, Md, 2001, Office of Disease Prevention and Health Promotion. Retrieved from *http://www.health.gov/healthypeople/Document/tableofcontents.htm*

U.S. Department of Health and Human Services (USDHHS): *Substance use during pregnancy: 2002 and 2003 update,* Rockville, Md, 2005, USDHHS.

U.S. Department of Health and Human Services (USDHHS): *Tenth special report to the U.S. Congress on alcohol and health,* Rockville, Md, 2000, USDHHS.

Alcohol

American College of Obstetricians and Gynecologists: At-risk drinking and illicit drug use: ethical issues in obstetric and gynecologic practice, *ACOG Committee Opinion,* No. 294, 2004.

Avner M, Nulman I: Attempts at more specific and practical diagnostic criteria for fetal alcohol spectrum disorders, *JFAS Int* 3:e12, 2005.

Barbour B: Alcohol and pregnancy, *J Nurse Midwifery* 35(2):78–85, 1990.

Bradley K and others: Alcohol screening questionnaires in women: a critical review, *JAMA* 280(2):166–171, 1998.

Ebrahim S and others: Alcohol consumption by pregnant women in the United States during 1988–1995, *Obstet Gynecol* 92(2):187–192, 1998.

Ewing J: Detecting alcoholism: the CAGE questionnaire, *JAMA* 252(14):1905–1907, 1984.

Fleming M and others: Brief physician advice for problem alcohol drinkers: a randomized controlled trial in community-based primary care practices, *JAMA* 277(13): 1039–1045, 1997.

Gardner J: Living with a child with fetal alcohol syndrome, *MCN Am J Matern Child Nurs* 25(5):252–257, 2000.

Gauthier T and others: Maternal alcohol abuse and neonatal infection, *Alcohol Clin Exp Res* 29(6):1035–1043, 2005.

Goodlett C, Johnson T: Temporal windows of vulnerability to alcohol during the third trimester equivalent: why "knowing when" matters. In Hannigan J and others, editors: *Alcohol and alcoholism,* Hillsdale, NJ, 1999, Lawrence Erlbaum Associates.

Hankin J, Sokol R: Identification and care of problems associated with alcohol ingestion in pregnancy, *Semin Perinatol* 19(4):286–292, 1995.

Hoyme H and others: A practical clinical approach to diagnosis of fetal alcohol spectrum disorders: clarification of the 1996 institute of medicine criteria, *Pediatrics* 115(1): 39–47, 2005.

Institute of Medicine (IOM), Food and Nutrition Board, Subcommittee on Nutritional Status and Weight Gain During Pregnancy: *Nutrition during pregnancy: weight gain,* Washington, DC, 1990, National Academy Press.

Lawrence R, Lawrence M: *Breastfeeding: a guide for the medical profession,* ed 6, Philadelphia, 2005, Mosby.

Mason E, Lee R: Drug abuse. In Barron W, Lindheimer M: *Medical disorders during pregnancy,* ed 2, St Louis, 1995, Mosby.

National Center on Birth Defects and Developmental Disabilities, Centers for Disease Control and Prevention, Department of health and Human Services: *Fetal alcohol syndrome: guidelines for referral and diagnosis,* Atlanta, Ga, 2004, NCBDDD, CDC.

Phillips K: When mom drinks, baby suffers, *Childbirth Instructor,* July/August, 20, 2000.

Sokol R, Martier S, and Ager J: The T-ACE questions: practical prenatal detection of risk drinking, *Am J Obstet Gynecol* 160(4):863–868, 1989.

Stratton K, Howe C, and Battaglia F: *Fetal alcohol syndrome: diagnosis, epidemiology, prevention, treatment,* Washington, DC, 1996, National Academy Press.

Taylor P, Zaichkin J, and Bailey D: *Substance abuse during pregnancy: guidelines for screening,* Olympia, Wash, 2002, Maternal and Child Health. Retrieved from *http://www.doh.wa.gov*

U.S. Department of Health and Human Services (USDHHS): *Substance use during pregnancy: 2002 and 2003 update,* Rockville, Md, 2005, USDHHS.

U.S. Department of Health and Human Services (USDHHS): *Tenth special report to the U.S. Congress on alcohol and health,* Rockville, Md, 2000, USDHHS.

U.S. Surgeon General: *Advisory on alcohol use in pregnancy,* News Release, 2005, USDHHS.

Methamphetamines

Andres R: Effects of therapeutic, diagnostic, environment agents and exposure to social and illicit drugs. In Creasy R, Resnik R, and Iams J editors: *Maternal-fetal medicine: principles and practice,* ed 5, Philadelphia, 2004, Saunders.

Drug Enforcement Administration: *Methamphetamine Fact Sheet,* Alexandria, VA, 2006, DEA. Retrieved from *http://www.usdoj.gov/dea/concern/meth_factsheet.html*

Medical Study News: Exposure to methamphetamine in the womb causes adverse developmental effects, 2004. *News-Medical.Net.*

Smith L and others: Effects of prenatal methamphetamine exposure on fetal growth and drug withdrawal symptoms in infants born at term, *J Dev Behav Pediatr* 24(1):17–23, 2003.

Cocaine

American Academy of Pediatrics: Neonatal drug withdrawal, Committee on Drugs, *Pediatrics* 101(6):1079–1088, 1998.

American College of Obstetricians and Gynecologists: At-risk drinking and illicit drug use; Ethical issues in obstetric and gynecologic practice, *ACOG Committee Opinion* No. 294, 2004.

Bada H and others: Gestational cocaine exposure and intrauterine growth: maternal lifestyle study, *Obstet Gynecol* 100(5 Pt 1):916–924, 2002.

Bandstra E and others: Intrauterine growth of full-term infants: impact of prenatal cocaine exposure, *Pediatrics* 108(6):1309–1319, 2001.

Bateman D, Chiriboga C: Dose-response effect of cocaine on newborn head circumference, *Pediatrics* 106(3):E33, 2000.

Beers M, Berkow R: *The Merck manual of diagnosis therapy.* Chapter 250. High risk pregnancy, 2005, Merck and Co, Inc. Retrieved from *http://www.merck.com/mrkshared/mmanual/home.jsp*

Buehler B, Conover B, and Andres R: Teratogenic potential of cocaine, *Semin Perinatol* 20(2):93–98, 1996.

Dolkart L, Plessinger M, and Woods J: Effect of alpha receptor blockade upon maternal and fetal cardiovascular responses to cocaine, *Obstet Gynecol* 75(5):745–751, 1990.

Drug Facts and Comparisons: *Topical local anesthetics,* St. Louis, 2004, Facts and Comparisons.

Fajemirokun-Odudeyi O, Lindow S: Obstetric implications of cocaine use in pregnancy: a literature review, *Eur J Obstet Gynecol Reprod Biol* 112(1):2–8, 2004.

FIRST Consult: Clinical Information for Quality Care, St Louis, 2006, Mosby. Retrieved from *http://www.firstconsult.com*

Frank D and others: Growth, development, and behavior in early childhood following prenatal cocaine exposure: a systematic review, *JAMA* 285(12):1613–1625, 2001.

Hepburn M: Substance abuse in pregnancy, *Clin Obstet Gynaecol* 14(6):419, 2004.

Kain Z and others: Cocaine-abusing parturients undergoing cesarean section. A cohort study, *Anesthesiology* 85(5):1028–1035, 1996.

Kuczkowski K: Anesthetic implications of drug abuse in pregnancy, *J Clin Anesth* 15(5): 382–394, 2003.

Lawrence R, Lawrence M: *Breastfeeding: a guide for the medical profession,* ed 6, Philadelphia, 2005, Mosby.

Lynch M, McKeon V: Cocaine use during pregnancy: research findings and clinical implications, *J Obstet Gynecol Neonatal Nurs* 19(4):285–292, 1990.

March of Dimes: *Illicit drug use during pregnancy,* professionals and researchers, White Plains, NY, 2004, MOD.

Plessinger M, Woods J Jr: Cocaine in pregnancy: recent data on maternal and fetal risks, *Obstet Gynecol Clin North Am* 25(1):99–118, 1998.

Potter S and others: Adverse effects of fetal cocaine exposure on neonatal auditory information processing, *Pediatrics* 105(3):E40, 2000.

Schiller C, Allen J: Follow-up of infants prenatally exposed to cocaine, *Pediatr Nurs* 31(5):427–436, 2005.

Singer L and others: Cognitive and motor outcomes of cocaine-exposed infants, *JAMA* 287(15):1952–1960, 2002.

Ursitti F, Klein J, and Koren G: Confirmation of cocaine use during pregnancy: a critical review, *Ther Drug Monit* 23(4):347–353, 2001.

Vidaeff A, Mastrobattista J: In utero cocaine exposure: a thorny mix of science and mythology, *Am J Perinatol* 20(4):165–172, 2003.

Wagner C and others: Substance abuse in pregnancy, *Obstet Gynecol* 25(1):169–194, 1998.

Yazigi R, Odem R, and Polakoski K: Demonstration of specific binding of cocaine to human spermatozoa, *JAMA* 266(14):1956–1959, 1991.

Heroin

Andres R: Effects of therapeutic, diagnostic, environment agents and exposure to social and illicit drugs. In Creasy R, Resnik R, and Iams J editors: *Maternal-fetal medicine: principles and practice,* ed 5, Philadelphia, 2004, Saunders.

Archie C: Methadone in the management of narcotic addiction in pregnancy, *Curr Opin Obstet Gynecol* 10(6):435–440, 1998.

Kendig S: Substance abuse in pregnancy, *Childbirth Instructor* 6(3):18, 1996.

Lee R: Drug abuse. In Burrow G, Ferris T, editors: *Medical complications during pregnancy,* ed 4, Philadelphia, 1995, Saunders.

Little B and others: Patterns of multiple substance abuse during pregnancy: implications for mother and fetus, *South Med J* 83:507, 1990.

National Institute on Drug Abuse: *How does heroin abuse affect pregnant women?* Bethesda, 2005, NIH. Retrieved from *http://www.nida.nih.gov*

Robins L, Mills J: Effects of in utero exposure to street drugs, *Am J Public Health* 83(Suppl):1–32, 1993.

Nursing Management

Archie C: Methadone in the management of narcotic addiction in pregnancy, *Curr Opin Obstet Gynecol* 10(6):435–440, 1998.

Morse B, Gehshan S, and Hutchins E: *Screening for substance abuse during pregnancy: improving care, improving health,* Arlington, VA, 1997, National Center for Education in Maternal and Child Health. Retrieved from *http://www.ncemch.org*

Marijuana

Beers M, Berkow R: *The Merck manual of diagnosis therapy,* Chapter 250. High risk pregnancy, 2005, Merck and Co, Inc. Retrieve from *http://www.merck.com/mrkshared/mmanual/home.jsp*

Drug Prevention Network of the Americas (DPNA): *Marijuana,* Washington, DC, 2004, National Institute on Drug Abuse and National Institute of Health.

Faden V, Graubard B: Maternal substance use during pregnancy and developmental outcome at age three, *J Subst Abuse* 12(4):329–340, 2000.

Fergusson D, Horwood L, and Northstone K: Maternal use of cannabis and pregnancy outcome, *BJOG* 109(1):21–27, 2002.

Fried P, Smith A: A literature review of the consequences of prenatal marihuana exposure: an emerging theme of a deficiency in aspects of executive function, *Neurotoxicol Teratol* 23(1):1–11, 2001.

Hubbard J, Franco S, and Onaivi E: Marijuana: Medical implications, *Am Fam Physician* 60(9):2583–2588, 1999.

Lee M: Marihuana and tobacco use in pregnancy, *Obstet Gynecol Clin North Am* 25(1): 65–83, 1998.

Maynard E, Amoruso L, and Oh W: Meconium for drug testing, *Am J Dis Child* 145(6): 650–652, 1991.

Wu T and others: Pulmonary hazards of smoking marijuana as compared with tobacco, *N Engl J Med* 318(6):347–351, 1988.

Tobacco

American College of Obstetricians and Gynecologists (ACOG): Smoking cessation during pregnancy, *ACOG Educ Bulletin,* No. 260, 2000.

Bradley J and others: Severity of respiratory syncytial virus bronchiolitis is affected by cigarette smoke exposure and atopy, *Pediatrics* 115(1):e7–e14, 2005.

Centers for Disease Control and Prevention: Treating tobacco use and dependence, *Clin Practice Guidelines,* 2000, U.S. Department of Health and Human Services. Retrieved from *http://www.cdc.gov/tobacco/statehi/statehi.htm*

Cleveland Clinic: *Smoking cessation,* Cleveland, OH, 2004, Author. Retrieved from *http://www.clevelandclinic.org/emergencymedicine/smoking.htm*

Dobson R: Smoking in late pregnancy is linked to lower IQ in offspring, *BMJ* 330:499, 2005.

Haste F and others: Nutrient intakes during pregnancy: observations on the influence of smoking and social class, *Am J Clin Nutr* 51(1):29–36, 1990.

Lawrence R, Lawrence M: *Breastfeeding: a guide for the medical profession,* ed 6, Philadelphia, 2005, Mosby.

Li Y and others: Maternal and grandmaternal smoking patterns are associated with early childhood asthma, *Chest* 127(4):1232–1241, 2005.

Lumley J and others: Interventions for promoting smoking cessation during pregnancy, *Cochrane Database Syst Rev* Issue 3, 2004.

Maloni J: *The prevention of preterm birth: research-based practice, nursing interventions, practice scenarios,* Washington, DC, 2000, AWHONN.

Maloni J: Preventing low birth weight: how smoking cessation counseling can help, *AWHONN Lifelines* 5(1):32–35, 2001.

March of Dimes (MOD): *Smoking during pregnancy,* Professionals and Researchers, White Plains, NY, 2004, MOD.

Melvin C and others: Recommended cessation counselling for pregnant women who smoke: a review of the evidence, *Tob Control* 9(Suppl 3):III80–III84, 2000.

Todd S, LaSala K, and Neil-Urban S: An integrated approach to prenatal smoking cessation interventions, *MCN Am J Matern Child Nurs* 26(4):185–190, 2001.

U.S. Department of Health and Human Services (USDHHS): *Healthy People 2010: understanding and improving health: Maternal, infant, and child health,* Rockville, Md, 2002, Office of Disease Prevention and Health Promotion (ODPHP). Retrieved from: *http://www.health.gov/healthypeople/Document/tableofcontents.htm*

U.S. Department of Health and Human Services (USDHHS): *Substance use during pregnancy: 2002 and 2003,* update, Rockville, Md, 2005, USDHHS.

U.S. Department of Health and Human Services (USDHHS): *The health consequences of smoking: a report of the Surgeon General,* Atlanta, Ga, 2004, CDC, Office on Smoking and Health.

U.S. Department of Health and Human Services (USDHHS): *Treating tobacco use and dependence,* Rockville, Md, 2000, USDHHS.

Vik T and others: Pre- and post-natal growth in children of women who smoked in pregnancy, *Early Hum Dev* 45(3):245–255, 1996.

Wardlaw G, Smith A: *Contemporary nutrition,* ed 6, Boston, 2006, McGraw Hill.

VII

Alterations in the Mechanism of Labor

S uccessful completion of pregnancy heralded by labor requires the harmonious interplay of the uterus, placenta, fetus, and pelvis. Disruptions can result if labor is not stimulated on time, the uterus contracts ineffectively, the fetus is larger than the pelvis, or the fetus is in a position that makes it impossible to pass through the pelvis. When a disruption in the mechanism of labor develops, early detection, active medical management, and timely nursing interventions are important to facilitate the best maternal and fetal outcome. A variety of nursing measures to facilitate progress in labor can significantly reduce the need for obstetric and surgical interventions.

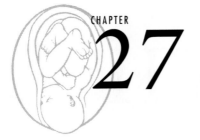

CHAPTER

27

Labor Stimulation

There are two classifications of labor stimulation: induction and augmentation. *Induction of labor* is any attempt to initiate uterine contractions before their spontaneous onset to facilitate a vaginal delivery. Before an induction, the ability of the cervix to be induced is determined. Artificial ripening of an unripe cervix is usually beneficial.

Augmentation of labor is any attempt to stimulate uterine contractions during the course of labor to facilitate a vaginal delivery. It is frequently used for certain types of uterine dysfunction. A labor should not be augmented until noninvasive interventions have been tried, such as the following:

- Making sure the bladder is empty
- Encouraging ambulation if possible or changing of position
- Allaying anxiety because epinephrine decreases uterine efficiency
- Making sure the patient is properly nourished and hydrated

Labor stimulant methods considered in this chapter include pharmacologic and mechanical cervical ripening methods and natural methods of labor induction and augmentation. Pharmacologic methods include using oxytocin; physiologic means include using amniotomy and stripping of fetal membranes.

INCIDENCE

Use of a labor stimulant for either inducing or augmenting labor varies among countries, cities, and hospitals. Rates between 10% and 25% are common in industrialized countries (RCOG, 2001). In the United States, according to the National Center for Health Statistics for 2003 (Martin and others, 2005), approximately 37% of all labors are stimulated; 20.5% are induced and 16.7% are augmented.

INDICATIONS

Common indications for induction of labor follow:

- Postterm
- Maternal diseases such as diabetes, renal disease, and cardiac disease

- Hypertensive disorders
- Premature rupture of membranes (PROM)
- Oligohydramnios
- Suggested fetal stress such as intrauterine growth restriction or chorioamnionitis

About 25% of all inductions are elective (Martin and others, 2005). Fetal maturity must be confirmed for all elective inductions. If one of the American College of Obstetricians and Gynecologists (ACOG, 1999) criteria for gestational dating (as outlined in Table 27-1) is met, amniocentesis to determine fetal lung maturity is not necessary.

CRITERIA

Criteria for an induction of labor are listed:
- Engaged presenting part
- No previous classic uterine incision
- No fetopelvic disproportion
- No nonreassuring fetal heart rate (FHR) patterns
- No major bleeding from an abruptio placentae
- No placenta previa or vasa previa
- No active herpes

Cervical ripening, induction of labor, and augmentation of labor are currently being questioned for a vaginal birth after previous cesarean.

Criteria for augmentation of labor are the same as for induction. There must also be definite signs that the progress of labor is slowing down.

Labor is seldom induced or augmented (1) on a grand multipara more than five parity, (2) on a multiple pregnancy, or (3) in the presence of polyhydramnios because of the increased risk for uterine rupture related to uterine overdistention.

Table 27-1   ACOG Criteria for Gestational Dating

Test	Results
Fetal heart rate	• Documented for 20 weeks with a fetoscope or 30 weeks with a Doppler evaluation
Pregnancy test	• It has been 36 or more weeks since a positive serum or urine human chorionic gonadotrophin pregnancy test, performed by a reliable laboratory
Ultrasonography	• Ultrasound measurement of the crown-rump length, obtained between 6 and 12 weeks, indicates gestation of at least 39 weeks • Ultrasound scan between 13 and 20 weeks confirms the clinical history and physical examination gestational age of at least 39 wks

Modified from American College of Obstetricians and Gynecologists: Induction of labor, *ACOG Practice Bulletin*, No. 10, Washington, DC, 1999, ACOG.

PREDICTORS OF SUCCESS

The success of the induction or augmentation usually depends on a ripe cervix. A cervix is considered ripe when it is soft, anterior, effaced more than 50%, and dilated 2 cm or more. Bishop (1964) developed a 13-point scoring system to predict the responsiveness of a patient to an induction. When the pelvic score totals 8 or more, induction is usually successful (Table 27-2) (ACOG, 1999). When the score is 6 or less, cervical ripening is usually considered prior to induction (SOGC, 2001).

RISKS

The need for other interventions increase (Simpson and Atterbury, 2003) such as:

- Intravenous line
- Activity limitation
- More frequent monitoring
- Increased need for epidural analgesia related to more painful contractions
- Increased need for other interventions such as instrumental or cesarean delivery

PHYSIOLOGY OF UTEROTROPINS AND UTEROTONINS

Many substances interplay to prepare for and promote labor. Prostaglandins are formed enzymatically from phospholipids and arachidonic acid in most tissues of the body. They act as a local hormone by exerting their action primarily at the site of production. The biosynthesis of reproductive tissue prostaglandins varies among tissue. The myometrium is the primary source of prostacyclin (PGI_2) (PGE_2), and the decidua is the primary source of prostaglandin F_2a (PGF_2a).

During pregnancy, PGI_2 helps the uterus remain quiet by inhibiting the formation of gap junctions and the release of phospholipase A, and PGI_2 blocks calcium movement into cells. Progesterone further regulates the myometrial activity throughout pregnancy by inhibiting the formation of oxytocin receptors and gap junctions (Olson, Mijovic, Sadowsky, 1995). Estrogen promotes this process.

Table 27-2   Bishop Prelabor Scoring System

	Score			
	0	1	2	3
Dilation (cm)	0	1–2	3–4	5–6
Effacement (%)	0–30	40–50	60–70	80
Station	−3	−2	−1/0	+1/+2
Consistency of cervix	Firm	Medium	Soft	
Cervical position	Posterior	Median	Anterior	

Reference: Bishop, E: Pelvic scoring for elective induction, *Obstet Gynecol* 24:266–268, 1964.

During the prelabor phase or preparation phase just before true labor, production of PGE_2 by the amnion increases; this increase is normally induced by the fetus (Olson, Mijovic, Sadowsky, 1995). During this phase, the body is prepared for labor by the following occurrences:

- Increasing myometrial receptors for estrogen but not progesterone (Olson, Mijovic, Sadowsky, 1995)
- Softening and ripening of the cervix caused by enzymatic rearrangement of the collagen fibers into smaller, more flexible fibers and increasing synthesis of hyaluronic acid, thereby facilitating water absorption by the cervix (Leppert, 1995), leading to a softer, more stretchable cervix
- Increasing elastin in the cervix, which gives the cervix its ability to recoil and regain its shape after birth
- Increasing the frequency of Braxton-Hicks contractions
- Developing gap junctions in the myometrium that are cell-to-cell contact areas to coordinated myometrium contractions
- Increasing the number of oxytocin receptors in the myometrium and decidua; myometrium receptors gradually increase during the latter part of pregnancy peaking at the end of the first stage of labor, whereas decidua receptors increase during labor and peak at birth (Simpson and Poole, 1998)

As true labor is initiated, PGF_2a production increases significantly by the decidua, which continues to promote the responses that PGE_2 initiated, as well as increasing the contractile responsiveness of the myometrium by moving calcium into the cells. Production of prostacyclin is suppressed during labor because of high levels of cortisol (MacKenzie and others, 1988).

Oxytocin levels in the plasma may not increase significantly until labor begins with a significant increase during second stage of labor, when oxytocin appears to maximize uterine contractions (Arias, 2000). Oxytocin is ineffective in promoting myometrial contractions until oxytocin receptors are present in the myometrium and then the decidua. High levels of estrogen, PGF_2a, and PGE_2 (Olson, Mijovic, Sadowsky, 1995) stimulate these receptors.

According to Clayworth (2000), there are three important variables that influence the body's response to oxytocin:

1 Oxygen status of the uterus
2 Availability of glucose for uterine energy
3 Number of oxytocin receptors present in the uterus

PHARMACOLOGIC METHODS FOR CERVICAL RIPENING: PROSTAGLANDINS E_2-DINOPROSTONE

Dinoprostone is the most commonly used medication for ripening the cervix, the first step in labor induction. It causes dissolution of the cervical collagen bundles and increases cervical submucosal water content, stimulates smooth muscle contraction of the cervix and uterus, and increases gap junction formation (Rayburn and others, 1994; Witter, 2000; Sanchez-Ramos and Delke, 2006).

Cervidil and Prepidil are U.S. Food and Drug Administration (FDA)-approved for labor stimulation.

Dosages

Table 27-3 presents a comparison of the most commonly used forms of PGE_2.

Advantages

The advantages of prostaglandin-initiated cervical ripening as demonstrated by research reviewed in the *Cochrane Review* (Kelly, Kavanagh, and Thomas, 2003) follow:

- Enhanced cervical ripening
- Decreased need for oxytocin for induction
- Decreased oxytocin induction time, when used
- Reduced amount of oxytocin needed for a successful induction

The effectiveness of cervical ripening before labor induction with prostaglandins has been compared with low-dose oxytocin. According to Pollnow and Broekhuizen (1996), prostaglandin was superior to low-dose oxytocin. This was demonstrated by the incidence of higher Bishop scores, higher rate of successful inductions, and shorter labors. Morbidity and cesarean delivery rates were similar in both groups.

Risks

Uterine Hyperstimulation

Uterine hyperstimulation is seen in approximately 1% to 5% of the patients, with the greatest risk following administration of prostaglandins through the intravaginal route or vaginal insert (ACOG, 1999). *Uterine hyperstimulation* is defined as five or more contractions in 10 minutes, or a single contraction lasting more than 2 minutes either with or without signs of fetal stress such as late decelerations or fetal bradycardia. When uterine hyperstimulation occurs, it is effectively reversed with the use of beta$_2$-adrenergic tocolytic therapy, such as intravenous or subcutaneous terbutaline, 250 mcg (ACOG, 1999). When a vaginal insert is being used, removal helps reverse uterine hyperstimulation.

Nonreassuring Fetal Heart Rate Pattern Changes

A nonreassuring pattern, such as severe variable decelerations or bradycardia, is very uncommon in patients during prostaglandin labor stimulation. When associated FHR changes occur because of uterine hyperstimulation, they are responsive to the standard treatment protocol, such as position change, increasing intravenous (IV) fluids, and administering oxygen at 10 L/min.

Other Side Effects

Gastrointestinal side effects such as nausea, vomiting, and diarrhea are negligible for patients being treated with low-dose prostaglandins (Sanchez-Ramos and Delke, 2006). Rarely, an infection, a fever, or headache occurs.

Table 27-3   Comparison of Commonly Used Pharmacologic Cervical Ripening Products

Drug	Route	Dosage	Considerations
Dinoprostone (Cervidil) Vaginal insert: a thin, flat, polymer chip in a polyester mesh net with attached cord Prostaglandin E$_2$ agent	Insert into vaginal posterior fornix	10 mg, which is released slowly (approximately 0.3 mg/hr for maximum of 12 hr)	Can be inserted by a perinatal nurse Stored at −20°C but does not require warming Oxytocin can be administered 30–60 min after removal of insert Can be removed when labor starts or when hyperstimulation occurs FDA-approved Not messy
Dinoprostone (Prepidil) prostaglandin E$_2$ gel Prefilled syringe applicator with 10 mm or 20 mm endocervical catheter	Intracervical: one syringe application inserted into cervical canal	2.5 ml gel with 0.5 mg dinoprostone May repeat every 6 hr Maximum of three doses per 24 hr (1.5 mg)	Inserted by physician or midwife FDA-approved Required refrigeration and must be warmed to room temperature before catheter administration Prompts minimal uterine activity Product reliable Quite expensive Efficiency decreased with rupture of membranes Must wait 6–12 hr to start oxytocin induction per package insert Has been used for outpatient management

Continued

Table 27-3 Comparison of Commonly Used Pharmacologic Cervical Ripening Products—cont'd

Drug	Route	Dosage	Considerations
Misoprostol (Cytotec) Synthetic PGE_1 analog tablet	Posterior vaginal fornix	25 mcg (¼ of a 100-mcg tablet) (ACOG, 2003b). May repeat in 3–6 hr for a maximum of 6 doses Comes in 100- or 200- mcg tablet	FDA-approved in 2002 Inexpensive Stable at room temperature Effective in presence of rupture of membranes Not to be used in patients with a history of previous cesarean or prior uterine surgery because of the increased risk for uterine rupture Oxytocin can be administered 4 or more hr after the last dose

FDA, Food and Drug Administration; *PGE_1*, prostaglandin E_1; *PGE_2*, prostaglandin E_2.

Nursing Interventions

Preadministration

- Obtain an informed consent following an informative discussion as to the procedure, reasons for the procedure, what it means to the patient, and potential side effects and risks.
- Determine the cervical Bishop score (see Table 27-2), which is a standard of predicting inducibility. A score of 4 or less indicates an unfavorable cervix that could benefit from prostaglandin softening.
- Assess for any contraindications of prostaglandin use such as an active pelvic infection, vaginal bleeding, active cardiopulmonary disease, known hepatic or renal disease, or an allergy to the drug (Weiner and Buhimschi, 2004).
- Assess amniotic membrane status because the intravaginal route is usually used after rupture of membranes (ROM).
- Obtain a baseline FHR tracing per protocol.
- Analyze the baseline tracing for any nonreassuring signs, such as bradycardia or late decelerations.
- Obtain baseline readings of blood pressure, temperature, pulse, and respiration rate.
- Assess for uterine activity.

Administration

- Assess blood pressure, temperature, pulse, and respiratory rate before each PGE_2 gel application.
- Prepare medication and equipment for insertion.
- Instill gel per protocol with patient in a dorsal lithotomy position.
- Provide ongoing emotional support, and encourage relaxation.
- Have patient turn on her side and rest in bed for 30 to 60 minutes after each PGE_2 gel application.
- Monitor for hyperstimulation uterine activity and nonreassuring FHR changes per protocol.
- Be prepared to treat uterine hyperstimulation and any nonreassuring FHR change with the standard treatment protocol, such as changing patient's position, increasing IV fluids, and administering oxygen at 10 L/min. Have a beta$_2$-adrenergic tocolytic drug readily available to give on physician's order. The dosage is usually 250 mcg of terbutaline administered subcutaneously or IV (ACOG, 1999).
- Assess for the development of any side effects, such as diarrhea, nausea, or vomiting, which occur most often during the first 30 minutes after administration.
- Permit ambulation after the assessment phase until the next dose, in most cases.
- Reassess the Bishop score after completion of the prostaglandin protocol.

PHARMACOLOGIC METHODS FOR CERVICAL RIPENING: PROSTAGLANDIN E$_1$-MISOPROSTOL

Misoprostol (Cytotec) is a synthetic PGE$_1$ analog that is FDA-approved for the prevention and treatment of gastric and duodenal ulcers. Although it is not FDA-approved for obstetric use, it is widely used for cervical ripening and induction of labor. Various research studies (Buser and others, 1997; Sanchez-Ramos and others, 1997; Sanchez-Ramos and others, 1998; Blanchette, Nayak, and Erasmus, 1999; Nunes, Rodrigues, and Meirinho, 1999) have demonstrated benefits to misoprostol, such as increased cervical ripening, decreased oxytocin use, shortened labor, and decreased cost. These studies did show an increased risk for uterine hyperstimulation, which can cause uterine rupture and meconium-stained amniotic fluid. According to ACOG (2000), it is a safe effective agent for cervical ripening and labor induction except in vaginal births after previous cesarean. There is an increased risk for uterine rupture in women with a prior cesarean or major uterine surgery.

However, according to the *Cochrane Review* (Hofmeyr and Gulmezoglu, 2003), the increase in uterine hyperstimulation is of concern and the studies did not exclude the possibility of serious adverse effects such as uterine rupture with or without previous cesarean. These researchers concluded that further research is needed to establish safety, and therefore some health care providers do not prescribe its use because of the concern about its effect.

If misoprostol is prescribed, see Table 27-3 for administration protocols.

MECHANICAL METHODS FOR CERVICAL RIPENING: LAMINARIA OR SYNTHETIC DILATORS

Laminaria tents, such as *Laminaria digitata* or *Laminaria japonica,* are natural cervical dilators made from seaweed. Synthetic alternatives are currently being used more frequently. Two common synthetic dilators are Dilapan, a hygroscopic cervical dilator, and Lamicel, an alcohol polymer sponge impregnated with 450 mg of magnesium sulfate and compressed into a tent. A 30-ml Foley catheter placed in the cervical canal prior to inflation may also be used.

Physiology

The dilators are inserted into the full length of the cervical canal, where they absorb cervical fluids and swell, dilating the cervix slowly (Sanchez-Ramos and Delka, 2006).

Advantages

Dilators are used primarily for labor induction in the presence of minimal cervical effacement.

Risks

Chorioamnionitis

Infection is a risk of using dilators. It is caused primarily by beta-hemolytic streptococci. Because of the faster expansion time (4 hours as compared with 12 to 16 hours), the synthetic dilators pose less of a risk for an infection than the *Laminaria* dilators, but the presence of any foreign body may allow vaginal flora to ascend into the uterus (Chua and others, 1997; Sanchez-Ramos, 2005).

Premature Rupture of Membranes
Because the tents must be placed into the full length of the cervical canal, including the internal os, there is a risk for PROM if the cervix is short.

Cervical Trauma
Cervical trauma is related to insertion technique.

Nursing Interventions
- Prepare the patient and assist the physician with the preinsertion assessment, which includes ruling out ruptured membranes; inspecting the cervix and vagina for an infection, especially for beta-streptococcus or *Neisseria gonorrhoeae;* assessing fetal size, position, amniotic fluid volume, and placental position with ultrasound; and assessing for fetal well-being with a biophysical profile or a contraction stress test.
- Prepare the patient, and assist the physician with the insertion procedure, which includes a vaginal examination to assess cervical anatomy and cervical status; insertion of a sterile speculum so that the cervix can be visualized, stabilized with a ring forceps, and painted with povidone-iodine (Betadine); lubricate with a bacteriostatic cream or jelly; insert four to nine tents to fill the cervix; and pack the upper vagina with 4- × 4-inch sponges to hold the tents in place.
- Instruct the patient that she might experience mild cramping during the insertion.
- Document the number of dilators and sponges placed.
- Continue to assess urinary output following insertion because pressure on the bladder may cause urinary retention.
- Continually assess for ROM, uterine tenderness or pain, or uterine bleeding. If any of these signs occur, assess for signs of fetal compromise and notify the physician so that tents can be removed.

PHARMACOLOGIC LABOR INDUCTION METHOD: OXYTOCIN
Oxytocin, a normal hormone secreted from the posterior pituitary gland, is chemically related to vasopressin antidiuretic hormone (ADH). It promotes smooth muscle contractions of the uterus by activating the myometrium. The effect of oxytocin is enhanced in the presence of high levels of estrogen. This is why oxytocin has little effect on the pregnant uterus until near term; this is when estrogen levels are high and adequate oxytocin receptors are present in the myometrium.

Oxytocin is administered in synthetic form as Pitocin. It is available in solution form for IV or intramuscular injections. It cannot be administered orally because the digestive enzyme trypsin inactivates it. IV administration of dilute oxytocin is the preferred route because the absorption rate is predictable and the absorption of the drug can be stopped at any time by discontinuing the IV infusion. Its effect on the body usually ceases quickly after the drug is discontinued; the pregnant woman's plasma, near term, contains a high concentration of the enzyme pitocinase.

Physiology

When labor must be initiated by oxytocin, the preparation for labor that normally takes place during the prelabor phase may not have occurred. Therefore, the initial oxytocin-induced uterine contractions must promote these activities by causing a myometrial cell inflammatory response that frees arachidonic acid so that it is converted to prostaglandins. Once enough prostaglandins have been synthesized and myometrial gap junctions formed so that the uterus can respond in a coordinated manner, the active phase of labor begins.

By the middle of the active phase of labor, adequate oxytocin receptors are formed so that the dosage of oxytocin may be decreased. It can frequently be discontinued when 7 to 8 cm of dilation is reached because of adequate endogenous prostaglandins and oxytocin production.

Pharmacologic Characteristics

Individualized Uterine Response to Oxytocin

The uterine response to oxytocin is individualized (Perry and others, 1996).

Sensitivity to Oxytocin Changes During Various Phases of Labor

Sensitivity to oxytocin increases as labor advances related to the development of gap junctions and oxytocin receptors (Dawood, 1995), peaking during the second stage of labor (Shyken and Petrie, 1995).

Oxytocin Secretion in Pulses and by the Fetus

During normal labor, oxytocin has been found to be secreted in pulses or spurts (Shyken and Petrie, 1995). The fetus is thought to secrete oxytocin in response to maternal oxytocin at a rate of 3 mU/min (Simpson and Poole, 1998).

Maximum Uterine Contractile Effect of Oxytocin

A uterine response occurs to oxytocin in 3 to 5 minutes with a half-life of approximately 10 minutes. It takes approximately 40 minutes for a steady serum plasma state to be reached after oxytocin administration (Gonser, 1995; Shyken and Petrie, 1995). However, according to Perry and others (1996), serum plasma levels of oxytocin may not be important in determining dosing of the drug.

Uterine Response to Oxytocin

A triphasic uterine response to oxytocin occurs. During the incremental phase, the uterine response increases evenly as oxytocin dose increases. In the stable phase, the uterine response is unchanged even when oxytocin doses are increased. During the third phase, uterine contractions increase in frequency but intensity decreases, leading to an ineffective uterine contraction pattern. This change in uterine response may be gradual or abrupt (Dawood, 1995).

Dosages

There is a wide discrepancy among health care providers as to the most effective protocol for administering oxytocin. Currently, there are three schools of thought.

Low-Dose Management: Physiologic Approach

Low-dose management in oxytocin administration is based on research by Seitchik and others (1982, 1985), who recommended starting oxytocin at 1 mU/min and increasing the dosage by 0.5 to 1 mU/min every 30 to 60 minutes. The effects that conservative management has on outcome variables of labor has been studied by Blakemore and others (1990), Chua and others (1991), Mercer, Pilgrim, and Sibai (1991), Muller, Stubbs, and Laurent (1992), and Shyken and Petrie (1995). The findings of these four studies include decreased hyperstimulation, decreased fetal compromise, and significantly less oxytocin needed without affecting the duration of labor or cesarean rate. Table 27-4 lists examples of current low-dose oxytocin management.

High-Dose (Active) Management: Pharmacologic Approach

Current high-dose oxytocin protocols are based on the active management by O'Driscoll, Meagher, and Robson (2004), who recommended starting oxytocin at 6 mU/min and increasing the dosage by 6 mU/min every 15 minutes. The goal is strong uterine contractions leading to shortened labor and delivery. The effect that active management has on outcome variables of labor has been studied by Lopez-Zeno and others (1992), Xenakis and others (1995), Peaceman and Socol (1996), Crane and Young (1998), and Merrill and Ziatnik (1999). The findings of these studies include decreased length of labor, rate of forceps delivery, and rate of cesarean birth for dystocia, with increased hyperstimulation and cesarean birth for fetal stress. However, Frigoletto and others (1995) found active management to shorten labor to some degree and decrease risk for maternal fever but not to decrease cesarean delivery rate.

Table 27-4   Examples of Low-Dose and High-Dose Oxytocin Management for Labor Stimulation

Oxytocin	Starting Dose (mU/min)	Incremental Increase (mU/min)	Dosage Interval (in minutes)	Maximum Dose (mU/min)
Low dose	0.5–1.0	1	30–40	20
	1–2	2	15	40
High dose	6	6, 3, 1	20–40	42
	6	6	15	40

Modified from American College of Obstetricians and Gynecologists: Induction of labor, *ACOG Practice Bulletin*, No. 49, Washington, DC, 2003, ACOG.

According to O'Driscoll, Meagher, and Robson (2004), there are other components to the active management protocol beyond just high-dose oxytocin. Most American obstetricians emphasize the high-dose oxytocin and fail to incorporate all other components.

Components of active management in O'Driscoll, Meagher, and Robson are:

- *Childbirth education.* The patient is taught what to expect in labor and that it will not last more than 12 hours.
- *Criterion for diagnosis of labor.* The Dublin criterion is complete effacement. The healthy primigravida is not admitted until this criterion is met.
- *Amniotomy.* On admission, the membranes are artificially ruptured if still intact. If the amniotic fluid is clear, FHR is auscultated. If the amniotic fluid is meconium-stained, a continuous electronic monitor is used.
- *Criterion for early diagnosis and treatment of dystocia.* The Dublin criterion is 1 cm of progress per hour. If the patient's progress is slower than the standard, high-dose oxytocin (6 mU) is started immediately. It is increased every 15 minutes by 6 mU until the patient dilates 1 cm/hour. In their patients in 2000, 24% were induced (O'Driscoll, Meagher, and Robson, 2004). If the patient's contraction pattern cannot be stimulated to accomplish a dilation rate of 1 cm/hour in a reasonable time, a cesarean delivery is done. The cesarean birth rate in Dublin was 14% in 2000 (O'Driscoll, Meagher, and Robson, 2004).
- *Continual presence of a personal nurse.* One nurse is assigned to one patient, and the nurse remains with the patient until her delivery. According to Thornton and Lilford's review and meta-analysis (1994) of published studies on active labor management, the personal nurse who provides constant emotional and physical support is the only component associated with shorter labors and lower cesarean rates (see Table 27-4 for examples of current high-dose oxytocin management in the United States.)

Pulsatile Oxytocin Management

Oxytocin is administered by some health care providers in 10-minute pulsed infusions as opposed to a continuous IV infusion. According to Willcourt and others (1994), significantly less oxytocin and infusion fluid is used without loss of effectiveness.

Maternal Side Effects

Uterine Hyperstimulation

Uterine hyperstimulation can cause strong tetanic contractions that occur more often than four times in a 10-minute period, last longer than 90 seconds without a period of relaxation, or have an increased uterine resting tone above 20 mm Hg. This type of uterine contraction pattern can cause abruptio placenta or uterine rupture, as well as fetal stress. This is seen more often with high-dose regimens and more frequent dose increases.

Uncoordinated, Unproductive Uterine Activity

Unproductive uterine activity may be defined as an increase in frequency with a decrease in intensity of the contractions. This type of activity is related to the cessation of uterine blood flow during a contraction, causing accumulation of metabolites and hypoxia, which renders the muscle ineffective.

Antidiuretic Effect: Water Intoxication

Because oxytocin has a weak antidiuretic property, large doses can cause the kidneys to increase the reabsorption of water, decreasing urinary output. Antidiuretic effect is seen more frequently when the oxytocin infusion rate is 40 mU/min or more. This condition is enhanced if large amounts of electrolyte-free dextrose solution are used to administer the oxytocin (Sanchez-Ramos, 2005). Possible signs of water intoxication are decreased urine output, hypotension, tachycardia, headache, and nausea and vomiting.

Cesarean Birth

Cesarean birth rate is increased for nonreassuring fetal status or failed induction.

Failed Induction

According to Stubbs (2000), failed induction is the most common risk and is directly related to the degree of cervical ripening.

Fetal and Neonatal Effects

Iatrogenic Prematurity

Any time labor is induced, there is a risk for prematurity. Therefore fetal maturity should always be assessed before an induction unless it is being performed because of medical indications when the benefits of delivery outweigh the risks of prematurity.

Fetal Stressors

Labor contractions normally impede uterine blood flow. A healthy fetus that has an adequate oxygen reserve can withstand this stress. However, if the frequency, intensity, duration, or resting tone of the contractions is increased by a labor stimulant, this can further impede the uterine blood flow and can cause fetal compromise, resulting in a nonreassuring FHR pattern.

Nursing Interventions

Because of the individualized response to oxytocin, the variations of practice philosophy supported by research, and variable resources unique to each institution, the following oxytocin protocol is generic:

- Ensure an informed consent has been obtained by providing information about the indication, the agents and methods, alternative options, and risk such as repeat induction and cesarean delivery (JCAHO, 2003).
- Initiate oxytocin induction or augmentation only after a physician who can perform a cesarean delivery and who is readily available has evaluated the

patient, determined a medical indication, provided documentation of fetal maturity, and obtained an informed consent from the patient. The consent must include indication for, risks, and methods to be used and possible alternatives.

- Have an appropriate nurse-to-patient ratio on the unit—1:1 or 1:2 (AAP and ACOG, 2002).
- Have a unit- or hospital-based validation program established for the registered labor nurse to prepare the nurse to safely administer and monitor labor stimulants (Simpson and Atterbury, 2003).
- Explain the procedure and what to expect to the patient and her coach.
- Assess the response of the patient and her coach to labor stimulation. Often, they feel as if they have failed when such an intervention is needed. An explanation as to the reason can help to alleviate these feelings.
- Assess the patient's level of fear associated with labor-induced contractions. Many patients have heard alarming reports about oxytocin. The nurse should inform the patient and her coach that stimulated contractions are usually very similar to normal, active labor contraction. An induced labor usually has a shorter latent phase, with contractions that may be more uncomfortable than those occurring with a spontaneous latent phase do, but the active phase is not usually altered.
- Apply an external fetal monitor or assist with the placement of an internal fetal monitor, and determine a baseline for maternal vital signs, FHR, and uterine activity for 10 to 20 minutes before initiation.
- Perform a vaginal examination to determine cervical effacement and dilation, fetal presentation, and station.
- Prepare the oxytocin solution according to hospital policy, and label properly. Usually, 10 units of oxytocin are mixed with 1000 ml of an IV isotonic electrolyte solution.
- Have the patient positioned on her side or sitting up to avoid the vena cava syndrome.
- Administer the solution by way of a continuous infusion device to ensure precise control over the amount of medication administered.
- Piggyback the oxytocin solution into a well-functioning infusion line next to the infusion site so that oxytocin can be discontinued and restarted as necessary while maintaining an open vein for any emergency.
- Start the pump, usually at a low setting, per hospital protocol or physician's order and patient response. Frequency of uterine contractions, progression of labor, and fetal tolerance are all part of the patient response (Clayworth, 2000).
- The dose is gradually increased per hospital protocol or physician's orders until a desired contraction pattern is established or the instituted maximum dose is reached. The licensed maximum dose is 20 mU/min, but some controlled trial studies are evaluating regimens up to 32 mU/min. In the majority of cases, an adequate contraction pattern is usually achieved at around 12 mU/min (RCOG, 2001).

- When labor has progressed to 5 to 6 cm of dilation, oxytocin may be reduced by 1 to 2 mU/min every 30 to 60 minutes.
- The goal of oxytocin is to establish an adequate uterine contraction pattern that promotes cervical dilation of approximately 1 cm per hour once active labor is established. Usually, this contraction pattern consists of three contractions every 10 minutes, each lasting 40 to 60 seconds with an intensity of 25 to 75 mm Hg intrauterine pressure. This produces between 150 and 350 Montevideo units, in which the uterus returns to baseline (resting tone, which does not exceed 20 mm Hg) for at least 1 minute between each contraction.
- Check the patency of the IV infusion frequently so that backup of the oxytocin solution into the IV tubing does not result in a bolus of oxytocin.
- Assess the FHR and uterine contractions for resting tone, intensity, frequency, and duration according to the institution's policy. According to the Association of Women's Health, Obstetric, and Neonatal Nurses (Simpson and Atterbury, 2003), the frequency of FHR and uterine contractions assessment is based on the condition of the mother and the fetus' response to labor with a minimum standard of assessment before every dose increase. The American Academy of Pediatrics and the American College of Obstetricians and Gynecologists (2002) recommend monitoring for low risk patients during first stage of labor at least every 30 minutes and during second stage of labor at least every 15 minutes, preferably just following a contraction. When risk factors are present or the fetus response to labor indicates, the FHR should be assessed every 15 minutes during first stage and every 5 minutes during second stage. However, the Royal College of Obstetricians and Gynecologists (2001) recommends continuous monitoring similar to that for any high risk pregnancy.
- Assess vital signs per institution's policy.
- Perform periodic vaginal examinations to determine cervical dilation and fetal descent. To evaluate the progress of labor, check cervical dilation and descent of the presenting part (station). A 1-cm/hour cervical dilation indicates sufficient progress and adequate oxytocin.
- Drug doses, times of increase, maternal vital signs, and FHR should be charted on a flow sheet.
- Assess the patient's level of pain frequently. Determine the effectiveness of distraction tools. If the distraction tools are ineffective for her level of discomfort, the physician should be notified. An analgesic may decrease the pain so that distraction tools are effective and the patient can stay in control. Allow the patient a choice in this regard.
- Encourage the patient and her coach by giving them frequent positive reinforcement. This can help alleviate some of the negative feelings associated with a stimulated labor.
- Ensure adequate hydration to enhance effective contractions and avoid dehydration and exhaustion. A fluid bolus may be requested before initiating oxytocin, and fluid should usually infuse at a minimum of 125 ml/hour.
- Keep an accurate intake and output record.

- Assess for signs of fluid retention such as decreased urine output, bounding pulse, peripheral edema, increasing blood pressure, shortness of breath, or crackles.
- Decrease or discontinue oxytocin if a hyperstimulation contraction pattern is noted, and notify the attending physician. Hyperstimulation contractions (1) occur more often than four every 10 minutes, (2) last 90 seconds or more without a period of relaxation, and (3) have an increased uterine resting tone above 20 mm Hg pressure.
- Discontinue oxytocin, administer oxygen, position patient on her side, and notify the attending physician if a nonreassuring FHR pattern is noted, such as late or variable decelerations, loss of long- or short-term variability, tachycardia, or bradycardia. The oxytocin infusion may be restarted after careful assessment by the attending physician of the uterine contraction pattern and the FHR. It may be advantageous to lower the dose and lengthen the dose interval. If oxytocin has been stopped for longer than 30 minutes, it may be necessary to restart from the initial ordered dose (Clayworth, 2000).
- If uterine hyperstimulation persists, be prepared to give terbutaline or another tocolytic.
- Make sure the attending physician is close to the labor and delivery area to manage any complication that might arise.
- Discontinue the induction if labor has not started or no progress is made within 2 to 3 hours.
- Follow the health care facility's chain of command if you disagree with the physician's plan.

PHYSIOLOGIC METHODS OF LABOR INDUCTION: AMNIOTOMY

An *amniotomy* is artificial ROM with an amniohook. It is used to induce or augment labor. According to the *Cochrane Review* (Fraser and others, 2000), amniotomy is associated with birth risks and benefits and should be reserved for women with abnormal labor progress.

Physiology

Arachidonic acid release increases with its conversion into prostaglandins following amniotomy (Tenore, 2003). Before 4-cm dilation, amniotomy may modestly shorten labor if the cervix is ripe. There is an increased risk for chorioamnionitis and cord compression (UK Amniotomy Group, 1994; Mercer and others, 1995). After 4 cm, amniotomy may improve an uncoordinated uterine contraction pattern related to increased prostaglandin release or enhance a normal uterine contraction pattern because of the dilating wedge of the fetal head on the cervix with no adverse fetal or neonatal effect (Fraser and others, 1993; Garite and others, 1993; Rouse and others, 1994; UK Amniotomy Group, 1994). However, according to *The Cochrane Review*, inadequate data prevents a conclusion as to its safeness and effectiveness (Howarth and Botha, 2001).

Advantages

Amniotomy has two advantages. First, it decreases the length of some labors without the use of oxytocin. Second, it allows for amniotic fluid assessment for meconium and permits internal fetal and uterine contraction monitoring.

Risks

One risk of amniotomy is that once the fetal membranes are ruptured, delivery is expected within a reasonable and safe period of time. Unresolved variable decelerations may progress to a nonreassuring pattern, are more likely to occur at an early stage of labor, and are more likely to be unresponsive to position change. This is the most common risk and can be treated with amnioinfusion.

The risk for an intraamniotic infection increases with the duration of the rupture. Umbilical cord prolapse and change in fetal presentation are two additional risks that can occur with amniotomy.

Fetal stressors can be related to decreased amniotic fluid that results from the rupture in amniotomy or from a prolapsed cord.

If the fetal vessels transfuse through the membranes that lie over the cervix (vasa previa), these may rupture when the membranes are ruptured. If there is an undiagnosed placenta previa, membrane rupture can also cause bleeding.

Caput succedaneum related to direct pressure on the presenting part as it acts as a dilating wedge may occur with amniotomy.

Nursing Interventions

- Amniotomy should be done only where an emergency delivery can be performed nearby.
- Assess for engagement of the presenting part before amniotomy (ROM). (The presenting part must be engaged for an amniotomy to be done.) The health care provider who is rupturing the membranes should assess for fetal blood vessels under fetal membranes before rupture is carried out.
- Check FHR before ROM.
- Assist health care provider with rupture. According to AWHONN, an amniotomy is to be performed by a physician or midwife. If it is performed by a perinatal nurse, the institution must have a policy and protocol based on the respective state's scope of practice (Simpson and Poole, 1998).
- During the amniotomy, gentle fundal and suprapubic pressure may be applied, if needed, to decrease risk for cord prolapse.
- Check FHR immediately following ROM. If an FHR change or non-reassuring pattern occurs, rule out cord prolapse, cord obstruction, or fetal bleeding.
- Assess amniotic fluid (amount, color [clear or meconium-stained]), and odor.
- Monitor the uterine contraction pattern following rupture. Oxytocin may be ordered if normal labor does not follow rupture.
- Assess maternal temperature after rupture every 4 hours, or more frequently if signs and symptoms of infection occur.

- If fetal compromise develops from a prolapsed cord, apply and maintain pressure to the presenting part; with other hand, push abdomen up; call for help; notify physician; instruct helper to put bed in a Trendelenburg position; evaluate FHR; start oxygen by mask at 10 L/min; and start an IV line with an 18-gauge intracatheter if not already started.

PHYSIOLOGIC METHODS OF LABOR INDUCTION: STRIPPING OF FETAL MEMBRANES

During membrane stripping, the chorionic fetal membrane is separated from the decidua of the lower uterine segment.

Physiology

When the membrane is stripped from the decidua, a local deciduitis results, causing the local release of phospholipase A_2 and prostaglandins in the area and may increase the systemic release of oxytocin (Sanchez-Ramos and Delke, 2006). Membrane stripping has been shown to increase spontaneous labor, decrease the incidence of postdate gestations, and reduce the need for other induction methods and without increasing complications (McColgin and others, 1990; El-Torkey and Grant, 1992; Allott and Palmer, 1993; Krammer and O'Brien, 1995). However, according to the *Cochrane Review* (Boulvain, Stan, Irion, 2005), the decreased use of other induction methods needs to be balanced against the discomfort and other risks of the procedure.

Risks

Risks with stripping the fetal membranes include (1) increased maternal discomfort during the examination, (2) PROM at the time they are stripped, and (3) bleeding if there is an undiagnosed placenta previa.

Interventions

- Firm documentation must be made that the fetus is at or older than 37 weeks of gestation.
- No medical contraindications such as an abnormal fetal presentation or a low-lying placenta may exist.
- During the procedure, the health care provider digitally separates 1 to 2 cm of the chorionic membrane from the decidua of the lower uterine segment.

COMPLEMENTARY THERAPIES: BREAST STIMULATION

Breast stimulation is a physiologic labor stimulant method that offers an alternative method to pharmacologic induction or augmentation. It has been demonstrated through research to initiate or enhance labor and to shorten, especially the latent phase of labor (Chayen and others, 1986; Mastrogiannis and Knuppel, 1995; Kavanagh, Kelly, and Thomas, 2005).

Physiology

Nipple stimulation causes the spontaneous release of oxytocin by the posterior pituitary gland.

PROCEDURE

Manual or Warm Compress Breast Stimulation

- The patient gently rolls or brushes one nipple through her clothes or with a warm moist clothe for 10 minutes with a 5-minute rest. She then gently rolls or brushes the other nipple for 10 minutes.
- Discontinue stimulation during a contraction or after no observable effect occurs after 1 hour (Curtis and others, 1999).

Breast Pump Stimulation

- Patient stimulates one breast at a time for 10 minutes with the electric breast pump on moderate suction.
- Patient stops pumping for 10 minutes following one cycle of stimulation.
- The cycle just described may be repeated up to five times (Young and Poppe, 1987).

Risks

Uterine Hyperstimulation

Research has documented the risk for hyperstimulation from breast stimulation (Adair, 2000).

Nipple Soreness and Engorgement

Nipple soreness and engorgement occur in approximately 25% to 30% of cases of breast stimulation (Young and Poppe, 1987).

Fetal Compromise

Research has documented the risk for fetal compromise from breast stimulation to be comparable to oxytocin (Curtis and others, 1999; Kavanagh, Kelly, and Thomas, 2001).

Nursing Interventions

- Discuss the benefits of breast stimulation such as increased patient control, early milk production for the breastfeeding mother, lack of expense, and avoidance of invasive measures. Discuss the possible adverse side effects listed earlier.
- Explain the appropriate technique to the patient and her coach.
- Assess the response of the patient and her family to the procedure.
- Determine a baseline for maternal vital signs, FHR, and uterine activity for 10 to 20 minutes before having the patient begin.
- Perform a vaginal examination to determine cervical effacement and dilation, fetal presentation, and station.
- Have the patient lie on her side or sit to avoid supine hypotension from obstruction of the vena cava.
- Evaluate uterine contractions for quality, frequency, duration, and resting tone every 15 to 30 minutes.

- Assess FHR response to uterine contractions every 15 to 30 minutes.
- During periods of no stimulation, encourage patient to void, ambulate, and drink fluid unless contraindicated.
- Have the patient discontinue stimulation if a hyperstimulation contraction pattern occurs. Notify the attending physician, and be prepared to administer a tocolytic. Hyperstimulation contractions are contractions that (1) occur more often than four every 10 minutes, (2) last 90 seconds or more without a period of relaxation, or (3) have a suspected increased uterine resting tone above 20 mm Hg pressure.
- Have the patient discontinue stimulation, administer oxygen, and lie on her side; notify the attending physician if a nonreassuring FHR pattern is noted, such as late or nonreassuring variable decelerations, loss of long- or short-term variability, tachycardia, or bradycardia.
- Have the patient discontinue stimulation, and notify the physician if labor has not started after five cycles of stimulation.

OTHER COMPLEMENTARY THERAPIES

Various complementary measures have been shown to enhance cervical ripening of a thick, unripe cervix or to induce labor if the cervix is ripe. A few such measures are as follows:

- *Herbal preparations.* Blue cohosh, black cohosh, evening primrose oil, raspberry leaves, or another safe herbal preparation taken orally may promote prostaglandin or oxytocin production (Hunter and Chern-Hughes, 1996; Woolven, 1997; Belew, 1999; McFarlin and others, 1999). Evening primrose oil is usually taken in the form of three capsules every day for 1 week or more (Adair, 2000). The dosage of blue cohosh tincture is 3 to 8 drops in a glass of warm water or tea; it may be repeated every 30 minutes for several hours until regular contractions occur (Hunter and Chern-Hughes, 1996). Black cohosh tincture dosage is 10 drops sublingual hourly until cervical changes occur, usually within 3 to 4 hours (Adair, 2000).
- *Orgasm.* Associated oxytocin or prostaglandin release stimulates uterine contractions.
- *Sexual intercourse.* Semen contains prostaglandin, which may hasten cervical ripening and orgasm stimulates the uterine as well. There is a plethora of evidence to support the belief that sexual intercourse enhances ripening of the cervix (Howarth and Halligan, 2000). This method would be contraindicated in the presence of ROM.
- *Acupuncture or electric transcutaneous electrical nerve stimulation (TENS).* Stimulation of the nerve loci of the uterus with needles or TENS has been demonstrated to initiate labor (Adair, 2000). The issues of efficacy and safety need to be studied before their general use (Smith and Crowther, 2004).
- *Bowel stimulation.* Stimulation of the bowel with castor oil, bath, and/or enema increases prostaglandin production, which may facilitate cervical ripening. According to the *Cochrane Review* (Kelly, Kavanagh and Thomas,

2001), further research is needed to determine the effectiveness of bowel stimulation in facilitating induction of labor. According to the AHRQ evidence report (2002), castor oil given at term has a positive effect in promoting labor but consistently causes maternal nausea.

CONCLUSION

The use of labor stimulants enables many patients to have a vaginal delivery. However, risks are associated with their use. The primary role of the nurse is to closely monitor the labor progress, the uterine contraction pattern, and fetal well-being. Developing complications can then be recognized early so that the labor stimulant can be stopped before a negative development occurs. A labor stimulant should never be used simply to speed up labor or to initiate a labor for convenience.

BIBLIOGRAPHY

Adair C: Nonpharmacologic approaches to cervical priming and labor induction, *Clin Obstet Gynecol* 43(3):447–454, 2000.

Agency for Healthcare Research and Quality: Management of prolonged pregnancy, Evidence Report/Technology Assessment, No 23, Durham, NC, 2002, AHRQ. Retrieved from *http://www.ahrq.gov*

Alfirevic Z: Oral misoprostol for induction of labour, *Cochrane Database Syst Rev* Issue 2, 2001.

Allott H, Palmer C: Sweeping the membranes: a valid procedure in stimulating the onset of labour? *Br J Obstet Gynaecol* 100(10):898–903, 1993.

American Academy of Pediatrics and American College of Obstetricians and Gynecologists: *Guidelines for perinatal care,* ed 5, Elk Grove Village, Ill, 2002, AAP/ACOG.

American College of Obstetricians and Gynecologists: Dystocia and augmentation of labor, *ACOG Practice Bulletin,* No. 49, Washington, DC, 2003a, ACOG.

American College of Obstetricians and Gynecologists: Induction of labor, *ACOG Practice Bulletin,* No. 10, Washington, DC, 1999, ACOG.

American College of Obstetricians and Gynecologists: New US food and drug administration labeling on cytotec (Misoprostol) use and pregnancy, *ACOG Committee Opinion,* No. 283, Washington, DC, 2003b, ACOG.

American College of Obstetricians and Gynecologists: Response to Searle's drug warning on misoprostol, *ACOG Committee Opinion,* Washington, DC, 2000, ACOG.

Arias F: Pharmacology of oxytocin and prostaglandins, *Clin Obstet Gynecol* 43(3):455–468, 2000.

Belew C: Herbs and the childbearing woman: guidelines for midwives, *J Nurse Midwifery* 44(3):231–252, 1999.

Bishop E: Pelvic scoring for elective induction, *Obstet Gynecol* 24:266, 1964.

Blakemore K and others: A prospective comparison of hourly and quarter-hourly oxytocin dose increase intervals for the induction of labor at term, *Obstet Gynecol* 75(5): 757–761, 1990.

Blanchette H, Nayak S, and Erasmus S: Comparison of the safety and efficacy of intravaginal misoprostol (prostaglandin E_1) with those of dinoprostone (prostaglandin E_2) for cervical ripening and induction of labor in a community hospital, *Am J Obstet Gynecol* 180(6 Pt 1):1551–1559, 1999.

Boulvain M, Stan C, and Irion O: Membrane sweeping for induction of labour, *Cochrane Database Syst Rev* Issue 1, 2005.

Buser D and others: A randomized comparison between misoprostol and dinoprostone for cervical ripening and labor induction in patients with unfavorable cervices, *Obstet Gynecol* 89(4):581–585, 1997.

Chayen B, Tejani N, and Verma U: Induction of labor with an electric breast pump, *J Reprod Med* 31(2):116–118, 1986.

Chua S and others: Oxytocin titration for induction of labour: a prospective randomized study of 15 versus 30 minute dose increment schedules, *Aust N Z J Obstet Gynaecol* 31(2):134–137, 1991.

Chua S and others: Preinduction cervical ripening: prostaglandin E₂ gel vs. hygroscopic mechanical dilator, *J Obstet Gynaecol Res* 23(2):171–177, 1997.

Clayworth S: The nurse's role during oxytocin administration, *MCN Am J Matern Child Nurs* 25(2):80–84, 2000.

Crane J, Young D: Meta-analysis of low-dose versus high-dose oxytocin for labour induction, *J Soc Obstet Gynaecol Can* 20:1215, 1998.

Curtis P and others: A comparison of breast stimulation and intravenous oxytocin for the augmentation of labor, *Birth* 26(2):115–122, 1999.

Dawood M: Pharmacologic stimulation of uterine contraction, *Semin Perinatol* 19(1): 73–83, 1995.

Edwards R, Richards D: Preinduction cervical assessment, *Clin Obstet Gynecol* 43(3): 440–446, 2000.

el-Torkey M, Grant J: Sweeping of the membranes is an effective method of induction of labour in prolonged pregnancy: a report of a randomized trial, *Br J Obstet Gynaecol* 99(6):455–458, 1992.

Foong L and others: Membrane sweeping in conjunction with labor induction, *Obstet Gynecol* 96(4):539–542, 2000.

Fraser W and others: Effect of early amniotomy on the risk of dystocia in nulliparous women, *N Engl J Med* 328(16):1145–1149, 1993.

Fraser W and others: Amniotomy for shortening spontaneous labour, *Cochrane Database Syst Rev* Issue 1, 2000.

French L: Oral prostaglandin E2 for induction of labour, *Cochrane Database Syst Rev* Issue 2, 2001.

Frigoletto F and others: A clinical trial of active management of labor, *N Engl J Med* 333(12):745–750, 1995.

Garite T and others: The influence of elective amniotomy on fetal heart rate patterns and the course of labor in term patients: a randomized study, *Am J Obstet Gynecol* 168(6 Pt 1):1827–1831, 1993.

Gonser M: Labor induction and augmentation with oxytocin: pharmacokinetic considerations, *Arch Gynecol Obstet* 256(2):63–66, 1995.

Hadi H: Cervical ripening and labor induction: clinical guidelines, *Clin Obstet Gynecol* 43(3):524–536, 2000.

Hofmeyr G, Gülmezoglu A: Vaginal misoprostol for cervical ripening and induction of labour, *Cochrane Database Syst Rev* Issue 1, 2003.

Howarth E, Halligan A: Induction of labor. In Kean L, Baker P, and Edelstone D, editors: *Best practice in labor ward management,* Philadelphia, 2000, Saunders.

Howarth G, Botha D: Amniotomy plus intravenous oxytocin for induction of labour, *Cochrane Database Syst Rev* Issue 3, 2001.

Hunter L, Chern-Hughes B: Management of prolonged latent phase labor, *J Nurse Midwifery* 41(5):383–388, 1996.

Joint Commission on Accreditation of Healthcare Organizations: *Comprehensive accreditation manual for hospitals,* Oak Park, IL, 2003, Author.

Kavanagh J, Kelly AJ, and Thomas J: Breast stimulation for cervical ripening and induction of labour, *Cochrane Database Syst Rev* Issue 3, 2005.

Kavanagh J, Kelly AJ, and Thomas J: Sexual intercourse for cervical ripening and induction of labour, *Cochrane Database Syst Rev* Issue 2, 2001.

Kelly AJ, Kavanagh J, and Thomas J: Castor oil, bath and/or enema for cervical priming and induction of labour, *Cochrane Database Syst Rev* Issue 2, 2001.

Kelly AJ, Kavanagh J, and Thomas J: Vaginal prostaglandin (PGE2 and PGF2a) for induction of labour at term, *Cochrane Database Syst Rev* Issue 4, 2003.

Kelly AJ, Tan B: Intravenous oxytocin alone for cervical ripening and induction of labour, *Cochrane Database Syst Rev* Issue 3, 2001.

Krammer J, O'Brien W: Mechanical methods of cervical ripening, *Clin Obstet Gynecol* 38(2):280–286, 1995.

Leppert P: Anatomy and physiology of cervical ripening, *Clin Obstet Gynecol* 38(2):267–279, 1995.

Lopez-Zeno J and others: A controlled trial of a program for the active management of labor, *N Engl J Med* 326(7):450–454, 1992.

Luckas M, Bricker L: Intravenous prostaglandin for induction of labour, *Cochrane Database Syst Rev* Issue 4, 2000.

Ludmir J, Sehdev H: Anatomy and physiology of the uterine cervix, *Clin Obstet Gynecol* 43(3):433–439, 2000.

MacKenzie L and others: Prostacyclin biosynthesis by cultured human myometrial smooth muscle cells: dependency on arachidonic or linoleic acid in the culture medium, *Am J Obstet Gynecol* 159(6):1365–1372, 1988.

Martin J and others: Birth: final data for 2003, *Natl Vital Stat Rep* 54(2):1–120, 2005.

Mastrogiannis D, Knuppel R: Labor induced using methods that do not involve oxytocin, *Clin Obstet Gynecol* 38(2):259–266, 1995.

McColgin S and others: Stripping membranes at term: can it safely reduce the incidence of post-term pregnancies? *Obstet Gynecol* 76(4):678–680, 1990.

McFarlin B and others: A national survey of herbal preparation use by nurse-midwives for labor stimulation, *J Nurse Midwifery* 44(3):205–216, 1999.

Mercer B and others: Early versus late amniotomy for labor induction: a randomized trial, *Am J Obstet Gynecol* 173(4):1321–1325, 1995.

Mercer B, Pilgrim P, and Sibai B: Labor induction with continuous low dose oxytocin infusion: a randomized trial, *Obstet Gynecol* 77(5):659–663, 1991.

Merrill D, Zlatnik F: Randomized, double-masked comparison of oxytocin dosage in induction and augmentation of labor, *Obstet Gynecol* 94(3):455–463, 1999.

Muller P, Stubbs T, and Laurent S: A prospective randomized clinical trial comparing two oxytocin induction protocols, *Am J Obstet Gynecol* 167(2):373–380, 1992.

Nunes F, Rodrigues R, and Meirinho M: Randomized comparison between intravaginal misoprostol and dinoprostone for cervical ripening and induction of labor, *Am J Obstet Gynecol* 181(3):626–629, 1999.

O'Driscoll K, Meagher D, and Robson M: *Active management of labor,* ed 4, St Louis, 2004, Mosby.

Olson D, Mijovic J, and Sadowsky D: Control of human parturition, *Semin Perinatol* 19(1):52–63, 1995.

Peaceman A, Socol M: Active management of labor, *Am J Obstet Gynecol* 175(2):363–368, 1996.

Perry R and others: The pharmacokinetics of oxytocin as they apply to labor induction, *Am J Obstet Gynecol* 174(5):1590–1593, 1996.

Pollnow D, Broekhuizen F: Randomized, double-blind trial of prostaglandin E_2 gel versus low-dose oxytocin for cervical ripening before induction of labor, *Am J Obstet Gynecol* 174(6):1910–1913, 1996.

Ramsey P, Ramin K, and Ramin S: Labor induction, *Curr Opin Obstet Gynecol* 12(6):463–473, 2000.

Rayburn W and others: A model for investigating microscopic changes induced by prostaglandin E_2 in the term cervix, *J Matern Fetal Investig* 4:137, 1994.

Rouse D and others: Active-phase labor arrest: a randomized trial of chorioamnion management, *Obstet Gynecol* 83(6):937–940, 1994.

Royal College of Obstetricians and Gynaecologists: *Evidence-based clinical guideline for induction of labors,* Regents' Park, London, 2001, RCOG Press. Retrieved from *http://www.rcog.org.uk/guidelines/labour.html*

Sanchez-Ramos L and others: Labor induction with prostaglandin E_1 misoprostol compared with dinoprostone vaginal insert: a randomized trial, *Obstet Gynecol* 91(3):401–405, 1998.

Sanchez-Ramos L and others: Misoprostol for cervical ripening and labor induction: a meta-analysis, *Obstet Gynecol* 89(4):633–642, 1997.

Sanchez-Ramos L, Delke I: Induction of labor pregnancy termination for fetal abnormality. In James D and others, editors: *High risk pregnancy: management options,* ed 3, Philadelphia, 2006, Saunders.

Sanchez-Ramos L, Kaunitz A: Misoprostol for cervical ripening and labor induction: a systematic review of the literature, *Clin Obstet Gynecol* 43(3):475–488, 2000.

Sanchez-Ramos L: Induction of labor, *Obstet Gynecol Clin North Am* 32(2):181–200, 2005.

Seitchik J, Amico J, and Castillo M: Oxytocin augmentation of dysfunctional labor, V: an alternative oxytocin regimen, *Am J Obstet Gynecol* 151(6):757–761, 1985.

Seitchik J, Castillo M: Oxytocin augmentation of dysfunctional labor. I. Clinical data, *Am J Obstet Gynecol* 144(8):899–905, 1982.

Shyken J, Petrie R: Oxytocin to induce labor, *Clin Obstet Gynecol* 38(2):232–245, 1995.

Simpson K, Atterbury J: Trends and issues in labor induction in the United States: Implications for clinical practice, *J Obstet Gynecol Neonatal Nurs* 32(6):767–779, 2003.

Simpson K, Poole J: *Cervical ripening and induction and augmentation labor,* Washington, DC, 1998, AWHONN.

Smith CA, Crowther CA: Acupuncture for induction of labour, *Cochrane Database Syst Rev* Issue 1, 2004.

Smith CA: Homoeopathy for induction of labour, *Cochrane Database Syst Rev* Issue 4, 2003.

Stubbs T: Oxytocin for labor induction, *Clin Obstet Gynecol* 43(3):489–494, 2000.

Tenore J: Methods for cervical ripening and induction of labor, *Am Fam Physician* 67(10):2123–2128, 2003.

UK Amniotomy Group: A multicentre randomized trial of amniotomy in spontaneous first labour in term, *Br J Obstet Gynaecol* 101(4):307–309, 1994.

Weiner C, Buhimschi C: *Drugs for pregnant and lactating women,* Philadelphia, 2004, Churchill Livingstone.

Willcourt R and others: Induction of labor with pulsatile oxytocin by a computer-controlled pump, *Am J Obstet Gynecol* 170(2):603–608, 1994.

Wilson C: The nurse's role in misoprostol induction: a proposed protocol, *J Obstet Gynecol Neonatal Nurs* 29(6):574–583, 2000.

Witter F: Prostaglandin E_2 preparations for preinduction cervical ripening, *Clin Obstet Gynecol* 43(3):469–474, 2000.

Woolven L: Alternative therapies for pregnancy, labor and delivery, *Childbirth Instructor* 7(2):40, 1997.

Xenakis E and others: Low-dose versus high-dose oxytocin augmentation of labor—a randomized trial, *Am J Obstet Gynecol* 173(6):1874–1878, 1995.

Young J, Poppe C: Breast pump stimulation to promote labor, *MCN Am J Matern Child Nurs* 12(2):124–126, 1987.

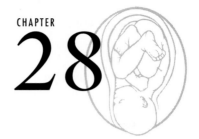

CHAPTER

28

Dysfunctional Labor

onditions can exist or develop that interfere with normal labor progress. An abnormal or difficult labor is usually termed *dysfunctional labor*
or *dystocia*. Management of labor based on evidence and best practice
can significantly reduce the incidence of dysfunctional labor and thereby decrease the incidence of preventable cesarean and instrument-assisted delivers.
Nurses must be willing to make a paradigm shift away from a routine, familiar,
task-oriented labor care approach to an open-minded, individualized, evidence-
based research approach to care (Kardong-Edgren, 2001; Sakala, 2005). This
chapter presents evidence-based practices when available.

INCIDENCE

Dysfunctional labor occurs in approximately 8% to 11% of all deliveries and is
the leading cause of cesarean deliveries (Bowes and Thorp, 2004; Ness, Goldberg,
and Berghella, 2004). In 2003 in the United States, 27.4% of all deliveries were by
cesarean, up from 26.1% in 2002 (USDHHS, 2005). Repeat cesarean delivery
rate is up to 90.4%, and primary cesarean birth rate is at 19% (USDHHS,
2005). Dysfunctional labor accounted for 60% of all cesarean deliveries
(ACOG, 2003a), repeat cesarean birth for 25%, and malpresentations for
12%. Only 16% of cesarean births were done for fetal compromise (Dickinson,
2006).

The continual rise in cesarean deliveries is related to the following:
- Increasing trend in the restrictive use of vaginal birth after cesarean
  (VBAC)
- Current trend in the substantial use of induction as a means of timing
  delivery
- Underuse of care that promotes the natural progress of labor
- The fear of litigation

Dysfunctional labor that occurs in stage two often leads to delivery with
vacuum extractor or forceps. The incidence of instrument-assisted delivery is
10% to 15% (Patel and Murphy, 2004).

ETIOLOGY

Dysfunctional labor is influenced by 13 essential labor forces (VandeVusse, 1999). These forces, commonly referred to as the 13 Ps, are the original internal involuntary body processes listed below:

- *Power or uterine contractions.* Ineffective uterine activity or contractions can lead to uterine dystocia. Some issues that appear to increase one's risk for developing uterine dystocia follow: overweight, short stature, advanced maternal age, infertility difficulties, prior version, masculine characteristics, congenitally abnormal uterus, overdistended uterus as in multiple pregnancy or polyhydramnios, lack of reflex stimulation of the myometrium related to malpresentations (e.g., posterior positions; face, brow, or breech presentations; or transverse lie), fetopelvic disproportion (FPD), overstimulation of the uterus with oxytocin, extreme maternal fear or exhaustion causing the adrenal medulla to secrete catecholamines that interfere with uterine contractility, dehydration, electrolyte imbalance, administration of an analgesic too early in labor, or use of continuous epidural analgesia (Thorp and others, 1993; Morton and others, 1994; Ramin and others, 1995; Lau and others, 1997; Fraser and others, 2002; Sheiner and others, 2002).
- *Passenger or the fetus.* An abnormal fetal presentation or position, such as face, brow, or breech; posterior occiput presentation; or transverse lie can lead to fetal dystocia. Fetal anomalies, such as hydrocephalus, abdominal enlargement, tumors, conjoined twins, or excessive fetal size, usually greater than 4000 g (9 lb), can cause fetal dystocia as well.
- *Passageway or pelvis.* A small pelvic inlet, midpelvis, or pelvic outlet as the result of heredity, previous pelvic fracture, or disease can lead to pelvic dystocia.
- Physiologic involuntary experience by the mother.
- Psychologic state of the mother who wants to control her labor and delivery experience.
- Preparation of the mother for the birth.
- Position during labor.
- Professional providers' (especially the nurse's) attitudes, helpfulness, flexibility, support, consideration of individualized needs, communication skills in providing information and explanations, and comfort measures provided.
- Place of birth.
- Procedures performed such as electronic fetal monitoring (EFM), intravenous (IV) infusions, episiotomies, and internal examinations.
- People present other than the professional team such as office staff, family members, friends, and other patients.
- Politics defined as societal influences or expectations of appropriate labor behavior.
- Pressure interface regarding decision making.

NORMAL PHYSIOLOGY

Normal uterine contractions have two phases: contraction (systole) and relaxation (diastole). A pacemaker situated at the uterine end of the right fallopian tube initiates the contraction phase. The contraction phase, like a wave, moves downward to the cervix and upward to the fundus of the uterus. At the acme (peak) of the contraction, the entire uterus is contracting, with the greatest intensity in the fundal area. The relaxation phase follows and occurs simultaneously in all parts of the uterus. The round ligaments contain muscle and are stimulated to contract as the uterus contracts, thereby anchoring the uterus and promoting a downward force on the presenting part.

Uterine contractions of an intensity of 30 mm Hg or greater initiate cervical dilation. During active labor, the intensity usually reaches 50 to 80 mm Hg. During the second stage of labor, the intensity can peak at 100 mm Hg. Resting tone is normally between 5 and 10 mm Hg in early labor and between 12 and 18 mm Hg in active labor.

Normal labor usually begins with a latent phase, which is characterized by the cervix slowly dilating to about 4 cm. The average duration of this phase for the nullipara is 6½ hours; for the multipara, 5 hours. An active phase follows and is identified as the time when dilation takes place more rapidly. It is characterized by a period of acceleration and then a period of maximum slope followed by a period of deceleration (Fig. 28-1).

The deceleration phase, often referred to as *transition,* is not associated with decreased uterine activity, but during this phase, the cervix is being retracted around the fetal presenting part. The normal rate of cervical dilation during the active phase should be at least 1.2 cm/hr in nulliparas and 1.5 cm/hr in multiparas (Friedman, 1995). Except for prelabor engagement, fetal descent generally does not begin until the active phase of dilation and starts to reach its maximum slope during the deceleration phase of active labor, which continues

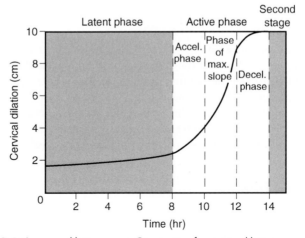

Figure 28-1 Average dilation curve. Composite of average dilation curves for nulliparous labor based on analysis of data derived from patterns traced by large, nearly consecutive series of primigravidas. First stage is divided into relatively flat latent phase and rapidly progressive active phase. Active phase has three identifiable components: acceleration phase, linear phase of maximum slope, and deceleration phase. (From Friedman EA: *Labor: clinical evaluation and management,* ed 2, New York, 1978, Appleton & Lange.)

throughout the second stage of labor. The normal rate of descent is at least 1 cm/hr in nulliparas and 2 cm/hr in multiparas (Friedman, 1995).

Recent research on the current relevance of Friedman's work supports its clinical usefulness with some adaptations. Zhang, Troendle, and Yancey (2002) and Cesario (2004) observed a current pattern:

- A more gradual transition from latent to active phase labor
- No deceleration phase at the end of stage one of labor
- A wider normal range in the length of the first stage of active labor
- A longer second-stage labor

PATHOPHYSIOLOGY

Uterine Dystocia

Two types of abnormal uterine activity lead to uterine dystocia. First, there is hypotonic uterine activity, in which the rise in uterine pressure during a contraction is insufficient (<25 mm Hg) to promote cervical effacement and dilation. The force provided by voluntary contractions of the abdominal musculature, facilitated by the urge to push, may be insufficient to facilitate fetal descent and delivery. Second, there is hypertonic or uncoordinated uterine activity, in which the contractions are frequent and painfully strong but ineffective in promoting effacement and dilation. They can be ineffective because the uterine pacemakers arise in other areas of the uterus. This causes the myometrium to contract spasmodically and frequently but ineffectively, and the presenting part is not forced downward.

Fetal Dystocia

Several factors may influence the progress of labor, such as fetal lie, size, presentation, and number. The presence of anomalies may interfere with labor progress as well.

The fetus can move through the birth canal with the greatest ease when the head is sharply flexed so that the chin rests on the thorax and the occipital area of the skull (vertex) is presenting anterior to the mother's pelvis. Thus the smallest diameter of the fetal head enters the mother's pelvis, and the most flexible part of the fetal body, the back of the neck, adapts to the curve of the birth canal. At times, the fetus assumes other presentations, making labor difficult or impossible. These presentations are discussed in the following sections.

Occiput Posterior Presentation

Occiput posterior presentation occurs in approximately 15% of labors in the latent phase, and 5% are in this position at delivery (Stitely and Gherman, 2005). The occiput of the fetus is in the posterior portion of the pelvis instead of in the anterior portion (Fig. 28-2). As the fetus moves through the birth canal, the occiput bone presses on the mother's sacrum. Severe back pain usually results from this presentation. The occiput must also rotate 135 degrees. This rotation can occur during fetal descent, causing slow progress in the active

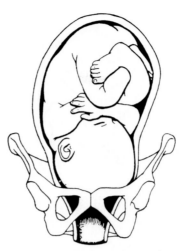

Figure 28-2 Occiput posterior presentation. (From *The normal female pelvis: clinical education aid*, No 8, Columbus, Ohio, Ross Laboratories.)

phase or a persistent anterior cervical lip. Most often, it does not occur until the occiput reaches the pelvic floor. Therefore the second stage of labor is usually prolonged.

Face Presentation

Face presentation, or mentum, occurs approximately once in every 500 to 600 deliveries (Simm and Woods, 2004) when the fetal head is in extension instead of flexion as it enters the pelvic inlet (Fig. 28-3). If the mentum is in an anterior position, the labor usually progresses very close to normal and vaginal delivery results without much difficulty. This is because the widest diameter of the presenting part is similar in size to an occiput presentation and the neck can glide around the short symphysis pubis with ease. When the mentum is in a posterior position, approximately 70% of the time it rotates to an anterior face presentation, making vaginal delivery possible but causing the labor to be prolonged. If the posterior position persists, cesarean delivery is necessary because the neck is too short to stretch the long distance of the sacrum.

Brow Presentation

A brow presentation occurs approximately once in every 1000 to 1500 deliveries (Simm and Woods, 2004) when the fetal head presents in a position midway between full flexion and extreme extension (Fig. 28-4). This causes the largest diameter of the fetal head to engage. Vaginal delivery depends on the successful conversion to an occiput or a face presentation by varying degrees of flexion or extension, which occurs in 70% to 90% of the cases. A brow presentation may be present when descent of the presenting part is prolonged or a long second-stage labor develops. Cesarean birth is indicated if this malpresentation fails to convert.

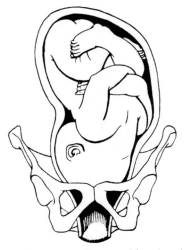

Figure 28-3 Face presentation. (From *The normal female pelvis: clinical education aid*, No 8, Columbus, Ohio, Ross Laboratories.)

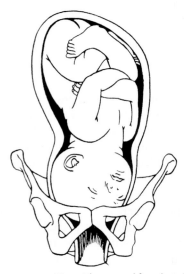

Figure 28-4 Brow presentation. (From *The normal female pelvis: clinical education aid*, No 8, Columbus, Ohio, Ross Laboratories.)

Shoulder Presentation

Shoulder presentation occurs approximately once in every 300 deliveries (Simm and Woods, 2004) when the fetal spine is lying vertical to the mother's spine (Fig. 28-5). Because of the high mortality risk from prolapsed cord, cesarean delivery is usually the best management. However, if placenta previa and FPD are not present, external cephalic version has been successful in controlled circumstances.

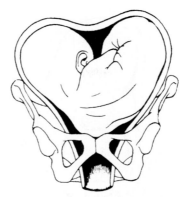

Figure 28-5 Shoulder presentation. (From *The normal female pelvis: clinical education aid*, No 8, Columbus, Ohio, Ross Laboratories.)

Compound Presentation

Compound presentation occurs approximately once in every 1000 deliveries (Simm and Woods, 2004) when one or more of the fetal extremities accompany the presenting part. An arm presenting along with the head is the most common compound presentation. Vaginal delivery is usually possible unless cord prolapse occurs or labor fails to progress. Then, an emergency cesarean delivery is done. Attempts should not be made to replace the prolapsed fetal part.

Breech Presentation

Breech presentation occurs in approximately 3% to 4% of all deliveries (Simm and Woods, 2004) when the buttocks of the fetus present. The breech can present in three different attitudes. It is termed a *frank breech* when the thighs are flexed and the legs lie alongside the fetal body; a *complete breech* when the legs are flexed at the thighs allowing the feet to present with the buttocks; and a *footling breech* when one foot (single footling) or both feet (double footling) present before the buttocks (Fig. 28-6).

Prematurity, multiple gestation, and advancing maternal age are causes of breech presentation (Simm and Woods, 2004). Other causes are uterine relaxation associated with parity greater than 5 and decreased fetal capability to move within the uterus associated with diminished muscle tone of the fetus, neuromuscular disorders, or decreased uterine space. Infrequent causes are placenta previa, polyhydramnios, and hydrocephalus.

A breech presentation is considered high risk for the following reasons:
- Prolapse of the cord is more likely to occur, especially in a footling breech, because the buttocks do not fit as snugly into the cervix as does the fetal head.
- Dysfunctional labor is much more likely to result because the buttocks are soft and make a poor dilating wedge against the cervix.
- Birth trauma is more likely to occur because the head does not have time to mold and it must pass through the birth canal quickly. The premature fetus is even more prone to birth trauma from an incompletely dilated cervix.

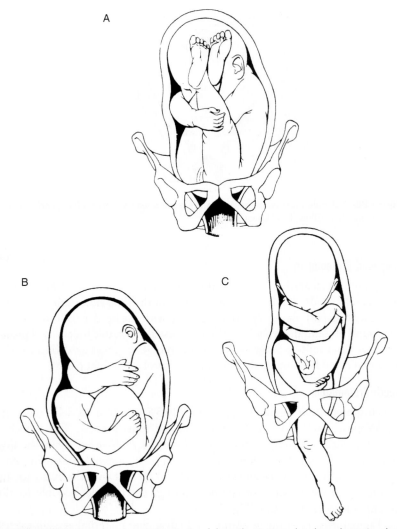

Figure 28-6 Breech presentation. **A,** Frank breech. **B,** Complete breech. **C,** Single footling breech. (From *The normal female pelvis: clinical education aid,* No 8, Columbus, Ohio, Ross Laboratories.)

Today's trend, based on the Term Breech Trial (Hannah and others, 2000), is to attempt external version at 37 or more weeks of gestation. If the version is unsuccessful, a scheduled cesarean delivery is discussed. Scheduled cesarean birth can decrease perinatal and neonatal mortality with modest increase morbidity risk to the mother according to a *Cochrane Review* (Hofmeyr and Hannah, 2003). Once labor is established, cesarean birth further increases maternal morbidity. The American College of Obstetricians and Gynecologists recommends cesarean delivery for all women with persistent term breech presentation (ACOG, 2001). However, the woman's preferences should be considered in the plan of management once risks and benefits have been shared. Vaginal delivery is the safest if it is a frank or complete breech with adequate neck flexion, symmetric fetal body proportions, clinically adequate pelvis as indicated by pelvic radiography or prior delivery, and an estimated fetal weight 3800 g or less (Edelstone, 2000; Bowes and Thorp, 2004).

Pelvic Dystocia

The shape and dimensions of the pelvis influence the progress of labor. The bony pelvis is composed of the inlet, midcavity (or canal), and the outlet. Pelvic dystocia is related to a contraction of one or more of the three planes of the pelvis.

Inlet Contraction

The pelvic inlet normally has a larger transverse diameter than anteroposterior diameter. No matter what the pelvic size measures, most obstetricians allow the patient to go into labor. Descent and engagement of the fetal head would indicate an adequate pelvic inlet.

Midcavity Contraction

Contraction of the midcavity is more common than an inlet contraction and often causes an arrest of descent. It is more difficult to determine manually. Possible indicators are (1) prominent ischial spines, (2) convergent pelvic side walls, and (3) a narrow sacrosciatic notch.

Outlet Contraction

The outlet of the pelvis normally has a larger anteroposterior diameter than transverse.

The final outcome of any labor depends on the interrelation of the size and shape of the pelvis; the size, presentation, and position of the fetus; and the quality of uterine contractions. Therefore dystocia can rarely be diagnosed until labor has progressed for a time. If the fetus is too large to pass through the pelvis or the pelvis is too small for the fetus to pass through, the condition is usually referred to as *fetopelvic disproportion* (FPD) or *cephalopelvic disproportion (CPD)*.

SIGNS AND SYMPTOMS

Cervical dilation, effacement, and fetal descent occur progressively during labor. In an abnormal labor (1) contractions slow or fail to advance in frequency, duration, or intensity; (2) the cervix fails to respond to the uterine contractions by dilating and effacing; or (3) the fetus fails to move downward. Thus labor does not progress normally.

MATERNAL EFFECTS

Any time the birth canal is too small to accommodate the presentation of the fetus, uterine rupture can result. This can lead to maternal death related to hemorrhage. However, the incidence is rare; an obstructed labor is not usually allowed to continue. The greatest risk to the mother with a dysfunctional labor is associated with maternal exhaustion and a cesarean delivery.

Cesarean birth is associated with 4 to 13 times more maternal risks than is vaginal birth (Edelstone, 2000). These risks include postoperative complications of hemorrhage, endomyometrial and incision infections, urinary tract infection, aspiration pneumonitis, amniotic fluid embolism, anesthesia complications, thrombophlebitis, bowel and bladder trauma, anemia, and psychologic stress (Edelstone, 2000; Enkin and others, 2000; Bernstein, 2005). According to the Drudge Report (2001), the need for an emergency hysterectomy is 30 times more likely as a complication of a cesarean delivery. Approximately one third to one half of maternal deaths of cesarean patients are related to the procedure itself (Harper and others, 2003; Wen and others, 2004). In a pregnancy following a cesarean birth, the risk for placenta previa is increased three times (Ananth, Smulian, Vintzileos, 1997). In the presence of a placenta previa, the risk for an invasive placenta is 35 times higher in those with a uterine scar from a prior cesarean than in those with an unscarred uterus (Miller, Chollet, Goodwin, 1997).

FETAL AND NEONATAL EFFECTS

Fetal and infant mortality are usually related to hypoxia or birth trauma. Hypoxia is often the result of intense uterine contractions that lead to uteroplacental insufficiency or cord prolapse related to malpresentation. A malpresentation can also cause such birth traumas as cranial or neck compression; fracture of the trachea, larynx, or shoulder; and spinal cord injury during an attempted vaginal delivery. The various interventions to facilitate delivery also increase the risk to the fetus of hypoxia and trauma.

According to an extensive review of literature, increased cesarean rate has not decreased the rate of neurologic disorders or cerebral palsy (Enkin and others, 2000). Cesarean birth does increase the risk for respiratory difficulties (Levine and others, 2001), trauma related to surgical cuts (Dessole and others), 2004, more breastfeeding problems (Towner and others, 1999), and later risk for developing asthma (Bager and others, 2003; Hakansson and Kallen, 2003). Furthermore, continuous EFM does not provide an advantage over periodic auscultation (Thacker, Stroup, and Chang, 2001; ACOG, 2003a; see Chapter 3).

DIAGNOSTIC TESTING

During the prenatal period, the health care provider determines general pelvic size and configuration and fetal position and presentation. This is done by abdominal palpation and vaginal examination. The Leopold maneuver is an effective way to screen for a fetal malpresentation.

Diagnostic prediction of the outcome of labor is rarely possible before labor. This is because it depends not only on the size and shape of the pelvis but also on the size, presentation, and position of the fetus and the quality of uterine contractions. Therefore dystocia can rarely be diagnosed until labor has progressed for a time. The diagnosis is then based on clinical findings during labor such as the uterine contraction pattern or the progression of labor as indicated by cervical dilation and effacement and fetal descent.

Labor progress historically has been evaluated according to Friedman normal labor curves or the labor line of active labor. These evaluation tools provide a visual picture of some basic labor patterns, but they fail to address extrinsic factors, such as the emotional and sensory reality of birth. Recent research on the current relevance of Friedman's work supports its clinical usefulness with some adaptations. Zhang, Troendle, and Yancey (2002) and Cesario (2004) observed current labor pattern variations:

- A more gradual transition from latent to active phase labor
- No deceleration phase at the end of stage one of labor
- A wider normal range in the length of the first stage of active labor
- A longer second-stage labor

A graphic representation of the patient's progress in labor plotted against the labor curve can assist in early identification of abnormal labor patterns (Bowes and Thorp, 2004; ICSI, 2005). Therefore the Friedman labor curve and the labor line of active labor or another type graphic representation should be used with the above variations in mind. The World Health Organization (WHO, 2002) currently recommends the use of a partograph to observe labor trends. The partograph incorporates cervical dilation and fetal descent, along with maternal and fetal factors such as contractions pattern, maternal position, maternal vital signs, fetal heart rate, fluids, medications, and amniotic fluids.

Labor Line of Active Labor

The labor line of active labor is based on the assumption that after 4-cm dilation, a woman in active labor normally dilates at a rate of 1 cm/hour or more. Therefore for this method, the vertical side of square-ruled graph paper should be numbered from 1 to 10 in ascending order to indicate centimeters of dilation. Horizontally across the bottom, it is numbered from 0 to 10 to indicate hours in labor. The labor line is then drawn diagonally from the lower left corner to the upper right corner (Fig. 28-7). The admission time is the first interval entered on the graph so that the cervical dilation at admission is marked on the vertical axis that corresponds with zero hour. Each time a vaginal examination is performed, the dilation is recorded on the corresponding hour's vertical axis on the graph. According to O'Driscoll, Meagher, and Robson (2004), the labor line indicates the slowest rate of progress necessary to achieve delivery. If the patient's pattern of dilation falls below the labor line, a dysfunctional labor is diagnosed and oxytocin is initiated.

Some obstetricians have modified the minimal labor line by drawing alert and action lines 2 and 4 hours to the right, respectively (see Fig. 28-7). If the patient's progress is slow and crosses the alert line, the health team should be alerted to the possibility of an abnormal labor. If the labor progress is slowed enough to cross the action line, definitive measures of oxytocin or cesarean delivery should be taken (Martin and Hutchon, 2004; O'Driscoll, Meagher, and Robson, 2004).

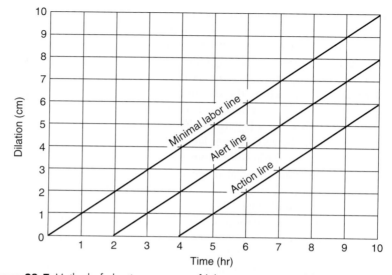

Figure 28-7 Method of charting progress of labor against minimal labor line. (Modified from O'Driscoll K, Meagher D, Robson M: *Active management of labour*, ed 4, Edinburgh, 2004, Mosby Ltd.; World Health Organization [WHO]: *Managing complications in pregnancy and childbirth: a guide for midwives and doctors*, Switzerland, 2002, Department of Reproductive Health and Research [RHR].)

Labor Curve

According to best practice, Friedman's analyses of normal labor patterns remain the most useful available tool (Gee, 2006); however, this must be considered as only one variable and all other relevant data must be considered as well (Fig. 28-8). If the labor curve is chosen as the method of assessment, the amount of dilation and the fetal station found on examination should be graphed on the normal labor curve. Friedman (1995) developed this evaluation tool after graphically plotting the relationship of time to station and dilation of many patients in labor. He developed a normal labor curve for nulliparas and one for multiparas.

The labor curve method of evaluation can be instituted using square-ruled graph paper. Across the top, number the hours the patient is in labor from left to right using hourly intervals. The vertical side should be numbered from 1 to 10 in ascending order to indicate dilation in centimeters and from 1 to 5 in descending order to indicate station. Dilation is usually indicated by small circles and station by small x's, each connected with a straight line (Friedman, 1995). The normal labor curve for a nullipara and a multipara should appear on the graph for easy comparison (Fig. 28-9). On admission, the patient is asked when regular contractions began, and this time is the first interval entered on the graph. Each time a vaginal examination is performed, the dilation and station are recorded under that hour on the graph.

Friedman (1995) classified the various deviations from the normal labor curve as follows:

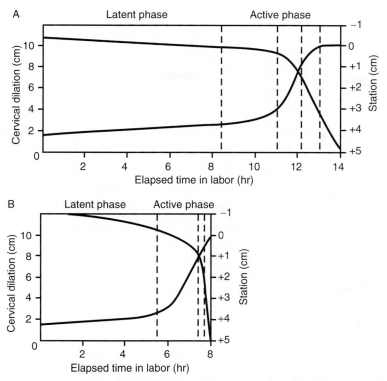

Figure 28-8 Normal labor patterns. **A,** Normal labor pattern for nullipara. **B,** Normal labor pattern for multipara. (From Friedman E: An objective method of evaluating labor, *Hosp Pract* 5[7]:82, 1970. Artist: Albert Miller.)

- Prolonged latent-phase disorders (Fig. 28-10)
- Protraction disorders, which include protracted active-phase dilation and protracted descent disorders (Fig. 28-11)
- Arrest disorders, which include secondary arrest of dilation, arrest of descent, and failure of descent disorders (Fig. 28-12)
- Precipitous labor disorders (Fig. 28-13)

USUAL MEDICAL MANAGEMENT AND PROTOCOLS FOR NURSE PRACTITIONERS

Labor Management to Decrease Cesarean Rate

The current focus is on managing labor more effectively to decrease primary cesarean rate. Because elective induction of labor is associated with significantly increased risk for primary cesarean, especially in nulliparous women (Seyb and others, 1999; Drudge Report, 2001), this practice should be evaluated. In the presence of a dysfunctional labor without FPD or other contraindication for labor augmentation, oxytocin should be used. Cesarean delivery has great

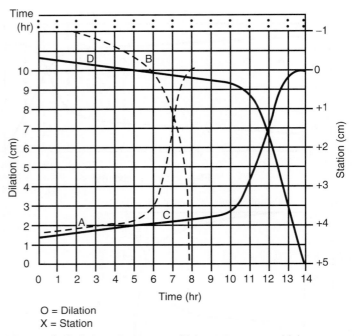

Figure 28-9 Method of charting progress of labor against normal labor curves. Normal dilation for multigravida *(A)*. Normal fetal descent for multigravida *(B)*. Normal dilation for primigravida *(C)*. Normal fetal descent for primigravida *(D)*. (Modified from Friedman E: An objective method of evaluating labor, *Hosp Pract* 5[7]:82, 1970.)

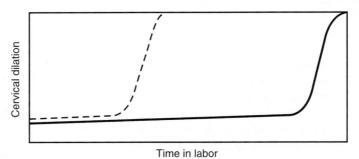

Figure 28-10 Prolonged latent-phase pattern *(solid line)* is only disorder thus far objectively diagnosable in preparatory division of labor. It is an abnormality characterized by latent-phase duration exceeding established critical limits, shown with typical elongation of lower initial arm of sigmoid curve of cervical dilation. It is followed by a normal active phase here, as is usually the case. Average dilation curve for nulliparas *(broken line)* is shown for comparison. (From Friedman EA: *Labor: clinical evaluation and management*, ed 2, New York, 1978, Appleton & Lange.)

potential benefits if indicated. However, it should be the last option because it is of higher maternal risk. Cesarean delivery also has increased risks for the newborn such as respiratory distress and lower breastfeeding rates. The timing of a planned cesarean should be based on fetal lung maturity.

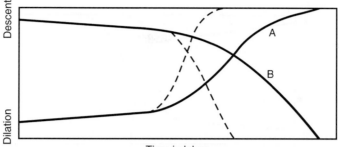

Figure 28-11 Protraction disorders of labor. Protracted active-phase dilation pattern with abnormally slow maximum slope of dilation (A). Protracted descent pattern with maximum slope of descent less than prescribed critical limits of normal (B). These labor aberrations are similar to each other in many ways and frequently occur together in same patient. They are clearly different from average normal dilation and descent patterns (broken lines). (From Friedman EA: *Labor: clinical evaluation and management,* ed 2, New York, 1978, Appleton & Lange.)

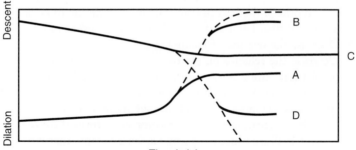

Figure 28-12 Arrest disorders of labor. Secondary arrest of dilation pattern with documented cessation of progression in active phase (A). Prolonged deceleration-phase pattern with deceleration-phase duration greater than normal limits (B). Failure of descent in deceleration phase and second stage (C). Arrest of descent characterized by halted advancement of fetal station in second stage (D). These four abnormalities are similar in etiology, response to treatment, and prognosis, being readily differentiated from normal dilation and descent curves (broken lines). (From Friedman EA: *Labor: clinical evaluation and management,* ed 2, New York, 1978, Appleton & Lange.)

The most common medical indications for a planned cesarean follow:
- Fetus with known meningomyelocele: cesarean may improve later motor function
- Macrocephaly for improved later mechanical function
- Active herpes and positive HIV status in certain situations
- Known placenta previa
- Previous classic uterine incision
- Family preference in the case of a prior cesarean

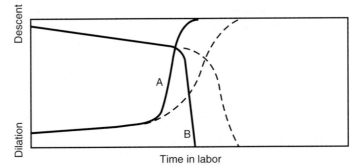

Figure 28-13 Precipitate labor patterns. Precipitate dilation (A) and precipitate descent (B) are defined by their excessively rapid rates of progressive cervical dilation and fetal descent, respectively, which distinguish them from course of normal labor (broken lines). (From Friedman EA: *Labor: clinical evaluation and management,* ed 2, New York, 1978, Appleton & Lange.)

To reduce the number of preventable primary cesarean deliveries, labor protocols should be based on the best available evidence. According to DeMott (2000) and others, the best practice factors include the following:
- View and treat labor as a normal physiologic event in low risk patients.
- Decrease the overuse of technology.
- Decrease the reliance on electronic fetal heart rate (FHR) monitoring to predict fetal stress because it has led to increased cesarean deliveries with no proven benefit (Thacker, Stroup, and Chang, 2001).
- Avoid elective inductions and manage inductions more effectively.
- Provide information to obtain a complete informed consent.
- Provide realistic expectations by teaching parents that it is not possible to have a perfect outcome with every pregnancy.
- Consider alternatives to cesarean delivery for breech presentation, such as external version and possible vaginal delivery.
- Remember that prolonged latent phase of labor, according to ACOG (2003a), is not indicative of dystocia, and failure to progress should not be diagnosed until the cervix has dilated to a least 4 cm.
- Use forceps or vacuum delivery carefully, when appropriate (Patel and Murphy, 2004).
- Revise the 2-hour limit for stage two of labor, as recommended by Association of Women's Health, Obstetric, and Neonatal Nurses (AWHONN) (Mayberry and others, 2000; Sampselle and others, 2005; Simpson and James, 2005), thus allowing the second stage of labor to continue as long as there is progress in descent without fetal compromise.
- When epidural pain management is considered, instruct regarding the possible effects on labor progress, increased risk for oxytocin use and instrumental delivery, increased risk for serious perineal laceration, and greater risk for maternal intrapartum fever resulting in evaluation and treatment of their infant for suspected sepsis (Thorp and others, 1993;

Morton and others, 1994; Lieberman and O'Donoghue, 2002; Anim-Somuah, Smyth, Howell, 2005;).

- Use one-to-one labor support, when possible, which has been shown by research to decrease the rate of cesarean and the rate of instrument-assisted vaginal delivery (Enkin and others, 2000; Hodnett and others, 2003).

VBAC is still an appropriate way to decrease the repeat cesarean delivery rate. Both repeat cesarean delivery and VBAC are associated with maternal and fetal risks (ACOG, 2004). Uterine rupture is the greatest risk for VBAC but occurs in less than 1% of VBAC attempts (Mozurkewich and Hutton, 2000; Kieser and Baskett, 2002). Failed VBAC trial of labor carries the greatest risk for operative complications, hysterectomy and increase neonatal mortality (Kieser and Baskett, 2002; Chauhan and others, 2003). Factors that increase this risk are need for oxytocin, maternal obesity, gestational age greater than 40 weeks of gestation, birth weight greater than 4000 g, and time since prior delivery less than 19 months (ACOG, 2004; Goodall and others, 2005; SOGC, 2005). Multiple cesarean births cause cumulative increase maternal risks (Mankuta and others, 2003). Epidural is safe to use in a VBAC labor (ACOG, 2004). Therefore according to ACOG (2004), women with a history of one previous low-transverse cesarean may be offered VBAC after discussion of the risks and benefits. Immediate availability of a physician and anesthesia during the trial of labor are essential to the labor care.

To further lower the primary cesarean delivery rate, consideration should be given to external version as an appropriate treatment of a breech presentation. More than 50% of all attempted external versions are successful with a 2% reversion rate (Lau and others, 1997; Simm and Woods, 2004).

Instrument-assisted delivery with either vacuum extraction or forceps is indicated for shortening second-stage labor caused by factors such as the following (O'Grady, Pope, and Patel, 2000):

- Maternal paralysis
- Heavy motor block epidural
- Indication of fetal stress
- Maternal exhaustion

According to the *Cochrane Review* (Johanson and Menon, 2000), the use of a vacuum extractor as compared with forceps reduces maternal morbidity, but a forceps delivery is less likely to cause newborn cephalhematoma, hyperbilirubinemia, and retinal hemorrhages. A forceps, however, is more likely to cause facial and cranial injuries as well as maternal soft tissue injury.

Dysfunctional Labor Disorders

Significant slowing of any phase of labor should be individually evaluated as to the possible cause or causes. Table 28-1 summarizes the types, possible causes, and possible management plans for each dysfunctional labor pattern.

Fetal Malpresentations

The manner in which the fetus presents also influences the outcome and manner of treatment. Table 28-2 outlines the various fetal malpresentations and the appropriate treatment.

Table 28-1 Summary of Abnormal Labor Patterns

Type	Definition	Etiology	Management
Prolonged latent phase or "prelabor"	*Nullipara.* Latent phase of labor continues for longer than 20 hr (Friedman, 1995) *Multipara.* Latent phase of labor continues for longer than 14 hr (Friedman, 1995) *Diagnosis.* After 6–8 hr of little progress, assessment can be made May be false labor	Unripe cervix at onset of labor—thick, uneffaced, rigid cervix Anxiety or fear Inhibitory effect of early administration of narcotic Early administration of regional anesthesia Abnormal position of fetus FPD	Best treated by explanation, reassurance, and allowing time for cervical changes to occur (Gee, 2006). Encourage adequate fluid and small, frequent meals. If analgesia or anesthetic has been used, let it wear off. If rest is needed, give oral zolpidem 5–10 mg to take home or morphine 15–20 mg if hospitalized (Ness, Goldberg, and Berghella, 2004) Administer labor stimulant if delivery is indicated.
Protraction disorders Protracted active-phase dilation Protracted descent Arrest of dilation Arrest of descent	*Nullipara.* Rate of dilation in active phase <1.2 cm/hr or rate of descent <2.0 cm/hr (Friedman, 1995) *Multipara.* Rate of dilation in active phase <1.5 cm/hr or rate of descent <2.0 cm/hr (Friedman, 1995) *Current standard.* <1 cm/1–2 hr (Zhang, Troendle, and Yancey,	No specific cause Ineffective uterine contractions FPD Excessive sedation Fetal malpresentation Early conduction anesthesia ROM before onset of labor Inadequate nutrition Maternal exhaustion	Rule out obvious FPD. If FPD, patient will deliver by cesarean Amniotomy Augmentation with oxytocin to achieve 3–5 contractions/10 min Assess for uterine hyperstimulation Ongoing fetal assessment Dx. FPD, if no cervical change after 2 hours of oxytocin (ACOG, 2003) Initiate or continue the following nursing

labor stops before full dilation occurs and continue for 2 hr or longer (Friedman, 1995)

and reassure regarding possible reasons for slow progress
- Encourage patient to keep bladder empty
- Provide physical and emotional support
- Let her know you are there for her and that you have confidence in her ability
- Allay anxiety
- Encourage position change
- Assess fluid and electrolyte needs and administer IV as ordered

Precipitous labor

Nullipara. Cervix dilates faster than 5 cm/hr or descent faster than 1 cm per 12 min

Multipara. Cervix dilates faster than 10 cm/hr or descent faster than 1 cm per 6 min

Abnormally low cervical resistance

Abnormally strong uterine or abdominal muscular contractions

Tocolytic agents, such as magnesium sulfate or terbutaline, may be used in attempt to slow down progress of labor.

FHR, Fetal heart rate; FPD, fetopelvic disproportion.

Table 28-2 Fetal Malpresentations

	Occiput Posterior	Face	Brow	Shoulder	Compound Presentation	Breech
Definition	Fetal occiput lies in either right or left posterior quadrant of mother's pelvis	Presenting head completely extended	Presenting head midway between full flexion and extreme extension	Fetal spine lies vertical to mother's spine	One or more fetal art extremities accompany presenting part	Buttocks of fetus present in one of three attitudes: • *Frank:* thighs flexed and legs lie along side fetal body • *Complete:* legs flexed at thighs, allowing feet to present with buttocks • *Footling:* one or both thighs extended and present before buttocks
Presenting part Incidence **Diagnosis:** Leopold maneuver	Occiput 10%–25% Patient will often complain of severe back or suprapubic pain; differentiation by Leopold maneuver is difficult	Chin (mentum) 0.2% Absence of smooth, flexed spine; prominent extremities and head	Brow 0.2% No differentiation	Scapula 0.33% Abdomen may look wider than long; head can be palpated on one side of mother's abdomen and buttocks on other	0.01% No differentiation	Sacrum 4% Fetal heart tones heard best above umbilicus; fetal head palpated in upper part of uterus
Vaginal examination	Anterior fontanel can be felt in anterior quadrant of mother's pelvis and posterior fontanel in	Nose, eyes, and mouth can be felt	Anterior fontanel can be felt in center of cervical opening with eyes on one side	Scapula can be felt or no presenting part reached since it is often high	Fetal extremity felt alongside presenting part	Soft presenting part felt

spontaneously to anterior position and are delivered vaginally; in 10% that do not rotate completely, rotation usually done with forceps or vacuum extraction

If posterior position persists without progress, cesarean delivery is done

anterior rotation of chin occurs

Cesarean delivery if chin is directed posteriorly and progress stops

brow presentation converts by flexion to occiput presentation or extension to face presentation

Cesarean delivery if brow presentation persists

prolapse with ROM during labor

Cesarean delivery if version fails; external cephalic version can be attempted under very controlled circumstances if placenta previa or FPD not present after 37 weeks

unless cord prolapses or labor fails to progress

Immediate cesarean delivery if prolapsed cord develops or progress stops

assess amniotic fluid volume, placental site, position of fetal extremities and neck in relation to the umbilical cord

External version may be attempted after 37 weeks

If external version fails, a planned cesarean birth is recommended by the *Term Breech Trial* (Hannah and others, 2000) and ACOG (2001)

If mother requests, vaginal delivery for a frank or complete breech, with adequate neck flexion, gestational age greater than 36 weeks, and estimated fetal weight between 2000 and 4000 g

Vaginal birth increases risk for perinatal mortality and morbidity by 3%

FPD, Fetopelvic disproportion.

NURSING MANAGEMENT

Prevention

Managing labor by considering all of the 13 Ps is the art and science of labor nursing. The nurse can have a significant influence on the progress and outcome of labor as shown in a research study by Radin, Harmon, and Hanson (1993). In their research, some patients of specific nurses had a low cesarean birth rate, whereas patients of other nurses had a high rate. The nurses' use of a variety of therapeutic techniques to facilitate labor and their ability to instill confidence in the laboring patient can make a significant difference.

Time of Admission

Unless maternal or fetal status indicates, delay admission of low risk patients until they are dilated 4 cm or more. This policy prevents misdiagnosis of the preparatory status of prelabor versus true labor and thus decreases unnecessary interventions including cesarean delivery. Instead of admission, encourage ambulation with periods of rest and reevaluate in several hours (DeMott, 2000; Lauzon and Hodnett, 2001; Ness, Goldberg, Berghella, 2004).

Continuous Emotional Support

Continuous professional labor support is an important function of the intrapartum nurse (Miltner, 2000; Jackson and others, 2003) and is probably the most important aspect of effective care (ACOG, 2003a). According to the *Cochrane Review* (Hodnett and others, 2003), the Cochrane Pregnancy and Childbirth Group (Enkin and others, 2000), and AWHONN (2000), continuous labor support has been demonstrated to shorten labors, decrease the need for analgesia and anesthesia, reduce the cesarean birth rate, reduce the rate of instrumental deliveries, reduce the need for oxytocin, decrease oxytocin use, and decrease the number of infants with Apgar scores lower than 7 at 5 minutes. Maternal labor satisfaction is also increased.

There are five dimensions to labor support: emotional, teaching or informational support, physical, partner, and advocacy (Sleutel, 2000). Labor units should conduct classes to certify nurses in labor support as they do in EFM.

Empowerment and Control

To give the woman more control over labor practices, to treat with respect and affirm, to provide positive encouragement, and to support the woman's natural abilities is the art of nursing that empowers the laboring woman to give birth, decreasing dystocia (Fowles, 1998; Jackson and others, 2003).

Movement

Experimental studies clearly show that position and frequency of position change have a profound effect on uterine activity and efficiency. The maternal pelvic joints are flexible, and the baby's head will mold if given time, decreasing the risk for dystocia. (For specifics, refer to the nursing interventions in the Activity and Position Pattern section under Interventions to Enhance Labor

Progress Through Each of the 11 Functional Health Patterns to Decrease Risk for Dystocia, Epidural Anesthesia, and Instrumental Delivery.)

Empty Bladder

A full bladder interferes with fetal descent and may lead to a dysfunctional labor pattern.

Nutrition

According to the Cochrane Pregnancy and Childbirth Group (Enkin and others, 2000) and Hodnett (1996), simple measures such as encouraging movement and allowing women to eat and drink as desired may be as effective as oxytocin for a sizable portion of laboring women considered to be in need of labor augmentation. However, because of the rare but possibly devastating consequences of gastric aspiration in the event of general anesthesia, many labor and delivery units have a policy that the laboring patient should take nothing by mouth except sips of water or ice chips. Because the routine policy of giving the laboring patient nothing to eat or drink has not been scientifically substantiated and may affect her progress in labor, labor and delivery medical personnel should seriously evaluate this policy. This statement is based on the following:

- The policy of giving nothing by mouth (NPO) or giving ice chips came into practice only because of anecdotal reports of aspiration related to general anesthesia, not because of evidence-based research (McKay and Mahan, 1988; Roberts and Ludka, 1994; Newton and Raynor, 2000).
- The risk for aspiration is almost entirely associated with general anesthesia (Enkin and others, 2000; Newton and Raynor, 2000).
- Gastric emptying time is rarely delayed in early labor. A large volume of food and dietary fat slow gastric emptying time (Roberts and Ludka, 1994), as do narcotic medications (Keppler, 1988; McKay and Mahan, 1988; Newton and Raynor, 2000).
- Fasting does not ensure an empty stomach or lowered gastric acidity (O'Sullivan, 1994; Enkin and others, 2000). According to Crawford (1986), aspiration-related maternal deaths rose after the dietary restriction in labor was implemented. It appears that gastric acidity decreases during pregnancy (Smith and Bogod, 1995).
- The major reason that aspiration of gastric contents causes maternal mortality is improper anesthetic technique. This has been shown repeatedly through research (McKay and Mahan, 1988; Elkington, 1991; Enkin and others, 2000).

Maternal mortality risk related to aspiration is small, and fasting has not been shown to be an effective preventive strategy. According to an analysis by the British Department of Health following their investigation of two maternal deaths from aspiration, fasting during labor was ineffective in prevention of these deaths (Sharp, 1997). Data from developing countries indicate that a more liberal policy on food and fluids during labor does not result in greater maternal risk (Berry, 1997; Scheepers and others, 2001).

The key factor in preventing aspiration deaths is proper administration of general anesthesia by an anesthesiologist or nurse anesthetist trained in perinatal anesthesiology. This includes application of cricoid pressure, in which a trained assistant pushes the cricoid cartilage against the esophagus. Next, a cuffed endotracheal tube is correctly placed to seal the airway. Then proper placement of the endotracheal tube is checked before releasing the cricoid pressure (Douglas, 1988; McKay and Mahan, 1988; CNM Data Group, 1999).

Research indicates that when low risk women are allowed to eat and drink during labor, 85.5% choose to eat more in early labor and taper off during active labor. Women who were allowed to eat required less pain medication and less oxytocin, their labors were shorter, and their nausea, vomiting, or aspiration risk did not increase (Roberts and Ludka, 1994; Sleutel and Golden, 1999; Tranmer and others, 2005).

Restricting food and fluid during labor can cause dehydration and ketosis, which do not occur in those who are allowed to consume isotonic "sport" drinks or eat (Scrutton and others, 1999; Kubli and others, 2002). During exercise, fasting leads to accelerated fatigue. There is some evidence to suggest that dehydration, ketosis, and fatigue can turn a normal labor into a dysfunctional one in some women (Roberts and Ludka, 1994; Newton and Raynor, 2000; Scheepers and others, 2001).

Water-soluble vitamins, such as vitamins C and B complex, are quickly excreted from the body when the woman is given nothing to eat. Vitamin B_1 is important for the metabolism of carbohydrates that are used by the contracting uterine muscle (Newton and others, 1988).

Enforced hunger and routine IV insertion can be stressful for the laboring woman (Simkin, 1986a, 1986b; Newton and others, 1988; VandeVusse, 1999). An IV apparatus interferes with movement.

Routinely enforcing an NPO status, starting IV fluids, and placing a laboring mother in bed psychologically imply sickness, which can interfere with the normal progress of labor and set the mother up for labor augmentation or failure to progress (Broach and Newton, 1988).

Perinatal Massage

According to the *Cochrane Review* (Beckmann and Garrett, 2006), perinatal massage during pregnancy decreases the likelihood of perineal trauma during delivery.

Interventions to Enhance Labor Progress Through Each of the 11 Functional Health Patterns to Decrease Risk for Dystocia, Epidural Anesthesia, and Instrumental Delivery

Health-Perception and Health-Management Pattern

- Assess the woman's risk for dystocia.
- Assess the woman's progress in labor.
- Ask the patient and her coach about their birth plan. Parents have varying needs and expectations of care. As long as it does not affect the health of the

mother or baby, to promote and carry out the plan is therapeutic. Birth plans can decrease the family's anxiety and increase their feeling of control while facilitating communication with the health care team (Springer, 1996). However, during the prenatal care, families must be instructed that although a birth plan is a manner in which they sort out what will make their birth experience satisfying, it must be open to change when unexpected events develop (Jannke, 1995).

Nutritional and Metabolic Pattern (Preconception)

- Educate women about the importance of attaining an appropriate body weight before conception.
- Educate underweight women about the importance of eating appropriate nutritional foods in each of the food groups and avoiding empty-calorie foods that are high in fat and refined sugar, before and during pregnancy. (Being underweight increases the risk for a small-for-gestational-age fetus and preterm labor, which increases the risk for a breech presentation and cesarean delivery.)
- Educate women who are overweight before conception about the importance of a nutritious, weight-control, lifestyle diet change as opposed to an extreme quick weight loss program that usually leads to weight gain and depletes the nutritional stores needed for a healthy pregnancy. Weight reduction is contraindicated during pregnancy. (Being overweight is related to an increased risk for gestational diabetes and large-for-gestational-age infants, which increases the risk for cesarean birth.)
- Educate women with diabetes about the importance of achieving normal blood sugar levels before conception and maintaining this control throughout conception with diet, exercise, insulin if needed, and self-monitoring of blood glucose. This decreases the risk for congenital anomalies and a large- or small-for-gestational-age fetus, which increases the risk for a cesarean delivery.

Nutritional and Metabolic Pattern (Intrapartum)

During labor, unless there is a medical or obstetric contraindication, allow the patient to eat, if hungry, high-carbohydrate, low-residue, low-fat foods (e.g., frozen yogurt, lightly cooked eggs, crisp toast, plain biscuits, canned fruit) and drink fluids with electrolytes (e.g., Gatorade, fruit juices, tea with honey, clear broth) as she desires. This protocol is supported by the Better Birth Global Initiative (2000), a new initiate to promote humane evidence-based childbirth care and by the Cochrane Pregnancy and Childbirth Group (Enkin and others, 2000).

If opiate analgesic medication becomes necessary, if the patient is at high risk for requiring general anesthesia, or if she is experiencing gastric upset, allow clear fluids only. IV fluids may then be therapeutic. However, there appears to be no association between delayed gastric emptying and epidural opioids (Zimmerman and others, 1996; Kelly and others, 1997). Intrathecal, spinal, and systemic narcotics decrease gastric emptying.

Question a hospital or birthing center labor policy that requires routine use of IV fluids. Ringer's lactate, a nonglucose-based solution, provides no energy. IV dextrose during labor has been shown to increase the risk for hypoglycemia, hyperbilirubinemia, lactic acid, and hyponatremia in the newborn (Hazle, 1986; Ludka and Roberts, 1993; Tourangeau and others, 1999; Enkin and others, 2000). Lactated Ringer's solution has been shown to cause fewer problems if it is used when IV fluids are indicated during labor (Sleutal and Golden, 1999). If dehydrated, intravenous fluid has been shown to shorten labor (Garite and others, 2000)

If IV fluids are ordered only to keep a vein open, determine whether a heparin lock could be used instead.

Elimination Pattern

Encourage the patient to void every 2 hours. A full bladder interferes with fetal descent, and the sense of a full bladder is depressed related to pressure by the fetus.

Assess when the patient had her last bowel movement and whether she has been experiencing the natural diarrhea that frequently precedes labor. Administering routine enemas and shaving pubic hair are ineffective and should not be a part of routine labor management (Enkin, 2000).

Activity and Position Pattern

Antepartum. Educate pregnant women as to the benefits of a consistent, low-impact exercise program, such as walking, swimming, bicycling, or low-impact aerobics. Fitness during pregnancy reduces such discomforts as back pain and fatigue and fosters a more normal labor and delivery (Wong and McKenzie, 1987; Clapp, 1990). Varrassi, Bazzano, and Edwards (1989) found that plasma beta-endorphin levels are elevated in women who exercise during pregnancy as compared with expectant women who do not exercise. A higher endorphin level means a higher pain threshold.

Intrapartum: stage one. During labor, provide opportunities for position changes every 30 minutes and encourage position changes. Choice of position change should be based on maternal preference, safety, comfort, effective progress, and knowledge of hemodynamics (Romond and Baker, 1985; Rossi and Lindell, 1986; Fenwick and Simkin, 1987; ACOG, 2003a; Ness, Goldberg, Berghella, 2004). Malpresentations are frequently associated with increased pain. Allowing the mother to obtain a position she finds more comfortable frequently facilitates a favorable fetal rotation by altering the alignment of the presenting part with the pelvis. As the mother continues to change position based on comfort, the optimum presentation is maintained (Fenwick and Simkin, 1987; Enkin and others, 2000; Ness, Goldberg, Berghella, 2004).

Supine positions are avoided because they cause compression of the vena cava and decrease blood return to the heart.

During stage one of labor, the lateral recumbent and upright positions such as kneeling forward or doing the lunge on a birth ball (Fig. 28-14, *A-F*) increase

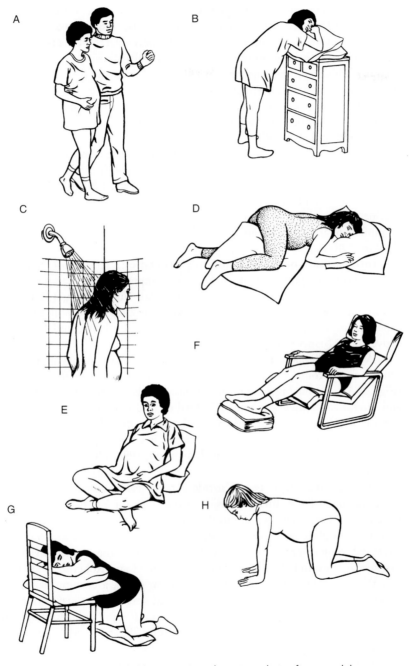

Figure 28-14 Various maternal positions during first-stage labor.

uterine intensity, decrease frequency, and decrease vena caval compression (Roberts and others, 1983; McKay and Roberts, 1989; Enkin and others, 2000). Therefore the uterine contractions are more effective because the upright position permits relaxation of the abdominal wall, allowing the fundus to fall forward. This facilitates engagement of the fetal head and descent. As the fetal head is pushed against the cervix, the uterus receives increased stimulation to contract (McKay and Roberts, 1989). Walking during labor may provide comfort and has been shown to neither enhance nor impede labor progress (Bloom and others, 1998).

The recumbent and sitting positions interfere with labor progress and fetal descent, decrease uterine intensity and frequency, and increase analgesic needs and malpresentation of the fetus (Roberts and others, 1983; Chen and others, 1987; McKay and Roberts, 1989; Mayberry and others, 2000). Therefore uterine contractions are not as effective. These positions may cause poor alignment of the fetal presenting part to the pelvic inlet as well (Fenwick and Simkin, 1987).

Intrapartum: occiput posterior presentation. Assess for signs of an occiput posterior presentation, such as (1) complaining of suprapubic pain or back pain, (2) feeling the urge to push before full dilation, (3) having an abdominal contour that shows a depression around the umbilical area, (4) experiencing early decelerations during latent phase labor, and (5) arresting active labor (Biancuzzo, 1993).

When the fetus is in an occiput posterior presentation, having the woman assume an "all fours" or kneeling (Fig. 28-14, *G*) and leaning-forward position (Fig. 28-14, *H*) may promote rotation to an anterior presentation. Pelvic rock and lateral abdominal stroking may further facilitate head rotation. The abdominal stroking is performed in the direction toward which the fetal head should rotate. For rest periods, the woman is encouraged to lie on the side toward which the baby should turn (Biancuzzo, 1993; Hodnett, 1996; Roberts and Woolley, 1996).

Intrapartum: stage two. Provide care for second-stage labor based on understanding of the three phases of second stage of labor: (1) *latent phase,* a time to rest when there is a lull in the contractions; (2) *active phase,* when fetal descent takes place facilitated by maternal pushing; and (3) *transition or perineal phase,* which just precedes birth and during which the mother needs active support to relax and let the birth occur (Aderhold and Roberts, 1991; Roberts and Woolley, 1996). If no anesthetic has been given, a burning perineal pain frequently characterizes this phase as the head stretches the perineum.

According to the Cochrane Review Group, (Gupta and Hofmeyr, 2004), an upright, slightly curled forward position (Fig. 28-15, *A* and *B*) decreases the length of second-stage labor, FHR abnormalities, instrument-assisted births, episiotomies, and pain perception because of decreased release of stress-related hormones with only a small increase in second degree perineal tears and blood loss. Squatting is the best upright position and can be achieved by using the squatting bar (Fig. 28-15, *C*) or sitting in bed curled forward (Fig. 28-15, *D*) (Shermer and Raines, 1997; McCartney, 1998; Mayberry and others, 2000).

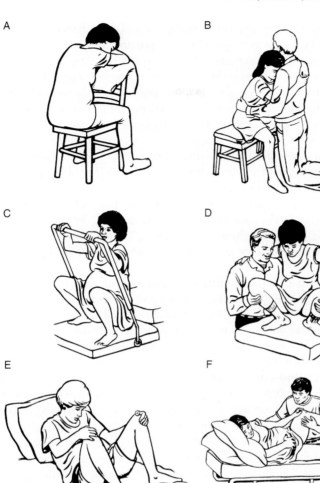

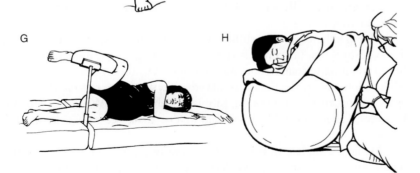

Figure 28-15 Various maternal positions during second-stage labor.

Squatting increases the pelvis size 0.5 to 2.0 cm (Fenwick and Simkin, 1987; Golay, Vedam, and Sorger, 1993). Squatting may increase the bearing-down sensation and enhance effective pushing as well (Kurokawa and Zilkoski, 1985). Therefore, it has been shown to shorten second-stage labor, lessen the need for oxytocin, decrease the need for mechanical-assisted deliveries, and decrease the need for episiotomy (Golay, Vedam, and Sorger, 1993; Roberts and Woolley, 1996). *Note:* Squatting is contraindicated for patients with epidural analgesia.

The reclining-back, sitting position puts pressure on the sacrum, restricting posterior movement and reducing the pelvic size (Fig. 28-15, *E*) (Fenwick and Simkin, 1987; Paciornik, 1990).

Avoid the supine position during the second stage of labor because in this position, gravity works against the woman's pushing efforts (Fenwick and Simkin, 1987; Johnson, Johnson, and Gupta, 1991). Also, this position has been shown to decrease fetal artery pH (Johnstone, Aboelmagd, and Harouny, 1987).

In low risk patients, intermitted FHR monitoring may be used in place of continuous monitoring to increase mobility and decrease unnecessary interventions (Tracker, Stroup, and Chang, 2001).

Encourage the woman to push in response to her body's urges rather than to sustain bearing-down efforts while holding her breath unless there is an obstetric indication to facilitate an immediate delivery (Aldrich and others, 1995; Mayberry and others, 2000; Sampselle and others, 2005; Simpson and James, 2005). This type of pushing initiated by the woman in response to an irresistible sensation is usually accompanied by expiratory grunting or vocalization and is less fatiguing to the mother and has less effect on umbilical cord blood gases (Cosner and deJong, 1993; Fuller, Roberts, and McKay, 1993; Parnell and others, 1993). Sustained, breath-holding bearing down can impose a hypoxic environment for the fetus and may conflict with the patient's own body sensations and increase the risk for perineal trauma (McKay, Barrows, and Roberts, 1990; Aderhold and Roberts, 1991; Paine and Tinker, 1992; Parnell and others, 1993; Thomson, 1993).

Manage the urge to push before full dilation by assessing if (1) cervix is dilated 8 to 9 cm, (2) cervix is soft and retracting with contractions, (3) fetal head is rotating to transverse or anterior position, and (4) station is at least one. Then allow the patient to push at the peak of the contraction if she is experiencing an irresistible urge to push (Roberts and Woolley, 1996; Vause, Congdon, Thornton, 1998; Fraser and others, 2000; Petrou, Coyle, and Fraser, 2000).

Manage complete dilation and no urge to push by (1) first assessing the fetal position, fetal station, and FHR and (2) then encouraging the mother to rest until she feels the urge to push, which is the result of the presenting part stimulating the stretch receptors of the pelvic floor (Roberts and Woolley, 1996).

Do not set an arbitrary time limit such as 2 hours on the length of second stage of labor, (Rouse, Owen, and Hauth, 1999; Mayberry and others, 2000;

Rouse and others, 2001; ACOG, 2003a). This does not improve outcomes; it only increases instrument-assisted deliveries.

The lateral recumbent position (Fig. 28-15, *F* and *G*) may be beneficial during the transitional phase of stage two labor when less bearing-down force is needed to help control the speed of the delivery and decrease the risk for perineal lacerations (Golay and others, 1993; Roberts and Woolley, 1996).

Rest and Relaxation Pattern

Encourage use of visualization, patterned breathing, attention focusing, quiet voice, and music in active labor. These stimuli affect the thalamus part of the brain and influence the limbic system, which governs emotional responses as well as inhibition of pain transmission (Simkin, 1987; Di Franco, 1988; Pugh and others, 1998; Hottenstein and Brit Pipe, 2005). The limbic system has been shown to increase pain tolerance by reducing anxiety, decreasing catecholamine response, and decreasing muscle tension. It enhances blood flow to the uterus as well (Watson, 1999).

Cognitive Pattern

- If involved with childbirth education, provide not only realistic information about the birth process but also activities that will instill confidence to control pain and deal with childbirth-related fears.
- Assess the patient's and her coach's understanding of labor, delivery, and effective tools. Determine which childbirth education method the couple plans to use, if any.
- Assess the woman's level of confidence in her and her coach's ability to use the techniques they learned in their childbirth class. Increased confidence and decreased labor pain are related (Lowe, 1991).
- Fill in the patient and coach's knowledge gaps between contractions.
- Teach the patient and coach to pace themselves, as if in a race, and not to use all their tools at first.
- Keep the patient and her coach informed of the progress.
- Allow participation in decision making.

Perceptual Pattern

- Assess patient's level of pain, location of pain, and degree of distress it is causing her (Lowe, 1996). A 10-point scale is an effective tool to use (1 = no pain or distress, 10 = worst pain or distress imaginable).
- Assess for leg cramps.
- Assess for back discomfort.
- Assess how the patient and her coach feel they should respond to pain because of any cultural or personal values.
- Encourage appropriate comfort measures.
- Provide back rubs and counterpressure for back labor.
- Apply cool washcloth to the forehead if feeling hot or nauseated.
- Offer hydrotherapy through baths and showers. This activates body-wide tactile receptors, which transport pleasant stimuli over the pathways that

pain stimuli must travel, thus closing the gate to pain and reversing the fight-or-flight responses that frequently occur during labor while increasing uterine activity (Simkin, 1995b).

- Suggest a Whirlpool bath. According to the *Cochrane Review* (Cluett and others, 2004), this decreases analgesia needs and the rate of instrument-assisted delivery while enhancing maternal satisfaction and confidence with no increased risk for infection. However, it is contraindicated in the presence of thick meconium, oxytocin infusion, bleeding, or heavy bloody show (Rush and others, 1996). No conclusive evidence can be made related to limited research at this time (Cluett and others, 2004), but no significant adverse affects have been detected.
- Apply superficial heat and cold with packs, which activate local tactile receptors, thus closing the gate to some pain stimuli.
- Offer massage, which facilitates relaxation and bombards the brain with another stimulus, decreasing the amount of pain sensation being perceived.
- Provide acupressure at acupoints. This facilitates pain control when done by a professional trained in acupressure. One example is to apply intense pressure during contractions by wrapping four fingers around the balls of the feet, the quarter-moon area from where the toes join the foot to the furthest end of the ball of the foot (Stephens, 1997). Cook and Wilcox (1997) and Gentz (2001) provided more acupoints that can be located by trained labor nurses.
- Encourage position change and motions such as rocking or walking (Lowe, 1996).
- Apply double hip squeeze, knee press, and counterpressure. These can decrease back pain (Simkin, 1995b).
- Encourage moaning because it decreases pain and medication need by releasing endorphins (Threlfall-Mase, 1997).
- Provide lip balm for dry lips, and keep the linen clean and dry to decrease extraneous uncomfortable sensations and thereby reducing the total amount of pain experienced.
- Provide effleurage of the abdomen to promote relaxation of the abdominal muscle, allowing the uterine muscle to be unrestrained.
- Use transcutaneous electrical nerve stimulation (TENS) to stimulate peripheral nerve endings, thereby decreasing the transmission of painful impulses and stimulating the production of natural endorphins (Phillips, 1998).
- Alleviate leg cramps by stretching the cramping muscle instead of massaging it.
- Value the doula, if present, as an important member of the health care team.
- Keep the patient clean and dry to promote comfort and decrease infection risk.
- Portray to her a deep sense of empathy and caring that transmits confidence so that she is enabled to trust her own body and relax more completely (Lowe, 1991).

- Help her use appropriate techniques so that her need for anesthesia or analgesia is less. An epidural analgesia may increase the incidence of oxytocin use, instrumental delivery, episiotomy and antibiotic use because of fever (Newman, Lindsay, and Graves, 2001; Goetzl and others, 2003; Anim-Somuah, Smyth, and Howell, 2005)
- Know when pharmacologic interventions are needed and use them effectively.
- Administer narcotic analgesic, narcotic agonist-antagonist, or analgesic potentiators during the peak of a contraction and titrate them to desired effects, not to a specific dose.
- Provide pain relief using various methods. Epidural analgesia is the most effective method of providing pain relief, but as with all procedures, there are accompanying risks that should be discussed with the expectant mother, ideally during a prenatal visit. Refer to the section later in this chapter on epidural anesthesia.
- Manage pain with intrathecal narcotics (injection of narcotics in the subarachnoid space), another form of pain management during labor (Manning, 1996).

Self-Perception and Self-Concept Pattern
- Assess attitude toward pregnancy, labor, and delivery.
- Provide ongoing labor support.
- Ensure modesty at all times throughout the birth experience.
- Facilitate a positive body image by helping the laboring woman maintain body control. This can be promoted if the nurse understands the laboring woman's behaviors and provides appropriate nursing interventions (Richardson, 1984).
- During the latent phase of labor, the woman is usually excited, anxious, and very distractible. This is an ideal time to gather an assessment and educate as indicated.
- During the accelerated and maximum-slope dilation phases of active labor, the laboring woman needs to focus because of the increasing inner body tension. The woman should not be distracted during a contraction but encouraged to focus on previously learned patterned breathing, using mind focusing, relaxation, and diminished verbal and gross motor activities. Between contractions, questions, instructions, and socializing are distracting and appropriate.
- During the deceleration phase of active labor (transition), the laboring woman is vulnerable. Because of the pain intensity, focusing is no longer effective. Rhythmic and repetitive verbal and gross motor activities are more effective in displacing tension. The woman may moan, chant, rock her body, or pedal her feet to maintain body control. Soft, repetitive, encouraging verbal contact from the coach or nurse can be helpful. Tactile intrusiveness or verbal demands only increase tension. Between contractions, the woman frequently desires rest instead of social interaction.

Role-Relationship Pattern

- Assess role expectations of all participants during the birth process.
- Assess economic needs and concerns.
- Assess cultural practices that influence the various roles of the participants.
- Promote family members' involvement, according to their birth plan, if possible.
- Provide therapeutic interventions for the support person or persons by evaluating their comfort in the labor situation, orienting them to the environment and equipment being used, asking whether they have any special requests, acknowledging their physical and psychologic needs, providing times for nutritional snacks, encouraging them to actively participate, and providing a welcome environment.

Coping and Stress-Tolerance Pattern

- Assess the patient's and coach's fears and concerns.
- Assess level of emotional tension compared with level of effective coping. Maintain an equilibrium, if possible, among comfort measures, effective labor support, and appropriate use of medications. Some anxiety is therapeutic for the birth process because increased catecholamines prepare the body for action, facilitate the oxygen conservation of the fetus, stimulate the adsorption of fluid from the newborn's lungs, facilitate neonatal respiratory function by stimulating surfactant release, and promote alertness in the neonate for the first 30 to 60 minutes of life (Copper and Goldenberg, 1990). However, excessive catecholamines are not therapeutic and can decrease efficiency of uterine contractions, causing dystocia, decreasing uteroplacental blood flow, and increasing the possibility of poor neonatal adjustment.
- Offer ongoing encouragement and avoid comments that may worry the patient.
- Minimize common stressors of labor such as restriction of activity, vaginal examinations, and administration of IV fluids.
- Teach the woman and her coach how to deal with unexpected changes in their birth plan through empowerment.
- Ask whether this is an emergency or whether there is time to discuss the situation.
- If it is not an emergency, ask questions that help the woman and her coach understand the situation.
- Ask questions to learn the risks and benefits of the suggested intervention.
- Ask questions to determine alternatives to the suggested intervention.

Interventions to Accomplish Early Detection and Treatment of a Dysfunctional Labor

- Determine onset of true labor.
- Evaluate the uterine contraction pattern every 30 to 60 minutes, or more often if needed, for frequency, duration, intensity, and resting tone.

- Assess state of cervix as to soft or hard, effaced or long, dilatable or resistant, and amount of dilation as indicated (depending on phase of labor). Use the Bishop system or a comparable scoring system.
- Assess fetal position, station, and status of the presenting part.
- Assess for a malpresentation by doing the Leopold maneuver to help decide maternal positioning.
- Evaluate the woman's labor progress in active labor using the simple rule of 1 cm per hour, or plot and compare the patient's labor using the Friedman labor graph or the labor line of active labor.
- Assess for discomfort and tension.
- Assess for signs of dehydration and electrolyte imbalance.
- Assess for signs of hypoglycemia. A prolonged difficult labor depletes the mother's energy and glucose stores.
- Encourage patient to void every 1 to 2 hours.
- Catheterize for distended bladder if unable to void.
- Encourage patient to verbalize anxieties and fears.
- Encourage patient to try various position changes to facilitate labor progress (see Figs. 28-14 and 28-15).
- Monitor for effective use of breathing and relaxation techniques.
- Provide continuous support. Be supportive of coping methods and provide help with new ones as needed.
- Provide support to the labor coach.
- Encourage rest between contractions.
- If labor begins to progress slower than normal, encourage ambulation and alternative positioning if not contraindicated.
- Be prepared to administer a labor stimulant as ordered (see Chapter 26).
- If it is necessary to withhold analgesia or anesthesia, explain the need to the patient and her coach.
- Keep the attending physician informed of labor progress.
- If a dysfunctional labor pattern develops, outline the treatment plan so that the patient and her coach are prepared for what might occur. Stress the normalcy of patient's physiologic response to labor.

Management of Shoulder Dystocia

- Be familiar with the management plan of shoulder dystocia. Shoulder dystocia is unpredictable (Nocon, 2000; Minkin, 2004), and there are no reliable indicators according to research. It is often suspected in macrosomia, but the majority of the time when shoulder dystocia occurs, the fetus weighs less than 4000 g (Ouzounian and Gherman, 2005).
- Assess labor progress closely and use the squatting method when appropriate to increase pelvic capacity.
- An early indication of shoulder dystocia is when the fetal head retracts against the mother's perineum as soon as the head is delivered (Baxley and Gobbo, 2004). The most common risk factor for shoulder dystocia is instrumental delivery (ACOG, 2002).

- When shoulder dystocia is diagnosed, the nurse can be prepared to assist by staying calm and calling for added assistance (an anesthesiologist or nurse anesthetist and a pediatrician or intensive care nursing team).
- Be prepared to catheterize the patient to ensure a completely emptied bladder.
- Be prepared to assist in the recommended shoulder dystocia manipulations as the health care provider instructs. Refer to Table 28-3 for various sequential maneuvers or assist with the Gaskin maneuver. With this maneuver, the mother immediately assumes the "all fours" position (on her hands and knees). This is believed to increase the pelvic size and make use of the forces of gravity (Bruner and others, 1998; Jukelevics, 2000). The McRoberts maneuver can be done in this position.
- Fundal pressure alone is to be avoided because of the potential neurologic complications (Nocon, 2000; Simpson and Knox, 2001; Minkin, 2004).
- Superpubic pressure may be applied over the fetal shoulder.
- Be prepared to assist the patient to roll to all-fours position if instructed.
- Following the delivery, assess the baby's Moro reflex, check for a fractured clavicle or humerus, and if ordered, obtain cord blood for pH. A complete symmetric Moro response usually indicates no brachial plexus injury, which is the most common serious resulting injury (Benedetti, 1991; Nocon, 2000). Increased intracranial pressure and hypoxia occur less often.
- If an injury occurred, be prepared to discuss the possible outcomes with the parents after the pediatrician has spoken with them. Approximately 80% of these injuries resolve and cause no permanent damage with appropriate treatment (Baxley and Gobbo, 2004).
- Assess for postpartum hemorrhage because this is the greatest risk to the mother from a shoulder dystocia. The hemorrhage is usually related to uterine atony or vaginal or cervical lacerations (Gherman, 2006). Other maternal trauma can include bladder injury, vaginal hematoma, uterine rupture, or endometritis.

Management of External Version
Preprocedural

- Evaluate the patient's and her coach's understanding of the procedure. Greater than 50% of all attempted external versions are successful with a very low reversion rate (Simm and Woods, 2004).
- Evaluate the patient's and her coach's understanding of the advantage and the risks of version. The advantage is decreased cesarean birth rate. Potential risks include failed version, reversion, fetal stress related to cord entanglement or abruption, ruptured uterus, and abruptio placentae (Edelstone, 2000).
- Evaluate the patient's and her coach's understanding of alternatives to version. Postural exercises, visualization, and taped music or voices have been effectively used as alternatives to version. Assuming an upright, forward leaning position at times during the day and sleeping with pillows

Table 28-3   Sequential Shoulder Dystocia Maneuvers

Name	Benefits and Risks	Maneuver
McRoberts maneuver (Fig. 28-16)	Noninvasive Safe Straightens sacrum and decreases angle of incline of symphysis pubis Dislodges impacted shoulder 90% of time (Gonik and others, 1989)	Assist by grasping mother's posterior thighs and flexing them against her abdomen Fundal pressure is usually inappropriate because it may further affect anterior shoulder against symphysis and increase risk of a brachial plexus injury (Gherman and Gudwin, 1998; Simpson and Knox, 2001)
Suprapubic pressure (Figs. 28-17 and 28-18)	Noninvasive Second maneuver to be used because it may cause a clavicular fracture	Assist by exerting firm downward or oblique pressure on anterior shoulder just above symphysis pubis Instruct mother to push during this maneuver
Woods screw maneuver (Fig. 28-19)	Invasive technique Thought to attempt to unscrew fetus like a bolt is unscrewed from a nut (Horger, 1995)	Health care deliverer intravaginally applies pressure against posterior shoulder, rotating it to an anterior position Health care deliverer may request suprapubic pressure during maneuver to help keep anterior shoulder adducted (Naef and Martin, 1995)
Rubin rotational maneuver or reverse Woods screw maneuver (Fig. 28-20)	Invasive technique	Health care deliverer intravaginally applies pressure against scapula of anterior shoulder and rotates it forward 180° Health care deliverer may request suprapubic pressure during maneuver to help keep anterior shoulder adducted (O'Leary, 1992)
Delivery of posterior arm (Fig. 28-21)	Invasive Requires a large episiotomy Risk of humerus fracture	Health care deliverer intravaginally applies pressure at antecubital fossa, which causes fetal arm to flex, at which time it is grasped and drawn across chest and toward opposite side of fetal face
Cephalic replacement	Last resort	Health care deliverer returns fetal head to maternal pelvis, followed by an emergency cesarean birth

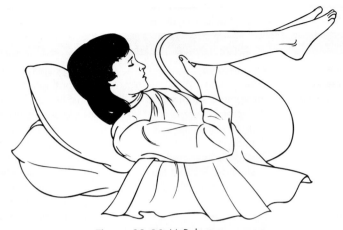

Figure 28-16 McRoberts maneuver.

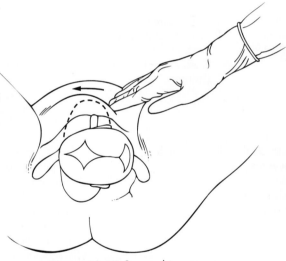

Figure 28-17 Suprapubic pressure.

behind the back and the top leg resting forward may facilitate occiput anterior (OA) fetal presentation (Sutton and Scott, 1996; Founds, 2005). Instruct the patient to relax during the exercise and visualize the baby turning. Music can be played on the lower abdomen to encourage the baby to turn. Without any random controlled trial studies, the effectiveness of these alternative practices is unknown. Moxibustion, a form of Chinese medicine that involves burning herbs close to the skin, has shown some possibility of converting a breech presentation to cephalic. According to a Cochrane Review, further study is needed (Coyle, Smith, and Peat, 2005).

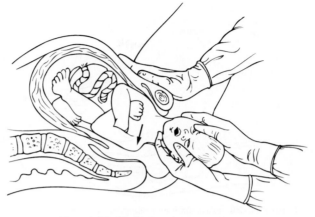

Figure 28-18 Suprapubic pressure.

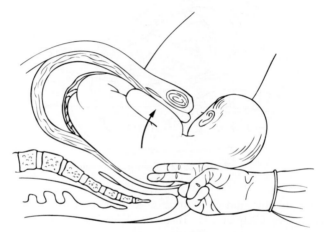

Figure 28-19 Woods screw maneuver.

- Advise the parents that even if the version is successful, the fetus is more likely to develop signs of fetal stress during labor and there is a greater risk for labor dystocia and need for a cesarean delivery (Edelstone, 2000). This may be related to factors that caused the fetus to present breech.

Intraprocedural

- Obtain a baseline FHR strip for 15 to 30 minutes before the procedure.
- Assist with a preliminary ultrasound examination to locate placenta, fetal lie, estimated size, volume of amniotic fluid, and presence of fetal anomalies. In the presence of a nuchal cord, version is not attempted.
- Start an IV infusion, as ordered, with an 18-gauge intracatheter.
- Be prepared to administer piggyback tocolytic agent before and continuously throughout the procedure. The solution usually is prepared in the

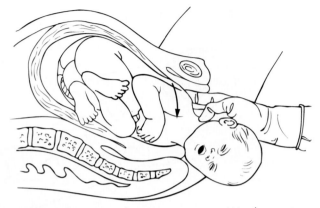

Figure 28-20 Rubin rotational maneuver or reverse Woods screw maneuver.

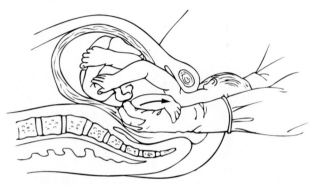

Figure 28-21 Delivery of posterior arm.

same manner and concentration as that used for tocolysis in premature labor (see Chapter 21). Tocolytics have been shown to improve success (Hofmeyr and Gyte, 2004)

- Monitor the FHR every few minutes during the procedure with a Doppler instrument.
- If fetal compromise develops, be prepared to assist with an emergency cesarean delivery.

Postprocedural

- After the procedure, discontinue the tocolytic agent and reapply FHR and contraction monitors. Monitor FHR and uterine contraction pattern approximately 30 to 60 minutes after the version.
- Be prepared to administer RhD immune globulin (RhoGAM; HypRho-D) following the procedure if the mother is D-negative.

Intrapartum Care

- Consider the patient high risk and monitor carefully for dystocia and fetal stress following a version.

Antepartum Management of Vaginal Birth After Cesarean

- Discuss the risks and benefits of a VBAC with every pregnant woman who had a previous lower segment transverse incision cesarean delivery to attempt a vaginal delivery (ACOG, 2004; Dodd and others, 2004).
- Teach the pregnant woman who had prior cesarean delivery and her family early in the current pregnancy regarding the positive chances of a vaginal delivery (60% to 80%) (Bujold and Gauthier, 2001; Hibbard and others, 2001; Chauhan and others, 2003).
- Help the woman and her partner weigh their options, identify the reasons for their choice, and then support their choice (Roberts and others, 1997; Zwelling, 2001; ACOG, 2004).
- Participate in the formation of support groups and childbirth classes for couples planning a VBAC.
- Be involved with childbirth education training to increase childbirth educators' awareness and knowledge regarding VBAC, to emphasize the importance of appropriate adequate nutrition, and to improve the outcome of the pregnancy, labor, and delivery.

Intrapartum Management of Vaginal Birth After a Cesarean–Trial of Labor

- Note that VBAC-TOL standards are to include an available physician immediately and to respond to acute emergency by performing a cesarean within a short time (ACOG, 2004).
- Individualize the management of care based on a family assessment of physical and psychologic factors.
- Determine the family's birth plan for vaginal delivery and a contingency plan in the event that complications arise.
- Use effective physiologic techniques for promoting labor.
- Use effective psychologic techniques to promote labor. Determine first what the family's perception of the previous cesarean birth experience is, their concerns, and their expectations. Determine whether their expectations of themselves are realistic. It is important to prevent the patient from feeling like she failed or is less of a woman if she is unable to deliver vaginally.
- Evaluate the terminology used, such as "successful VBAC" or "failed trial of labor," when talking to the patient and her family.
- Assess FHR according to ACOG's standard of practice for a normal labor patient (see Chapter 3).
- Create IV access and make blood products available if that is the protocol for the institution and the status of the patient requires it.
- Assess for signs of scar separation. The most common sign is a variable FHR deceleration that evolves into a late deceleration or bradycardia and blood-stained amniotic fluid (ICSI, 2005). Other less common signs are hematuria, vaginal bleeding, alterations in uterine contractions, and abdominal pain that continues in between contractions.

- Use epidural anesthesia, if needed; it has not been found to be contraindicated (ACOG, 2004; ICSI, 2005).
- Notify the attending physician immediately of any signs of fetal compromise or uterine scar separation.
- Use oxytocin during labor if there is an obstetric indication for it; it is not contraindicated, as once thought, in the patient attempting a VBAC. Close monitoring, however, is important to prevent hyperstimulation, which can increase the risk for uterine rupture (ACOG, 2004; ICEA, 2005). Because of the increased risk for uterine rupture with prostaglandin use, it is not recommended.
- Progress of labor during the trial of labor should progress according to the norm of 1 cm/hr in active labor and second-stage labor not to last longer than 2 hours. A delay indicates a more aggressive intervention than for a normal low risk patient (Gee, 2000; Gee, 2006).
- Repeat cesarean may become necessary for failure to progress, fetal distress, maternal complication, or uterine rupture.
- As a patient advocate, the nurse may be the spokesperson for women experiencing a VBAC. For example, routine manual exploration of the uterus following a VBAC delivery is usually painful, it may increase the risk for a postpartum infection, and its routine benefit has not been demonstrated by research (Enkin and others, 2000; ICSI, 2005).

Management of Instrumental Delivery with Forceps or a Vacuum Extractor

- Promote preventive nursing management during labor to lower the need for assisted vaginal delivery. This includes the following:
- Provide continuous labor support.
- Encourage use of the upright position.
- Encourage delay in initiating pushing during second-stage labor unless there is an urge to push (Cargill and others, 2004).
- Revise the 2-hour limit for stage two to longer if there is no indication of fetal stress.
- Use fetal scalp blood sampling in the presence of nonreassuring fetal status to determine real need for assisted delivery.
- Provide supportive techniques in labor to decrease the need for epidural anesthesia. Epidural anesthesia increases the frequency of instrument-assisted delivery (Thorp and Breedlove, 1996; Anim-Somuah, Smyth, and Howell, 2005). If an epidural is indicated, allow time for it to wear off before encouraging pushing.
- When delayed progress in second stage or decreased head rotation is noted, (1) encourage the patient to try various positions such as "all fours" or squatting, (2) check for maternal hydration, (3) check for a full bladder, and (4) assess pushing techniques, to decrease the need for forceps or vacuum use or if necessary make the procedure easier (Roberts and Woolley, 1996).

- Provide educational opportunities for expectant parents to learn about the technique of forceps or vacuum extraction and reasons for their use to decrease anxiety in the event either is needed. The most common reasons for instrument use are delayed progress in second-stage labor, a nonreassuring FHR pattern in late second-stage labor, or medical factors prohibiting effective maternal pushing.

- Provide supportive care in the event that instrument assistance is needed by encouraging the mother to remain active in the birth process by continuing to push with each contraction unless there is a medical contraindication.

- Encourage the patient to continue to feel in control by verbally reassuring her that she is continuing to facilitate the delivery by her pushing efforts.

- Assist with appropriate anesthesia for forceps delivery. Anesthesia may not be necessary for a vacuum extraction.

- Following the delivery, encourage parents to express their feelings about the procedure to resolve any negative feelings.

- Following forceps delivery, observe the infant for facial nerve trauma, ecchymoses, and forceps marks. Assure the parents that these are only temporary effects and tell them when they can expect them to disappear. Other more series birth injuries may include brachial plexus injury, intracranial hemorrhage, or spinal cord injury. The risk is lowest with low-outlet forceps and increases with midforceps deliveries.

- After a vacuum delivery, assess the infant for caput succedaneum or cephalhematoma. If either is present, reassure the parents that it usually disappears in 3 to 5 days. After a cephalhematoma, teach the parents to observe their infant for hyperbilirubinemia, signs of infection, and cerebral irritation and to report any signs to their pediatrician. Discuss signs of cerebral irritation: vomiting, high-pitched cry, and neck and spine rigidity.

- Assess for a clavicle fracture during the infant's routine physical examination. Positive findings are edema, crepitus, and lack of movement of the affected limb.

- After an instrumental delivery, observe the mother for soft tissue trauma such as birth canal and perineal lacerations, bladder dysfunction, and vaginal hematoma (Evans and Edelstone, 2000).

- If the neonate is sleepy and sucks poorly, explain to the parents that this is a normal response following a difficult delivery and does not indicate any problem.

Management of Intrapartum Epidural
Preprocedural

- Ensure that information is provided, preferably before labor, regarding the procedural steps of epidural administration, maternal and fetal risks and benefits, alternative methods of pain relief, costs, and expected restrictions in movement related to the epidural.

- According to the *Cochrane Review* (Anim-Somuah, Smyth, and Howell, 2005), epidural anesthesia is the most highly effective method of pain relief for labor and delivery but it is not without potentially adverse side effects. A prolonged labor caused by anxiety may be speeded up. Hypotension is the most common side effect of an epidural and is nearly always preventable with a fluid load. However, an epidural may increase the length of first and second stages of a normal labor, increasing the need for oxytocin. It may also decrease the bearing-down reflex, thereby increasing the need for episiotomy or forceps or vacuum extraction. There is an increased incidence of maternal fever as well (Newman, Lindsay, and Graves, 2001; Alexander and others, 2002; Goetzl and others, 2003; Anim-Somuah, Smyth, and Howell, 2005).
- Undesired effects on the newborn include irritability, inconsolability, uncoordinated suck, and decreased responsiveness (Simkin, 1991; Ransjo-Arvidson and others, 2001). These effects have been show to interfere with the newborn's spontaneous breastseeking and breastfeeding behaviors (Ransjo-Arvidson and others, 2001; Baumgarder and others, 2003).
- Provide information regarding other medical interventions that often accompany use of an epidural. Those that are always necessary include IV therapy, continuous FHR monitoring, and frequent blood pressure monitoring. Medical interventions that are frequently needed are oxytocin to augment labor contractions and urinary catheterization.
- Facilitate use of other methods of pain relief by the laboring woman and attempt to delay epidural placement until active phase of labor (Gregory, 2000; Smith and others, 2003). Recognize when the patient needs an epidural analgesia (ACOG, 2004). Become familiar with alternative techniques such as low dose epidural analgesia without heavy motor block, a patient-controlled epidural, intrathecal narcotic analgesia (Youngstrom, Baker, and Miller, 1996; Shermer and Raines, 1997; Hughes and others, 2003).
- Start an IV infusion and administer a preload of 500 to 1000 ml of fluid as ordered to decrease the risk for hypotension (ACOG, 2003a; Hofmeyr, Cyna, Middleton, 2004).
- Obtain baseline maternal vital signs and an FHR tracing.
- Have patient empty her bladder just before the procedure.
- Prepare emergency equipment at the bedside, such as oxygen and suction equipment.
- Make sure that resuscitation bag and mask and resuscitation drugs are readily available (ACOG, 1996).

Procedure

- Position the patient in either a lateral decubitus or a sitting position with head and hips flexed and shoulders and hips squared to facilitate the insertion by a licensed anesthesia provider (AWHONN, 2001).
- Provide ongoing emotional support and information to the patient.

Postinjection

- Position patient on her side with head of bed elevated 30 degrees. Encourage position change at least every 30 minutes.
- Continuously monitor FHR.
- Check for signs of respiratory depression related to accidental administration of the medication into the spinal space. (Similar medications are used for spinal anesthesia, but much smaller doses are used.)
- Check blood pressure every 15 minutes following an epidural, until delivery, because maternal hypotension can occur resulting from vasodilation.
- If hypotension develops, turn patient on left side, elevate her legs, increase the IV fluid, administer oxygen, notify the anesthesiologist or nurse anesthetist, and be prepared to administer ephedrine if ordered.
- Assess temperature.
- Keep an accurate intake and output record. Encourage the laboring patient to void every 2 to 4 hours. (Epidural anesthesia blocks sensations of a full bladder.)
- Assess for other side effects such as toxicity to the drugs, breakthrough pain, and dural puncture that can cause a postdural headache.
- If ambulatory epidural or intrathecal analgesia is used, evaluate for ambulation safety that includes no postural hypotension, normal leg strength as demonstrated by performance of a partial knee bend while standing, and assistance with ambulation at all times.
- Delay pushing after full dilation if fetal descent is less than +1 and there is a lack of the Ferguson or bearing-down reflex. This delay will lower the need for instrumental deliveries (Enkin and others, 2000).

Management of Postpartum Epidural Analgesia

Preprocedural

- Evaluate patient's understanding of epidural analgesia if it is to be used in the event of a cesarean birth or fourth-degree laceration during vaginal delivery. Usual procedure is 4 or 5 mg of morphine analgesic injected through the epidural catheter at the close of the surgical repair. Maternal benefits include prolonged pain relief for 24 hours, ambulation, interaction with infant with minimal discomfort, and earlier recovery. Some patients experience side effects of respiratory depression, itching, nausea, vomiting, or urinary retention, but these side effects are generally mild.
- Assist in obtaining an informed consent.

Postprocedural

- Assess respiratory rate often. A typical assessment routine may be every 15 minutes for 2 hours, every 30 minutes for 6 hours (total of 8 hours after injection), and every 1 hour for 16 hours (total of 24 hours after injection).

- Assess for itching and nausea or vomiting per observational check while patient is awake.
- Keep accurate intake and output record.
- If a Foley catheter is present, do not remove it for 14 to 16 hours after delivery. If urinary retention occurs, it usually develops early and is resolved by 14 to 16 hours after administration of medication.
- Be prepared to administer naloxone (Narcan), 0.04 to 0.40 mg, as ordered, if side effects develop.
- A low naloxone dose of 0.04 mg frequently alleviates mild side effects and does not diminish the analgesic effect.
- Notify physician of the development of side effects and responsiveness to ordered treatment.

Management of Cesarean Birth

Preoperative

In accordance with *Healthy People 2010* objectives (USDHHS, 2000), decrease the incidence of primary cesarean delivery among low risk full-term singleton vertex presentations by maintaining a positive attitude toward the laboring woman, supporting normal physiologic processes of labor, and implementing a variety of nontechnologic nursing interventions. (See nursing diagnosis on interventions to enhance labor progress through each of the 11 functional health patterns.)

- Be prepared to manage the family that refuses a cesarean delivery in the presence of fetal or maternal medical indicators and the family that demands a cesarean without any medical indication.
- If cesarean delivery becomes medically or obstetrically necessary, assess the couple's understanding of the reason for the cesarean and advocate for a complete informed consent.
- Involve the couple in as much of the decision-making process as possible to increase feeling of control.
- Support the coach in being able to provide support during the cesarean delivery.
- Emphasize that cesarean delivery is an "alternative birth method," and encourage "family-centered options" where possible.
- Start an IV infusion with an 18-gauge intracatheter.
- Shave the abdomen from the xiphoid process to about 5 cm (2 in) below the pubic hairline.
- Insert a Foley catheter, and connect it to continuous drainage to decrease the risk for bladder trauma during the surgery. This frequently can be inserted after the administration of the anesthetic to decrease the discomfort of the procedure.
- Check to see whether laboratory work has been done, such as complete blood count, blood typed and cross-matched for two units, and urinalysis.
- Preferred anesthesia is regional.
- Have equipment available for monitoring a pulse oximetry.

Postoperative

- Be prepared to administer prophylactic antibiotics. They are frequently started just after the clamping of the umbilical cord. Endomyometritis is the most common complication following a cesarean delivery, occurring in 35% to 40% of women; prophylactic antibiotics reduce the risk to approximately 5% (DeMott, 2000; ACOG, 2003b). A narrow-spectrum antibiotic such as a first-generation cephalosporin, should be used for prophylaxis (ACOG, 2003b).

- Keep in mind that the patient is foremost a new mother. Help her find success in her mothering role within postsurgical limits.

- Assess for signs of hemorrhage by recording blood pressure, pulse, and respirations according to protocol. A typical assessment routine may be every 15 minutes for eight times, every 30 minutes for two times, every 4 hours for two times, and then routinely. Check firmness of uterus and vaginal flow with each vital signs check. Keep a pad count.

- Manually massage a relaxed, boggy fundus very gently until firm, and maintain oxytocin and IV fluids as ordered.

- Assess for signs of an infection by checking temperature every 4 hours for 48 hours; if higher than 38° C (100.4° F), check every 2 hours. Check lochia every shift for odor.

- Encourage abdominal tightening exercises and early ambulation to decrease the risk for gas pains.

- Give patient nothing to eat or drink until bowel sounds are present. Then give patient full liquids until she passes flatus. Then a soft or regular diet can be given.

- Encourage coughing and deep breathing to decrease the risk for respiratory infection.

- Measure the first two voidings after the Foley catheter is removed. Assess for burning on urination and blood in the urine.

- Initiate prophylaxis against thromboembolism by early ambulation and adequate hydration. If the woman is at increase risk, she should be on prophylactic heparin therapy. If she is at high risk, she should also wear graduated stockings.

- Notify physician if uterus fails to contract or stay contracted with massage, temperature is over 38° C, lochia develops an odor, the incision site shows signs of an infection, or the patient complains of burning on urination.

- During the woman's postpartum hospital stay, encourage the couple to verbalize their feelings about the cesarean delivery. The mother who experiences an unexpected cesarean delivery often relates a feeling of guilt or failure because she was unable to achieve a vaginal delivery (Murphy and others, 2003).

- Reassure the couple they did not fail and reiterate the reason for the alternative birth method.

- If the couple expresses extreme failure, refer to a local cesarean birth support group or to therapy.

CONCLUSION

The ultimate goal for any patient during labor is normal labor progression with absence of nonreassuring fetal responses. The nurse can have a significant influence on the progress of labor by using evidence-based practice, imparting confidence in the patient's ability to deliver vaginally and using a variety of therapeutic, nontechnologic techniques to facilitate labor (Radin, Harmon, and Hanson, 1993). Other factors beyond the nurse's control, however, can impede labor. The nurse must assess these factors and report them to the attending health care provider immediately. The medical team should then work together to facilitate the labor and delivery for the best maternal and neonatal outcome.

BIBLIOGRAPHY
Breech Management: External Version and Selected Vaginal Breech Delivery

American College of Obstetricians and Gynecologists: Mode of term singleton breech delivery, *ACOG Committee Opinion*, No. 265, Washington, DC, 2001. Author.

Coyle ME, Smith CA, and Peat B: Cephalic version by moxibustion for breech presentation, *Cochrane Database Syst Rev* Issue 2, 2005.

Edelstone D: Breech presentation. In Kean L, Baker P, and Edelstone D, editors: *Best practice in labor ward management*, Philadelphia, 2000, Saunders.

Founds S: Maternal posture for cephalic version of breech presentation: a review of the evidence, *Birth* 32(2):137–144, 2005.

Hannah M and others: Planned caesarean section versus planned vaginal birth for breech presentation at term: a randomized multicentre trail, *Lancet* 356(9239):1375–1383, 2000.

Hofmeyr GJ, Gyte G: Interventions to help external cephalic version for breech presentation at term, *Cochrane Database Syst Rev* Issue 1, 2004.

Hofmeyr GJ, Hannah ME: Planned caesarean section for term breech delivery, *Cochrane Database Syst Rev* Issue 2, 2003.

Hutton EK, Hofmeyr GJ: External cephalic version for breech presentation before term, *Cochrane Database Syst Rev* Issue 1, 2006.

Lau T, Lo KW, and Rogers M: Pregnancy outcome after successful external cephalic version for breech presentation at term, *Am J Obstet Gynecol* 176(1 Pt 1):218–223, 1997.

Sutton J, Scott P: *Understanding teaching optional fetal positioning*, Tauranga, New Zealand, 1996, Birth Concepts.

Thacker S, Stroup D, and Chang M: Continuous electronic heart rate monitoring for fetal assessment during labor (Cochrane Review). In *The Cochrane Library*, Issue 2, Oxford, 2001, Update Software.

Cesarean Delivery

American College of Obstetricians and Gynecologists: Dystocia and the augmentation of labor, *ACOG Practice Bulletin*, No. 49, Washington, DC, 2003a, ACOG.

American College of Obstetricians and Gynecologists: Prophylactic antibiotics in labor and delivery, *ACOG Practice Bulletin*, No. 47, Washington, DC, 2003b, ACOG.

Ananth C, Smulian J, and Vintzileos A: The association of placenta previa with history of cesarean delivery and abortion: A meta-analysis, *Am J Obstet Gynecol* 177:1071–1078, 1997.

Bager P and others: Mode of delivery and risk of allergic rhinitis and asthma, *J Allergy Clin Immunol* 111(1):51–56, 2003.

Bernstein P: Complications of cesarean deliveries, *Medscape*, September 15, 2005.

Dessole S and others: Accidental fetal lacerations during cesarean delivery: experience in an Italian level III university hospital, *Am J Obstet Gynecol* 191(5):1673–1677, 2004.

DeMott R: Cesarean birth. In Kean L, Baker P, and Edelstone D, editors: *Best practice in labor ward management*, Philadelphia, 2000, Saunders.

Dickinson J: Cesarean section. In James D and others, editors: *High risk pregnancy: management options,* ed 3, Philadelphia, 2006, Saunders.

Drudge Report: *The demise of natural childbirth,* June 13, 2001.

Enkin M and others: *A guide to effective care in pregnancy and childbirth,* ed 3, New York, 2000, Oxford University Press.

Friedman E: Dystocia failure to progress in labor. In Flamm B, Quilligan E, editors: *Cesarean section: guidelines for appropriate utilization,* New York, 1995, Springer-Verlag.

Gamble J, Creedy D: Women's preference for a cesarean section: incidence and associated factors, *Birth* 28(2):101, 2001.

Gifford D and others: Lack of progress in labor as a reason for cesarean, *Obstet Gynecol* 95(4):589–595, 2000.

Gregory K: Monitoring, risk adjustment and strategies to decrease cesarean rates, *Curr Opin Obstet Gynecol* 12(6):481–486, 2000.

Hakansson S, Kallen K: Caesarean section increases the risk of hospital care in childhood for asthma and gastroenteritis, *Clin Exp Allergy* 33(6):757–764, 2003.

Harper M and others: Pregnancy-related death and health care services, *Obstet Gynecol* 102(2):273–278, 2003.

Hayashi R: Obstetric collapse. In Kean L, Baker P, and Edelstone D, editors: *Best practice in labor ward management,* Philadelphia, 2000, Saunders.

Kacmar J and others: Route of delivery as a risk factor for emergent peripartum hysterectomy: A case-control study, *Obstet Gynecol* 102(1):141–145, 2003.

Levine E and others: Mode of delivery and risk of respiratory disease in newborns, *Obstet Gynecol* 97(3):439–442, 2001.

Miller D, Chollet J, and Goodwin T: Clinical risk factors for placenta previa-placenta accreta, *Am J Obstet Gynecol* 177(1):210–214, 1997.

Radin T, Harmon J, and Hanson D: Nurses' care during labor: its effect on the cesarean birth rate of healthy, nulliparous women, *Birth* 20(1):14–21, 1993.

Seyb S and others: Risk of cesarean delivery with elective induction of labor at term in nulliparous women, *Obstet Gynecol* 94(4):600–607, 1999.

Towner D and others: Effect of mode of delivery in nulliparous women on neonatal intracranial injury, *N Engl J Med* 341(23):1709–1714, 1999.

U.S. Department of Health and Human Services: *Healthy People 2010: understanding and improving health,* Washington, DC, 2000, USDHHS.

Wen S and others: Comparison of maternal mortality and morbidity between trial of labor and elective cesarean section among women with previous cesarean delivery, *Am J Obstet Gynecol* 191(4):1263–1269, 2004.

U.S. Department of Health and Human Services: *Women's health USA 2005,* Rockville, Md, 2005, USDHHS.

Dysfunctional Labor

American College of Obstetricians and Gynecologists: Dystocia and the augmentation of labor, *ACOG Practice Bulletin,* No. 49, Washington, DC, 2003a, ACOG.

Bowes W, Thorp J: Clinical aspects of normal abnormal labor. In Creasy R, Resnik R, and Iams J, editors: *Maternal-fetal medicine: principles and practice,* ed 5, Philadelphia, 2004, Saunders.

Cammu H, Van Eeckhout E: A randomised controlled trial of early versus delayed use of amniotomy and oxytocin infusion in nulliparous labour, *Br J Obstet Gynaecol* 103(4):313–318, 1996.

Cesario S: Reevaluation of Friedman's labor curve: a pilot study, *J Obstet Gynecol Neonatal Nurs* 33(6):713–722, 2004.

Fraser W and others: Risk factors for difficult delivery in nulliparas with epidural analgesia in the second stage of labor, *Am J Obstet Gynecol* 99:409–418, 2002.

Fraser WD and others: Amniotomy for shortening spontaneous labour, *Cochrane Database Syst Rev* Issue 1, 2000.

Friedman E: Dystocia failure to progress in labor. In Flamm B, Quilligan E, editors: *Cesarean section: guidelines for appropriate utilization,* New York, 1995, Springer-Verlag.

Gee H: Abnormal patterns of labor prolonged labor. In Kean L, Baker P, and Edelstone D, editors: *Best practice in labor ward management,* Philadelphia, 2000, Saunders.

Gee H: Poor progress in labor. In James D and others, editors: *High risk pregnancy: management options,* ed 3, Philadelphia, 2006, Saunders.

Lau T and others: Predictors of successful ECV at term, *BJOG* 104:798–802, 1997.

Liao J, Buhimschi C, and Norwitz E: Normal labor: mechanism and duration, *Obstet Gynecol Clin North Am* 32(2):145–164, 2004.

Martin W and Hutchon S: Mechanism and management of normal labour, *Curr Obstet & Gynecol* 14(5):301–308, 2004.

Morton S, William M, Keeler E: Effect of epidural analgesia for labour on the cesarean delivery date, *Obstet Gynecol* 83:1045, 1994.

Myles T, Santolaya J: Maternal and neonatal outcomes inpatients with a prolonged second stage, *Obstet Gynecol* 102(1):52–58, 2003.

Ness A, Goldberg J, and Berghella V: Abnormalities of the first and second stages of labor, *Obstet Gynecol Clin North Am* 32(2):201–220, 2004.

O'Driscoll K, Meagher D, and Robson M: *Active management of labour,* ed 4, Edinburgh, 2004, Mosby Ltd.

Rouse D, Owen J, and Hauth J: Active-phase labor arrest: Oxytocin augmentation for a least 4 hours, *Obstet Gynecol* 93(3):323–328, 1999.

Rouse D and others: Active phase labor arrest: revisiting the 2 hour minimum, *Obstet Gynecol* 98(4):550–554, 2001.

Sheiner E and others: Risk factors and outcome of failure to progress during the first stage of labor: a population based study, *Acta Obstet Gynecol Scand* 81(3):222–226, 2002.

Simm A, Woods A: Fetal malpresentation, *Curr Obstet Gynecol* 14(4):231–238, 2004.

Stitely M, Gherman R: Labor with abnormal presentation and position, *Obstet Gynecol Clin North Am* 32(2):165–179, 2005.

Thorp J and others: The effect of intrapartum epidural analgesia on nulliparous labor: a randomized, controlled, prospective trial, *Am J Obstet Gynecol* 169:851, 1993.

VandeVusse L: The essential forces of labor revisited: 13 P's reported in women's stories, *MCN Am J Matern Child Nurs* 24(4):176–184, 1999.

Zhang J, Troendle J, and Yancey M: Reassessing the labor curve in nulliparous women, *Am J Obstet Gynecol* 187(4):824–828, 2002.

Epidural Analgesia and Anesthesia: Intrapartum Management

American College of Obstetricians and Gynecologists: Pain relief during labor, *ACOG Committee Opinion,* No. 295, Washington, DC, 2004, ACOG.

Alexander J and others: Epidural analgesia lengthens the Friedman active phase of labor, *Obstet Gynecol* 100(1):46–50, 2002.

American College of Obstetricians and Gynecologists: Obstetric analgesia and anesthesia, *ACOG Technical Bulletin,* No. 225, 1996.

Anim-Somuah M, Smyth R, and Howell C: Epidural versus non-epidural or no analgesia in labour, *Cochrane Database Syst Rev* Issue 4, 2005.

Association of Women's Health, Obstetric, and Neonatal Nurses: *Evidence-based clinical practice guideline: nursing care of the woman receiving analgesia/anesthesia in labor,* Washington, DC, 2001, AWHONN.

Baumgarder D and others: Effect of labor epidural anesthesia on breast-feeding of healthy full-term newborns delivered vaginally, *J Am Board Fam Pract* 16(1):7–13, 2003.

Emmett RS and others: Techniques for preventing hypotension during spinal anaesthesia for caesarean section, *Cochrane Database Syst Rev* Issue 3, 2002.

Enkin M and others: *A guide to effective care in pregnancy and childbirth,* ed 3, New York, 2000, Oxford University Press.

Goetzl L and others: Maternal epidural analgesia and rates of maternal antibiotic treatment in a low-risk nulliparous population, *J Perinatol* 23(6):457–461, 2003.

Gregory K: Monitoring, risk adjustment and strategies to decrease cesarean rates, *Curr Opin Obstet Gynecol* 12(6):481–486, 2000.

Gupta JK, Hofmeyr GJ: Position in the second stage of labour for women without epidural anaesthesia, *Cochrane Database Syst Rev* Issue 1, 2004.

Hofmeyr GJ, Cyna AM, and Middleton P: Prophylactic intravenous preloading for regional analgesia in labour, *Cochrane Database Syst Rev* Issue 4, 2004.

Hughes D and others: Combined spinal-epidural versus epidural analgesia in labour, *Cochrane Database Syst Rev* Issue 4, 2003.

Lieberman E, O'Donoghue C: Unintended effects of epidural analgesia during labor: a systematic review, *Am J Obstet Gynecol* 186(5 Suppl Nature):S31–S68, 2002.

Morton S and others: Effect of epidural analgesia for labor on the cesarean delivery rate, *Obstet Gynecol* 83(6):1045–1052, 1994.

Newman M, Lindsay M, and Graves W: The effect of epidural analgesia on rates of episiotomy use and episiotomy extension in an inner-city hospital, *J Matern Fetal Med* 10(2):97–101, 2001.

Ransjo-Arvidson A and others: Maternal analgesia during labor disturbs newborn behavior: effects on breastfeeding, temperature, and crying, *Birth* 28(1):5–12, 2001.

Rush J and others: The effects of whirlpool baths in labor: a randomized, controlled trial, *Birth* 23(3):136–143, 1996.

Shermer R, Raines D: Positioning during the second stage of labor: moving back to basics, *J Obstet Gynecol Neonatal Nurs* 26(6):727–734, 1997.

Simkin P: Weighting the pros and cons of the epidural, *Childbirth Forum*, pp 1, 3, Fall, 1991.

Smith CA and others: Complementary and alternative therapies for pain management in labour, *Cochrane Database Syst Rev* Issue 2, 2003.

Thorp J and others: The effect of intrapartum epidural analgesia on nulliparous labor: a randomized, controlled, prospective trial, *Am J Obstet Gynecol* 169:851, 1993.

Torvaldsen S and others: Discontinuation of epidural analgesia late in labour for reducing the adverse delivery outcomes associated with epidural analgesia, *Cochrane Database Syst Rev* Issue 4, 2004.

Vause S, Congdon H, and Thornton J: Immediate and delayed pushing in the second stage of labour for nulliparous women with epidural analgesia: a randomized controlled trial, *Br J Obstet Gynaecol* 105(2):186–188, 1998.

Youngstrom P, Baker S, and Miller J: Epidural redefined in analgesia and anesthesia: a distinction with a difference, *J Obstet Gynecol Neonatal Nurs* 25(4):350–354, 1996.

Instrumental Delivery: Forceps and Vacuum

American College of Obstetricians and Gynecologists: Operative vaginal delivery, *ACOG Practice Bulletin*, No. 17, Washington, DC, 2000, ACOG.

Evans W, Edelstone D: Instrumental delivery. In Kean L, Baker P, and Edelstone D, editors: *Best practice in labor ward management*, Philadelphia, 2000, Saunders.

Johanson R, Menon V: Soft versus rigid vacuum extractor cups for assisted vaginal delivery, *Cochrane Database Syst Rev* Issue 2, 2000.

O'Grady J, Pope C, and Patel S: Vacuum extraction in modern obstetric practice: a review and critique, *Curr Opin Obstet Gynecol* 12(6):475–480, 2000.

Patel R, Murphy D: Forceps delivery in modern obstetric practice, *BMJ* 328(7454): 1302–1305, 2004.

Nursing Management

Aderhold K, Roberts J: Phases of second stage labor, *J Nurse Midwifery* 36(5):267–275, 1991.

Aldrich C and others: The effect of maternal pushing on fetal cerebral oxygenation and blood volume during the second stage of labour, *Br J Obstet Gynecol* 102:448, 1995.

Association of Women's Health, Obstetric, and Neonatal Nurses: *Issue: professional nursing support of laboring women*, Washington, DC, 2000, AWHONN.

Beckmann M, Garrett A: Antenatal perineal massage for reducing perineal trauma, *Cochrane Database Syst Rev* Issue 1, 2006.

Berry H: Feast or famine?. Oral intake during labour: current evidence and practice, *Br J Midwifery* 5:413, 1997.

Better Births Global Initiative: *Changes to obstetric practice*, Liverpool School of Tropical Medicine, UK, 2000, International Collaborative Group. Retrieved from *http://www.liv.ac.uk/lstm/bbimain-page.html*

Biancuzzo M: How to recognize and rotate an occiput posterior fetus, *Am J Nurs* 93(3): 38–41, 1993.

Biancuzzo M: The patient observer: does the hands and knees posture during labor help to rotate the occiput posterior fetus? *Birth* 18(1):40–47, 1991.

Bloom S and others: Lack of effect of walking on labor and delivery, *N Engl J Med* 339(2):76–79, 1998.

Broach J, Newton M: Food and beverages in labor, Part II: the effects of cessation of oral intake during labor, *Birth* 15(2):88–92, 1988.

Cargill YM and others: Clinical Practice Obstetrics Committee. Guidelines for operative vaginal birth, *J Obstet Gynaecol Can* 26(8):747–761, 2004.

Chen S and others: Effects of sitting position on uterine activity during labor, *Obstet Gynecol* 69(1):67–73, 1987.

Clapp J: The course of labor after endurance exercise during pregnancy, *Am J Obstet Gynecol* 163(6 Pt 1):1799–1805, 1990.

Cluett ER and others: Immersion in water in pregnancy, labour and birth, *Cochrane Database Syst Rev* Issue 2, 2002.

CNM Data Group: Oral intake in labor: trends in midwifery practice, *J Nurse Midwifery* 44(2):135–138, 1999.

Cook A, Wilcox G: Pressuring pain: alternative therapies for labor pain management, *AWHONN Lifelines* 1(2):36–41, 1997.

Copper R, Goldenberg R: Catecholamine secretion in fetal adaptation to stress, *J Obstet Gynecol Neonatal Nurs* 19(3):223–226, 1990.

Cosner K, deJong E: Physiologic second stage labor, *MCN Am J Matern Child Nurs* 18(1):38–43, 1993.

Crawford J: Maternal mortality from Mendelson's syndrome, *Lancet* 1(8486):920–921, 1986.

Di Franco J: Music for childbirth, *Childbirth Educator,* p 36, Fall, 1988.

Douglas M: The case against a more liberal food and fluid policy in labor, *Birth* 15(2):93–94, 1988.

Elkington K: At the water's edge: where obstetrics and anesthesia meet, *Obstet Gynecol* 77(2):304–308, 1991.

Enkin M and others: *A guide to effective care in pregnancy and childbirth,* ed 3, New York, 2000, Oxford University Press.

Fenwick L, Simkin P: Maternal positioning to prevent or alleviate dystocia in labor, *Clin Obstet Gynecol* 30(1):83–89, 1987.

Fowles E: Labor concerns of women two months after delivery, *Birth* 25(4):235–240, 1998.

Fraser W and others: Multicenter, randomized, controlled trial of delayed pushing for nulliparous women in the second stage of labor with continuous epidural analgesia: the PEOPLE study group, *Am J Obstet Gynecol* 182(5):1165–1172, 2000.

Fuller B, Roberts J, and McKay S: Acoustical analysis of maternal sounds during the second stage of labor, *Appl Nurs Res* 6(1):8–12, 1993.

Garite T and others: A randomized controlled trial of the effect of increased intravenous hydration on the course of labor in nulliparous women, *Am J Obstet Gynecol* 183(16):1544–1548, 2000.

Gentz B: Alternative therapies for the management of pain in labor and delivery, *Clin Obstet Gynecol* 44(4):704–732, 2001.

Gilder K and others: Maternal positioning in labor with epidural anesthesia: results from a multi-site survey, *AWHONN Lifelines* 6(1):40–45, 2002.

Golay J, Vedam S, and Sorger L: The squatting position for the second stage of labor: effects on labor and on maternal and fetal well-being, *Birth* 20(2):73–78, 1993.

Gupta J, Hofmeyr G: Position in the second stage of labour for women without epidural anaesthesia, *Cochrane Database Syst Rev* Issue 1, 2004.

Hansen S, Clark S, and Foster J: Active pushing versus passive fetal descent in the second stage of labor: a randomized controlled trial, *Obstet Gynecol* 99(1):29–34, 2002.

Hazle N: Hydration in labor: is routine intravenous hydration necessary? *J Nurse Midwifery* 31(4):171–176, 1986.

Hodnett E and others: Continuous support for women during childbirth, *Cochrane Database Syst Rev* Issue 3, 2003.

Hodnett E: Nursing support of the laboring woman, *J Obstet Gynecol Neonatal Nurs* 25(3): 257–264, 1996.

Hofmeyr G, Kulier R: Hands and knees posture in late pregnancy or labour for fetal malposition (lateral or posterior), *Cochrane Database Syst Rev* Issue 2, 2005.

Hottenstein S, Brit PipeT: Continuous labor support, *AWHONN Lifelines* 9(3):242–247, 2005.

Institute for Clinical Systems Improvement (ICSI): *Health care guideline: management of labor,* 2005, ICSI. Retrieved from *http://www.icsi.org*

Jackson D and others: Outcomes, safety, and resource utilization in a collaborative care birth center program compared with traditional physician-based perinatal care, *Am J Public Health* 93(6):999–1006, 2003.

Jannke S: Birth plans, *Childbirth Instructor Magazine* 5(3):26, 1995.

Johnson N, Johnson V, and Gupta J: Maternal positions during labor, *Obstet Gynecol Surv* 46(7):428–434, 1991.

Johnstone F, Aboelmagd M, and Harouny A: Maternal posture in second stage and fetal acid base status, *Br J Obstet Gynaecol* 94(8):753–757, 1987.

Jukelevics N: Big myths about big babies, *Childbirth Instructor* May/June, 18–23, 2000.

Kardong-Edgren S: Using evidence-based practice to improve intrapartum care, *J Obstet Gynecol Neonatal Nurs* 30(4):371–375, 2001.

Kelly M and others: A comparison of the effect of intrathecal and extradural Fentanyl on gastric emptying in laboring women, *Anesth Analg* 85(4):834–838, 1997.

Kennell J and others: Continuous emotional support during labor in a U.S. hospital: a randomized controlled trial, *JAMA* 265(17):2197–2201, 1991.

Keppler A: The use of intravenous fluids during labor, *Birth* 15(2):75–79, 1988.

Kubli M and others: An evaluation of isotonic sport drinks during labor, *Anesth Analg* 94(2):404–408, 2002.

Kurokawa J, Zilkoski M: Adapting hospital obstetrics to birth in the squatting position, *Birth* 12(2):87–90, 1985.

Lauzon L, Hodnett E: Caregivers' use of strict criteria for diagnosing active labour in term pregnancy (*Cochrane Review*). *The Cochrane Library,* Issue 3, Oxford, 2001, Update Software.

Lowe N: Maternal confidence in coping with labor: a self-efficacy concept, *J Obstet Gynecol Neonatal Nurs* 20(6):457–463, 1991.

Lowe N: The pain and discomfort of labor and birth, *J Obstet Gynecol Neonatal Nurs* 25(1):82–92, 1996.

Ludka L, Roberts C: Eating and drinking in labor: a literature review, *J Nurse Midwifery* 38(4):199–207, 1993.

Mackey M: Use of water in labor and birth, *Clin Obstet Gynecol* 44(4):733–749, 2001.

Manning J: Intrathecal narcotics: new approach for labor analgesia, *J Obstet Gynecol Neonatal Nurs* 25(3):221–224, 1996.

Maternity Center Association: *What every pregnant woman needs to know about cesarean section,* New York, 2004. Author. Retrieved from *http:www.maternitywise.org/cesareanbooklet*

Mayberry L and others: Maternal fatigue: implications of second stage labor nursing care, *J Obstet Gynecol Neonatal Nurs* 28(2):175–181, 1999.

Mayberry L and others: *Second stage labor management: promotion of evidence-based practice and a collaborative approach to patient care,* Washington, DC, 2000, AWHONN.

McCartney P: The birth ball-are you using it in your practice setting? *MCN Am J Matern Child Nurs* 23(4):218, 1998.

McKay S, Barrows T, Roberts J: Women's views of second stage labor as assessed by interviews and videotapes, *Birth* 17(4):192, 1990.

McKay S, Mahan C: Modifying the stomach contents of laboring women: why and how; success and risks, *Birth* 15(4):213–221, 1988.

McKay S, Roberts J: Maternal position during labor and birth: what have we learned? *IJCE* 13(2):9, 1989.

Miltner R: Identifying labor support actions of intrapartum nurses, *J Obstet Gynecol Neonatal Nurs* 29(5):491–499, 2000.

Minato J: Is it time to push?. examining rest in second stage labor, *AWHONN Lifelines* 4(5):20–23, 2001.

Murphy D and others: Women's views on the impact of operative delivery in the second stage of labour: qualitative interview study, *BMJ* 327(7424):1132, 2003.

Newton N, Newton M, and Broach J: Psychologic, physical, nutritional, and technologic aspects of intravenous infusion during labor, *Birth* 15(2):67–72, 1988.

Newton C, Raynor M: Routine intrapartum care. In Kean L, Baker P, and Edelstone D, editors: *Best practice in labor ward management,* Philadelphia, 2000, Saunders.

O'Sullivan G: The stomach-fact and fantasy: eating and drinking during labor, *Int Anesthesiol Clin* 32(3):31–44, 1994.

Paciornik M: Commentary: arguments against episiotomy and in favor of squatting for birth, *Birth* 17(2):104–105, 1990.

Paine L, Tinker D: The effect of maternal bearing-down efforts on arterial umbilical cord pH and length of the second stage of labor, *J Nurse Midwifery* 37(1):61–63, 1992.

Parnell C and others: Pushing method in the expulsive phase of labor: a randomized trial, *Acta Obstet Gynecol Scand* 72(1):31–35, 1993.

Petrou S, Coyle D, and Fraser W: Cost-effectiveness of a delayed pushing policy for patients wit epidural anesthesia: the PEOPLE study group, *Am J Obstet Gynecol* 182(5): 1158–1164, 2000.

Phillips K: Medical update: TENS during labor, *Childbirth Educator* 24, September/ October, 1998.

Pugh and others: First stage labor management: an examination of patterned breathing and fatigue, *Birth* 25(4):241, 1998.

Radin T, Harmon J, and Hanson D: Nurses' care during labor: its effect on the cesarean birth rate of healthy, nulliparous women, *Birth* 20(1):14–21, 1993.

Roberts C, Ludka L: Food for thought: the debate over eating and drinking in labor, *Childbirth Instructor* 4(2):24, 1994.

Roberts J, Mendez-Bauer C, and Wodell D: The effects of maternal position on uterine contractility and efficiency, *Birth* 10(4):243–249, 1983.

Roberts J, Woolley D: A second look at the second stage of labor, *J Obstet Gynecol Neonatal Nurs* 25(5):415–423, 1996.

Romond J, Baker I: Squatting in childbirth: a new look at an old tradition, *J Obstet Gynecol Neonatal Nurs* 14(5):406–411, 1985.

Rossi M, Lindell S: Maternal positions and pushing techniques in a nonprescriptive environment, *J Obstet Gynecol Neonatal Nurs* 15(3):203–208, 1986.

Rush J and others: The effects of whirlpool baths in labor: a randomized, controlled trial, *Birth* 23(3):136–143, 1996.

Sakala C: Current resources for evidence-based practice, *J Obstet Gynecol Neonatal Nurs* 34(5):625–628, 2005.

Sampselle C and others: Provider support of spontaneous pushing during the second stage of labor, *J Obstet Gynecol Neonatal Nurs* 34(6):695–702, 2005.

Scheepers H and others: Eating and drinking in labor: the influence of caregiver advice on women's behavior, *Birth* 28(2):119–123, 2001.

Scrutton M and others: Eating in labour: a randomised controlled trial assessing the risks and benefits, *Anaesthesia* 54(4):329–334, 1999.

Sharp D: Restrictions of oral intake for women in labour, *Br J Midwifery* 5:408, 1997.

Shermer R, Raines D: Positioning during the second stage of labor: moving back to basics, *J Obstet Gynecol Neonatal Nurs* 26(6):727–734, 1997.

Simkin P: Active management of labor, *Childbirth Instructor* 5(4):8, 1995a.

Simkin P: Comfort measures for labor and how they work, *IJCE* 11(1):57, 1987.

Simkin P: Reducing pain enhancing progress in labor: a guide to nonpharmacologic methods for maternity caregivers, *Birth* 22(3):161–171, 1995b.

Simkin P: Stress, pain, catecholamines in labor, part 1: a review, *Birth* 13(4):227–233, 1986a.

Simkin P: Stress, pain, catecholamines in labor, part 2: stress associated with childbirth events: a pilot survey of new mothers, *Birth* 13(4):234–240, 1986b.

Simpson K, James D: Effects of immediate versus delayed pushing during second-stage labor on fetal well-being: a randomized clinical trial, *Nurs Res* 54(3):149–157, 2005.

Simkin P: The labor support person: latest addition to the maternity care team, *IJCE* 16(1):19, 1992.

Sleutel M: Intrapartum nursing care: a case study of supportive interventions and ethical conflicts, *Birth* 27(1):38–45, 2000.

Sleutel M, Golden S: Fasting in labor: relic or requirement, *J Obstet Gynecol Neonatal Nurs* 28(5):507–512, 1999.

Smith I, Bogod D: Feeding in labour, *Bailliere's Clin Anaesthesiol* 9:735, 1995.

Springer D: Birth plans: the effect on anxiety in pregnant women, *IJCE* 11(3):20, 1996.

Stephens S: Body work and childbirth, proven wonders, *IJCE* 12(4):20, 1997.

Thacker SB, Stroup D, and Chang M: Continuous electronic heart rate monitoring for fetal assessment during labor, *Cochrane Database Syst Rev* Issue 2, 2001.

Thomson A: Pushing techniques in the second stage of labour, *J Adv Nurs* 18(2):171–177, 1993.

Threlfall-Mase A: The moaning option, *Childbirth Instructor* 7(2):43, 1997.

Tourangeau A and others: Intravenous therapy for women in labor: implementation of a practice change, *Birth* 26(1):31–36, 1999.

Tranmer J and others: The effect of unrestricted oral carbohydrate intake on labor progress, *J Obstet Gynecol Neonatal Nurs* 34(3):319–328, 2005.

Varrassi G, Bazzano C, and Edwards W: Effects of physical activity on maternal plasma B-endorphin levels and perception of labor pain, *Am J Obstet Gynecol* 160(3):707–712, 1989.

Vause S, Dongdon H, and Thornton J: Immediate and delayed pushing in the second stage of labour for nulliparous women with epidural analgesia: a randomized controlled trial, *Br J Obstet Gynecol* 105(2):186–188, 1998.

Watson J: *Postmodern nursing beyond,* Edinburgh, UK, 1999, Churchill Livingstone.

Wong S, McKenzie D: Cardiorespiratory fitness during pregnancy and its effect on outcome, *Int J Sports Med* 8(2):79–83, 1987.

World Health Organization: *Managing complications in pregnancy and childbirth: a guide for midwives and doctors,* Switzerland, 2002, Department of Reproductive Health and Research (RHR).

Zimmerman D, Breen T, and Fick G: Adding fentanyl 0.002% to epidural bupivacaine 0.125% does not delay gastric emptying in parturients, *Anesth Analg* 82(6):612–616, 1996.

Shoulder Dystocia

American College of Obstetricians and Gynecologists: Shoulder dystocia, *ACOG Practice,* Bulletin, No 40, Washington, DC, 2002, ACOG.

Baxley E, Gobbo R: Shoulder dystocia, *Am Fam Physician* 69:1707–1714, 2004.

Benedetti T: Dystocia: causes, consequences, correct response, *Contemp OB/GYN* 36(special issue):37, 1991.

Bruner J and others: All fours maneuver for reducing shoulder dystocia during labor, *J Reprod Med* 43(5):439–443, 1998.

Gherman R: Shoulder dystocia. In James D and others, editors: *High risk pregnancy: management options,* ed 3, Philadelphia, 2006, Saunders.

Gherman R, Goodwin T: Shoulder dystocia, *Curr Opin Obstet Gynecol* 10:459, 1998.

Gonik B, Allen R, Sorab J: Objective evaluation of the shoulder dystocia phenomenon: effect of maternal pelvic orientation on force reduction, *Obstet Gynecol* 74:44–48, 1989.

Horger E: Shoulder dystocia, *Female Patient* 20(12):12, 1995.

Jukelevics N: Big myths about big babies, *Childbirth Instructor* May/June, p 18, 2000.

Minkin M: A no-fault approach to shoulder dystocia, *Contemp OB/GYN* 49(12): 11–12, 2004.

Naef R, Martin J: Emergent management of shoulder dystocia, *Obstet Gynecol Clin North AM* 22: 247, 1995.

Nocon J: Shoulder dystocia macrosomia. In Kean L, Baker P, and Edelstone D, editors: *Best practice in labor ward management,* Philadelphia, 2000, Saunders.

Nocon J: Shoulder dystocia: managing risk to avoid negligence, *Contemp OB/GYN* 36(special issue):15, 1991.

Oleary J: *Shoulder dystocia and birth injury: Prevention and treatment,* Boston, 1992. McGraw-Hill.

Ouzounian J, Gherman R: Shoulder dystocia: are historic risk factors reliable predictors? *Am J Obstet Gynecol* 192(6):1933–1935, 2005.

Simpson K, Knox G: Fundal pressure during the second stage of labor, *MCN Am J Matern Child Nurs* 26(2):64–70, 2001.

Vaginal Birth After Cesarean

American College of Obstetricians and Gynecologists: Vaginal delivery after previous cesarean birth, *ACOG Practice Bulletin,* No 54, Washington, DC, 2004, ACOG.

Bujold E, Gauthier R: Should we allow a trial of labor after a previous cesarean for dystocia in the second stage of labor? *Obstet Gynecol* 98(4):652–655, 2001.

Chauhan S and others: Maternal and perinatal complications with uterine rupture in 142, 075 patients who attempted vaginal birth after cesarean delivery: a review of the literature, *Am J Obstet Gynecol* 189:408–417, 2003.

Dodd J and others: Planned elective repeat caesarean section versus planned vaginal birth for women with a previous caesarean birth, *Cochrane Database Syst Rev* Issue 4, 2004.

Enkin M and others: *A guide to effective care in pregnancy and childbirth,* ed 3, New York, 2000, Oxford University Press.

Gee H: Abnormal patterns of labor prolonged labor. In Kean L, Baker P, and Edelstone D, editors: *Best practice in labor ward management,* Philadelphia, 2000, Saunders.

Goodall P and others: Obesity as a risk factor for failed trial of labor in patients with previous cesarean delivery, *Am J Obstet Gynecol* 192(5):1423–1426, 2005.

Hibbard J and others: Failed vaginal birth after a cesarean section: how risky is it? *Am J Obstet Gynecol* 184(7):1365–1371, 2001.

Institute for Clinical Systems Improvement: *Health care guideline: Management of labor,* 2005, ICSI. Retrieved from *http://www.icsi.org*

Kieser K, Baskett T: 10-year population-based study of uterine rupture, *Obstet Gynecol* 100(4):749–753, 2002.

Mankuta D and others: Vaginal birth after cesarean section: trial of labor or repeat cesarean section?. a decision analysis, *Am J Obstet Gynecol* 189(3):714–719, 2003.

Mozurkewich E, Hutton E: Elective repeat cesarean delivery versus trial of labor: a meta-analysis of the literature from 1989–1999, *Am J Obstet Gynecol* 183(5):1187–1197, 2000.

Roberts R and others: Trial of labor or repeated cesarean section: the woman's choice, *Arch Fam Med* 6(2):120–125, 1997.

Society of Obstetricians and Gynaecologists of Canada: Guidelines for vaginal birth after previous caesarean birth, *Clinical Practice Guidelines,* No 155, 2005.

Zwelling E: VBAC revisited: a declining trend? *Childbirth Forum* Spring/Summer, p 1, 2001.

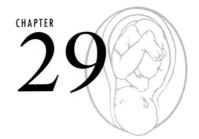

CHAPTER

29

Prolonged Pregnancy

*P*ostterm or *prolonged pregnancy* is one that lasts a gestational period of 42 completed weeks (294 days) or more from the first day of the last menses, if the menstrual cycle is 28 days. *Postmaturity* refers to the abnormal condition of the fetus or newborn resulting from a prolonged pregnancy.

INCIDENCE

The incidence of prolonged pregnancy is approximately 7% (Martin and others, 2003). However, others have found the incidence to be 1% to 3% when a reliable menstrual history and ultrasound criteria were used (Resnik and Resnik, 2004).

ETIOLOGY

The actual physiologic cause of prolonged pregnancy is still obscure. There is some evidence that the initiation of labor is triggered by sequential changes beginning within the fetal brain and influencing the hypothalamus, pituitary gland, adrenal gland, lungs, and kidneys, resulting in hormonal changes in the placenta and amniotic fetal membranes. A placental estrogen deficiency or decreased release of prostaglandins by the decidua and fetal membranes are possible causes.

When there is insufficient estrogen, there is decreased production and storage of prostaglandin precursors and decreased stimulation to form oxytocin receptors in the myometrium. These physiologic processes are important in the initiation of labor. (Refer to the Normal Physiology section of Chapter 22.) Occasionally, estrogen deficiency can result from fetal pituitary or adrenal insufficiency. Lack of secretion of the precursor hormone dehydroisoandroster-one sulfate, which is necessary for the placenta to produce increasing amounts of estriol, may also partially explain the fetal contribution to causing prolonged pregnancy. Genetics may influence the length of gestation (Olesen, Bosso, and Olsen, 2003)

695

NORMAL PHYSIOLOGY
Amniotic Fluid

The normal physiology of amniotic fluid (its volume and functions) is relevant to understanding the pathologic complications in prolonged pregnancy.

Volume

Amniotic fluid is derived from the following sources:
- Maternal circulation, primarily from placental sufficiency
- Amniotic membrane
- Fetal plasma via lungs and kidneys

The volume changes by (1) the fetal contribution through excretion of urine and fetal lungs, (2) fetal use of the fluid for nourishment by swallowing the fluid and sending it into the gastrointestinal tract, (3) movement of water and solutes back into fetal blood across fetal membranes and placenta, and (4) movement of water and solutes directly into maternal blood.

The volume of amniotic fluid gradually increases until it reaches its maximal level of 800 to 1200 ml at approximately 34 weeks of gestation, at which time it begins to decrease normally. By 40 weeks, the level is approximately 500 to 1000 ml. In contrast, by 42 and 43 weeks, the levels are 400 and 300 ml, respectively (Brace, 2004; Cunningham and others, 2005).

Functions

The following functions of amniotic fluid are relevant to prolonged pregnancy:
- Cushions the fetus and umbilical cord from direct pressure and injury
- Allows the fetus to move and exercise freely
- Assists the fetus in respiratory efforts
- Facilitates fetal lung development and surfactant production

Placenta
Exchange

The placenta provides a large surface area through which materials can be exchanged across the placental membrane between the fetal and maternal circulations. From the maternal blood, the fetus obtains nutrients and oxygen. Waste products formed by the fetus are transferred back across the placental membrane into the intervillous space.

Functions

The placenta has an optimal functional period of about 40 to 42 weeks. There appear to be no significant morphologic changes in the postterm placenta until about 42 weeks (Cunningham and others, 2005). After 43 to 44 weeks, the placenta begins aging, as noted by the increased size of areas of infarction and deposition of calcium and fibrin within its tissue, decreasing its reserve (Proud and Grant, 1987; Gribbin and Thornton, 2006).

PATHOPHYSIOLOGY
Amniotic Fluid
Decreased Amniotic Fluid

Decreased amniotic fluid, or *oligohydramnios*, is the factor most frequently associated with prolonged pregnancy (Cunningham and others, 2005). Decreased amniotic fluid below 400 ml can reduce the cushioning effect of the fluid. As a result, it becomes far more likely that the fetus will entrap or compress its own cord, shutting off blood flow to and from itself for intermittent intervals.

Meconium Contamination

Meconium in the amniotic fluid occurs in prolonged pregnancies 12% to 22% of the time (Cunningham and others, 2005). When the fetus is postterm, the expulsion of meconium into the already diminished volume of amniotic fluid causes the meconium to thicken, inhibits the normal antibacterial properties of the amniotic fluid, and pulls fluid from Wharton jelly, promoting stiffening of the cord.

Placenta and Umbilical Cord
Placental Dysfunction

When the placenta ages, depositing fibrin and calcium, intervillous hemorrhagic infarcts occur and the basal membrane of the placental blood vessels thickens and degenerates, affecting diffusion of oxygen. These changes have been noted in the postterm placenta. Whether or not these placental changes affect the fetal outcome in the prolonged pregnancy is unknown at this time because most fetuses continue to grow.

Decreased Wharton Jelly

As aging takes place, water content is lost from the Wharton jelly encasing the umbilical cord, decreasing the amount of Wharton jelly. As the amount of Wharton jelly decreases, the cord stiffens and becomes firm rather than remaining flexible and pliable.

Decreased Umbilical Cord Blood Flow

As a result of umbilical cord stiffening, susceptibility to pressure on the cord and to bending of the cord is increased. If the cord bends or kinks, much like a sun-baked garden hose, increased resistance to fetal blood flow can result in serious neurologic damage or sudden intrauterine fetal death.

SIGNS AND SYMPTOMS

A number of obstetric warning signs in conjunction with a pregnancy continuing past the estimated due date (EDD), including the following, can alert caregivers to potential problems.

Maternal Weight Loss

In the last weeks of pregnancy, a weight loss in excess of 3 pounds per week, caused by a decreased amount of amniotic fluid, may warn of a prolonged pregnancy.

Decreased Uterine Size

Decreased amniotic fluid (<400 ml) frequently correlates with maternal weight loss and with a decrease in uterine size.

Meconium-Stained Amniotic Fluid

Meconium in the amniotic fluid can represent a normal physiologic event in the maturation of the fetal gastrointestinal tract, can be the result of vagal stimulation from transient umbilical cord compression that results in increased peristalsis or can be the direct result of fetal hypoxia (Cunningham and others, 2005).

Advanced Bone Maturation

Advanced bone maturation can be detected by palpation of an excessively hard fetal head. It can lead to a lack of cephalic molding and a high arrest of the fetal head with potential for failure to progress, prolongation of the active phase of labor, and failure to complete the transitional phase of labor.

Prolonged Labor

A macrosomic fetus, failure of cephalic molding, or decreased uterine sensitivity to oxytocin can cause prolonged labor.

MATERNAL EFFECTS

Physical Exhaustion

Many women report extreme fatigue if their pregnancy is prolonged.

Psychologic Depression

Women express a great deal of frustration with the prolongation of the pregnancy and a feeling of total lack of personal control in bringing it to an end. Feelings of inadequacy emerge because of their inability to complete the process of the pregnancy "like everyone else." Women often blame themselves for prolonging the pregnancy by working too hard, working too long into the pregnancy, or not seeking adequate help with everyday tasks.

Relationships with those people closest to the pregnant woman become strained. Resentment is expressed because friends and relatives repeatedly check on the woman's progress and condition. Physical discomfort becomes an intolerable burden, which in turn decreases the ability to continue caring for the home and other family members in the accustomed manner. Women describe feeling awkward, big, and ugly. They comment that they have lost their "glow" and feel generally unattractive. A woman's negative feelings about herself may be projected as feelings of resentment toward the baby for not cooperating or for being a "stubborn" child.

Realistic fears are commonly shared about the continued well-being of the baby. Women report fears that the baby is "stuck" and will somehow be harmed or that something is very wrong and that the baby has decided not to be born.

Other Maternal Risks

Most other risks are related to labor dystocia such as increased risk for perineal injury related to macrosomia or treatment to prevent prolong pregnancy, such as complications related to induction or cesarean delivery (Grant, 2006).

FETAL AND NEONATAL EFFECTS

When 42 weeks of gestation is exceeded, oligohydramnios increases substantially, and intrapartum perinatal risk is increased (Cunningham and others, 2005). This is related to a wide range of features.

Macrosomia

Macrosomia is defined as a birth weight greater than 4000 to 4500 g (Baschat, 2006). In the United States about 10% of newborns weigh more than 4000 g, and 1.5% weigh more than 4500 g. The risk for macrosomia increases from 1.4% at term to 2.2% if gestational age exceeds 42 weeks (Cunningham and others, 2005). Macrosomia poses a risk to the postdate fetus because it can lead to shoulder dystocia and birth trauma.

Dysmaturity Syndrome

Dysmaturity syndrome occurs in approximately 20% of postdate fetuses (ACOG, 2004) because of a compromised environment. This syndrome is characterized by degrees of skin change with or without loss of subcutaneous fat and muscle mass and meconium staining dependent on severity of cord compression and placental dysfunction. Dysmaturity syndrome was initially classified by Clifford (1954) and was later revised by Vorherr (1975). However, most of these infants regain their weight quickly and exhibit few long-term neurologic problems (Resnik and Resnik, 2004).

First Stage

In the first stage of dysmaturity syndrome, the skin becomes desquamated due to the loss of the protective effects of vernix caseosa. It is characterized by a dry, cracked, parchmentlike peeling, with or without loss of subcutaneous fat and muscle mass. The nails are usually long.

Second Stage

The second stage of dysmaturity syndrome includes first-stage characteristics and also green meconium-stained fetal skin and umbilical cord.

Third Stage

The third stage of dysmaturity syndrome includes the first two stages plus yellow staining of the skin and the umbilical cord. This yellow staining is related to meconium being passed several days before. The bile in the meconium, as it breaks down, turns the fluid yellow.

Fetal Hypoxia

Fetal hypoxia can be caused by placental deprivation or oligohydramnios (decreased amniotic fluid) that leads to cord compression (Resnik and Resnik, 2004).

Meconium Aspiration Syndrome

Meconium-stained amniotic fluid is more common in postterm deliveries. If amniotic fluid is diminished, the risk for meconium-stained amniotic fluid can be as high as 71% (Resnik and Resnik, 2004). From 2% to 8% of infants with meconium-stained amniotic fluid develop meconium aspiration syndrome (Glantz and Woods, 2004).

The fetus normally moves fluids into and out of the lungs in utero by two breathing patterns. Shallow, regular breathing comprises 90% of fetal respirations, and deep, irregular breathing comprises the other 10%. An abnormal pattern of breathing may be stimulated in the presence of hypoxia, which is characterized by compensatory gasping respirations. Aspiration of meconium from the amniotic fluid into the lungs occurs if gasping respirations are stimulated by asphyxia, and a small amount may occur during the normal deep respiration breathing. If meconium aspiration occurs, it is normally cleared through the pulmonary circulation in the same manner as amniotic fluid is normally cleared from the lungs. If pulmonary vascular damage has occurred because of asphyxia, the mechanism of clearing the lung fields of fluid is affected and meconium aspiration syndrome results (Steer and Danielian, 2006).

Hypoglycemia

Acute episodes of hypoxia related to cord compression result in anaerobic glycolysis, which exhausts carbohydrate reserves. Placental deterioration can lead to chronic fetal nutritional deficiency and further depletion of the carbohydrate reserves.

Polycythemia

The fetus increases production of red blood cells as a compensatory response to hypoxia. The polycythemia can be a significant problem in the newborn period, contributing to hyperbilirubinemia from destruction of no longer needed red blood cells.

DIAGNOSTIC TESTING

When a pregnancy extends beyond 7 days past the EDD, the prenatal chart should be reviewed for confirmation of the due date. Parameters for review include the following aspects.

Gestational Length Variables

Based on the Nägele rule, the length of gestation is 280 days. However, the length of gestation has been shown to vary among women. Parity may influence gestational length. One study has shown that 287 days is the mean gestation for the primigravida and 281 days is the mean for the multigravida (Nichols, 1985). Other studies have shown that there may be ethnic variances (Mittendorf and others, 1990). The average length of gestation for white primiparas is 288 days; for white multiparas it is 283 days; for Japanese women it is 278 days; and for African American women it is 277½ days.

Menstrual Cycle Length

If the woman has a prolonged preovulatory phase, the EDD should be appropriately adjusted to a later date.

Contraceptive Use

Oral contraceptives may delay ovulation.

Quickening

Pregnant women should be asked prospectively to note the date they felt their fetus move for the first time (quickening). For the primigravida, this usually occurs when the fetus is approximately 18 to 20 weeks of gestational age. For the multigravida, it usually occurs around 16 to 18 weeks of gestation.

Audible Fetal Heart Sounds

The fetal heart sounds can be heard with the Doppler ultrasound at around 10 to 12 weeks of gestation and with the fetoscope at 16 to 18 weeks.

Fundal Growth

Between 20 and 32 weeks of gestation, fundal height measurement, assessed with the mother's bladder empty, from the symphysis pubis to the top of the fundus, should approximate gestational age within 2 weeks.

Diagnostic Ultrasound Findings

For accurate dating, ultrasound measurements should be done before 20 weeks of gestation. An early crown-rump length, between 4 and 10 weeks of gestation (ACOG, 2004; Resnik and Resnik, 2004), offers the most accurate means. By averaging the biparietal diameter, head circumference, abdominal circumference, and femur length between 14 and 20 weeks, diagnostic ultrasound is 90% accurate in determining the EDD within ±1 weeks (Manning, 2004).

After 26 weeks, and particularly during the last 10 weeks of gestation, accuracy of estimating gestational age is progressively limited. For these reasons, in the presence of a questionable last menstrual period, ultrasound is used as early as possible—preferably before 20 weeks to prevent confusion regarding diagnosis of prolonged pregnancy once the EDD is past (Bicker and Neilson, 2000).

In estimating fetal weight, Leopold's maneuver with fundal height measurements have similar accuracy as compared with ultrasound measurements. However, both methods are subject to significant errors (Liao, Buhimschi, Norwitz, 2004).

USUAL MEDICAL MANAGEMENT AND PROTOCOLS FOR NURSE PRACTITIONERS

The antepartum intervention of a prolonged pregnancy is still controversial. The first major issue is when to initiate intervention, at 41 or 42 weeks of gestation. The second issue is what intervention should be implemented: labor induction or expectant management using antepartum fetal testing with selective labor induction. In the presence of oligohydramnios or fetal stress, delivery should be initiated. From the many randomized control trial studies and evidence-based research reviews, there is no conclusive evidence that one protocol affords greater benefit or greater risk in low risk patients. To date no randomized control trial studies have indicated that any single antepartum fetal test has been shown to be better than another (Hannah and others, 1992; Crowley, 1997; Alexander and others, 2000; AHRQ, 2002; ACOG, 2004; Resnik and Resnik, 2004; Briscoe and others, 2005; Cunningham and others, 2005; Grant, 2006).

According to ACOG recommendations (2004), between 41 and 42 weeks of gestation, if the cervix is ripe, an induction is generally initiated; however, if the cervix is unfavorable, fetal surveillance or cervical ripening can be implemented. Therefore without a defined protocol, women should be informed of the benefits and risks for induction of labor and expectant management. The woman's preferences should be considered in the plan of management. Individualize the plan of care with the goal of not pushing nature too soon, but do not allow variables to develop that will decrease tolerance to labor, such as decreased, meconium-stained amniotic fluid, a hard fetal head, and macrosomia.

Active Management with Induction of Labor

Any of the interventions of labor stimulation outlined in Chapter 27 can be used to induce a prolonged pregnancy. Stripping fetal membranes has been shown to decrease the incidence of postdate gestations without increasing complications (AHRQ, 2002). Cervical ripening, with a cervical ripening agent, is usually attempted before oxytocin induction is started. If the cervix is ripe, with a Bishop score of 8 or greater, labor induction with oxytocin is usually initiated.

Expectant Management with Fetal Surveillance

Daily fetal movement counts may be started around term. Antenatal fetal surveillance is to be initiated by 42 weeks if induction is not attained (ACOG, 2004). These studies continue until the cervix becomes ripe, spontaneous labor is started, an antepartum fetal test becomes abnormal, or induction is done at the completion of 42 weeks (Cunningham and others, 2005).

A single means of fetal surveillance or a combination of two studies may be used. Usually, twice weekly amniotic fluid index is used as one of two methods of fetal surveillance when twice weekly nonstress tests or weekly contraction stress tests are used as the principal means of evaluating fetal well-being (ACOG, 2004). Biophysical profile may be used, but it is more costly. According to the Agency for Healthcare Research and Quality Evidence Report (AHRQ, 2002), a combination of fetal heart rate monitoring and amniotic fluid volume appear to have the highest levels of sensitivity.

Labor Management

Because of the increased risk for fetal hypoxia when the pregnancy is prolonged, it is ideal to do a nonstress test on admission to labor. If accelerations are absent with the use of acoustic stimulation, even if the fetal heart rate (FHR) strip is otherwise normal, this may indicate a fetus that is maintaining antenatal oxygenation but not adequate oxygen levels during the stress of uterine contractions. Close FHR monitoring is indicated.

Continuous intrapartum electronic fetal monitoring is preferable along with close monitoring of the labor progress related to the possibility of a large-for-gestational-age infant. If baseline variability is less than 5 amplitudes, if baseline FHR is less than 100 beats/min or greater than 150 beats per minute, or if late decelerations are noted, immediate cesarean delivery is considered (Steer and Danielian, 2000).

According to the *Cochrane Review* (Hofmeyr, 2002) and a meta-analysis of randomized control trials (Pitt and others, 2000), benefit has been shown when amnioinfusion is used during intrapartum to treat severe variable decelerations or meconium-stained amniotic fluid in the presence of oligohydramnios. Beneficial effects are decreased incidence of meconium aspiration below the vocal cords and decreased reduction in cesarean delivery for fetal distress. However, a more recent large randomized control trial showed no benefit with the treatment of amnioinfusion to prevent meconium aspiration syndrome (Fraser and others, 2005; Fraser and others, 2006).

NURSING MANAGEMENT

Antepartum Nursing Interventions if Pregnancy Goes Beyond the Due Date

- Encourage the patient and her family to openly express their frustrations, feelings regarding the extreme fatigue and unattractiveness, and fears related to fetal well-being with professional health care providers and each other.
- Discuss the meaning of the EDD with the patient and her family. The EDD is merely a midpoint in a 1-month range between 38 and 42 weeks of gestation during which 90% of women will deliver (Nichols, 1987; Rehns, 2004).
- Provide opportunities for the patient to listen to the FHR and see evidence of FHR reactivity during fetal surveillance studies.
- Assist in planning alternative arrangements for help in the home for the present and postpartum periods because of fatigue.
- Discuss the benefits and risks of induction of labor and expectant management using antepartum fetal testing with selective labor induction. The woman's preference should be considered in the management plan.

- Instruct the patient about the importance of and how to assess for daily fetal activity.
- Prepare the patient for the reason for weekly cervical examinations to determine cervical ripening.
- Prepare the patient for potential medical interventions, such as induction of labor, instrument-assisted delivery, cesarean birth, and fetal surveillance studies.
- Refer to available and appropriate support services, such as social service, high risk pregnancy support group, home health aides, visiting nurse, and church or other supportive community resource.

Intrapartum Nursing Management

- Admit patient when she is in early labor or when she is due for induced labor.
- Use pain medications and sedatives cautiously and only after other alternative methods of coping have been determined to be inadequate alone.
- Use continuous fetal monitoring to recognize early evidence of a nonreassuring FHR change.
- Manage the labor in a facility that can provide a cesarean birth or instrument-assisted delivery so that if either of these becomes necessary, they can be performed. Also, make sure the personnel qualified for infant resuscitation can be immediately summoned.
- When rupture of membranes occurs, assess FHR and note the amount and color of amniotic fluid. (Minimal amniotic fluid on amniotomy is predictive of meconium 50% of the time, even if obvious meconium is not immediately observed.)
- Be prepared to assist with fetal scalp blood gas analysis, if desired, before delivery. Be prepared to collect cord pH sample from umbilical artery immediately after delivery.
- Be prepared to manage a saline amnioinfusion if multiple variable decelerations occur related to decreased amniotic fluid or combined with thick meconium on rupture of membranes.
- Notify the physician at the first signs of a nonreassuring FHR change.

Intrapartum Nursing Interventions for Amnioinfusion

- Chart the purpose for an amnioinfusion if used.
- Rule out cord prolapse.
- Assess patient's understanding of the procedure and obtain her consent.
- Educate patient about the reasons for the procedure.
- Assess baseline maternal vital signs, FHR, and uterine activity.
- Obtain a 1000-ml bag of normal saline or lactated Ringer's solution that has been stored in a heating unit or warmed with a blood warmer.
- Connect the warmed solution to the intrauterine pressure catheter by way of intravenous tubing.
- Give an initial bolus of 500 to 800 ml or per protocol.

- If variable decelerations persist, notify health care provider for possible amniotic fluid index. When less than 8 cm, additional bolus of 250 to 500 ml may be ordered.
- Then continue 150 to 180 ml/hour infusion if fluid continues to leak onto the chux. This rate can be accomplished without an infusion pump by hanging the saline bag 3 to 4 feet above the uterus, but it is preferable to use an infusion pump when available.
- Continue infusion until the variable decelerations resolve or intolerable side effects develop, such as an increasing uterine resting tone, nonreassuring signs of fetal compromise, or uterine tenderness.
- If fluid does not continue to leak onto the chux, discontinue and notify the health care provider.
- Monitor FHR and uterine activity continuously with a separate or solid, multiple-lumen intrauterine pressure catheter.
- Check temperature every 2 hours.
- Measure and mark fundal height and reassess every hour.
- Monitor the patient's comfort or pain.
- Keep the patient as dry as possible by changing the pads often.
- Notify the physician if nonreassuring variable decelerations are not resolved with a total of 800 ml of warmed solution or when signs of maternal or fetal response are not reassuring or intrauterine pressure is greater than 25 mm Hg.
- Document the amount of uterine input, amount and character of vaginal discharge, uterine activity including resting tone, FHR, and vital signs.
- Notify pediatric personnel for presence if meconium is noted in the amniotic fluid so that prompt resuscitation and oxygenation can be administered as needed. Visualization of the vocal cords and deep suction of the trachea to clear the airway of meconium before the infant takes its first breath may be required.

CONCLUSION

The etiology and pathophysiology of prolonged pregnancy are not completely understood, but early and ongoing prenatal care is essential, and the importance of assignment of an accurate EDD is clearly evident. When prolonged pregnancy can be diagnosed without significant shades of doubt, the nurse can then collaborate with the other health care team members in developing an effective plan of care to prevent undue maternal anxiety, reduce sources of fears, and lower infant mortality and morbidity.

BIBLIOGRAPHY

Agency for Healthcare Research and Quality: *Management of prolonged pregnancy, Evidence Report/Technology Assessment,* No. 23, Durham, NC, 2002, Duke Evidence-Based Practice Center.

Alexander J, McIntire D, and Leveno K: Forty weeks and beyond: pregnancy outcomes by week of gestation, *Obstet Gynecol* 96(2):291–294, 2000.

American College of Obstetricians and Gynecologists: Management of postterm pregnancy, *ACOG Practice Bulletin,* No 55, Washington, DC, 2004, ACOG.

Baschat A: Fetal growth disorders, In James D and others, editors: *High risk pregnancy: management options*, ed 3, Philadelphia, 2006, Saunders.

Boulvain M and others: Sweeping of the membranes to prevent post-term pregnancy and to induce labour: a systematic review, *Br J Obstet Gyanecol* 106(1):481–485, 1999.

Brace R: Amniotic fluid dynamics. In Creasy R, Resnik R, and Iams J, editors: *Maternal-fetal medicine: principles and practice*, ed 5, Philadelphia, 2004, Saunders.

Bricker L, Neilson J: Routine ultrasound in late pregnancy (after 24 weeks gestation), *Cochrane Database Syst Rev* Issue 1, 2000.

Briscoe D and others: Management of pregnancy beyond 40 weeks' gestation, *AAFP* 71(10):1935–1941, 2005.

Clifford S: Postmaturity with placental dysfunction: clinical syndrome and pathologic findings, *J Pediatr* 44(1):1–13, 1954.

Crowley P: Interventions for preventing or improving the outcome of delivery at or beyond term, *Cochrane Database Syst Rev* Issue 1, 1997.

Cunningham G and others: *Williams' obstetrics*, ed 22, New York, 2005, McGraw-Hill Professional.

Fraser W and others: Amnioinfusion for the prevention of the meconium aspiration syndrome, *N Engl J Med* 353(9):909–917, 2005.

Fraser W and others: Amnioinfusion for the prevention of the meconium aspiration syndrome, *Obstet Gynecol* 61(2):80–81, 2006.

Gribbin C, Thornton J: Critical evaluation of fetal assessment methods, In James D and others, editors: *High risk pregnancy: management options*, ed 3, Philadelphia, 2006, Saunders.

Glantz C, Woods J: Significance of amniotic fluid meconium. In Creasy R, Resnik R, and Iams J, editors: *Maternal-fetal medicine: Principles and practice*, ed 5, Philadelphia, 2004, Saunders.

Grant J: Prolonged pregnancy, In James D and others, editors: *High risk pregnancy: management options*, ed 3, Philadelphia, 2006, Saunders.

Hannah M and others: Induction of labor as compared with antenatal monitoring in post-term pregnancy: a randomized controlled trial, *N Engl J Med* 326(24):1587–1592, 1992.

Hofmeyr G: Amnioinfusion for meconium-stained liquor in labour, *Cochrane Database Syst Rev* Issue 1, 2002.

Liao J, Buhimschi C, and Norwitz E: Normal labor: mechanism and duration, *Obstet Gynecol Clin N Am* 32(2):145–164, 2004.

Manning F: General principles applications of ultrasonography. In Creasy R, Resnik R, and Iams J, editors: *Maternal-fetal medicine: principles and practice*, ed 5, Philadelphia, 2004, Saunders.

Martin J and others: Births: final data for 2002, *Natl Vital Stat Rep* 52(10):1–113, 2003.

Mittendorf R and others: The length of uncomplicated human gestation, *Obstet Gynecol* 75(6):929–932, 1990.

Nichols C: Dating pregnancy: gathering and using a reliable data base, *J Nurse Midwifery* 32(4):195–204, 1987.

Nichols C: The Yale Nurse-Midwifery Practice: addressing the outcomes, *J Nurse Midwifery* 30(3):159–165, 1985.

Olesen A, Basso O, and Olsen J: Risk of recurrence of prolonged pregnancy, *BMJ* 326(7387):476, 2003.

Pitt C and others: Prophylactic amnioinfusion for intrapartum oligohydramnios: a meta-analysis of randomized controlled trials, *Obstet Gynecol* 96(5 Pt 1):861–866, 2000.

Proud J, Grant A: Third trimester placental grading by ultrasonography as a test of fetal wellbeing, *BMJ* 294:1641–1647, 1987.

Rehns M: The trouble with due dates, *CBE reporter* 3:1–2, 2004.

Resnik J, Resnik R: Post-term pregnancy. In Creasy R, Resnik R, and Iams J, editors: *Maternal-fetal medicine: Principles and practice*, ed 5, Philadelphia, 2004, Saunders.

Steer P, Danielian P: Fetal distress in labor. In James D and others, editors: *High risk pregnancy: management options*, ed 3, Philadelphia, 2006, Saunders.

Vorherr H: Placental insufficiency in relation to postterm pregnancy fetal postmaturity: evaluation of fetoplacental function; management of the postterm gravida, *Am J Obstet Gynecol* 123(1):67–103, 1975.

Index

Page numbers followed by *b* indicate boxed material; *f* indicate figures; *t*, tables.